Mark Pellowski Ph.D. CCC-SLP
Department of Communication
Sciences and Disorders
Towson University

Stuttering

Stuttering

Foundations and Clinical Applications

Ehud Yairi

University of Illinois at Urbana-Champaign
Tel Aviv University

Carol H. Seery

University of Wisconsin-Milwaukee

PEARSON

Boston   Columbus   Indianapolis   New York   San Francisco   Upper Saddle River
Amsterdam   Cape Town   Dubai   London   Madrid   Milan   Munich   Paris   Montreal   Toronto
Delhi   Mexico City   São Paulo   Sydney   Hong Kong   Seoul   Singapore   Taipei   Tokyo

Vice President and Editor in Chief: Jeffery W. Johnston
Executive Editor and Publisher: Stephen D. Dragin
Editorial Assistant: Jamie Bushell
Vice President, Director of Marketing: Quinn Perkson
Senior Marketing Manager: Christopher Barry
Senior Managing Editor: Pamela D. Bennett
Project Manager: Kerry Rubadue
Senior Operations Supervisor: Matthew Ottenweller
Senior Art Director: Diane Lorenzo
Cover Designer: Ali Mohrman
Full-Service Project Management: Thistle Hill Publishing Services, LLC
Composition: Integra Software Services
Printer/Binder: Courier/Westford
Cover Printer: Lehigh-Phoenix Color/Hagerstown
Text Font: Utopia

Credits and acknowledgments borrowed from other sources and reproduced, with permission, in this textbook appear on appropriate page within text.

Every effort has been made to provide accurate and current Internet information in this book. However, the Internet and information posted on it are constantly changing, so it is inevitable that some of the Internet addresses listed in this textbook will change.

Library of Congress Cataloging-in-Publication Data

Yairi, Ehud.
   Stuttering : foundations and clinical applications / Ehud Yairi, Carol H. Seery.
     p. ; cm.
   Includes bibliographical references and index.
   ISBN-13: 978-0-13-157310-9 (casebound)
   ISBN-10: 0-13-157310-1 (casebound)
   1. Stuttering.   I. Seery, Carol H.   II. Title.
[DNLM: 1. Stuttering.   WM 475 Y14s 2011]
RC424.Y35 2011
616.85'54—dc22

                               2010001488

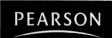

www.pearsonhighered.com

10 9 8 7 6 5 4 3 2 1
ISBN 10:   0-13-157310-1
ISBN 13: 978-0-13-157310-9

To my wife, Janie.

—E. Yairi

To my husband, Tom, and son, David.

*To my mother, Frances, and the memory of
my father, David F. Hubbard.*

—C. Seery

About the Authors

Ehud Yairi, Ph.D. (Iowa), CCC-SLP
University of Illinois at Urbana-Champaign

Professor Yairi is an internationally recognized expert on stuttering. A recipient of several major grants from the National Institutes of Health, his research and clinical work on many aspects of the disorder throughout the age range, especially in children, has incorporated both environmental and genetic factors. Yairi is the recipient of the Honors of the Association (the highest award of the American Speech-Language-Hearing Association), the Researcher Award of Distinction (from the International Fluency Association), and the Malcolm Fraser Award for excellence in the field of stuttering (from the Stuttering Foundation of America). He is the author (with Nicoline Ambrose) of *Early Childhood Stuttering* (2005), as well as of numerous scientific articles.

Carol Hubbard Seery, Ph.D. (UW-Seattle), CCC-SLP
University of Wisconsin-Milwaukee

Professor Seery has engaged in teaching, research, and clinical service related to stuttering for more than 25 years. She has worked professionally in school, hospital, and university settings. Seery has been a board-certified specialist in fluency disorders and has made presentations on stuttering to clinicians in various settings. She received National Institutes of Health grant support, has authored and coauthored multiple articles in scientific journals, has been an editorial consultant for several scientific journals, and serves on the editorial board for the *Journal of Communication Disorders*.

Brief Contents

Contents

3   When and How Does Stuttering Begin? How Does It Develop?   47

6   Is Stuttering Psychological? Psychoemotional, Psychobehavioral, and Psycholinguistic Theories   123

13 Assessment of Stuttering in Early Childhood   337

14 Treatment of Preschool-Age Children Who Stutter   373

15 Other Fluency Disorders and Multicultural/Bilingual Issues   405

Foreword

We wrote *Stuttering: Foundations and Clinical Applications* to serve both instructors and students in speech-language disorders and related fields as a single main text for a general course on stuttering. It is composed of three parts: the nature of stuttering, the explanation of stuttering, and the clinical management of stuttering. Many textbooks on stuttering are dedicated primarily to one or two of these subjects, but few address all three of them equally. We have undertaken to provide a balanced presentation across all three areas.

In addition, we also offer a balanced perspective with regard to stuttering etiology, assessment, and treatment methods. We provide a comprehensive coverage of the options from the various viewpoints and relate them to specific age groups.

Finally, we sought a balance in using a written style that is easy to read yet deals with concepts and scientific material with appreciable depth. Whenever appropriate, we have shared examples from our own scholarly, clinical, and personal experiences to enrich the understanding of our readers.

We hope that reading this book enhances your knowledge, as it has ours in writing it.

Acknowledgments

Special thanks to Stephanie Johnson for her comments on nearly the entire book. Thanks are also extended to Hee-Cheong Chon, who provided technical assistance throughout.

Finally, we gratefully acknowledge the project management of Kerry Rubadue, the editorial oversight of Angela Urquhart, and the comments and suggestions made by the following reviewers:

Anne Bothe, University of Georgia, Athens
Thalia Coleman, Appalachian State University
C. Richard Dean, Ohio University
Rodney Gabel, Bowling Green State University
Regina Grantham, SUNY Cortland
Brent Gregg, University of Arkansas, Little Rock
Charlie Healey, University of Nebraska, Lincoln
Elisa Huff, University of South Dakota
Lisa LaSalle, University of Wisconsin–Eau Claire
Nancy Montgomery, Rockhurst University
Glyn Riley, California State University, Fullerton

Jean Sawyer, Illinois State University
Lisa Scott, Florida State University
Rosalee Shenker, McGill University
Ying-Chiao Tsao, California State University, Fullerton
Mandy Williams, University of South Alabama
Richard Zraick, University of Arkansas for Medical Sciences, Little Rock

Chapter 1: What Is Stuttering?

LEARNER OBJECTIVES

Readers will be able to:

- Discriminate definitions of stuttering in terms of speech phenomena or complex disorder.
- Analyze concepts and issues related to defining stuttering.
- Evaluate the significance and influence of various stuttering definitions.
- Examine the context of stuttering identification with respect to normal speech and normal disfluency.
- Analyze the meaning of stuttering from different points of view, and identify sources of definitional diversity.

Defining Stuttering: Bases and Aims

At first glance, stuttering appears to be a phenomenon that would be rather easy to define. When most people think of stuttering, they typically recall speech that everyone would recognize, like the repetitive hesitations of "I I I I um I um I um." Hence the common notion is that "everyone knows what stuttering is." Such, however, is not the case for scholars in the field. For them, the definition of stuttering is far from straightforward. To the contrary, as we shall see, the closer they have looked at stuttering, the more it has grown in complexity. But laypeople too may be confused. We had a case of a child brought to us by parents complaining about his stuttering. We concluded that the child exhibited cleft palate speech with no sign of stuttering. The parents concurred that what they called "stuttering" was the child's unusual articulation and voice quality.

In this chapter, we discuss the diversity of the viewpoints about stuttering held by scholars. Before attempting either to define stuttering or evaluate its definition, it is important to clarify the aim of this endeavor. According to *The New Oxford American Dictionary*, a definition is "a statement of the exact *meaning* of a word, . . . or, description of the *nature*, scope, or meaning of something . . . , or, the degree of *distinctness* in outline of an object or image" [italics added] (Jewell & Abate, 2001, p. 447). As professionals and researchers, we must clarify what we mean by the term *stuttering*, strive to agree on the scope of that term, and determine precisely when it applies.

Sometimes people use the term *stuttering* referring only to the overt (surface) features. Its overt features are the speech events. But are the observed speech events really the essence of stuttering? Another use of *stuttering* is referring to the covert (or hidden) features, particularly the speaker's experience of a loss of control and a host of negative emotional reactions. But must there be an underlying sense of helplessness every time? Finally, because stuttering encompasses both overt and covert features, there have been definitions intended to capture both aspects.

With some slight deviation from the *New Oxford American Dictionary*, we hold that a definition should be a statement that expresses what is the *essential* rather than the *exact* (comprehensive) nature or meaning of a matter, and the information must make it distinct from other similar or related concepts. Thus the aim of defining stuttering should be to state the necessary properties and set forth the limits of this phenomenon. It is tempting to believe that a thorough definition of stuttering is the goal. But for professional purposes that usually involve measurement, the most useful definition may not be the one that is most thorough. Instead, the most useful definition of stuttering is one that remains free from opinion, explanation, or theory. This point is illustrated by analogy through various definitions of "water." If *water* is defined as "a tasteless liquid," we encounter the problem that "taste" is a matter of opinion. Or, if water is defined as "a liquid compound of hydrogen and oxygen," the application is limited because most "water" contains many other constituent elements. But if people agreed that "water" is the liquid form of what falls from the sky as precipitation, then the concept is ready for discussion, study, and description, including its numerous and ever-changing properties.

We must point out that a definition is not the same as a set of diagnostic criteria. Trying to define stuttering and undertaking to diagnose it are two different endeavors. Whereas a definition attempts to delineate the meaning of a term, the function of a diagnosis is to determine whether the presenting communication pattern constitutes a clinical problem or a risk for becoming one. Arriving at a clinical diagnosis often involves use of specifications of the frequency or intensity of the parameters found in the definition. For example, if the parameter that defined stuttering was syllable repetitions, the diagnostician would still have to determine whether the number of repetitions raised a need for concern. Specifications, such as the number of repetitions that cause concern, may vary with factors of age, gender, time since onset, and so on. Researchers strive to study, identify, and enumerate these parameters with ever-increasing specificity.

Definitions of stuttering have varied for many reasons. Some have differed depending on the areas of expertise, interests, and needs of the definers. Others have been influenced by the many characteristics and dimensions of stuttering, typical age of onset, patterns of development, suspected etiology, and more. Across the years, many have boldly announced an answer, but to our knowledge no statement yet has attained the status of attracting majority agreement. Still we believe that the wide range of perspectives by the many who have tried to define it yield valuable information that may eventually help us solve the issue of what should be called "stuttering."

Thus a useful definition of stuttering needs to be free of opinion or explanation so that it enables researchers to explore its various forms and features, and generate, prove, or disprove theories of its causes, all without changing the definition. Unfortunately, many of the definitions of stuttering have lacked these desired qualities, and therefore have not been sufficiently rigorous in support of research. In this chapter we review many definitions of stuttering, consider their content, application, benefits, and limitations, so that students of stuttering can appreciate and critically evaluate the issues involved.

Why Be Concerned with Definition? Practical Implications

A recent study found that college students tend to pour single servings of beer and liquor that are larger than commonly used standards (White et al., 2005). One possible reason for the overpouring is students' lack of knowledge of the definition of standard serving sizes. This may have unfortunate health and other hazardous consequences. From scientific considerations, however, the implications are that the absence of knowledge of definitions of a serving size casts doubt on the accuracy of various studies of students' reports about their alcohol consumption. Critically, lacking a clear referent, they underestimate their drinking. This example highlights the potentially powerful influence of definitions.

Because definitions provide a reference and orientation to their conceptual topics, definitions of "what is stuttering" exert direct impact on theory, research, and clinical application. One method of specifying a phenomenon is to collect samples of cases people can agree on, and then determine features that the cases share in common. But if there has not been any clarity about which cases belong in the sample, then conclusions are apt to be misleading. Definitions impact the population identified, what is quantified, and ultimately how progress in treatment is evaluated. These three important functions of a definition are elaborated next.

Population Identification

This issue is encountered at the very early stage of systematic research of stuttering—identifying and counting the subpopulation of people who stutter. The specific definition, or the absence of one, can influence the findings concerning incidence and prevalence of stuttering (to be discussed in Chapter 2), regardless of the data collection method. Consider, for example, the potential inconsistency in a survey where hundreds of schoolteachers around the country are asked to report the number of stuttering children in their schools but are not provided with a definition of a child who stutters. Similarly, in the conduct of just about every study of stuttering, the investigator should follow some operational definition to determine who is qualified to be included as a participant who stutters. In comparative studies, it is also necessary to determine who does not stutter and thus qualifies as a control subject.

Unfortunately, many past studies failed to adhere to this basic requirement. For example, participants were included because they were "regarded" as stutterers without further elaboration of what they had to exhibit to be viewed as "stuttering." When such studies have clinical implications, the use of a vaguely defined population makes it difficult to apply their results.

Quantification and Measurement

The implications of a definition extend beyond the selection of potential clients and research participants. Definition is important to those who look at changes in the phenomena. Investigators and clinicians interested in the amount or characteristics of stuttered speech under various conditions must define, in advance, what the "stuttering" is—that is, what will be measured as the target. For example, Yairi and Ambrose (1999a) investigated changes in the frequency of stuttered speech events in preschool children over several years. They defined stuttering as consisting of three observable speech elements: (1) repetitions of parts of words, (2) repetitions of single-syllable words, and (3) sound prolongations and blocks. They referred to these as "stuttering-like disfluencies." Their definition was based on a long history of investigations revealing a valid and reliable set of overt speech behaviors typical of children who were judged by their parents and clinicians to exhibit stuttering. By contrast but no less valid, in a study of the effect of therapy on the speech of young children who stutter, J. Ingham and G. Riley (1998) defined stuttering in terms of what the experimenters *perceived* as stuttered syllables. No objective, observable characteristics were specified. Their definition was based on an extensive history of research experiments revealing that experienced, well-trained examiners can perceptually identify instances of "stuttering" (no further definition) with sufficiently valid and reliable judgments. Both sets of researchers have contributed significantly to the wealth of knowledge about stuttering, yet their scientific definitions were very different. Decisions about what stuttering is and how it will be measured affect which research can be consulted during clinical applications.

Evaluation of Clinical Progress

It should be clearer by now that definitions of stuttering have major implications in the clinical arena. Although the matter of diagnosis is separate from the issue of definition, critical decisions of whether a person is diagnosed as exhibiting stuttering and recommended for therapy on one hand, and, on the other hand, whether or not he or she has stopped stuttering and should be discharged, hinge on its formal definition as well as evaluative criteria. Such decisions are particularly difficult when the person in question exhibits a mild or a borderline case. Public consumers of clinical services need to be confident their concerns at all stages and levels are not overlooked because of insufficient definitions and diagnoses of the disorder. Several definitions a reader may encounter, such as "Stuttering is a transient disturbance in communicative, propositional, language usage," are not useful in practical situations. Clients and health-care agencies paying for treatment are entitled to insist on reasonable grounds for identification of the condition for which treatment is requested. Thus, in addition to theoretical, research, and clinical purposes, there is also a significant economic motive to establish a clear, acceptable definition of stuttering.

What to Define: Event or Disorder?

When the term *stuttering* or a derivative (e.g., *a stutter*) is used, the referent may either be to a speech event or to a disorder. In the statement "Last night he was *stuttering*," the term refers exclusively to the occurrence of the surface (overt) phenomena: interruptions of the flow of speech that are perceived as abnormal. By contrast, in the statement "She has had *stuttering* a long time," it has a much broader application. Here, stuttering refers to the whole disorder, involving other important aspects, such as physiology, emotion, cognition, and social facets that have persisted over time, not just with isolated occurrences of speech events. This is illustrated in Sheehan's (1958, p. 123) notion of the "stuttering iceberg" that what we perceive as stuttering events reveals only a small part of the disorder—that is, the tip of the iceberg.

Accordingly, "stuttering" has been defined or conceptualized by scholars as either event or disorder, although not always in a mutually exclusive manner. The stuttering literature, however, reveals far too many discussions that fail to establish what needs to be defined, overlooking the two conceptualizations of stuttering and leaving the student of the subject bewildered. Thus we contrast definitions of stuttering as an observable speech phenomenon with definitions of stuttering as a disorder. Taking this orientation, the definitional language referring to stuttering as a speech phenomenon generally describes what a person is *doing* when talking. The second, broader concept of stuttering, as a disorder, necessitates an entirely different focus. Here, the definitional language usually contains statements about what a person *is* or *has*.[1] We develop these two concepts of stuttering further, in the next sections.

Stuttering as a Speech Event

The event of stuttering only occurs in the context of attempting to speak. It is different from a hiccup that occurs whether a person is speaking or not. The most meaningful speech, like saying one's name, is more apt to be stuttered than a nonsense phrase made up of words in a mixed up order (Wingate, 1979). For many, the act of saying an isolated speech sound is far less apt to trigger stutter events than delivering a public address. For others, however, the mere attempt to make the sound of an isolated vowel will trigger stuttering. Stuttering is an involuntary disruption of the smooth execution of a speaker's intentional speech act. Because stuttering is so inextricably tied to the act of speaking, it will be beneficial to examine normal speech production and the concepts of speech fluency and disfluency, prior to defining stuttering.

---

[1] Johnson (1958) made comparisons between what a person is *doing* versus what a person *is or has*.

Normally Fluent Speech Production

Normal fluency is recognized by the ease and ongoing flow of speech muscular movement and the resultant speech sounds. Speech produced fluently consists of suitable
dimensions of (1) rate (i.e., appropriate timing within and across words), (2) continuity
(i.e., smooth connections within and across words), and (3) tension effort (i.e., appropriate regulation of exertion or force) (Starkweather, 1987). Hence various levels of the
speech system must function properly and in close coordination.

Levels and Systems

Speech originates in the speaker's brain and involves complex processes, including linguistic formulation of an intended message, selection and ordering of sounds, syllables,
and words, preparation of utterance rhythm, tempo, and vocal tone, and final transmission of coordinated neurological commands from the brain to the peripheral motor
and sensory mechanisms that produce the desired speech signals and movements. The
gross anatomical components of the peripheral speech system are the lungs, trachea,
larynx, pharyngeal cavity, oral cavity, and nasal cavity. The pharyngeal and oral cavities
are usually referred to as the *vocal tract*, beginning at the larynx and terminating at the
lips. The nasal cavity begins at the velum (soft palate) and ends at the nostrils.

At the motor physiological level, normally fluent speech requires a series of precisely coordinated movements of respiratory, phonatory, and articulatory muscles.
Prior to speaking, an optimal air volume within a certain range enters the lungs via
inhalation. The air is then expelled into the larynx and the vocal tract. As air rushes
from the lungs through the trachea, the vocal cords within the larynx approximate
(i.e., are positioned near midline) and are set into gentle vibration, interrupting
the air flow with quasi-periodic pulses that result in the sound that we call "voice."
In the next stage, the relatively simple acoustic properties of the sound are modu-
lated and filtered as the airwaves pass through the vocal tract and are then shaped
by the movement and positioning of the articulators, especially the tongue, lips, and
jaw, creating recognized speech sounds, such as vowels. When the velum is lowered,
the nasal cavities are acoustically coupled to the vocal tract to produce the nasal
sounds of speech. Other sounds are generated by varying the shape and size at various locations in the vocal tract. For example, some consonants (i.e., fricatives) are
formed by generating turbulent noise as the air is forced through various narrow
constrictions shaped in the oral cavity, whereas others, such as plosives (or stops),
are formed by quick releases of air pressure built up behind obstructions, such as
closed lips. Sounds are filtered and modified still further as they blend (e.g., for coarticulation) into syllables, words, and sentences. They are then further refined by
changes in rate, pitch, intonation, and loudness (which combine alterations of the
respiratory, phonatory, and articulatory systems). Thus speech output becomes
acoustically complex in both the frequency and time dimensions, and as a function
of the constantly varying length and cross-sectional area of the vocal tract, as well as
the position of the articulators and durations of their movements.

This account, which is probably familiar to many of you, is presented to make
the point that stuttering, at least as at the surface level, should be appreciated against
the larger complex structures and functions that are disrupted. It is the precise,

delicate, coordinated, and timed array of movements and resultant normal flow of speech that may be disrupted at just about any or all levels of the speech motor system: respiration, phonation, and articulation. The disruptions frequently appear as various disfluencies described later or as complete cessations of speech, inability to initiate words, respiratory and phonatory irregularities (e.g., running out of air for speech, pitch raising, glottal fry, etc.), and others. Additionally, there is growing evidence to suspect that disruptions underlying disfluency also occur at higher levels of speech planning and control in the brain, but we will save expansion of this topic to Chapter 7.

Normal Disfluency or Instances of Stuttering?

The various surface interruptions that occur in ongoing speech have been referred to as "disfluencies." For most practical purposes, these speech events have been categorized using linguistic terminology or other descriptors applied to speech events. Among the most commonly referred to disfluency categories are word repetition, part-word or syllable repetition, sound repetition, phrase repetition, sound prolongation, blockage,[2] interjection, and revision. Some of these (e.g., phrase repetition) minimally interrupt the continuity of speech, but they do slow down its progress.[3] A critical fact is that disfluencies occur not only in the speech of people who stutter but also in the speech of practically all speakers, especially young children (Davis, 1939; Johnson, 1961a; Yairi, 1981). It is important, therefore, to recognize from the outset that disfluency and stuttering, although related, are not synonymous. In most people and under most circumstances, disfluencies are not too frequent and are regarded as normal. But, under some circumstances, disfluent speech is regarded as abnormal or stuttering. Thus the term *disfluency* or *disfluencies* refers to speech disruptions regardless of whether they happen to be normal or abnormal (stuttered) speech events.

Alternate spellings of some terms are found in the stuttering literature. Examples are 'disfluencies' vs. 'dysfluencies,' or 'disrhythmic phonations' vs. 'dysrhythmic phonations.' Although not all writers use the distinction, the prefix 'dis' may be contrasted with 'dys' on purpose. Wingate (2002) explains that the prefix 'dis' is the Latin for 'not'; 'dys' refers to 'disorder.' Therefore when encountering 'dys,' you should understand that the referent may be more closely tied to the disorder of stuttering. By contrast, the prefix 'dis' commonly refers to all disruptions whether specifically stuttered or not.

The distinction between "normal disfluency" and "stuttering," sometimes blurred, stems from two sources, speech production and speech perception. From a production perspective there are abundant data showing that several disfluency types occur much more frequently in the speech of people who are regarded as exhibiting stuttering (Ambrose & Yairi, 1999; Johnson et al., 1959). Syllable repetition is a prime example. It is found in the speech of all speakers but much more frequently in the speech of

---

[2] The categories of sound prolongations and blocks are frequently merged in a single category, disrhythmic phonations.

[3] Disfluencies are described and discussed in more detail in Chapter 4.

people who stutter. Additionally, in many cases, disfluencies produced by people who stutter are not only more frequent but also different in other properties from the same type produced by normally speaking people. When a person who stutters repeats a syllable such as "an-an-and," the speed of the repetitions is much faster than repetitions produced by a normally speaking person (Throneburg & Yairi, 1994, 2001), the number of repetitions per instance is greater (Ambrose & Yairi, 1995), and their distribution (clustering) within speech is different (Hubbard & Yairi, 1988; Sawyer, 2005; Sawyer & Yairi, in press). From a perceptual perspective, the very same disfluency types also tend to be judged as "stuttering" by listeners. Of course, the frequency of occurrence is very influential. One or two syllable repetitions per 100 words of running speech may be perceived as normal, but five syllable repetitions in the same amount of speech are likely to be perceived as stuttering (Sander, 1963). Still, listeners vary in how they perceive the same disfluencies as "normal" or "stuttering" (Young, 1984).

Concerning disfluency types, all conventionally recognized and defined disfluencies found in people who stutter also occur in the speech of normally fluent children. But disfluency types that are most typical to stuttering have been dubbed as "core behaviors" (Van Riper, 1971). Yairi and Ambrose (1992a) distinguished between these stuttering-like disfluencies, or SLD ("stuttering-like" indicates that they are not exclusive to stuttering), and other disfluencies, which are regarded as more typical to normally fluent speakers. These are listed in Table 1.1.

Perceptible differences may distinguish many moments of stuttering from normal disfluency, but some listeners may find it difficult to determine if a disfluency they have heard is normal or stuttered (Curlee, 1981; Martin & Haroldson, 1981). Listeners seem to operate with different perceptual thresholds in regard to *"how much is too much?"* That is, how much disruption does it take to evoke the person's judgment that a repetition is "stuttering" rather than "normal disfluency"? (Martin & Haroldson, 1981). Factors potentially affecting listener judgment include the type, duration, and intensity of the disfluency, as well as the context, past experience, and characteristics (e.g., gender) of the listener (Kawai, Healey, & Carrell, 2007). For example, a person who has relatives who stutter may be more sensitive to disfluencies and exhibit a lower threshold.

Table 1.1: Types of Disfluency

Stuttering-Like Disfluency	Examples
Part-Word Repetition	Bu-bu-but
Single Syllable Word Repetition	An-an-and
Disrhythmic Phonation	Mo—mmy

Other Disfluencies	Examples
Phrase Repetition	I like to—I like to . . .
Revision	It was, I mean . . .
Interjection	Uhm, well, er

From the speaker's perspective, the reason(s) underlying the behavior are also important. A normal speech disruption is usually associated with reasons that the speaker recognizes, such as word-finding, a sentence-formulation decision, a reconsideration of message content, a distracting event nearby, and so on. When the speaker recognizes the reason for the speech disruption, he or she is apt to acknowledge it as a "normal disfluency." The experience of normal disfluency for reasons such as these is shared by the nonstutterer and stutterer alike. By contrast, when the word(s) to be said are fully decided and the speaker is intent to engage in speaking, but the production becomes "stuck" for what seems to be no apparent reason, it is then that the experience by the speaker is apt to fit the label of "stuttering."

Defining the Event of Stuttering

The preceding discussion revealed a precedent for categorizing instances of speech disruption into primary (or "core") disfluency types commonly evident as the overt symptoms of stuttering and secondary[4] (or "other") disfluency types, evident when a speaker hesitates or reformulates for reasons that may or may not relate to stuttering. This two-class structure has been confirmed with empirical research (Lewis, 1991), and not surprisingly, a number of scientists have offered definitions of stuttering from the standpoint of criteria based on behavioral observations.

Examples of Definitions of Stuttering as an Event

As early as 1931, Travis defined stuttering objectively as "a disturbance in the rhythm of speech; an intermittent blocking; a convulsive repetition of a sound." This definition, proposed at the beginning of the modern era of speech pathology, appears to have influenced Travis's students to coin the term *moment of stuttering*. Among them, Wendell Johnson was probably the person most responsible for the widespread usage of the concept of "moments of stuttering" (Johnson, 1955, p. 13). This terminology suggests that immediately before and immediately after the perceived stuttering, speech was normal, a questionable assumption. In our opinion the term *stuttering event* is preferable because it reflects the concept of *activity* rather than *time*.

Wingate (1964a, 1988) offered one of the most well-known definitions of stuttering as events. At first, he provided a lengthy three-part definition where the first part, focused on core speech features, was as follows: "The term stuttering means (a) disruption in the fluency of verbal expression, which is (b) characterized by involuntary, audible or silent, repetitions or prolongations in the utterance of short speech elements, namely, sounds, syllables and words of one syllable. These disruptions (c) usually occur frequently or are marked in character and (d) are not readily controllable" (Wingate, 1964a, p. 488). Later, however, he argued that the essence of stuttering consisted of "silent or audible elemental repetitions and prolongations"

---

[4] The term *accessory* has also been applied to this class of disfluencies.

(Wingate, 1988, p. 9). Although present also in the speech of normally fluent people, they are, by contrast, only rarely uttered. It is the frequent occurrence of these events in a person's speech that conveys the impression of stuttering. Wingate's latter definition was helpfully succinct and it has been applied frequently in research.

More recently, Guitar (1998) proposed that stuttering consists of "an abnormally high frequency or duration of stoppages in the forward flow of speech. These stoppages usually take the form of (a) repetitions of sounds, syllables or one-syllable words, (b) prolongations of sounds, or (c) 'blocks' of airflow or voicing in speech. . . . Moreover, they often use excessive physical and mental effort to speak" (pp. 10–11). These statements offer additional characteristics not mentioned in Wingate's definition. The last phrase, however, extends the definition beyond the realm of overt features of speech.

The American Speech-Language-Hearing Association has addressed the definition of stuttering in a technical paper prepared for its Special Interest Division 4, *Fluency and Fluency Disorders*, by the Task Force on Terminology (1999). They discuss the issue of definition at greater length, but among their statements is "Stuttering refers to speech events that contain monosyllabic whole-word repetitions, part-word repetitions, audible sound prolongations, or silent fixations or blockages. These may or may not be accompanied by accessory (secondary) behaviors (i.e., behaviors used to escape and/or avoid these speech events)" (1999, p. 31). This definition also extends beyond pure speech characteristics to include secondary physical characteristics.

Yairi and Ambrose (2005) considered the fact that also normally fluent speakers produce, at times, some disfluent speech. Therefore, they defined stuttering based on the statistical probability that certain speech patterns will be either produced by people who stutter or will be so perceived by listeners. In their words,

> [W]e consider those speech characteristics that young children who stutter tend to produce, and those that are *likely* to be judged by listeners as stuttering. Thus, children considered to stutter are inclined to exhibit interruptions in the flow of speech in the form of repetition of parts of words (e.g., sounds and syllables) and monosyllabic words, as well as by disrhythmic phonations—prolongations of sounds and arrests of speech (blocks). We have referred to these overt speech phenomena as Stuttering-Like Disfluency (SLD). These are the most common disfluencies produced by children who stutter, as well as the speech events most *likely* to be perceived as stuttering. (Yairi & Ambrose, 2005, p. 20)

They go on to say that these elements are similarly listed in the definition suggested by the American Speech-Language-Hearing Association of 1999.

Finally, offering our own opinion, we propose that stuttering events are evident when speech is characterized by periods of frequent and/or intense disruptions to the integration of syllable elements or syllables as components of spoken utterances.[5]

---

[5] The concept of stuttering as a disruption to the integration of syllables was developed and supported most thoroughly by Wingate (1988).

At its minimum, such interruptions consist of repeated and/or elongated segments, including sound, syllable, or a single-syllable words. Examples of intense disruptions include repetitions that are fast in tempo and prolongations that are longer than one-half second.

Fluent Speech of People Who Stutter

It is well recognized that a substantial percentage, often the majority, of the speech of people who stutter is fluent. On the average, only 10% of words in oral reading were found to be stuttered by adults (Bloodstein, 1944). Similarly, a mean of 11.84% stuttered words was found in conversation/storytelling or conversation/reading contexts for 76 children ages 5 through 12 (G. Riley & J. Riley, 1980). An inevitable question is whether or not the stutterer's fluent speech is also abnormal in other speech parameters. If yes, should this be considered in the definition? In fact, for several decades there has been growing evidence that the fluent portions of the speech of a person who stutters differ from the fluency of normally fluent speakers. For example, when all disfluent segments were removed from tape-recorded speech samples, listeners could still correctly identify the speech of stutterers from matched samples of nonstutterers (Wendahl & Cole, 1961). Although replications of this work yielded negative or mixed results (Young, 1964), research of the acoustic and physiologic properties of the fluent speech of stutterers has reported more convincing support. Vowel duration measures (Zimmermann, 1980a), second formant transitions (Robb & Blomgren, 1997), and vocal fold vibrations (Hall & Yairi, 1992) produced by stutterers in their fluent speech are different from those produced by normal speakers. These findings have been used in support of arguments against limiting stuttering definitions to disfluent speech characteristics. So far, however, the characteristics of fluent speech of people who stutter have not been incorporated into definitions of stuttering. The challenge remains for future scientists to determine how best to incorporate this aspect.

Overall, in spite of difficulties arising from a certain amount of overlap between normal disfluency and stuttering, speech-oriented definitions appear to be in a reasonably close agreement on the essential elements (disfluency features) that should be included in definitions of stuttering. Experimenters and clinicians are in a position of being able to apply some principles in formulating working definitions for their specific studies or clinical needs. Still, reflecting the incomplete state of knowledge, there are inconsistent applications, and definitions have failed to refer to fluent speech characteristics of people who stutter. Focusing on speech, they disregard other important aspects of stuttering and therefore may not cover certain cases such as people with covert stuttering.

Stuttering as a Disorder

Multidimensional Characteristics of the Stuttering Disorder

The backdrop for defining stuttering as a disorder is its multidimensionality. It involves much more than the overt dimensions of disfluent speech. The multifaceted nature is apparent from the very first contact of a speech-language clinician with an adult who stutters who exhibits lip tremor during stuttering and reports strong anxiety prior to and during talking. To this particular client, the fear associated with stuttered speech is as much of a problem, if not more, than the speech aspects. Also children who stutter may exhibit physical body tension and secondary movements during stuttered speech, as well as avoidance behavior and social withdrawal. The reactions of parents must also be addressed. The clinician realizes that all these have to be described, and if possible quantified.

Six major dimensions of the stuttering disorder are distinguished:

I. *Overt speech characteristics.* These are interruptions of the normal flow of speech that occur at the respiratory, phonatory, and articulatory levels but are evident acoustically as repetitions of sounds and/or syllables, prolongations of sounds, cessation of sound, and so on.

II. *Physical concomitants.* This dimension can be described as "tense" body movements, especially in the head and neck, but also in other parts of the body, that are often manifest in association with the disfluent speech events. These are known as "secondary characteristics." Thus they are not necessary for stuttering to occur or be diagnosed, but may appear as the person who stutters struggles through a stuttering event, attempting to move forward in communication.

III. *Physiological activity.* Stuttered speech is associated with changes in blood flow, skin reactions, pupil responses, brainwave activities, and other physiological changes. Many of these cannot be observed with the naked eye but have been well documented, and they continue to be studied by researchers.

IV. *Affective features.* It is quite common for people who stutter to develop strong emotional reactions about talking, especially fears of speaking in many situations. When these emotions become intense, leading to avoidance of speaking, the emotional dimension of the disorder could overshadow that of the abnormal speech. Even in young children, particularly those with sensitive temperaments, slow adaptation to change and problems with self-regulation, their difficulties speaking may yield speech avoidance, fear of speaking, sadness, and/or frustration.

V. *Cognitive processes.* Every professional familiar with stuttering has heard parents, teachers, relatives, or other listeners comment that the person who stutters is "thinking faster than he can talk." A parent may comment, "He has so much to say and he just can't get it all out at once." These assumptions could be valid. The cognitive underpinnings of the selection, planning, preparation, and execution of speech (i.e., what to say, how to say it, when to say it, etc.), may, in effect, present "overload" for the person who stutters, yielding stuttered speech. Second, the cognitive dimension also pertains to the level of awareness that a person has of his or her stuttering, perceptions during moments of stuttering, and perceptions of listeners' reactions to the stuttering. A third aspect is the concepts the person has about the nature of disorder and the language used to characterize it. For example, a person may relate his or her perception of stuttering as "words get stuck" in the throat, likening words to objects. Actually, muscular activity and movement is interrupted.

VI. *Social dynamics.* The disorder of stuttering can have devastating effects on interpersonal communication because the fear of stuttering contributes to various difficulties in social interactions. Examples include class participation, initiating conversations, answering the telephone, dating, adjustments to new environments, and making career choices.

Additionally, in complex ways, stuttering is also interwoven with the language and phonological development of some children. These aspects can have particularly important implications for clinical intervention during early childhood. Finally, all of the above are impacted by genetic factors, a topic we expand on in later chapters.

Diversity of Disorder-Oriented Definitions

When reviewing the plethora of definitions of the stuttering disorder, and the diversity encountered, it raises the question of whether the experts who offered them were addressing the same condition. It also becomes evident that not all definitions have adhered to the principles stated in the *New Oxford American Dictionary* regarding their role to clarify the meaning, scope, and application of a term. Some digress to explain stuttering or merely offer a point of view regarding its etiology; others constitute descriptions of a few selected features. Even those that provide descriptions have not offered a characterization that sufficiently distinguishes the disorder of stuttering from other speech problems (e.g., apraxic speech, aphasic speech, etc.). Before we proceed with examples of these definitions, it is important to better understand the potential sources of the diversity among them.

Within the *disorder* conceptual framework, a further division of the definitions must be noted. You will come across some definitions that are confined to a single domain, (e.g., neurologic factors), and other definitions with interactions among multiple domains (e.g., motoric and psychologic). Unfortunately, some scholars, perhaps hungry for a clear-cut definition that also promotes their theoretical inclination, have succumbed to the temptation of focusing on a single domain of the complex disorder of stuttering to the neglect, or insufficient consideration, of its other domains. When the satisfaction promised by these pronouncements proves to be short lived, however, the hunger and search for the meaning of stuttering resumes.

Until the 1940s, many professionals who expressed active interest in stuttering were psychiatrists, physicians representing other specialties, psychologists, and more. Understandably, these professionals operated from different knowledge bases, informational sources, general perspectives, entrenched conventions, and strong biases. Although they looked at many of the same facts, they arrived at different definitions that reflected their diverse backgrounds. They also were inclined to examine only one, or a few, pieces of the stuttering puzzle, those that were more in tune with their particular area of expertise. Having pointed this out, it is only fair to acknowledge that varying experiences and circumstances do indeed provide different types and amounts of information about any particular problem. For example, scholars and clinicians who work primarily with young children who stutter are likely to have a different perspective and understanding of the disorder than those working exclusively with adults. If, however, people with different areas of knowledge and expertise work together to solve the multidimensional puzzle of stuttering, understanding of the disorder will continue to grow.

Examples of Definitions of Stuttering as a Disorder

Because different frames of reference have influenced definitions of the stuttering disorder, they are organized here into five subcategories that roughly reflect various theoretical positions on the nature of stuttering. They include organic, psychopathogenic, psychosocial, learning-based orientations, and speaker-based perspectives (i.e., from the standpoint of the person who stutters). Examples of each are presented next.

Organic Orientations

During much of the first half of the 20th century, the view that stuttering is organically based was popular as seen in West, Nelson, and Berry's (1939) reflection that stuttering, like left-handedness, twinning, or other atypical subpopulation characteristics, rests on some common heritable factor of structure or biochemistry. Years later, West (1958) was more specific in stating that stuttering is "primarily an epileptic disorder that manifests itself in dyssynergies of the neuromotor mechanism for oral language" (p. 197). In our view, this provides a good example of an attempted definition that, instead, ought to be classified as an explanation. In relation to the previous discussion, note that it does not treat stuttering as a surface phenomenon but as a disorder. Further, as such, it is focused on a single etiological variable, faulty neurological system, viewed by West as the essence of the disorder. It does not define stuttering as a complex disorder.

Also representing the organic orientation is Van Riper's (1971) definition that highlights the timing of muscle movement. He proposed that "Stuttering is a disorder of timing . . . when a person stutters on a word, there is a temporal disruption of the simultaneous and successive programming of muscular movement required to produce one of the word's integrated sounds, or to emit one of its syllables appropriately" (p. 415). This definition treats stuttering as a disorder and focuses on a single variable. In the same source, however, Van Riper stated that "stuttering occurs when a forward flow of speech is interrupted by a motorically disrupted sound, syllable, or word or the speaker's reactions thereto" (p. 15). This definition has the advantage that it appreciates the reality that stutter events can take many different behavioral forms (i.e., prolonged sounds, repetitions, etc.). It acknowledges, however, that the inner experience of a person who stutters exceeds the usual momentary embarrassment of stumbled speech. By combining these two elements of surface and covert features, it treats stuttering as a truly complex disorder.

Finally, most stuttering cases fit the profile of the classic developmental speech disorder that originates in early childhood without apparent causal factors and, in some cases, continues for several or many years. For that reason, many definitions are like the one found in *Churchill's Illustrated Medical Dictionary*: "A speech disorder affecting the fluency of production, often characterized by repetitions of certain sounds, syllables, words, or phrases, and by the prolongation of sounds and blocking of the articulation of words. Severer forms may be associated with facial grimacing, limb and postural gestures, involuntary grunts, or impaired control of airflow. The severity of symptoms may vary with the speaker's situation and audience." And a statement is added: "It is unusual to find evidence of neurological dysfunction in the confirmed adolescent or adult stutterer" (Koenisberger, 1989, pp. 1802–1803).

Psychopathogenic Orientations

Also during the 20th century, especially its first half, viewing stuttering as a psychopathological disorder was similarly popular. Although this theoretical orientation has lost much ground, a brief review will serve to illuminate the diversity of opinions. Coriat (1943a, p. 28) conceived stuttering to be "a psychoneurosis caused by the persistence into later life of early pregenital[6] oral nursing, oral sadistic, and anal sadistic components." A quarter century later, Glauber (1958, p. 78) suggested that "Stuttering is a neurotic disorder in which personality disturbance is in part reflected in speech. . . . Stuttering is a symptom of a psychopathological condition classified as pregenital conversion neurosis." Similarly, Murphy and Fitzsimons (1960, p. 17) stated that "First, stuttering behavior is primarily a psychogenically motivated symptom which manifests itself most discernibly in oral function." Again, all three definitions are primarily explanations, viewing stuttering as an underlying psychological disorder but limited in scope to a single essential factor.

Psychosocial Orientations

Another take on stuttering is seen in the attempts to define it as a psychosocial problem. As Fletcher (1928, p. 226) conceived it, stuttering is "a morbidity of social consciousness, a hyper-sensitivity of social attitude, a pathological social response." The main factors that operate here are fear, anxiety, inferiority feelings, and so on, in terms of social relationships, all of which have their genesis in specific experiences. Thus the fears and anxiety are not general but in the anticipation of the necessity to speak under certain defined conditions that set off the pathological reactions. Another perspective of stuttering within the context of social interaction was offered by Eisenson (1958, p. 244), who proposed that "Stuttering is a transient disturbance in communicative propositional language usage." This concept of stuttering emphasizes its social impact as a breakdown in conveying meaning when communicating with others. This dimension is difficult to research, and the field has future work ahead to better incorporate it into our understanding of the disorder.

Learning Orientations

In the 1950s when psychological learning theories were popular, Johnson (1955a, pp. 23–24) opined that the essence of stuttering was "an anticipatory apprehensive hypertonic avoidance reaction." Although the definition lacks specific reference to

---

[6] Pregenital refers to the organization of the child's sexual development during the early infantile period, before the genital zone became its focus.

speech, Johnson's writings clearly point out speech as the cause of the anticipation. Accordingly, stuttering is a complex, although transient problem, that occurs when (based on past experience) a speaker anticipates stuttering and reacts by setting off an acquired (learned) array of cognitive, emotional, and tense physical responses that end up as struggled, stuttered speech. There is a circular, slightly troublesome, nature to this definition in that it necessitates another definition to characterize the stuttering events that prompted the initial reaction.

In this group of learning-oriented definition we also cite Brutten and Shoemaker (1967, p. 61), who defined stuttering as "a form of fluency failure that results from conditioned negative emotions." This definition, as the previous one, would hardly aid anyone attempting to identify stuttering. It is merely a statement concerning the authors' belief about its cause: certain acquired (learned) emotions that trigger fluency failure. One may infer that if fluency failures were caused by a different agent, it would not be stuttering.

Orientations Representing the Speaker's Perspective

Stemming from a difference in basic conceptualization, another factor has impacted the diversity of stuttering definitions. Whereas most definitions assume a *listener-observer's* frame of reference, a few are based on the *speaker's*, that is, the person who stutters, point of view (e.g., Perkins, 1990a). Related to this matter, there are people who stutter severely yet never miss an opportunity to speak, and people who stutter very mildly but hesitate to speak at all, revealing a wide contrast in the *speaker's* perceptions of their stuttering problem. It can be argued, therefore, that the personal point of view has major implications for describing, diagnosing, and treating stuttering, and hence, also in defining it.

One example of a succinct definition of stuttering that zeroes in on the speaker's perspective was offered by Perkins (1990a). He proposed that "loss of control of the ability to voluntarily continue a disrupted utterance is the essence of stuttering" (p. 376). Again from the perspective of the person who stutters, the speaker's feeling of loss of control of his or her speech is the key characteristic, but it is difficult to distinguish this problem from an apraxia of speech. This definition has little practical value for research purposes. It does not guide investigators as to what needs to be quantified as stuttering.

Another definition of stuttering from the speaker's point of view was adopted by the World Health Organization: "Disorders of rhythm of speech in which the individual knows precisely what he wishes to say, but at the time is unable to say it because of involuntary, repetitive prolongation or cessation of a sound" (World Health Organization, 1977). Here, considerable weight is given to the inner experiences of the person while it also includes the basic symptomatology. As is the case with the Perkins definition, however, it may be difficult to distinguish the defining characteristics from apraxia. The additional limitation of these definitions is that stuttering might constitute a variety of different experiences for different people who perceive themselves to stutter.

Other Views

One approach to overcoming the challenge of individual differences among those who stutter is seen in the model presented by Yaruss and Quesal (2004, 2006) (Fig. 1.1). They include components of body function and structure, personal and environmental factors, and activity/participation as a framework for describing the stuttering disorder. Their model, however, is more useful for consideration of what stuttering *involves*, as opposed to defining what stuttering *is*.

Overall, the few definitions just cited that address stuttering as a disorder are sufficient to demonstrate a wide diversity in the ways the supposed essence of stuttering has been captured, conceiving of it as an organic/motor disorder, psychiatric disorder, psychosocial disorder, learned disorder, and a disorder affecting a speaker's intentional control. The definitions differ so greatly that one might almost wonder if all of them refer to the same disorder. From a practical point of view, although each definition depicts one or several relevant parameters of stuttering, none of them is sufficiently specific (precise) to be useful in the identification of people who exhibit the disorder.

Our Point of View

In the preceding discussion of how to define stuttering as a disorder, we highlighted its multidimensional characteristics. In view of its complexity and the vast individual and age variations across multiple dimensions, it is nearly impossible to formulate a definition of stuttering to satisfy the desired criteria successfully. With these reservations in mind, we nevertheless propose this perspective (not a

Figure 1.1: **Model Representing the Stuttering Disorder (From Yaruss & Quesal, 2006)**

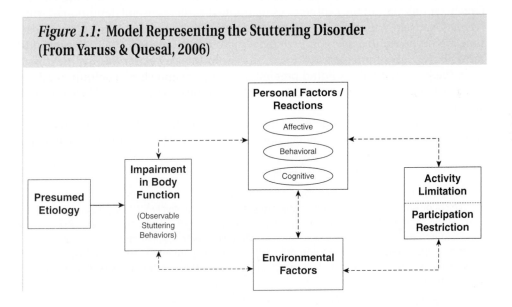

definition): Near its onset in young children, stuttering is a speech disorder (also known as "developmental stuttering" because of its childhood onset) in those who are prone to experience, for at least a period of time, intermittent disruptions in the form of one or all of the following: sound/syllable repetitions, sound/postural prolongations, and complete blockages of the vocal tract. It is genetically-based but highly responsive to environmental factors. When the disorder persists, its expands to acquire additional characteristics reflected in dynamic, multidimensional patterns of overt body tensions, motor-physiological adaptations, as well as emotional, cognitive, and social reactions. These additional characteristics intensify as the disorder persists and, to the person who stutters, may be more disturbing than the stuttered speech events.

Summary

The term *stuttering* may refer to certain speech events or to the complex disorder. Defining stuttering, especially as a disorder, has proved to be a difficult task that has not yet been successfully accomplished. This is not surprising considering the different meanings of stuttering and its multidimensionality as a disorder. Such diversity in how scholars have dealt with the basic matter of defining stuttering, and their continuous difficulties in agreeing on what stuttering is and who is qualified as a "stutterer" have had a strong impact on how the disorder has been understood, investigated, and treated. The current state of affairs is a source of concern because one wonders about the effect of such diversity in definitions and points of view, and the difficulties encountered in arriving at a reasonable agreement, on the overall progress in the field. Still, progress has been made as reflected in the World Health Organization's view of the problem. As mentioned earlier, a useful definition of stuttering for research purposes should endure even when multiple theories across time are proposed to explain it. Perhaps researchers should focus on defining stuttering in its purest and simplest form, similar to the way water has been defined essentially as what falls as liquid precipitation. A pure and simple definition might prove beneficial even if, just like water, stuttering is rarely encountered in a pure and simple form.

We agree with the preceding statement in contrast to the disorder-based definitions that have continued to reflect huge diversity. As we see it, there was an early

Regarding the role of speech-based definition, it was noted that "whatever else the clinical disorder of stuttering entails, there seems to be relatively little disagreement that the term 'stuttering' refers to the domain of motor speech production and its disruption by speech disfluencies. Physical, physiological, cognitive, and emotional components, regardless of how frequent or intense they might be, would not be labeled as 'stuttering' if they did not accompany a speaker's disfluent speech" (Yairi & Ambrose, 2005, p. 19).

tendency to present a confusing state of affairs when it came to speech characteristics, overemphasizing overlap between normal disfluency and stuttering. Encouraging progress has been made through continuing research to clarify the differences between what is normal and what is not, and in zeroing on the essential features of disfluency necessary for defining stuttering as speech events. Additional information about the fluent speech of people who stutter may strengthen future definitions.

STUDY QUESTIONS AND DISCUSSION TOPICS

1. What is the purpose of a definition of a phenomenon?
2. Why is a definition of stuttering important? List and explain at least three reasons.
3. What are the two main categories of definitions of stuttering? Explain. Refer to two examples of each category.
4. What are the sources of diversity in definitions of stuttering?
5. What are the similarities and differences between normal disfluency and stuttered speech?

WEB SITES

Stuttering at the Web site for the National Institutes on Deafness and Other Communication Disorders. Accessed May 12, 2009, at www.nidcd.nih.gov/health/voice/stutter.htm

Stuttering at the Web site of the American Speech-Language-Hearing Association. Accessed May 12, 2009, at www.asha.org/public/speech/disorders/stuttering.htm

SUGGESTED READINGS

Packman, A., & Attanasio, J. (2004). What should a theory of stuttering explain? In *Theoretical issues in stuttering* (pp. 55–68). Hove, East Sussex, UK: Psychology Press.

Van Riper, C. (1982). Stuttering: Its definition. In *The Nature of Stuttering* (2nd ed., pp. 11–31). Englewood Cliffs, NJ: Prentice-Hall.

Yaruss, S., & Quesal, R. (2004). Stuttering and the International Classification of Functioning, Disability, and Health (ICF): An update. *Journal of Communication Disorders*, *37*(1), 35–52.

Young, M. (1984). Identification of stuttering and stutterers. In R. Curlee & W. Perkins (Eds.), *Nature and treatment of stuttering: New directions*. Boston: College-Hill.

Chapter 2: Who and How Many Stutter?

LEARNER OBJECTIVES

Readers will be able to:

- Recognize the meanings of *incidence* and *prevalence* in general, and relate to stuttering in particular.
- Identify population characteristics (i.e., age, gender, etc.) that influence the incidence and prevalence of stuttering.
- Understand the various research methodologies employed in prevalence and incidence studies of stuttering and interpret results of these studies.
- Evaluate implications of incidence and prevalence data toward an understanding of stuttering and its possible etiologies.

Incidence and Prevalence

The question of how many people experience the disorder of stuttering is one of the first raised by the professionals who study and/or treat it. The answer is not simple, because the question can be approached from different angles or contexts. Customarily, scientists distinguish between *incidence*—the probability that new cases of any disorder will develop over a period of time, and *prevalence*—the estimate of all the cases of the disorder at a given time. To use a familiar example, many, perhaps all, individuals in the population at large have had at least one ear infection at some point in life. The percentage of individuals who have ever developed an ear infection would be an estimate of incidence, and if by "ever" we mean at any time in life, then this would be the *lifetime incidence*. By contrast, a smaller percentage of people are apt to have ear infections at the particular time a population is examined. This would be the *prevalence* of ear infections when a survey is conducted (e.g., of 6-month-olds at a day-care facility). Naturally, the percentages will vary by age and season; for example, young children have more ear infections than older ones, especially in the winter months.

Interpretation of Incidence and Prevalence Data

For stuttering, examples of these measures are found in a study by Andrews and Harris (1964), who reported both the *incidence* and *prevalence* of the disorder.

In their longitudinal survey of 1,000 children followed for 15 years after the time of birth, the incidence of developmental stuttering, in this case *lifetime* incidence,[1] was approximately 4.5% (i.e., about 45 cases had stuttering that lasted any duration). By contrast, the *prevalence* of stuttering among the children when surveyed at age 15 was approximately 1% (i.e., about 10 were currently stuttering). Because in the stuttering literature incidence estimates have frequently (and erroneously) addressed prevalence, the comparison just cited highlights the higher rates of stuttering incidence across the lifetime in contrast to the prevalence figures of all those who stutter at a given time. Still, keep in mind that had the study begun at age 15 and lasted for only 1 year, the prevalence would have been 1%, whereas the incidence would have been 0% because no children began to stutter at 15 years of age.

> Which is greater, the incidence or the prevalence? It all depends on the time period used as a basis for comparison. When compared within a limited duration, for example a 1-year span between the ages of 6 and 7, the incidence of new stuttering cases that develop will be lower than the prevalence that includes all of the continuing cases. But when compared for the span across all ages, the lifetime incidence, which is the number of people who have ever stuttered, exceeds the prevalence, or number of people who currently stutter.

The change in incidence and prevalence for 30 children followed longitudinally over a 3-year time span is illustrated in Figure 2.1. Recall that in a longitudinal study, data are collected from the same sample population at specified intervals over time. In this case, the data were collected once a year. Each square in the grid represents one child. A minimum of 2 months of stuttering was required to count the case. In year 1, there were three new cases of stuttering that began among the 30 children.

Figure 2.1: **An Example of Tracking the Incidence and Prevalence of Stuttering Cases**

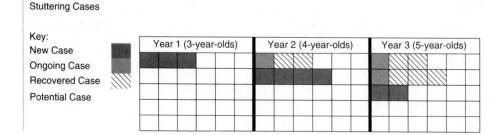

Stuttering Cases

Key:
New Case
Ongoing Case
Recovered Case
Potential Case

Year 1 (3-year-olds)   Year 2 (4-year-olds)   Year 3 (5-year-olds)

---

[1] The 15-year span is considered sufficient for "lifetime" incidence of developmental stuttering because it typically starts, and resolves for most, long before 15 years of age.

This represents an incidence of 10% (3 of 30). In year 2, four new cases began, for an incidence of 13.3% (4 of 30). Because two children recovered naturally among the three previous cases, the prevalence of the disorder for that year is 16.7% (5 of 30). Finally, in year 3, the incidence drops to 6.7% (2 of 30), and the prevalence drops to 13.3% (4 of 30) because three additional children recovered. The overall incidence of stuttering for the 3 years combined is 30% (9 of 30). The average incidence across the 3 years is 10% (3/30). This example shows there can be many ways of looking at incidence and prevalence data. It may be reported for specific periods, for the overall period, or as an average across periods. Appropriate interpretation and evaluation of the validity of estimates of incidence and prevalence depends on a firm grasp of their definitions and the time frame involved for the target population. Unfortunately, the two terms *incidence* and *prevalence* have frequently been confused; it is not uncommon to see the terms used interchangeably. Furthermore, the terms may be confusing when first encountered in research due to the overlap that may arise in the range of their estimates.

As with a number of other disorders (e.g., ear infections), cases of stuttering typically continue for a certain period of time and then subside. This additional dimension affects the estimates of incidence and prevalence and their interpretation. Researchers must specify the duration of the stuttering in individuals in order to be included in the count. Recall from earlier in this chapter that in the Andrews and Harris (1964) results, the lifetime incidence of stuttering was approximately 4.5%. This estimate was based on cases of stuttering that had lasted for *any* duration. By contrast, when the researchers examined only those cases that had lasted for *at least 6 months*, the estimate was only 3%. Thus estimates may be made on the basis of the length of time that the disorder lingers.

The Significance of Incidence and Prevalence

Information about the incidence and prevalence of stuttering with respect to factors such as age, gender, and/or different subpopulations (e.g., those with phonological delays/disorders), has direct implications for understanding the causation and dynamics of stuttering. It also provides essential guidance in clinical decision making related to diagnosis, prognosis, and treatment recommendations. Because incidence estimates reflect the rate of new stuttering cases, they are especially important to studies of how to *prevent* the disorder. Similarly, because prevalence estimates reflect the rate of currently existing cases, they are especially important to studies of how to evaluate and *treat* the disorder.

The implications of stuttering incidence and prevalence are significant in a wide range of areas. These areas include research and theory, professional training, clinical service delivery, and public awareness and funding.

Implications for Research and Theory

The incidence and prevalence of stuttering is a crucial consideration in both designing and evaluating the quality of research and theoretical propositions. The relative distribution of gender, age, development, skill domains, and natural recovery (recovery without clinical intervention) among the sample population can affect study results, depending on how these factors are considered. For example, investigators must be mindful of differences between males and females in the development of particular language skills or brain structures when selecting their participant groups. To be representative, sampled experimental groups need to include more males than females to reflect the gender ratio in the stuttering population. In the same vein, the gender disparity for stuttering changes with the ages of participants. Specifically, a representative sample of adults who stutter would be expected to include proportionately more males than would a sample of young (e.g., preschool) children. The knowledge that boys may lag behind girls in particular aspects of typical speech and language development, however, should also be considered when evaluating research methods and results obtained with young children who stutter. Samples with greater numbers of boys may lead to inaccurate conclusions that children who stutter are below the norms in this domain, unless similarly gender-balanced control groups also are studied.

> Changes in the prevalence of stuttering with age and gender, and the influence of the rate and timing of natural recovery from stuttering, must be considered when interpreting results of clinical efficacy studies conducted with preschool children. If the natural changes in the prevalence of stuttering are overlooked, the effects of natural recovery may be confused and misinterpreted as being the outcome of treatment. If the different rates of recovery across genders are not considered in sample populations that have uneven proportions of males and females, there may similarly be misinterpretations of treatment outcomes.

Incidence and prevalence information also possesses immense importance to the theoretical foundations of stuttering. From an etiological perspective, incidence and prevalence data related to gender distribution and percentage of natural recovery are essential for testing which of several genetic models best supports the notion that stuttering is hereditary. Furthermore, large deviations from the general incidence found in certain subpopulations may provide important clues for making hypotheses about the nature of stuttering. Several examples illustrate this point. The low incidence of stuttering among deaf people (Backus, 1938) draws attention to the role of auditory processes in stuttering. Similarly, a low or high incidence of stuttering in certain cultures, racial, or ethnic groups (Lemert, 1953; Stewart, 1960) may suggest the influence of environmental factors, such as high or low expectations of speaking skills. A high incidence of stuttering in other clinical subpopulations, such as people with Down syndrome (Preus, 1973), calls attention to a host of possible influences on stuttering, such as chromosomal abnormality, low intelligence level, low muscle tone, and discrepancies in language skills during the critical stages of oral skill development.

Implications for Professional Training

Information about the occurrence of stuttering may influence both educational and clinical domains. For example, decisions concerning undergraduate and graduate academic curricula for students aspiring to become speech-language clinicians as well as the amount of clinical practice required of them, are influenced by the incidence of the various disorders treated by these future professionals. Whereas many academic programs offer courses specifically devoted to language disorders in preschool children and language disorders in schoolchildren, such age-specific courses in stuttering may not be found. The relatively small size of the stuttering population was a reason the American Speech-Language-Hearing Association (ASHA) and many universities deemphasized academic and clinical training in fluency disorders required of students in speech-language pathology. For a period of several years, ASHA actually cancelled its traditional requirement for a minimum number of clinical practicum hours in the area of stuttering. It is encouraging that this professional/scientific organization resumed those requirements in the form of both knowledge and practical skill competencies so that future professional clinicians will be prepared to provide appropriate levels of service for individuals who stutter.

Incidence data impact the instructional content of courses taught on the topic of stuttering. The heightened occurrence of stuttering in early childhood, for example, would suggest the need to include parent counseling techniques in clinical curricula. Also, the focus of continuing education programs in stuttering mirrors the incidence of the disorder and its distribution. Not surprisingly, during the past two decades or so, there appear to be significantly more educational events focused on children than on adults who stutter.

Implications for Clinical Service Delivery

Information concerning the occurrence and distribution of stuttering, like that of many other disorders, is a major factor in both the planning of public and private clinical services and the availability of qualified personnel to treat the disorder. Considering the typical age of stuttering onset, which impacts the respective prevalence for that age range, health-care and educational systems should plan on providing more services for young children who stutter in early childhood centers and family community clinics, than in clinical facilities where the majority of people served are adults. Additionally, clinicians need to be aware of the gender ratio to be sensitive to cultural aspects of communication for those they serve. For example, in counseling parents from cultures where boys are more desired by parents, clinicians need to be prepared for the level of disappointment triggered by the parents learning that their son not only stutters but is at greater risk for persistence. This news may be received with more negative parental and societal reactions.

Incidence and prevalence data are also applicable in the interest of prognosis. The risk for persistent stuttering may be estimated based on demographic factors such as age, gender, and familial distribution of the disorder. The estimate for the probability (p) of the risk of chronic stuttering may be calculated by applying the following formula: $p(\text{risk}) = [p(\text{incidence}) \times p(\text{chronic})]$. The application can be demonstrated in an example of a mother concerned about the prognosis for her 2-year-old child who is stuttering. Suppose a lifetime incidence of 5%, an 80% chance of natural recovery, and a 20% chance for persistent (chronic) stuttering. Applying our formula, prediction of whether the child will stutter chronically is calculated as $p(\text{risk}) = [p(\text{incidence: 5\%}) \times p(\text{chronic: 20\%})] = 1\%$. Thus the child has a 1 in 100 chance of a lifetime of stuttering. Although these figures only approximate the estimates found in the literature, it should be no surprise that a common estimate of stuttering prevalence (from research, not mathematical deduction) also happens to be about 1%.

A similar prognostic application of prevalence and incidence data could be applied to answer the question about whether a 5-year-old boy who is not currently stuttering is at risk to exhibit stuttering. The *relative risk* of a disorder is a measure that may be derived from the longitudinal data of an outcome in a disorder-free control group compared with the identified cases of the disorder in the general population (Lubker, 1997). If 2% of the general population present the disorder after age 5, and if males comprise 75% of that group (a 3:1 male-to-female ratio), then the *relative risk* of the 5-year-old child developing stuttering would be $p(incidence$ for age 5 and up) $\times p(prevalence$ of male gender among cases age 5 and up), 2% $\times$ 75% = 1.5%. In other words, the 5-year-old boy would be estimated to have a 1.5 in 100 chance of stuttering at some time in his life.

Implications for Public Awareness and Funding

Public concern about various health issues has been influential in directing governmental agencies, as well as private foundations, as to the distribution of money for research and treatment programs. For example, the sharp increase in the incidence of AIDS during the recent decades combined with increasing public awareness through the work of activists, philanthropic groups, and the media, have led to the consequent increase in financial resources dedicated to detecting and treating this disease. In many ways, inadequate information about stuttering and misconceptions about the size of the stuttering population, namely the prevailing notion that "only" 1%, or even less, of the population stutters, has diminished both public and professional attention to this communication disability. The 1% figure has produced an incorrect impression that stuttering is a "small" problem, although in children the percentage is considerably higher. It has been an important reason why stuttering was temporarily deemphasized by ASHA and affiliated academic training programs, as mentioned earlier.

Research Methodology for Incidence and Prevalence

Speech-language clinicians may serve as both the users and collectors of data related to the occurrence of stuttering cases. When evaluating incidence or prevalence figures related to stuttering, special attention must be given to the research methods employed in obtaining the information. The fairly wide range of figures, 0.61% to 4.70% for prevalence, and 0.70% to 17.70% for incidence, reported across many studies (see review by Bloodstein, 1995; Bloodstein & Bernstein Ratner, 2008) can most likely be attributed to the differences in the respective research methods used. These differences resulted from design, characteristics of the sample investigated, the definition of stuttering, or who identified stuttering and/or counted individuals who stutter.

Approaches to Prevalence Research

What research methods are used to collect data about the occurrence of stuttering? By and large, prevalence research has been based on cross-sectional surveys of designated groups; for example, sampling schoolchildren in different grade levels. Recall that in a cross-sectional study, data are collected from target sample populations at a single point in time. The most common procedure in prevalence research relies on questionnaires returned by secondhand informers, such as schoolteachers, who are asked to list the children who stutter in their respective classes. Another method employs direct face-to-face examination of the participants by examiners who listen to their speech to identify stuttering. Although both the number of examiners and their professional experience with stuttering have varied, the face-to-face approach is expected to yield more valid and reliable information. Finally, a third approach is seen in several studies that applied multiple procedures, for example, using input from school personnel as well as individual screening by the investigators. It would be reasonable to assume that multiple inputs contribute to a higher degree of accuracy.

The accuracy of statistics on stuttering is further complicated by the variation among studies in aspects such as their target sample populations. Preschool children, just a single, narrow age group, were the focus of study by Proctor, Yairi, and Duff (2008). Others studied a slightly wider age range of school-age children, for example, looking at stuttering across grades 1 through 4 (Burdin, 1940) or in junior and senior high school students (Gillespie & Cooper, 1973). The most comprehensive studies include the widest age range from kindergarten to 12th grade (Brady & Hall, 1976). Generally, these investigations used samples that were convenient to survey instead of randomly selected. An exception can be found in the 2002 Craig, Hancock, Tran, Craig, and Peters study, which attempted a cross section of the entire population of certain areas in Australia. The variations in target populations just described can be expected to result in a wide range of prevalence figures.

In addition to age variability, several investigations have been conducted with specific subpopulations, such as African Americans (Proctor, Yairi, & Duff, 2008), individuals with cleft palate (Dalston, Martinkosky, & Hinton, 1987), individuals with cognitive impairment (Preus, 1973), and others. Ideally, studies are conducted in multiple sites reflecting diverse groups, settings, and/or geographic regions. It is important to conduct simultaneous sampling of the different groups and sites being surveyed, within a brief time frame, to obtain maximum uniformity in conditions. Still, variations abound, for example, Gillespie and Cooper (1973) obtained data on stuttering from just a single city.

Although cross-sectional prevalence studies using survey questionnaires have varied substantially in scope, on the whole, this method has made it possible to obtain large samples of participants. This is attractive because the sheer sample size may compensate for errors resulting from many possible uncontrolled variables. Examples of these large-scale studies that used questionnaires and teacher input are Schindler (1955) sampling nearly 23,000 children, Wallin (1916), covering 89,000, and Glogowski (1976) with its staggering sample of 875,000 children. Studies employing direct face-to-face observations, although potentially more valid and reliable, have been smaller in scope due to substantially increased costs for personnel, the required time for each interview, and difficulties in gaining entrance to schools and other institutions. Such studies include Gillespie and Cooper (1973), Mills and Streit (1942), and Proctor et al. (2002).

Approaches to Incidence Research

Data for stuttering incidence have been gathered by investigators who pursued one of two approaches: longitudinal studies and retrospective reports. With the first approach, the same group of individuals is followed for a period of time while being observed for newly emerging cases of stuttering. With the second approach, records are examined or informants surveyed to obtain information about past (retrospective) events. Unquestionably, the first method holds the best potential for providing accurate information. It is, however, costly, difficult to execute, and bound to be limited in terms of sample size and the number of years over which the research is conducted. Also, although these investigations pertain to incidence, for the most part the researchers conducting them cannot claim to have investigated the real *lifetime* incidence because, except for one study, they covered only portions of the lifespan.

The most famous longitudinal incidence study was carried out by Andrews and Harris (1964), who followed 1,000 children in the English city of Newcastle upon Tyne from the time of their birth to age 16. Through the entire study the children were visited at periodic intervals by health workers and speech therapists, who noted when a child began stuttering and when the stuttering ceased. The challenges and high costs involved in this type of study should be apparent. Although the first 16 years of life probably yield most of the information about stuttering incidence, any possible late onsets are missed. Another investigation that is unique was reported by Månsson (2000). His team assessed the incidence of stuttering by screening the *entire* population of 1,040 children who were born on the Danish island of Bornholm during 2 consecutive years. The children, however, were followed for only 5 years.

The second approach for gathering data on incidence, relying on retrospective reports, is illustrated in the Dickson 1971 study where parents of almost 4,000 children in kindergarten through Grade 9 were asked whether their children were stuttering at the time or if they had a history of previous stuttering. In the Craig et al. (2002) investigation, one of the most recent on this topic, nearly 4,689 families comprising over 12,000 individuals participated in telephone interviews. Whereas it was possible to assess current stuttering (prevalence) via the telephone, identification of past stuttering cases (part of incidence) depended solely on the recollection of family members or individuals who used to stutter.

Overall, studies that follow both longitudinal and retrospective approaches suffer from flaws related primarily to vague descriptions of procedures, content of questionnaires, referrals, details of the personal examination of participants or its length, and others. Surveys that are confined to school-age children can be expected to result in a lower stuttering incidence than surveys that are confined to preschool-age children, the period when stuttering typically begins. A survey conducted in an all-female dorm is likely to yield lower figures than a study conducted in an all-male dorm. If human races differ in respect to stuttering, a study conducted in schools where races are not proportionally represented will yield misleading overall figures. In very young ages when the stuttering is often intermittent, some children may be missed in direct examination if they happened to experience a fluent period at the time of the study. Large up-and-down fluctuations in stuttering are common in the early stage of stuttering. Considering all these influences, direct comparisons among many of the studies are impossible. Although their cumulative data are certainly useful in providing a reasonable idea of the range of the magnitude and distribution of the disorder of stuttering, ideally more carefully designed, executed, and reported research will be carried out in the future.

Approaches to Defining Stuttering

As alluded to in Chapter 1, varying definitions of stuttering employed in incidence and prevalence research may have had substantial impact on the outcome of studies and thus on the knowledge base of the profession. Consider the analogy of the challenges that arise when defining the common cold. There are colds with runny noses and sore throats, and there are colds with congestion and coughs. In turn, there may be differences in the prevalence or incidence of various colds reflected in the differences among cold symptoms. Similarly, not all stuttering is characterized by the same symptoms, and across research studies stuttering may not even be uniformly defined. For example, in the survey conducted by Loutit and Halls (1936), no guiding definition was provided. It was left open to the individual opinion of the many people who carried out the survey, allowing for broad interpretations that probably included all kinds of disfluent speech and/or other characteristics deemed "stuttering." Loutit and Halls recognized the problem in their honest statement that "The teacher's judgment is the basis of the raw figures, so our whole analysis must rest on this somewhat insecure foundation" (p. 74).

Gillespie and Cooper (1973) improved on this method by conducting questionnaire surveys supplemented with a face-to-face meeting with each of 5,054 junior and senior high school students. Judgment of a student's "stuttering" was based on conversational speech and reading. Other studies defined stuttering more carefully and uniformly, and they restricted their counts to cases that met behavioral criteria. Brady and Hall (1976) provided teachers participating in a questionnaire survey of stuttering with the following definition: "Stuttering is a communication disorder characterized by excessive involuntary disruptions or blocking in the flow of speech, particularly when such disruptions consist of repetitions or prolongations of a sound or syllable and when they are accompanied by avoidance struggle behavior" (p. 76). In yet another study, Dickson (1971, p. 100) defined stuttering as "repetitions of sounds and words and getting stuck on or between words." The questionnaires he used requested parents to provide specific information about disfluency as well as secondary stuttering characteristics. In the 2002 Craig et al. study, mentioned earlier, stuttering was defined as "repetitions of syllables, part or whole words or phrases; prolongations of speech; or blocking of sounds" (p. 1100). They also included information about secondary physical characteristics and the emotional components of stuttering referred to as "Associated symptoms such as embarrassment and anxiety" (p. 1100).

Approaches to Selecting Informants

The informants are the people who gather the raw data. They determine who stutters based on their own observations or indirect data provided by other sources, such as the family's oral history. These may be teachers, health professionals, parents, and/or other family members. The accumulated data about stuttering prevalence or incidence cover a long time period and have been gathered by people of different backgrounds and experience. Over the 70-year span between the studies of Loutit and Halls (1936), and Van Borsel, Moeyaert, Rosseel, Van Loo, and Van Renterghem (2006), many investigations have relied on the reports of schoolteachers, sometimes hundreds and thousands of teacher participants per study (e.g., White House Conference, 1931). Mostly, those teachers had no professional training in speech pathology, in identifying stuttering, or, for that matter, without even a brief preparatory training for the survey. The combined effects of so many people applying an individual perception of what constitutes stuttering without the benefit of a guiding definition, raise doubts about the validity and reliability of the findings.

In other studies, information was gathered from parents of children (e.g., Dickson, 1971; Glasner & Rosenthal, 1957) or from all the household members of the families surveyed (Craig et al., 2002). In this respect, it is interesting to note that parents' diagnosis of stuttering and rating of its severity was found by Yairi and Ambrose (2005) to closely align with that of experienced speech-language clinicians. One advantage of using parents as informants is that they are in a position to report an eruption of stuttering that lasted for a relatively short period. Such cases, occasionally quite severe, are typically missed by other methods, leading to underestimates of incidence or prevalence.

Another class of informants is that of professionals who conduct direct observations of all those included in the population sample under investigation. There are, however, appreciable differences in the qualifications of these informants and the number who tested each child. As early as 1942, Mills and Streit employed 10 examiners to conduct individual testing of children in their school survey. All examiners had at least a year of training in speech pathology, and at least two were present in the testing of each child. Still, this team managed to conduct individual testing for only 25% of the pupils. In the Andrews and Harris (1964) study, only one of several health-care workers visited the child's home. Those workers were inconsistent in that in some cases the examiners did not meet with the child; many had to rely only on a parent's report instead of on individual testing. Proctor et al. (2008) used multiple sources to identify each child, including day-care staff and parental reports, as well as direct speech screening by one of the team's speech-language clinicians. Stuttering was confirmed by the judgment of two clinicians. Corroboration by many informants strengthens the confidence in data validity.

Prevalence of Stuttering: Findings

Having reviewed a range of research methodology issues, the question is what has been found? We first review the relevant research by providing essential information about each study. The studies are then summarized in a table that allows better comparisons of the main findings.

Early Reports

Considering the many experimental hazards just summarized, it is quite intriguing that several early investigations of the school-age population yielded similar findings to better designed modern studies. More than 100 years ago, four separate studies conducted in a variety of geographic regions around the world revealed remarkably close results. Lindberg (1900) surveyed 212,000 Danish schoolchildren, finding a stuttering prevalence of 0.90%; Von Sarbo (1901) studied 231,468 Hungarian children, reporting a prevalence of 1.02%; Conradi (1904) surveyed approximately 87,440 schoolchildren in six American cities, yielding a prevalence of 0.87%; and Hartwell (1895) surveyed 129,060 schoolchildren in the Boston area, reporting a prevalence of 0.77%.

Information continued to come in during the first third of the 20th century. In 1916, Blanton reported 0.72% prevalence in Madison, Wisconsin, and Wallin (1916) found 0.7 % in St. Louis, Missouri. Twenty years later, Louttit and Halls (1936) reported 0.77% among almost 200,000 children in Grades 1 through 12. In Vienna, Austria, Watzl's (1924) survey of 136,000 children showed 0.60% of them to stutter. Finally, investigators working for the White House Conference on Child Health and Protection (1931) obtained data for various speech disorders in a whopping sample of 3,471,000 children from Grade 1 to Grade 12. This largest-of-all questionnaire-based survey yielded an overall prevalence of approximately 0.7 %. Unfortunately, the report is not clear because data presented in various tables are not fully compatible. A noticeable strength of this large project is the method used to establish reliability. To this end, speech-language clinicians conducted direct individual speech screenings of 10,033 pupils in the public schools of Madison, Wisconsin. Their findings were compared against data obtained from the nationwide questionnaire survey. In this face-to-face control study, approximately 0.68% of the pupil population was identified as stuttering, very close to the 0.70 in the general survey. The authors concluded that "differences between the Madison results and those shown by the questionnaire survey are probably not material" (p. 337).[2]

Later Studies

Prevalence studies conducted in the more recent past yielded a low of 0.35% and a high of 2.12% estimates, with a concentration of findings around 0.75%. Leavitt (1974) found 0.84% prevalence among 10,445 New York City pupils of Puerto Rican background, Grades 1 to 6. In 1976, Hall, Mielke, Willeford, and Timmons reported a survey of nearly 39,000 pupils, Grades K to 12, using a nationwide sample and also reported 0.80% prevalence. At the same time, however, Brady and Hall (1976) surveyed 187,420 schoolchildren, Grades K to 12, in Illinois and Pennsylvania with the resultant total prevalence of only 0.35%. In a much smaller study, Gillespie and Cooper (1973) used a double-stage strategy with an initial questionnaire-based survey followed by face-to-face interviews to examine the speech of 5,054 junior and senior high students. The results of the second stage were used by the investigators as the basis for making prevalence estimates. Their conclusion of 2.12% prevalence, however, should be viewed with some caution because of the imbalanced racial sample, which included more than 50% African American pupils. (We discuss the race factor in the incidence and prevalence of stuttering later in the chapter.) Similarly, Glogowski (1976) found 1.82% stuttering in a large sample of 875,000 Polish schoolchildren.

Four additional studies should be mentioned in this class of later investigations, all of which were conducted in other continents. Of the three studies carried out in Australia, the first (Harasty & Reed, 1994) found 1.8% prevalence for children 5 to 12 years old diagnosed by clinicians in two metropolitan Sydney schools. The second, more extensive study was conducted by Craig et al. (2002). This telephone survey involved 4,689 families comprising a representative sample of the whole population (the entire age range) in the Australian State of New South Wales. It yielded an overall prevalence of 0.72%. A third and most recently published Australian survey included over 10,000 primary school students from kindergarten to Grade 6 and was conducted based on teacher identification confirmed by the records of a speech-language pathologist (SLP). It yielded a very low stuttering prevalence of 0.33% (McKinnon, McLeod, & Reilly, 2007). Lastly, a survey carried out in Belgium by Van Borsel et al. (2006) by means of questionnaires distributed among teachers covered 21,000 pupils from regular schools, ages 6 to 20, with an overall prevalence of 0.58 %. Table 2.1 summarizes the incidence studies just reviewed.

---

[2] We wonder about Van Riper's (1971) statement (p. 34) that this survey found stuttering prevalence at 1.2%, almost twice the figure we extracted from the same source.

Table 2.1: Early and Later Reports of Stuttering Prevalence

Early Reports		Later Reports	
Lindberg (1900)	0.90%	Leavit (1974)	0.84%
Von Sarbo (1901)	1.02%	Hall et al. (1976)	0.80%
Conradi (1904)	0.87%	Brady & Hall (1976)	0.35%
Hartwell (1895)	0.77%	Gillespie & Cooper (1973)	2.12%
Blanton (1916)	0.72%	Glogowski (1976)	1.82%
Wallin (1916)	0.70%	Harasty & Reed (1994)	1.80%
Louttit & Hall (1936)	0.77%	Craig et al. (2002)	0.72%
Watzl (1924)	0.60%	Van Borsel et al. (2006)	0.58%
White House Conference (1931)	0.70%	McKinnon et al. (2007)	0.33%

Incidence of Stuttering: Findings

Estimates of the incidence of stuttering are likely to be less accurate than estimates of prevalence. This is because valid longitudinal or retrospective data are more difficult to obtain than cross-sectional data used in prevalence research. The ideal incidence estimates require prospective longitudinal studies that track large samples of children representative of the population at large, starting from *prior* to the typical age for stuttering onset, that is age 2 or so, in order to capture all cases before natural recovery occurs.

Most available data come from questionnaires or interview studies that rely on indirect or direct retrospective methods, such as informants reporting whether or not they, or members of their family, currently stutter or *have ever* stuttered. The accuracy of this type of data may be compromised by their secondhand nature, informants' use of different identification criteria, lost information about the familial history of stuttering, and lapses in memory. Therefore, the resultant risk estimates tend to suffer from underreporting, yielding conservative findings. We have selected three studies to present.

Glasner and Rosenthal (1957) interviewed parents of 996 children entering the first grade in 25 rural and urban schools in Maryland. Among others, parents were asked the critical question of whether their child had *ever* stuttered or stammered. One hundred and fifty-three children, 15.4% of the sample, were so reported, and most of them had already stopped stuttering. A very different outcome was reported in Sheehan and Martyn's (1970) study of more than 5,000 University of California students personally interviewed by four speech clinicians. Their speech was observed, and a history of past speech disorders was taken. Approximately 2.9% either exhibited or reported a past history of stuttering. Unfortunately, both studies covered a limited age range and relied on memory concerning past stuttering.

The most comprehensive lifespan incidence of stuttering investigation was carried out by Craig et al. (2002) and Craig and Tran (2005). In a telephone interview with one member of each of randomly selected families in the state of New South Wales,

Australia, interviewees were given a description of stuttering and asked if anyone residing in their home stuttered. Stuttering was identified on the basis of a recorded speech sample, and an affirmative answer to at least one of several follow-up questions. To obtain incidence across the lifespan, interviewees were also asked whether anyone in the household had ever stuttered, followed by corroborative questions. Adding the number of people who stuttered at the time of the interview to the number of those reporting past stuttering yielded an incidence of from 2.1% in adults (21 to 50 years of age), 2.8% in younger children (2 to 5 years), and 3.4% in older children (6 to 10 years).

To date, ideal controlled lifetime stuttering incidence data, encompassing the entire age range, do not exist. Nevertheless, a handful of prospective longitudinal studies have provided general estimates. Perhaps the most well known is the already mentioned study by Andrews and Harris (1964) with an initial sample of 1,142 babies, born and residing in the English city of Newcastle upon Tyne, who were tracked from birth to their 16th birthday (end of age 15). Tracking was conducted by health workers and speech clinicians through periodic home visits. No speech samples were recorded, and the evaluators had only brief contact with the child at each visit. Furthermore, quite often parental reports concerning the children's speech status substituted for the direct contact. Over the 16-year span, a total of 43 children were identified as exhibiting stuttering, amounting to 4.9%[3] of the participants.

Findings of the British study received strong support from the Danish investigator Hans Månsson (2000). Having a unique access to the birth records of *all* children born over a 2-year period on the Danish island of Bornholm with its 45,000 low-mobility population, the Månsson team conducted direct speech, language, and hearing screenings of nearly the entire population (98%) of 1,040 children born over 2 years, 1991 and 1992. This was done within a month or two following their third birthday. Månsson reported that 4.9% of the children exhibited stuttering, a figure identical to that found by Andrews and Harris (1964) in a sample of a similar size. He also reported that the figure rose several years later to 5.09% after two follow-ups were conducted. Månsson (2006) later repeated his incidence survey among preschoolers in Bornholm that included 928 children, comprising 92% of the island's newly born population during the years 1995 and 1996. The survey was conducted soon after the children's third birthday with Månsson employing extremely careful procedures, including identical diagnosis by parents and two speech-language clinicians of current cases, and detailed parent reports on past stuttering that could not have been more than 18 months prior to the survey. This time Månsson found a high incidence of 17.7%. His methods, though, were considerably more direct and verifiable than those employed in Craig et al.'s 2002 telephone survey and came close to those reported by Glasner

---

[3] The 4.9% percent was calculated for the average size of the group, 875, to account for attrition.

and Rosenthal (1957). Support for the high incidence was recently provided from a limited longitudinal investigation of early language conducted in Australia in which more than 1,600 children began participation from 8 months of age. When parents observed stuttering onset, expert diagnosis was necessary for confirmation. The team of investigators reported an 8.5% incidence by age 3 (Reilly et al., 2009).

In general, when the broad literature is reviewed, although estimates of the lifetime incidence of stuttering in the United States and western Europe vary greatly (Bloodstein, 1995), the central tendencies of the various reports, as well as their scientific merit, would seem to indicate that about 5% of the general population of these parts of the world has ever stuttered. Nevertheless, closer attention should be given to a few studies that closely focused on young children and came up with considerably higher figures using good methodologies. If valid, the higher incidence for early ages contrasted with a lower incidence for older ages adds credence to high levels of natural recovery. It is quite probable that many clinically significant cases of early stuttering recover naturally within a short time after onset and thus go unreported (Yairi & Ambrose, 1999a).

Biological Factors in Stuttering Prevalence and Incidence

Familiality

Stuttering tends to occur more frequently than average in specific types of families, those with members who already stutter. It is quite likely that a person who stutters has one, several, or many relatives who either currently stutter or had a past history of stuttering. Bryngelson and Rutherford (1937) were among the first to investigate this phenomenon, reporting that 46% of people who stuttered had a family history of stuttering compared with 18% in a control sample. This general pattern has recurred in many subsequent studies, although the specific percentages have varied greatly (Sheehan & Costley, 1977). In a more recent review of the scientific literature, Yairi, Ambrose, and Cox (1996) concluded that the majority of studies reported between 30% to 60% of people who stutter had a familial incidence of the disorder. In contrast, the majority of these studies found that fewer than 10% of normally fluent people had family members who stuttered. Thus it would appear that the risk for a family member of a person who stutters to also stutter is 3 to 4 times higher than the risk for the family member of a person who does not stutter. Although these studies did not account for differences in family size, and contain other methodological problems, the general picture is quite clear.

In the past, the familiality of stuttering received psychosocial explanations that supported learning theories of stuttering. For example, Johnson (1955b) suggested that families with stuttering histories may have developed concerns about stuttering that affect their reactions to their children's speech, reactions that eventually trigger stuttering. Currently, however, ample evidence indicates a strong genetic component to stuttering (Kidd, 1984; Suresh et al., 2006) (discussed in a later chapter). Note how incidence data can be, and have been, used to enhance theories of stuttering, as exemplified above.

Age

Age is among the strongest risk factors for stuttering mainly because in a very large proportion of cases the disorder erupts during the preschool period. The age factor is also seen in the decline of stuttering incidence and prevalence throughout the lifespan. An Australian investigation estimated prevalence across the lifespan at 0.72% with a substantial decline from 1.4% in young children to 0.53% in young adults to 0.37% in older adults (Craig et al., 2002). A more recent study in Belgium, confined to the school-age through high school population, found prevalence to decline with age from 0.78% in the 6- to 10-year age group, to 0.53% in the 11- to 15-year age group, to 0.27% in the 16- to 20-year age group (Van Borsel et al., 2006). Hence the overall prevalence figure, 1% (or our estimate of 0.75%), masks important information. In contrast, a face-to-face prevalence study confined to ages 2 through 5 years (Proctor, Duff, & Yairi, 2008) found that 2.6% of either African American or European American children stuttered. These statistics call for greater emphasis on preparing clinicians for working with early childhood stuttering.

The decline in stuttering prevalence with age is directly related to the reduction in stuttering onset with age and to natural recovery, which is discussed in Chapter 3. The mean age of onset across studies has been between 2 to 4 years (Bloodstein, 1995; Yairi & Ambrose, 2005). Few stuttering cases begin prior to age 2 and rarely after age 12. Natural recovery may occur within weeks after onset with most children exhibiting recovery within 4 years (Yairi & Ambrose, 1999a, 2005). Therefore, it is not surprising that the prevalence figures are highest among preschool- and school-aged children, decline with adolescence, and are lowest among adults. Theoretically, the high incidence between ages 2 and 4 would appear to suggest some relationship between rapid speech and language development and stuttering onset.

Gender

It has been widely recognized that the prevalence of stuttering differs substantially between the genders. Specifically, stuttering is more prevalent in males than in females. In one of the earliest studies, Conradi (1904) found a male-to-female ratio of 3:1. Thirty years later, Louttit and Halls (1936) reported a 3.1:1 ratio, and, after an additional 40 years passed, Brady and Hall's (1976) survey yielded, according to our calculations, a ratio of 3.63:1. (They mistakenly reported a ratio of 3.9:1.) Interestingly, all three studies covered schoolchildren from kindergarten to Grade 12. In his extensive review of the literature, Bloodstein (1995) concludes that the overall gender ratio is approximately 3:1, which seems reasonable to us. Craig and colleagues (2002) reported a similar, but lower overall estimate of 2.3 males to every female who stutters. However, the most recent relevant study (Van Borsel et al., 2006) yielded a male-to-female ratio of 4.6:1 for a school population of up to age 20.

There is an interesting interaction between gender and age in regard to stuttering. Some of the variations among the findings of different studies could probably be attributed to the fact that the gender ratio varies with age. For this reason, the specific ages targeted in incidence and prevalence studies influences their outcome. Most reports have shown a strong trend for the gender ratio to increase appreciably with age. Gender ratio estimates range from approximately 2:1 in preschool-age children (Yairi & Ambrose,1992b, 2005) to as high as 5.5:1 in 11th and 12th graders (Bloodstein, 1995, p. 118). The recent study by Craig et al. (2002) seems to uphold this trend, reporting a range from 2.3:1 in children under age 5 years to 4:1 in youth/young adults.

Why does the gender ratio increase with the advance of age? This may be attributed to a tendency for boys to begin stuttering later than girls as well as the greater occurrence of natural recovery among girls than boys (Yairi & Ambrose, 2005). There have been a few exceptions, however. Craig et al. (2002) found a gender ratio decline postadolescence. Also Van Borsel and colleagues (2006) found smaller male-to-female ratios in older groups within the age limits of their study.

The gender ratio is particularly interesting because it strongly suggests a genetic contribution to stuttering (Kidd, Kidd, & Records, 1978; Yairi & Ambrose, 2005). A study of the Illinois International Genetics of Stuttering Project (Suresh, Ambrose, Roe, et al., 2006) demonstrated that males and females who stutter had different chromosomes on which the strongest signs for the possible presence of genes underlying stuttering were found. It is worth noting that more males than females have been identified in various disabilities, and, generally, also in communication disorders (Broomfield & Dodd, 2004; Law, Boyle, & Harris, 2000; Shriberg, Tomblin, & McSweeny, 1999). Other potential factors contributing to gender differences, based in cultural practices, could be a tendency for males to be identified or referred to experts at higher rates than females, or that performance expectations may differ between the genders, with higher standards and more pressure placed on boys (Bloodstein, 1995; Schuell, 1947a, 1947b).

Geographic, Cultural, and Racial Factors

Geography

Stuttering is found worldwide and afflicts all races, and probably most, if not all, ethnic/cultural groups. Although race per se is biologically determined, it is discussed here because of its apparent close associations with geographic and cultural factors. Whereas previous sections in this chapter have focused on data from North America, Europe, and Australia, the professional literature testifies to the presence of the disorder in many geographic locations, including Asia, Africa, and South America. The October 18, 2005, issue of the *Asha Leader* featured several articles written by clinicians and investigators in India, Taiwan, Japan, Cameroon, Brazil, and other countries, describing the local status of the disorder and its treatment. Similarly, there have been some research-based publications of data obtained in these and other countries. Because of the strong evidence for genetic factors underlying stuttering, noticeable incidence differences among subpopulations, if found, should not be surprising. In particular small close groups with high levels of intermarriage may exhibit a higher percentage of stuttering if the disorder was present in the original founders of the group. Alternatively, theoretical perspectives oriented toward learning and environmental explanations of stuttering would also lead to the expectations of marked differences among culturally and socially different groups. Of course, cultural factors may contribute to variations in incidence/prevalence findings if there is a tendency for community beliefs and values to influence the extent to which people are willing to admit that they themselves or a family member stutters.

Viewing the geographic and cultural landscape, there has been a lack of relevant, sound research published outside of North America, parts of Europe, and Australia. From what has been done, however, the results approximate those found in the Western world. For example, a sample of 140,000 Japanese schoolchildren revealed a 0.82% prevalence (Toyoda, 1959); in a much smaller Japanese study, it was 0.98% (Ozawa, 1960). In Egypt, prevalence was reported at 0.93% (Okasha, Bishrey, Kamel, & Hassan, 1974). In South Africa, a survey of 6,581 pupils ages 5 to 21 yielded a stuttering prevalence of 1.26% (Aron, 1962). The single study (to our knowledge) reported for the whole of Latin America was carried out in Colombia. The investigators distributed questionnaires to nearly 1,900 college students of whom 2% reported stuttering (Ardila, Bateman, & Niño, 1994). The results, however, should be viewed with skepticism due to the many possibilities of procedural errors, including the likelihood that a good number of disinterested normally fluent students did not return their questionnaires. The equal gender ratio found among the Latin American students, which is quite unlike virtually all past studies on adults, reinforces this concern.

Culture

For a good number of years, a few speech-language clinicians and anthropologists argued that cultures that value competitiveness, social pressure, and attention to speech should exhibit more cases of stuttering and vice versa. Indeed, early reports claimed that certain Native American tribes, for example, the Bannock-Shoshone, did not stutter and had no word for stuttering (Johnson, 1944a, 1944b; Snidecor, 1947), whereas other tribes, such as the Salish, displayed a high incidence of stuttering (Lemert, 1953). Similar explanations for stuttering in Pacific societies were offered, for example, by Bullen (1945), Lemert (1962), and Stewart (1960), as well as African societies (Aron, 1962). In our opinion, this interpretation appears now to have been overly driven by anthropological and stuttering theories that were popular at the time. Several decades later, evidence for the disorder of stuttering, as well as for a word for it, in Native American tribes previously regarded as stuttering free, was published in 1983 by Zimmermann, Liljebald, Frank, and Cleeland.

In the 1940s, Johnson and Snidecor claimed they had found a society in which there was no stuttering. Based on interviews with the Bannock-Shoshone American Indians, they concluded that they had no word for it (stuttering) and had never seen anything like it (when modeled). Later, in the 1960s, Art Frank, an anthropologist, found conclusive evidence that the tribes had words for stuttering and that there had been people who stuttered present among them even when the earlier research was conducted. What was the source of the discrepancy? The people in the tribe needed to feel sufficiently safe and trusting of the outsiders before they would admit their knowledge and experience with stuttering. Thus the validity of data collected from cross-cultural interviews depends on investigator rapport with informants.

Bilingualism

The ability to speak colloquially in two languages is another cultural aspect that has received some attention in relation to stuttering. Does the introduction of a second language pose a risk factor for stuttering? The available data are scant and suffer from weaknesses identified earlier. Most of the past findings suggested that stuttering is more prevalent among bilingual than among monolingual speakers. Travis, Johnson, and Shover (1937) reported a prevalence of 2.8% and 1.8%, respectively, in 4,827 schoolchildren. In South Africa, stuttering prevalence among bilingual schoolchildren was 2.16% as compared to 1.66% among monolinguals (Stern, 1948). More recent studies that corroborate this trend are lacking. An Internet survey by Au-Yeung Howell, Davis, Charles, and Sackin (2000) of nearly 800 individuals from 40 countries did not corroborate the findings of Stern and Travis et al. The percentage of speakers reporting either current or past stuttering was almost identical among monolingual and bilingual speakers, 21.74% and 21.65%, respectively. The validity of this study, however, is questionable for several reasons, including the fact that the majority of the respondents were females, a very atypical sample of people who stutter. A recent study by Howell, Davis, and Williams (2009) sampled children who stutter, ages 8 to 12+ years, in southeast England. They reported that among 38 bilingual children who stuttered, 36 (95%) stuttered in both languages, and that among 23 children with bilingual development since birth, recovery was lower (25%) compared to the monolingual and bilingual children who did not start to develop the second language until they entered kindergarten. The results of this study must be viewed with caution due to several methodological and reporting deficiencies.

The cultural domain may also be expanded to include the stutterer's family's socioeconomic status, a factor that attracted some attention several decades ago. At the time, Morgenstern (1956) reported that among 29,500 Scottish schoolchildren, there was a statistically significant tendency for those coming from lower socioeconomic status groups, especially families of semiskilled workers, to be affected by a higher prevalence of stuttering than children from the middle or upper classes. A favorite explanation, fitting well within the then prevailing "diagnosogenic" theory (Johnson, 1942; Johnson et al., 1959) of the onset of stuttering, was that upward mobility pressure exerted in these social layers, that is, parents pressuring their children to do better than they have done, causes more children to stutter than in higher classes. These findings, however, have failed to gather much support, if at all.

Race

Until recently, only a few published studies were specifically interested in investigating stuttering in African American children (Carson & Kanter, 1945; Gillespie & Cooper, 1973; Goldman, 1967; Louttit & Halls, 1936). Others included African American children only as a part of the general participant population (Travis, Johnson, & Shover, 1937; Wallin, 1916, 1926). Additionally, there have been a few master's theses and doctoral dissertations that explored stuttering prevalence in African American children (Madding, 1995; Neely, 1960; Waddle, 1934). All surveyed elementary school children, except for Gillespie and Cooper (1973), who focused on prevalence in adolescents. Reviewing the findings, it is not surprising that a belief has prevailed that stuttering occurs more frequently in African American children than in European American children (Cooper & Cooper, 1998). This thinking, however, has recently changed, as we elaborate on later. Of course, all weaknesses we have attributed to prevalence research in stuttering in general also apply to research concerned with race: The studies are dated, contain many potential measurement errors, and the range of methodological variability creates difficulties in interpreting and comparing results. Additionally studies conducted prior to 1967 took place in racially segregated school systems, and it is highly probable that the children spoke African American English (AAE). In this dialect, several types of disfluencies, such as revisions, repetitions, and prolongations, represent distinct semantic functions that could have been mistakenly regarded as stuttering (Proctor, Yairi, Duff, & Zhang, 2008).

The belief regarding racial differences in the occurrence of stuttering has been recently challenged by Proctor et al. (2008) in the only study that zeroed in on preschool children, the age range when most stuttering cases have their onset. Using a three-pronged approach that included clinician screening of children, teacher identification, and parent identification, data were collected on 3,164 children between ages 2 and 5. Of these, 2,223 were African Americans and 941 were European Americans. The prevalence of stuttering was 2.6% for the African American children, and 2.44 for the European American children, with no statistically significant differences between the two groups.

Prevalence in Clinical Subpopulations

We turn now to very different subpopulations than the ones discussed in the previous section. Each of these is characterized by a certain abnormality, and their incidence and prevalence data also contribute relevant information to the understanding of stuttering. In a well-known review of the stuttering literature, Andrews et al. (1983) noted that various disorders, especially obvious neurological conditions such as cerebral palsy, are associated with a higher than expected prevalence of stuttering. They entertained the idea that more subtle central nervous system (CNS) dysfunctions may be causative factors of disfluent speech. Taking a different angle, several investigators have pointed out that stuttering tends to be associated with a host of other disorders (Arndt & Healy, 2001; Blood, Ridenour, Qualls, & Scheffner Hammer, 2003; Blood & Seider, 1981). That is, stuttering may be either a causative agent or a co-occurring disorder that shares a common cause. Regardless, we have emphasized the value of understanding incidence and prevalence differences in various groups. Either unusually high or unusually low figures could provide clues concerning causes, precipitating factors, and the treatment of stuttering. Several such groups are discussed next.

Hearing Impairment

One of the most interesting phenomenon within our topic of incidence and prevalence is that people who suffer substantial loss of their hearing sense exhibit little or no stuttering. If this finding holds, it could be important as indirect evidence regarding the nature and cause of stuttering. In other words, if sufficient auditory acuity is needed to stutter, one may infer that processes involving auditory self-monitoring of speech play a role in the disorder.

Two early teacher report-based surveys conducted in schools for the deaf (as these were called at the time), with a combined total student population of 28,000, yielded only 14 cases, which is 0.05%, or a 20th of 1% prevalence (Backus, 1938; Harms & Malone, 1939). It is important to point out that only oral communication was considered. Since then, Montgomery and Fitch (1988) carried out the last prevalence study in this population; they also sought information for stuttering in manual communication. Responses to a questionnaire survey from 77 schools for the hearing impaired with a total of 9,930 students enrolled revealed only 12 children who exhibited stuttering, 3 in the oral mode, 6 in the manual mode, and 3 in both modes. Stuttering in the manual mode occurs as repetitive or prolonged movements of the hands or arms while signing language. The prevalence of 0.12%, a fraction more than a 10th of 1%, is still considerably lower than that reported for the population at large. Of interest is the finding that the perceived manual disfluency was more prevalent than the oral disfluency. Silverman and Silverman (1971) too have reported on the presence of "manual stuttering" among deaf people.

> Anecdotal observations by professionals who had extensive contact with this group have supported the conclusion pertaining to the rarity of stuttering in deaf people. Gutzmann (1912) commented that this was a well-known fact, and Bleumel (1913) noted that Gallaudet, a famous educator of the deaf, had stated that in 50 years of experience he could not recall ever encountering a deaf person who stuttered. Thus a connection between stuttering and audition is strongly suspected.

The hypothesis of a stuttering–audition link has been reinforced because masking noise, which in effect reduces hearing, often results in a temporary reduction, or complete suppression, of stuttering, a phenomenon that has been applied in therapy. The theoretical views of the relation between stuttering and audition are discussed in Chapter 7.

Cleft Palate

Another clinical group with an apparent low occurrence of stuttering is that of individuals born with cleft palate, which typically renders them with hypernasal speech. Here again, if this finding is upheld, then it may have important implications for the underlying causal factors responsible for stuttering. The relevant literature, however, is limited. Bloodstein (1981) observed that stuttering in individuals with cleft palate is uncommon but did not provide substantiating data. Schwartz (1976) discussed a single case of a child with cleft palate who stuttered when wearing a corrective appliance. Blood and Seider (1981) reported that in a sample of 1,060 stutterers identified in the caseload of 358 speech-language clinicians, only 1% was composed of cleft palate patients. This finding, however, pertains to the occurrence of cleft palate among people who stutter, not the occurrence of stuttering in people with cleft palate. The only direct study on this population was conducted by Dalston, Martinkosky, and Hinton (1987) employing retrospective examinations of the records of 534 patients, ages 3 to 66 years, all with structural anomalies that affected the velopharyngeal closure. Only one person in the sample, less than 0.2% of the total, was identified by speech-language clinicians as manifesting stuttering. Such a low occurrence of stuttering in individuals likely to experience considerable parental intrusive behavior and concern about their speech (Long & Dalstrom, 1983) raises questions about theoretical positions that claim negative environmental reactions to speech cause stuttering (e.g., Johnson et al., 1959). The phenomenon, however, gives rise to physiological considerations, for example, the possible relation between the duration of intraoral pressure drop and speaking rate. It is known that the overall speaking rate of people with cleft palate is slower than normal. Slowing down the speaking rate also increases fluency in people who stutter.

Cognitive Impairment

Whereas those with cleft palate and those who are deaf or hard of hearing present less frequent rates of stuttering than the general population, on the other end of the spectrum lies the population of people with low mental abilities (called "mentally retarded" in past terminology) as classified by intelligence tests and other assessments. Several studies have reported considerably higher than normal stuttering cases in this population. In the general group of those with cognitive impairment, early studies indicated 14% to 17%[4] prevalence (Gottsleben, 1955; Schlanger & Gottsleben, 1957), whereas later findings suggested lower figures of 2.5% to 7.0% (Chapman & Cooper, 1973; Schaeffer & Shearer, 1968). Apparently the prevalence of stuttering increases with the severity of the cognitive impairment. According to Boberg, Ewart, Mason, Lindsay, and Wynn (1978), stuttering was twice as frequent among the trainable mentally retarded (TMR; IQs in the range of 25 to 50) compared to those who were educable mentally retarded (EMR; IQs in the range of 50 to 70). Similar results were reported by Brady and Hall (1976). They found 1.60% stuttering cases among 3,057 of those with relatively higher IQs; stuttering cases were twice as high, 3.08%, for 454 students with lower IQs.

---

[4] In a small study of only 74 children, Schlanger (1953) reported that more than 20% exhibited stuttering.

Most interesting are data pertaining to the Down syndrome subgroup, for whom surveys yielded prevalence estimates ranging from 15% (Schubert, 1966) to the extreme of 53.20% (Preus, 1973). Although some have argued that the high prevalence figures may have resulted from increasing diagnostic challenges, possibly confusing cluttering, hesitation, and various expressive language difficulties for stuttering (e.g., Weiss, 1964), others have maintained that stuttering characteristics exhibited by this subpopulation are similar to those observed in the population at large. Those with cognitive impairment who stutter, however, show low emotional reactivity to their stuttering (Preus, 1973, 1990). Otto and Yairi (1976) reported that children with Down syndrome, even if they are not regarded as exhibiting stuttering, produce very disfluent speech, including repetitions of syllables and words.

The high prevalence of stuttering in people with Down syndrome calls attention to a host of possible influences on stuttering e.g., chromosomal abnormality and/or motor deficiencies caused by low muscle tone during the critical stages of oral skills development. In the most recent study concerning the biological genetics of stuttering published by Suresh, Ambrose, Roe, et al. (2006), the strongest indications for possible genes underlying stuttering was found for females who stutter, and that sign came from an area located on chromosome 21, the chromosome that has also been implicated in Down syndrome. At the present, however, whether these two facts are related remains unknown. Additionally, the frequent occurrence of stronger vocabulary skills than expressive language abilities among children with Down syndrome provides clues that differences in the level of skills seen in certain areas of language proficiency may be an important factor in stuttering.

Although much of the available data concerning stuttering in the cognitively impaired population were collected more than 30 years ago, there has been recent support in a study that compared stuttering prevalence in regular and special education schools in Belgium. Among the 1,272 pupils attending special schools, including the so-called mentally handicapped, 2.28% were reported to stutter, four times more than the 0.58% of stuttering pupils in the regular schools (Van Borsel et al., 2006). This group, however, also included children with emotional and physical problems.

Other Groups

Scattered information has been published about other clinical groups showing either higher or lower prevalence than in the population at large. Higher than normal incidence was found for people with epilepsy (Gens, 1951), brain damage (Bohme, 1977), and psychosis (Freund, 1955). Lower than normal prevalence was found for people with diabetes (Boldon, 1955). Generally, however, all pertinent surveys are outdated, small, not well documented, and sometimes contradictory.

Summary

We learn about how many and who stutter by studying aspects related to the incidence and prevalence of stuttering. Prevalence and incidence data are very useful for understanding the nature and possible cause(s) of stuttering, guiding the preparation of clinicians to specific needs of subpopulations, overall planning of clinical services at the national and local levels, and for obtaining financial resources for both research and clinical purposes. Thus they are important to the development of both theory and treatment for stuttering.

Key points made in this chapter:

- *Incidence* is the rate or estimate of the chance of occurrence of any disorder. *Prevalence* is the rate or estimate of how many people exhibit the disorder at a specific time period. Data on these two parameters are essential for the design of many studies of people who stutter, the constructing of genetic models of stuttering, and for the understanding of its developmental trends.
- Appropriate interpretations of incidence and prevalence estimates require an appreciation of the varying methods that may have influenced the available data. Target populations have varied widely, and different approaches have been used, including cross-sectional, longitudinal, and retrospective studies.
- Methodological dissimilarities across studies have been related to the definition of stuttering, the specific technique of data collection (e.g., mailed questionnaires; direct examination), and the people providing the information of who stutters.
- Judging the accumulated data, their strengths and weaknesses, we are inclined to agree with past conclusions that the lifetime incidence of stuttering is approximately 5%.
- The overall prevalence of stuttering appears to be lower than the traditional 1% value and is probably closer to a 0.70% level. Most of the data reviewed were obtained in the United States. Several investigations, especially European (not all were reviewed here), tended to suggest a somewhat higher incidence.
- Children who stutter often are born into families that have other members who stutter. The strong familiality of stuttering has given rise to several interpretations of stuttering of which genetics has prevailed.
- Incidence and prevalence data reveal clear evidence for an age factor in stuttering. With possible slight variations, both incidence and prevalence decline across the lifespan.
- The age-related diminution in the number of people who stutter reflects the combined factors of declining new incidences of onset in older ages and the growing number of natural recovery cases.
- Among preschoolers, prevalence may be larger than 2%, nearly three times higher than the average prevalence across the lifespan. Therefore, it would seem justified to alter the common perception that stuttering is a "small" problem. From a practical point of view, more resources should be directed to the study of stuttering in young children and for the preparation of speech-language clinicians to treat them.

- Both the incidence and prevalence of stuttering are gender-influenced with males running twice the risk of females to exhibit the disorder initially; the risk for them to sustain stuttering over years or even for life is much greater.
- The male-to-female gender ratio is smallest in very young children, generally increasing with age (small ratio fluctuations between specific age brackets are possible). Overall, older age brackets include fewer stutterers, mostly males.
- The combined effect of the age and gender factors is to shrink the stuttering population as it matures and to greatly increase its male predominance. Such extensive changes in the composition of people who stutter should be kept in mind prior to reaching conclusions about the "nature of stuttering" when based on observations of a narrow population segment.
- Several clinical groups reveal large deviations, up or down, from the prevalence of stuttering in the population at large. Better understanding of such departures may provide relevant clues about the causes and nature of the disorder. Although there have been some indications for differences in the occurrence of stuttering in diverse cultural and racial populations spread over diverse geographic regions, much of the available information or reported impressions have not been adequately substantiated. Furthermore, it is not clear that, even if large differences exist, they are indeed due to cultural factors. That genetic factors underlie incidence in specific groups is a serious possibility.

STUDY QUESTIONS AND DISCUSSION TOPICS

1. Test your knowledge of incidence/prevalence by answering questions about hypothetical data, presented in the table here, from a combined longitudinal and cross-sectional study of children 3 to 5 years of age.

Hypothetical Cases of Stuttering in 3,400 Children Ages 3 to 5 Years in Each Year 2102 to 2104

	Age 3 years			Age 4 years			Age 5 years		
Year	Stuttering Cases	Pop. Sample	Percent	Stuttering Cases	Pop. Sample	Percent	Stuttering Cases	Pop. Sample	Percent
2102	20	400	5	15	600	2.5	15	900	1.67
2103	28	700	4	12	400	3	8	600	1.33
2104	32	800	4	14	700	2	6	400	1.5
Total	80	1,900	4.21	41	1,700	2.41	29	1,900	1.52

a. You will notice that one group of children was sampled longitudinally for all 3 years of the study (no attrition). How many children were in that group?

b. Does this table offer information about incidence or prevalence? Why?

c. What would you need to know in order to estimate the other kind of information (from Question C)?

d. How do the estimates change most, according to year or according to age?

2. What are the advantages and disadvantages of surveying reports of schoolteachers to study the prevalence of stuttering?

3. What is a retrospective study? What are the limitations of retrospective studies to gather incidence data?

4. Does stuttering vary across populations with the following characteristics? If so, how?
   a. Geographic region
   b. Gender
   c. Age
   d. Hearing impaired
   e. Cleft palate
   f. Cognitive impairment

5. Which figure is apt to be larger, prevalence or lifetime incidence of stuttering?

6. What are the research and clinical implication of incidence and prevalence data for stuttering?

7. What are plausible explanations for the variations in the sex ratio that occur with age in the stuttering population?

8. What factors may account for differences in the incidence of stuttering among cultures and races if, indeed, such differences are confirmed?

WEB SITES

Incidence and Prevalence of Speech, Voice, and Language Disorders in Adults in the United States: 2008 Edition at the American Speech-Language-Hearing Association Web site. Retrieved May 12, 2009, from www.nsslha.org/research/reports/speech_voice_language.htm

Research on Incidence and Prevalence of Stuttering at The Stuttering Foundation of America Web site. Retrieved May 12, 2009, from www.stutteringhelp.org/Default.aspx?tabid=418

SUGGESTED READINGS

Craig A., Hancock, K., Tran, Y., Craig, M., & Peters, K. (2002). Epidemiology of stuttering in the community across the entire life span. *Journal of Speech-Language-Hearing Research, 45*, 1097–1105.

Lubker, B. B. (1997). Epidemiology: An essential science for speech-language pathology and audiology. *Journal of Communication Disorders, 30*(4), 251–267.

Månsson, H. (2000). Childhood stuttering: Incidence and development. *Journal of Fluency Disorders, 25*, 47–57.

Proctor, A., Yairi, E., & Duff, M. (2008). Prevalence of stuttering in African American preschool children. *Journal of Speech, Language, and Hearing Research, 50*, 1465–1474.

Chapter 3: When and How Does Stuttering Begin? How Does It Develop?

Readers will understand:

- The features of stuttering onset with respect to gender, age, type of onset, and other factors.
- The characteristics of stuttering at onset in terms of disfluent speech, physical concomitants, emotional and physical health, and concomitant disorders.
- The potential developmental progressions and paths of stuttering.
- The phenomena of both natural recovery from and persistence in stuttering.
- Research related to the onset and development of stuttering.

Theoretical and Clinical Significance

Among the most challenging issues regarding stuttering has been its beginning, or "onset." The desire to know and understand the details of what, when, and how it begins is natural for speech-language clinicians and researchers alike. The potential theoretical significance of the onset event is seen in its relationship to the age factor. If stuttering typically began after age 25, then parental behavior and attitudes would be given minimal consideration as potential causative agents. However, because it typically begins in early childhood, when anatomical structures for speech are growing quickly and language-phonology systems are expanding sharply and quickly, possible influences of these processes on the child's fluency domain must be considered (Bernstein Ratner, 1997a; Yairi, 1983; Yairi & Ambrose, 1992b). As explained by the demands and capacities model, stuttering arises when various demands, both internal and external to the child, exceed his or her capacities (i.e., motor, linguistic, cognitive, and others) to sustain fluent speech (Adams, 1990). More about this model is explained in Chapter 6. It is understandable why early childhood is such a vulnerable period for stuttering onset. The act of coping with the taxing demands of anatomical growth, phonological and language learning, social development, and so on, depletes resources needed for mastering fluency and thus prompts the onset of stuttering. In a similar vein, we may look at what we call the *manner* of onset. Whereas sudden onsets may give rise to suspicions of organic or psychogenic agents being involved, gradual onset favors learning explanations of stuttering (e.g., Wischner, 1950) because habit-forming processes take time. Another possibility is that a sudden or gradual onset of stuttering represents a sudden or gradual shift into adopting a new speech motor strategy or new language structure. Other examples could be cited to illustrate why good scientific information on onset is pertinent for theories about the disorder of stuttering.

Similarly, professionals' strong interests are directed to what happens after stuttering has begun: the early features (symptomatology) of stuttering, how they change with time, and the duration of the disorder. Here too, several examples will illustrate how stuttering features at onset and early developmental paths have theoretical and practical significance. If very early symptomatology does not reveal psychological problems or emotional reactions (e.g., anxiety) specifically when the child stutters, then theories that propose emotional maladjustment or anxiety as the etiology of stuttering lose ground. This same evidence is also relevant for the kind of treatment selected (e.g., play psychotherapy versus speech therapy). Also, if in some children symptoms only run a short course and then recede and vanish, whereas in others they persist for a long time, it will be extremely helpful to identify these subgroups and distinguish them early on to facilitate clinical decision making. Furthermore, if stuttering persists, does it follow one or several courses? Is it possible that different patterns of onset and/or development indicate the presence of several stuttering subtypes? Information pertaining to these questions will have important theoretical and clinical implications.

In spite of the importance of issues involving the onset and development of stuttering and its symptoms, for many years they attracted only limited serious systematic research. One reason is that both topics have proved to be difficult to investigate due to a variety of factors discussed later. Still, encouraging progress has been made, especially in the past two decades.

Unlike disordered language and phonology that result from the child's failure to adequately develop those skills, and therefore have no identifiable onset, stuttering usually appears *after* the child has already demonstrated the skill of normal speech fluency (Yairi & Ambrose, 1992b, 2005). It is clear that major changes had occurred. The child actually suffered a loss: his or her fluency. This fact is significant because the loss of an important function is easily observable and has a dramatic effect. Parental alarm and panic reactions to the pronounced negative changes are common, adding a major element to the problem. There is also the possibility that the child is reacting to it, although unable to communicate this effectively. In contrast, children with disordered phonology did not possess good phonology that they then lost.

Onset

General Issues and Research Methods

As stated in Chapter 1, the great majority of developmental stuttering cases begin in early childhood. In this respect, it is one of several communication disorders affecting young children. There is, however, an important distinction in that many cases of stuttering have an onset observed by parents or others. The fact that there is a general recognition of an event called the "onset of stuttering," has justified scientific effort to investigate it.

Scientific studies of stuttering onset are difficult to execute because (1) stuttering afflicts a relatively small percentage of children, (2) there are no warning signs that onset is about to occur, and therefore (3) investigators cannot be present at the right place and time to objectively document the very earliest stuttering or secure data even shortly thereafter. Yes, there have been a few individual case study reports (e.g., Fogerty, 1930; Mowrer, 1998) where the investigator had access to the child close to the time of onset. These, however, vary in quality in terms of the detail of the recorded observations. They also failed to report quantified speech data among other points. Although they provide insight, the small number of cases and limited information make results insufficient to allow generalization. To improve the chances for closer observations, scientists in The Netherlands investigated onset in children from families where one or both parents have stuttered themselves. This was done because, due to genetics, their chance of having children who stutter is much higher than for the population at large (Kloth, Janssen, Kraaimaat, & Brutten, 1995). One weakness of this method is that those families may represent a biased sample of the stuttering population. Typically, fewer than 40% of those who stutter have a parent with a history of stuttering. In the Kloth et al. study, 100% of the children had at least one parent who stuttered.

An alternative research method would attempt to create stuttering onset intentionally in normally speaking individuals. This approach, however, would be unethical and a highly unlikely choice. A charge has been made that a master's thesis study conducted by Tudor (1939) under the mentorship of the late Wendell Johnson, a notable scientist in the field, attempted and succeeded at doing just this (Silverman, 1988). Years later, several U.S. newspapers repeated the accusation (e.g., the *San Jose Mercury News* in its June 10 and 11, 2001, editions). Subsequently, two independent scientists carefully scrutinized the text and data in Tudor's master thesis that was available to the public at the University of Iowa library. They (Ambrose & Yairi, 2002) concluded that the accusations that the objectives of the study were to turn normally speaking children into stutterers were unsupported by the materials. Furthermore, they found that the levels of stuttering-like disfluency (SLD), the speech interruptions most pertinent to stuttering, were not significantly altered from pre- to posttreatment testing. Neither were perceptual ratings of the level of disfluency changed by a group of judges. Hence no stuttering was effected by the study. All in all, the objectives, procedures, and outcomes show the accusations were moot (Ambrose & Yairi, 2002; Yairi, 2006). Unfortunately, Silverman (2004) continued to hold to his earlier charges, referring to newspapers and laypersons' opinions while completely ignoring the work of other scientists in this regard.

Considering the situation just described, the most common research approach has relied on retrospective reports, typically elicited in face-to-face, often lengthy interviews with parents of children who stutter. Questions such as the following have been typical: (1) When did your child first begin stuttering? (2) Who was the first to notice it? (3) What were the speech characteristics of the first stuttering (also mimic the early stuttering)? (4) Was the first stuttering associated with physical illness or emotional stress? (5) Was the early stuttering associated with physical tension? (6) How severe was the stuttering? This approach, too, runs several risks. First is the potential for biased participant samples when only children who have stuttered for a set minimum period of time were identified and recruited for the study. Because a majority of children who begin stuttering will stop within a short time after onset, participant selection criteria should not be eliminating these cases. Typically, this large subpopulation was not tapped in most past studies.

Second, often data were obtained from informants, usually parents, a long time after the onset. One study by the British team headed by Andrews and Harris (1964) used 80 children between 9 and 11 years of age. Because stuttering typically begins between ages 2 and 4, parents of participants had to remember details of events that occurred at least several years in the past. In the United States, Milisen and Johnson (1936) interviewed parents nearly 20 years after their children began stuttering. Apparently many parents prefer to adopt a wait-and-see strategy before seeking professional services of a speech-language clinician. Perhaps they listen to the pediatrician's advice telling them it will go away (Yairi & Carrico, 1992). The end result is that genuine early stuttering is rarely observed in these research participants. This raises the risk of obtaining low-accuracy data based on parents' vague, if not faulty, memory of significant details, for example: whether the first stuttering was composed of syllable repetitions or also of sound prolongations, how many times did the child repeat a syllable (two? four?), and whether secondary characteristics, such as eye closing, were noticed. Few may appreciate the fact that the difference between repeating a syllable twice or four times is indeed a large one in this context and has a very significant impact. At the time of onset, parents are not particularly tuned to such fine details. Being unaware of what is significant for stuttering when they first observe it, they cannot offer the most accurate information.

Studies Concerning Onset

Systematic research of stuttering onset probably began with a little known study by Taylor (1937) at the University of Iowa in which parents of 47 stuttering children, ages 3 to 7 years, were interviewed concerning the circumstances of the onset and the early characteristics of the stuttering. A series of three studies then followed, all conducted at the same university. In 1942, Johnson reported findings also based on retrospective interviews of parents of 46 stuttering children; so did Darley (1955) for parents of 50 stuttering and 50 nonstuttering children. The largest investigation was carried out by Johnson and his colleagues (1959) using an extensive 840-item questionnaire to interview both parents of 150 children who stuttered, ages 2 to 9, and their nonstuttering peers. The standard interviews in all three studies probed into the onset of stuttering, child development, health history and status, child rearing practices, home environment, and more. Their drawbacks were the wide age range of the children (2 to 9 years of age) and the long time gaps between the onset and the time when interviews were conducted (e.g., 50 months in the Darley 1955 study; 18 months in the Johnson et al., 1959 study). When memory for small details is relied on, such large intervals compromise data validity. Another significant study in this area was conducted in Britain with 80 children ages 9 to 11 (Andrews & Harris, 1964). It too suffers from similar problems. Limited information was also provided by Glasner and Rosenthal (1957), who interviewed parents of 153 young children who stuttered. They, however, asked only four questions.

Several decades later, parent interview studies of stuttering onset were carried out at the University of Illinois at Urbana-Champaign. The first one by Yairi (1983) included only 23 stuttering children. Results for a larger sample of 87 beginning stuttering children were reported in Yairi and Ambrose (1992b). Finally, in 2005 these two investigators presented data for 156 children. The Illinois investigations mark significant procedural improvements in that they were conducted directly with children (in addition to the parents) within a narrow age range (ages 2 to 5), and within 5 months, on the average, from the time of onset. The 5-month post onset was less than a third of the interval in the Johnson studies. Therefore, parents' reports were less colored by the passage of time. Recorded speech samples provided hard evidence about the stuttering, supplemented by data related to language and phonological skills.

The renewed interest in stuttering onset is also seen in European countries: Britain (Buck, Lees, & Cook, 2002), The Netherlands (Kloth, Janssen, Kraaimaat, & Brutten, 1995), and Denmark (Månsson, 2000, 2006). Each of the two Månsson studies surveyed nearly all newborn children on Bornholm, a Danish island, and included approximately 1,000 children born during 2 consecutive years (1990–1991 and 1995–1996). Soon after their third birthday, the children were examined and their parents interviewed concerning stuttering. The Danish studies, too, represent important improvements in procedures because entire populations, not just samples, participated, and direct observations, as well as parent interviews, were conducted close to the time of onset.

When Does Stuttering Begin?

In assessing research concerning the question of when stuttering begins, the age of the sample investigated must be considered. Samples of children under age 6 will miss some later onsets and therefore may tend to report a lower age at onset. In the Yairi (1983) study of 23 stuttering children younger than age 4, the mean age of onset was 28 months. Studies limited to school-age children and/or adults, however, yield older ages because they miss younger children. This is demonstrated in the Seider, Gladstien, and Kidd (1983) study reporting a mean age at onset of 62 months. Between these two options, we hold that the younger the sample, the more valid the data because of the extensive natural recovery (discussed later in this chapter) that occurs in early ages. Hence samples of older ages are apt to produce greater errors because they are bound to miss many cases of early natural recovery and also because of faulty memories of those who report a stuttering onset far in the past. Other factors, such as sample size and experimental procedures, should also be considered.

With the qualifications just listed in mind, reviewing data from studies that focused on onset, as well as from other surveys that included items pertinent to this question, it would appear that stuttering begins within a wide age range, from as young as 18 months (Milisen & Johnson, 1936; Yairi, 1983) and into the teenage period (Meltzer, 1935; Preus, 1981). Onsets in children older than age 9, however, are few. Rare onsets in adults are linked to either emotional traumas or brain damage (Mahr & Leith, 1992; Rosenbek, Messert, Collins, & Wertz, 1978; Van Borsel & Taillieu, 2001).

Table 3.1 presents data for mean age of onset taken from four studies, two conducted approximately 50 years ago and two in recent years. They illustrate our point concerning the influence of participants' age on the resultant mean age at onset; that is, studies of older children tend to yield an erroneous older mean age at onset.

Information about the age distribution is also of interest. For example, what is the age range in which the greatest concentration of stuttering onsets occurs? Some studies reported that 59% of onsets take place between 24 and 36 months of age, the 3rd year of life, increasing to 85% by 42 months of age and to 95% by age 48 months, the 4th birthday (Yairi & Ambrose, 2005). These data are relevant to other stuttering issues because in many cases the onset of stuttering parallels a critical period of fast growth of the child's speech mechanism as well as his or her speech and language skills. Indeed, links between stuttering and these factors have been suggested (Bernstein Ratner, 1997a).

The available research and clinical evidence indicates that the most stuttering onsets occur younger than age 5 or 6. Interestingly, in one study of 179 stuttering children only 5 had onset later than age 4 (Månsson, 2000). As for the mean age at onset, the overall mean for 11 investigations was calculated by Yairi (1997) to be 42 months. Many differences in sample sizes and procedural flaws, however, diminish the validity of this figure. Furthermore, as seen in Table 3.1, recent studies conducted with considerably greater rigor than past ones indicate a mean age at onset younger than 36 months. It also shows that gender does not seem to exert influence on the age at onset.

Table 3.1: Mean Age at Stuttering Onset

Study	Sample Size	Subjects' Age (years)	Mean Age at Onset (months)		
			Total	Boys	Girls
Johnson et al. (1959)	150	<9	42	42.4	41.2
Andrews & Harris (1964)	80	11–13	60		
Yairi & Ambrose (2005)	163	<6	33	33.6	32.9
Månsson (2006)	179	<4	30	30.9	30.5

How Does Stuttering Begin?

The view that stuttering always begins gradually, almost inconspicuously, with easy repetitions, no tension, and with the child being unaware of it, has been deeply entrenched in the our field (Bluemel, 1913; Froeschels, 1943; Johnson et al., 1959). Froeschels stated that only in rare cases did stuttering onset deviate from this pattern. Contradictory observations were ignored, perhaps under influences of learning theories that savor reinforcement dynamics. Nevertheless, sudden onset was reported by Van Riper (1971) for 10% of 114 cases and by Preus (1981) for 17% of 100 cases. In a very careful study of 87 children and parents soon after onset, Yairi and Ambrose (1992b) at the University of Illinois reported that for 44% of the children, onset was judged by parents as sudden, with 31% describing it as an abrupt change over a single day. Later, these authors found that nearly 30% of 163 children exhibited abrupt onset that took hold in a single day. Adding the onsets reported to occur over 2 to 3 days, the total sudden onsets exceeded 40%. Intermediate onsets (1 to 2 weeks) comprised 33% of the cases, with only 28% reporting gradual onset longer than 2 weeks. In other words, gradual onsets were found to be the *least*, not the most frequent, manner of onset. Males and females were distributed similarly also in respect to onset type.

In addition to variation in the manner of onset, some studies also contradicted the traditional view that early stuttering is characterized by mild, if not normal, repetitions. Far from this, the Illinois studies reported that most parents rated the early stuttering as moderate to severe, and they also said it was associated with some degree of force, even severe tension. More than 20% thought their child was aware of the problem (Yairi, 1983; Yairi & Ambrose, 1992b, 2005). The following letter received from a mother (several details were altered to protect privacy) vividly illustrates the above findings concerning abruptness of onset, severity of stuttering at onset, and early awareness of the stuttering. Also note the expressed parental anguish.

I am desperately trying to find help for my preschooler. Denise will be 4 years old in approximately two months and has always excelled at speaking. She is the oldest of three children, one of them is only one year younger. She suddenly developed severe stuttering a week ago. She never stuttered at all before this, nor was she slow in speech development in any way. It was as if someone had flipped a light switch, and her speech dramatically changed. She is very, very smart. I know that all parents think that their child is intelligent, but mine really is (Ha Ha.) Honestly though, I would get comments all of the time from complete strangers about how well she was talking and communicating. She stutters so severely now (and it has only been 7 days) that at times she will just quit trying to say the word she is stuck on and become silent. I will then say, "It's okay, baby, what were you saying?" And she will reply, "I can't." When she is stuck on a word, she will look at me with terrified eyes, and it is almost as though she CAN'T stop trying to say the word.

I have tried with great patience to follow all of the advice I can find from Web sites. They tell me not to acknowledge the stuttering, slow my speech, not finish her

(continued)

sentences, remain calm, etc. Nothing has helped in any way and it is dramatically worse even in these short 7 days. She asked me today, "Mommy, why can't I talk right?" (This question was a struggle that literally took at least a minute and a half to get through.) Her stuttering is so severe that it is literally robbing her of the ability to communicate with me. Although she diligently tries for a VERY long time to finish her thoughts, she is starting to quit talking and remain quiet.

I am desperate. I have an appointment today with her pediatrician and am thinking of enrolling her in speech therapy. However, with all of the conflicting reports out there, I don't know if I should ignore the stuttering and act as though it is not happening (I don't want to exacerbate the condition even more), or if I should proactively insist on speech therapy. The studies are totally conflicting. Although I do not show her my anxiety, I must tell you that I am completely overwhelmed and saddened. If you have any advice, I would be grateful to receive it. Please let me know what you have found to be helpful for a child in her situation. I cannot understand how this could literally start overnight and yet be so devastating.

Thank you so much for your time. Also, please let me know of any reference material that is beneficial.

Features of Early Stuttering

Having briefly discussed when and how stuttering begins, the next question is what are its early speech and other characteristics. What can the speech-language clinician expect? These are presented next.

Types and Frequency of Disfluencies

From the early research of stuttering onset and throughout, there has been considerable agreement about its most common features. Already in 1937 Taylor found that 85% of the parents reported repetitions, especially of whole words, as the only initial symptom. A few years later, Johnson (1942) revealed that 90% of parents reported the early stuttering as repetitions of parts of words, whole words, or phrases, typically at the beginning of speech attempts. Darley made a similar report in 1955. Johnson et al. (1959) stated that the most frequent features of early stuttering recounted by parents were syllable repetitions (60%) and word repetitions (50%). In the Yairi (1983) study, parents of 95% of the children recalled syllable repetitions at onset and 40% also recalled word repetitions. Nevertheless, the symptomatology at onset is not confined to repetitions as writers have emphasized for a long time (e.g., from Froeschels in 1943 to Packman, Code, & Onslow in 2007). The fact is that just about all investigators reported that a good number of children were described by parents to have other stuttering-like disfluencies. Between 8% and 16% of the children were reported to exhibit what was described as sound stoppages, complete blocks, prolongation, and articulatory fixations (Darley 1995; Johnson et al., 1959; Taylor, 1937). In the Yairi and Ambrose (1992b) study, parents reported 36% of the children had sound prolongations at the time of onset, 23% had conspicuous silent periods, and 14% had blocks.

Recall that the preceding descriptions are based on retrospective reports. Quantified objective information became available only in the past 25 years when Yairi and Lewis (1984) insisted on (1) recording speech for direct observation, (2) using children representing a narrow age range, and (3) identifying children close to stuttering onset. (Their participants were between 25 to 39 months of age and within 2 months after onset.[1]) They found large differences in the disfluencies produced by children who stuttered and normally fluent peers, especially in the quantities of part-word repetitions and sound prolongations, providing strong evidence that speech at onset is far from being normal as claimed by adherents to Johnson et al.'s (1959) theory of stuttering. Their findings were confirmed by other investigators (e.g., Schwartz, Zebrowski, & Conture, 1990), as well as in larger studies at the University of Illinois (Ambrose & Yairi, 1999; Yairi & Ambrose, 2005). Overlap between the two groups in critical types of disfluent speech was small.

Data on the frequency of disfluent speech output of children near onset of stuttering as compared with normally speaking children are shown in Table 3.2. As you can see, the gap between the two groups on the three disfluency types we call stuttering-like disfluency is large. The two groups, however, are very similar with respect to other disfluencies (i.e., interjections, revisions, phrase repetitions).

Length of Disfluencies

Because sometimes normally fluent speakers overlap with people who stutter in the number of disfluencies they produce in a given amount of speech, the length of each disfluency could make the distinction much clearer. Take two children, for example: Each repeats the word "and" on five different occasions within 100 words. One child repeats the word only one extra time ("and-and") on each occasion, whereas the second child repeats four extra times (and-and-and-and-and) on each occasion (each

Table 3.2: **Mean per 100 Syllables for Stuttering-Like Disfluencies and Other Disfluencies for Stuttering and Normally Fluent Children**

Disfluency Type	Stuttering Children, Mean (N = 103)	Normally Fluent Children, Mean (N = 52)
Part-word repetition	5.64	0.55
Single-syllable word repetition	3.24	0.79
Disrhythmic phonation	2.42	0.08
Total SLD	**11.30**	**1.41**
Other disfluencies	5.79	4.48

SLD = stuttering-like disfluencies.

Source: Adapted from Early Childhood Stuttering (p. 320) by E. Yairi and N. G. Ambrose (2005), Austin, TX: PRO-ED. Copyright 2005 by PRO-ED, Inc. Adapted with permission.

---

[1] Johnson et al. (1959) also provided valuable information based on analyses of recorded speech of 89 children but these were taken up to 3 years post-onset.

iteration is referred to as a "repetition unit"). Although the count of disfluent words, four, is the same, their disfluent speech is vastly different in quantity, and listeners will perceive it so. The first, the normally fluent child, would have uttered the word "and" a total of 10 times (5×2) as compared to 25 times (5×5) for the second child, the one who exhibits stuttering. Hence information on the frequency of disfluency alone may be insufficient. Both Johnson (1942) and Darley (1955), two well-known researchers of stuttering onset, commented that parents described the early stuttering as two to four iterations of syllables, words, or phrases. The investigators judged such disfluencies as "brief" and basically normal. This was quite unfortunate because two to four iterations is way above normal. In so doing, they overlooked the fundamental significance of the length factor.

Years later, objective data obtained by other investigators from careful analyses of tape-recorded speech samples revealed extremely important information in this regard. The mean number of iterations for children who stutter is less than two, that is, less than "you-you-you." The mean for normally fluent children is just above one repetition unit, translated as slightly more than "you-you" (Ambrose & Yairi, 1995; Johnson et al., 1959; Wexler, 1982; Yairi & Lewis, 1984). This is a big difference. Beyond single-unit repetition, there is little overlap between the two groups. Children who stutter do occasionally repeat three to five times, but such instances are not common for the normally fluent children. Hence Yairi and Lewis (1984) concluded that the extent of disfluency is a more powerful discriminant between children who stutter and their normally fluent peers than the number of disfluent events.

Physical Concomitants

The nonspeech body movements that accompany stuttering events have been referred to as concomitant (cooccurring) behaviors or, more often, "secondary" characteristics. For a long time, it was assumed that they appear late when the older child tries to cope with a stuttered event in an effort to "get the word out." Examination of past onset studies, however, question this assumption. The percentage of children reported by parents to exhibit secondary characteristics at onset, particularly head, face, and neck movement, varies from 11% in the Taylor (1937) study to 53% in the Yairi and Ambrose (2005) study. These investigators wrote that "Most parents (53%) of the 146 children we saw within one year of onset reported that their children exhibited at least one specific physical component at stuttering onset" (p. 69). Such parental reports were corroborated by frame-by-frame analyses of videotaped speech samples that identified and classified the different secondary characteristics (Conture & Kelly, 1991; Schwartz, Zebrowski, & Conture, 1990; Yairi, Ambrose, Paden, & Throneburg, 1996). Because a few secondary characteristics are often present from early on, even among children who later recover (Yairi et al., 1996), it is not unreasonable to entertain the thought that they may be an integral aspect of stuttering, not necessarily "secondary." Further research is needed to explore whether all secondary characteristics are integral components. For example, eye blinks may more frequently represent an integral or reflexive component of stuttering, whereas tongue protrusion might more often be a compensatory effort to release speech.

Emotional and Physical Health

The notion that stuttering onset is associated with specific emotional stresses and health problems has been around for a long time and has seen ups and down in the level of scientific support. According to an early estimate, 28% of a 1,000-child caseload suffered emotional antecedents, such as shock or fright, prior to onset (Makuen, 1914). Another investigator reported emotional shocks prior to onset in 27% of her caseload of 200 children (Katsovaskaia, 1962). Similarly, illness episodes prior to onset in 16% to 20% and in 35% of the children were reported by West, Nelson, and Berry (1939) and Katsovaskaia (1962), respectively. A very different picture is seen in the Iowa studies, which concluded that in only a few of the 246 stuttering children were there associations of onset with physical illness or emotional upheaval, and that the health histories revealed no more childhood diseases than those of normally fluent control children (Johnson et al., 1959). British investigators were in agreement, reporting no significant difference in the incidence of diseases between 80 stuttering children and their control peers (Andrews & Harris, 1964).

The past two decades have seen yet another turn in the information and views concerning physical emotional health issues associated with onset. For example, Poulos and Webster (1991) found that 37% of people who stutter *without* a family history of stuttering reported childhood incidences of anoxia, head injuries, and so on, that could have resulted in early brain damage. In contrast, such incidences occurred in only 2.6% stutterers *with* family stuttering. Also, the most recent pertinent investigation found that 14% of the children were reported to experience health problems, such as respiratory problems, surgery, or illness that required medical treatment just prior to onset. Over 40% experienced emotionally upsetting events such as: parents' divorce, death of a beloved pet, difficult day-care situations, and others. The authors opined that "If a child possesses predisposing (i.e., genetic) factors to stutter, aggravating physical or emotional stresses might very well trigger the onset" (Yairi & Ambrose, 2005, p. 63). So far, little, if any, in-depth research of health problems associated with the onset of stuttering has been done. The information could be useful to better understanding the role of biological and environmental forces to the emergence of stuttering.

Child temperament is another factor that may contribute to stuttering onset. Often based on parental questionnaires, the published data may have limited validity. Investigators have found several statistically significant differences in temperament traits between 31 young children who stutter and their age- and gender-matched controls (Anderson, Pellowski, Conture, & Kelly, 2003). A more meaningful, prospective study in Australia followed 1,911 children during their first 3 years of life. There were no significant differences between the 158 who began stuttering and those who did not on a temperament questionnaire administered to parents within 6 months prior to onset that may have been useful to predict stuttering onset (Reilly et al., 2009).

Phonology and Language

The scientific literature makes frequent references to a wide range of disorders that are present concomitantly with stuttering; those involving phonology/articulation and language skills are the most frequent. Much of the better incidence data have been reported for school-age children. A large survey of pupils who stutter revealed that 46% had articulation/phonology disorders and 26% had language disorders (Blood, Ridenour, Qualls, & Scheffner Hammer, 2003). Surveys of the status of language and phonology in the school population (see Chapter 4) have limited bearing on stuttering onset that typically occurs years earlier. The following discussion is limited to preschool children, especially near stuttering onset, if possible.

> The overlap between the most common period for the onset of stuttering and the period during which there is an explosion in speech and language development, between ages 2 and 4, raises the proposition of stuttering-language-phonology links. These potential links are of theoretical interest and are discussed in Chapter 6. If present, other speech-language difficulties during early stuttering are also relevant to clinicians' choice of a treatment regimen. For further study of the potential stuttering-language-phonology links, see Bernstein Ratner (1997a); Hall, Wagovitch, and Bernstein Ratner (2007); Paden (2005); Byrd, Wolk, and Davis (2007); and Watkins, 2005.

Disordered Phonology and Articulation

Are articulation or phonological disorders[2] present at the time of stuttering onset or shortly thereafter? The answer is not clear in reference specifically to the event of onset. It has not been our experience to commonly hear parents mentioning phonological issues when describing stuttering onset or problems that preceded it. More objective data for preschool children who stutter (ages 2 to 5) seem to suggest that a good number of them may have some problems, although the evidence is inconsistent as well as controversial.

A general observation of frequent speech articulation difficulties during the early stage of stuttering was reported by Van Riper (1971, 1982), especially in one subgroup that he designated as track II. This, however, was not the case in a study conducted in Scotland where comparisons of speech sound accuracy in single words were made over several years between 37 children who stutter and 113 control children who did not stutter (Morley, 1957). Unexpectedly, at the early testing, closer to stuttering onset, fewer children who stutter (CWS) had errors than children who did not stutter (CWNS), as summarized here:

- At 3:9, errors were present in 50% of the CWS and 58% of the CWNS.
- At 4:9, errors were present in 25% of the CWS and 36% of the CWNS.
- At 6:6, errors were present in 14% of the CWS and 5% of the CWNS.

In the United States, one study found no difference between 20 preschoolers who stuttered and normally fluent controls in scores on the Arizona Articulation Scale.

---

[2] For many years, the term *articulation disorder* was applied to inabilities to produce, or correctly produce, speech sounds. As of the 1980s, it is now reserved for disorders in which there is a clear motor involvement. The term *phonological disorder* or *phonological delay* is applied to the majority of difficulties in sound production during childhood where motor interference is not apparent. These difficulties are presumed to reflect delay in the child's subliminal awareness of the different classes of sounds and problems in central planning of speech (Paden, 2005).

Nevertheless, a few years later, five of the boys who stuttered needed phonological therapy (Ryan, 1971). Other investigators reported 40% of 30 CWS had phonological deficits compared to 7% in CWNS (Louko, Edwards, & Conture, 1990). Similarly, 37% of 99 CWS were found to have phonological disorders by Yaruss, LaSalle, and Conture (1998). No control group was employed. Also, it should be pointed out that the age of the participants in the last two studies extended to 6 and 7 years, beyond the preschool range. Regardless, if valid, these figures are substantially higher than the 2% to 6% expected in the general population (Beitchman, Nair, Clegg, & Patel, 1986).

The reports just cited, as well as other sources, are based on samples from local clinical centers and employed far too small samples for providing reliable prevalence data. Research in this area has also been criticized for its potential inflation of estimates due to several other methodological issues (Nippold, 1990, 2004). Supporting some of Nippold's concerns is a study by Throneburg, Yairi, and Paden (1994). Although it had a different focus, the investigators commented that among 75 preschool children ages 29 to 59 months who stutter, seen close to stuttering onset, none had profound phonological deficits and only 5 (7%) had severe phonological disorders. Similar results were found for their 50 normally fluent controls: None exhibited profound phonological deficits and only 3 (6%) had severe phonological disorders. These authors expressed skepticism about the notion of high prevalence of phonological disorders in preschool age children, stating, "If there is a strong relation between stuttering and disordered phonology it would be expected that a larger proportion of stutterers than nonstutterers would have severe and profound phonologic disorders" (p. 508). Their skeptical view is reinforced by studies that have failed to show relationships between the level of stuttering severity and the level of phonological skills (Gregg & Yairi, 2007; Wolk, Edwards, & Conture, 1993). Furthermore, the recent prospective study by Reilly et al. (2009), mentioned earlier, found that 158 children who began stuttering by the age of 3 years had a smaller proportion (14.6%) of speech-language-reading problems compared to those who did not start to stutter (19.7%). The direction of the difference is reminiscent of the Morely (1957) findings near onset. Because the Australian study did not report data for children past the age of 3, it is not known whether there may be differences for children with a later age of stuttering onset.

Overall, it appears to us that if the incidence and prevalence of phonological disorders associated with very early stuttering is higher than in the population's average, it is not as high as several scholars have claimed. Perhaps subgroups of children who stutter are more vulnerable in this respect. Indeed, a series of studies conducted at the University of Illinois, one with 36 children who stutter (Paden & Yairi, 1996) and one with 84 children who stutter (Paden, Yairi, & Ambrose, 1999), tested shortly after stuttering onset, showed that the mean phonological performance of the subgroup of children who later developed persistent stuttering lagged behind that of children who later recovered naturally as well as behind normally fluent controls in every measure. The differences, however, was a matter of slower acquisition, not of abnormal developmental pattern. One conclusion is that older children who stutter, those who persist, have a higher prevalence of phonological and articulation disorders, a conclusion supported by the Morely (1957) longitudinal data depicted earlier. This possibility is considered further in the later discussion of the development of stuttering.

Disordered Language

As stated earlier, the idea of links between stuttering and language factors in young children is intuitive due to the fact that stuttering onset coincides with a time of rapid expansion in expressive and receptive language ability in young children. Bloodstein (2002, p. 165) opined that "some children may reveal their tenuous grip on language . . . by stuttering." Does this link mean that stuttering is associated with language disorders? The perspective that children who stutter are likely to have language skills that are inferior to those of their normally fluent peers has been long-standing in the field. One literature review generalized that "stutterers performed more poorly than non-stutterers on some tests of language development" (Andrews, Craig, Feyer, Hoddinott, Howie, & Neilson, 1983, p. 230). Recall, however, that most large-scale surveys were conducted with school-age populations, with the most recent one reporting 26% of those who stutter also exhibited language disorders (Blood et al., 2003).

Credible incidence and prevalence data for language disorders in preschool children, especially near the onset of stuttering, however, is sparse. It is the product of a few small studies. Furthermore, current information presents an equivocal, or even opposite picture. In one study, 20 preschool children who stuttered scored lower than normally fluent controls on several language measures but they were still within normal range (Ryan, 1992). This investigator later reported a similar outcome for a sample that included a few new participants (Ryan, 2001a). Another small study compared 20 preschoolers who stuttered with control peers on several standardized language measures. The CWS scored lower and displayed a greater expressive-receptive discrepancy (Anderson & Conture, 2000). Generally, however, they performed within the average range of language abilities. This team had similar results with 16 CWS scoring lower than controls but within normal limits (Anderson & Conture, 2004). Also Miles and Bernstein Ratner (2001) reported average or above-average language test scores for 16 3-year-old CWS. Finally, as part of the Illinois studies, a substantially larger sample of 84 children, ages 2 to 5, tested near stuttering onset, provided intriguing language data based on spontaneous language analyses and one standardized test, the PLS (the Preschool Language Scale; Zimmerman, Steiner, & Pond, 1979). Most interestingly, the children's scores were at, or well above, norms. There were, however, greater variability and atypical patterns of language production in children whose stuttering persisted as compared to those who later exhibited natural recovery. On the PLS, scores were higher than normative on both comprehension and expression components (Watkins, Yairi, & Ambrose, 1999). Similarly, a team of scholars in Germany also found that their preschool-age participants who stuttered tended to have language skills at or above age expectations (Rommel, Hage, Kalehne, & Johannsen, 1999).

Overall, current data do not seem to indicate gross, or widespread, language deficiency associated with the onset of stuttering. One is left to ponder what factors might account for the discrepancy between more recent findings and interpretations regarding language abilities of young children who stutter. In a review of the literature, Watkins and Johnson (2004) concluded that much of the controversy may have been fueled by methodological issues, such as inadequate control groups or lack of comparison with normative data. We also suggest it is important to recognize that the global nature of measures and instruments used, such as the PLS, yields only superficial information about the participants' language abilities, particularly abilities in handling the online demands of language use in context. Perhaps closer examination of individual patterns of performance and finer language tasks may be important to clarifying the developmental relation between language proficiency and stuttering.

This section on the onset of stuttering is concluded with a rare, day-by-day, parental account of the event. It was recorded at the time by one of the authors (Yairi) as it was unfolding many years ago and involved the author's own son.

Micah (age 3 year, 6 months) began to show unusual disfluencies on December 20. December 21: Disfluencies continued, were quite frequent, and consisted of 6–7 repetitions of short words or just the initial syllable of a word. We noticed this with some concern.

December 22: Disfluent speech greatly increased. It is stuttering, at times severe. Short words, particularly /if/, /on/, /and/, and /in/ are often repeated 5–6 times, even up to 10–12 times. Also repetitions of initial syllables beginning with /l/ and /k/. There is a struggle behavior in that at times he closes his eyes. Most outstanding is Micah's reactions to the difficulties he had in talking. He would stop after a number of repetitions of a word and say "I cannot remember" and then just drop it. We are quite alarmed. The disfluencies do not always occur and there are sentences, and longer speech stretches, of only fluent speech. When disfluencies occur, they tend to be in groups. We decided to minimize his talking when severe disfluencies occurred (not asking questions, etc.) and be lax with demands and discipline. We also paid him more attention than usual. Except for the fact of my own, and my family's, history of stuttering, there was no apparent change in our life, or another reason of which we were aware, for the sudden stuttering onset.

December 23: There was considerable improvement. Spent much of the day in the nursery school. The babysitter who came in early evening reported later that his speech was rather fluent and that several instances of disfluency were quite mild. The nights of the 23rd and the 24th he wet the bed. This was the first time in several weeks. During the entire week he woke up at least once during each night, got out of bed, but went back to sleep.

December 24 and 25: We stayed at home. Disfluent speech was back. Up, but not as bad as on the 22nd. When disfluencies occurred, at times they gave a clear impression of stuttering because of the number of repetitions, 7–8, although no overt tension could be observed, nor closing of the eyes. Most of the speech was fluent and he talked slowly. The comment he made earlier "I cannot remember" was not repeated after December 22. We continue to make special efforts to reduce all pressure. Often talked to him slowly. I tried rhythmic speech, which he liked. Although it was Christmas week, we do not celebrate this holiday, so there was no unusual tension at home.

December 26: In the morning, speech was fluent except for a few instances of easy repetitions that contained 3–4 iterations. He spent 7 hours in the nursery school. Back at home, speech continued to be good during the early evening. Later, when

(continued)

we went out for dinner, he had severe stuttering in the car as well as in the restaurant. We felt that people were noticing him. When we returned home, speech was good again.

December 27: A good day in terms of speech with only occasional repetitions of a word or sounds, 3–4 iterations.

December 28: Speech was relatively good with several instances of repetitions of 3–5 iterations. More stuttering in the car was noticed again. On one occasion, however, he repeated 15 times. No apparent reaction on his part.

December 29: Micah had several instances of severe repetitions in the morning and early afternoon, with 10–15 units at times. These occurred consistently on groups of 3–4 words. He seemed to be reacting to a TV program where the animals were drowning in the water. Each attempt to say the word "animal" was very difficult. He kept talking about it for quite a while. I took him to the park for 2 hours. Speech was fine for the rest of the afternoon and evening. We are concerned and upset by the re-occurring of the stuttering even though most of the speech is normal.

December 30: Speech during the morning was normal. The nursery school teacher did not observe anything unusual except that he exhibited some jealousy of his younger brother (17 months younger). In the evening, though, and on December 31, there were random incidences of disfluent speech, primarily repetitions of 3–5 iterations but also 2–3 instances of over 10 units. At times he partially closed his eyes. Because most of the time his speech is fluent, we are not sure if he has a "stuttering problem."

January 1: We noticed Micah talking to himself (very slowly) for several minutes while playing in his room. This occurred several times. When talking to us, instances of stuttering, involving shutting of the eyes, were frequent. We were very concerned and tense about it. We began to do with him some rhythmic speech activities. Also, we began talking slowly to him and continued to avoid demands, relax discipline, and show more patience. On January 2, speech was very good all day. I took him out during early evening and let him do whatever he wanted to. Told him a story at bedtime. He was very affectionate and we were relieved. Speech was normal for 2 weeks or so.

January 18: Stuttering appeared again suddenly. Frequent excessive disfluencies. At times Micah stuttered on almost all words. This took the form of syllable (often beginning with consonants) repetitions, upward pitch shifts, closing eyes, and turning the head downward. He often stuttered on the same words: "marbles," "cookies," "Savta," and others. Struggle behaviors were very obvious; also his awareness of the speaking difficulties. He would stop without finishing the word, avoided words, and even substituted words. For example, he would try saying "marbles," repeating "ma-ma-ma-ma-ma-ma- ma- ma-" stops and say "the game." There were variations in the stuttering from situation to situation. Stuttering remained pretty consistent for the week with some day-to-day variations. The staff at the nursery school, as well as other people, also commented on the stuttering. We found out that one of the teachers reacted and told him to "stop mumbling," etc. She was advised to avoid all reactions, corrections, or suggestions."

Micah continued to stutter for approximately 10 weeks, during which he exhibited a wide range of stuttering severity. Stuttering stopped as quickly as it began and never occurred again. For the record, Micah's speech was relatively late to develop although his fine motor skills were excellent if not outstanding. According to notes taken at the time by his mother, a speech/language clinician, at 23 months of age expressive vocabulary was still mainly jargon with just a few words. Between 24 and 26 months of age, however, there was an apparent change. The notes indicate a sudden jump in expression, with many more single words. He finally began combining 2–3 word sentences. His language, however, was very advanced, and described as "wonderful." Indeed, receptive language test scores placed him at the 94th percentile. These observations are of interest in view of the controversy regarding possible links between stuttering onset and speech/language development.

Development

Once stuttering has emerged, what follows? This is an important question not only in regard to understanding the nature of the disorder but also for clinical purposes. A clinician examining a 3-year-old child who began stuttering a few weeks earlier should be able to provide educated answers to parents' typical questions like these: "What is going to happen with this stuttering?" "Will it stop before he goes to kindergarten?" "If he goes on stuttering, for how long? Will it improve or get worse?" The clinician should also be able to respond to these questions when examining a child who has already stuttered for 2 or more years. His or her answers, however, are likely to be different because, as we will soon see, stuttering may change extensively with time. Aside for parent counseling purposes, information about the development of stuttering may be critical for making clinical decisions, such as whether to initiate or postpone intervention, or what kind of intervention fits the particular status of the disorder at any given time.

Some information pertaining to the questions just posed and clinical needs has been provided through a variety of sources including clinical observations, cross-sectional retrospective research, and direct longitudinal studies.

Traditional Models of Developmental Progression

Similarly to the traditional portrayal of the onset of stuttering, the development of the disorder has also been pictured stereotypically. For a long time, the developmental outlines presented a unidirectional path of a disorder that begins mildly and then, in a stepwise succession, increases in abnormality. Froeschels (1921) offers a very detailed account that emphasizes the escalating tempo of the repetitions as stuttering persists. A classic depiction of this view is expressed in Robinson's (1964) statement that "Stuttering seldom remains static. It grows. And as it grows, it tends to change form and severity. Early patterns are replaced, obscured, or supplemented by more pronounced and abnormal behavior. Repetitions or prolongations become troublesome blocks" (p. 47).

The notion that stuttering progresses through prescribed stages in most individuals who exhibit the disorder has been particularly popular. Unfortunately, it emerged from unsystematic observations and subjective impressions by several influential clinicians such as Bluemel (1932). His developmental system included two phases: *primary stuttering*, which is a pure speech disorder characterized exclusively by easy repetitions, and *secondary stuttering*, marked by considerable physical tension in speech and the child's awareness of the stuttering that leads to fear and avoidance of speaking. Although the transition time from primary to secondary stuttering varies among individuals, all follow a similar developmental pattern. In 1954 Van Riper modified the Bluemel system by adding two intermediate stages. Essentially, however, he appears to have endorsed the concepts of primary and secondary stuttering. As indicated earlier in this chapter, however, recent data pertaining to onset negate the position that all early stuttering is "simple" repetitions, devoid of tension and emotional reactions. In our view, Bluemel's sharp stage dichotomy is not a valid depiction of the disorder.

A well-known four-phase developmental sequence was presented by Bloodstein (1960a, 1960b, 1961) based on changes in five parameters: type of disfluency, loci of disfluency, physical tension, cognitive awareness, and emotional reactions. He used information from diagnostic reports for 418 stuttering children who were evaluated at different ages. They were divided into 16 subgroups of 30 children, each representing 6-month age intervals between ages 2 and 16. Among the essential features of phase I (ages 2 to 6), for example, are (1) repetitions of syllables and words that occur primarily on functional short words at the initial position in phrases, (2) up-and-down cycles in the stuttering with possible complete amelioration for days or weeks followed by resumption of stuttering, and (3) little evidence of awareness and concern. During phases II and III, (1) stuttering becomes chronic, (2) the child identifies himself as a stutterer, (3) stuttered speech increases in complexity and severity to include sound prolongations and blocks, (4) stuttering occurs throughout the sentences and on other types of words (nouns, verbs, adjectives, adverbs), and (5) fears and anticipation of stuttering emerge. By phase IV (adolescence and adulthood), strong emotional reactions take over as individuals exhibit avoidance of speaking prior to stuttering and shame and embarrassment afterward.

In spite of Bloodstein's recognition of individual differences in the age and timing of the disorder's progression, its overall uniformity and linear directionality is cardinal to his model. That is, only one sequence is recognized in which the disorder is worsening. In our opinion, this system, which is based on cross-sectional data, is seriously flawed because the methodology employed is based on an erroneous premise that successively older subgroups represent all members of the youngest subgroup (the 2-year-olds) as they would have grown and their stuttering continues, although altered. Such a premise is acceptable in cross-sectional studies concerned, for example, with the development of height or weight for children in the general population. In these studies, it can be assumed that most 2-year-olds continue to live and grow in height and weight for years to come. Therefore a group of 16-year-olds can be considered to represent the 2-year-olds as they would be years later. Such a premise is not acceptable in a cross-sectional study of the development of stuttering, however, because so many of the children sampled in older age groups represent an entirely different subpopulation of people who stutter than the population used for the youngest group.

Unfortunately, Bloodstein neglected to consider the large natural recovery, 75% of all cases, that takes place. The fact is that the oldest group (phase 4) in his system represents only about 25% (probably appreciably less) of those who entered the study at age 2. Contrary to Bloodstein's conclusion, they do not present the typical development of stuttering (also true for his phases 2 and 3 groups). In other words, only a small percentage of people who stutter actually progress through the pre-scribed stages of increasing severity and complexity. Most stop stuttering within 2 to 4 years and never even enter into phase 2. This is illustrated in Figure 3.1. The older groups in the Bloodstein study were populated with highly biased samples of people who failed to recover. Hence the four phases may, at best, describe the development of the small minority of children who, as they grow up, develop chronic stuttering.

Figure 3.1: **Schematic Showing That Children Who Stutter Tested at Later Times Do Not Represent the Same Group Tested Earlier**

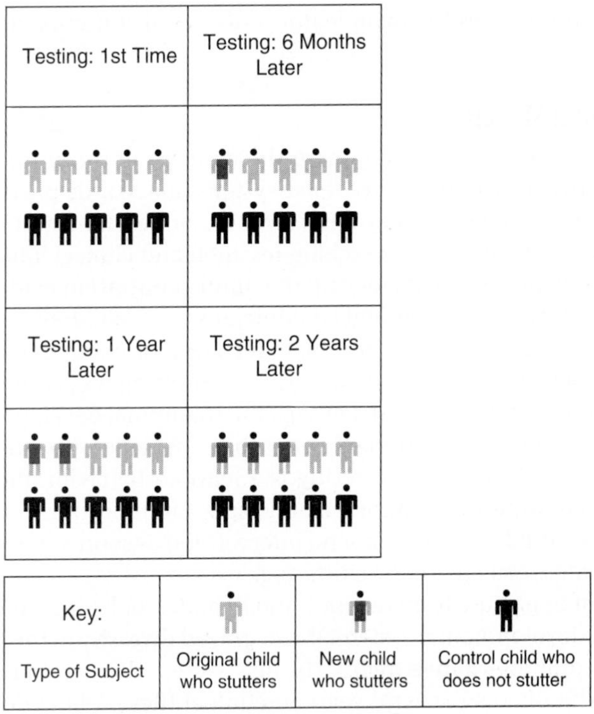

| Testing: 1st Time | Testing: 6 Months Later |
| Testing: 1 Year Later | Testing: 2 Years Later |

Key:			
Type of Subject	Original child who stutters	New child who stutters	Control child who does not stutter

Note: Previous children who stuttered and recovered had to be replaced by new ones from persistent stutterers. With time this group represents mostly those who persist, a small fraction of the stuttering population. Control children who do not stutter remained the same.

Table 3.3: Developmental Models of Stuttering That Described Sequential Stages

Source	Phase 1	Phase 2	Phase 3	Phase 4
Froeschels (1921)	Slow easy, even tempo "clonic" repetitions	Tense, fast tempo, irregular repetitions	Tense, forced, "tonic" postures, halted repetitions	Inhibited symptoms due to social pressures
Bleumel (1932)	"Primary" stuttering: easy repetitions of initial syllables	"Secondary" stuttering: tension, effort, awareness, fear	N/A	N/A
Van Riper (1954)	Slow easy, even repetitions and some prolongations	Faster, irregular repetitions; some prolongations; brief awareness	Tense, effortful stuttering; full awareness, fear, avoidance	N/A
Bloodstein (1960b)	Episodic; mostly repetitions of initial syllables; increases with excitement; little awareness or concern	Chronic; a variety of symptoms with more tension; still increases with excitement; aware but little concern	Chronic; complex symptoms; varies by sound, word, and situation; negative emotion but not fear; does not avoid talking	Chronic; complex symptoms; avoids sounds, words, and situations of talking; fear and shame; personal and social impact

N/A = not applicable.

Furthermore, even among these there are some whose stuttering remains steady or even decreases. Table 3.3 summarizes the main features of several stuttering development systems.

Differential Developmental Models

The developmental systems reviewed earlier share the concept of uniformity in upward progression of stuttering. Not only have these systems made little provision for alternative developmental sequences, they reinforced the notion that stuttering is a homogeneous disorder that has had far-reaching research and clinical implications. This way of thinking is puzzling considering the ample contrarian evidence that was probably observed by many experienced clinicians (e.g., children whose stuttering took the opposite path leading to complete recovery, or children whose stuttering changed little over time, or those whose initial stuttering was severe, or those who indicated awareness from early on). Perhaps the traditional developmental ideas were so strongly influenced by learning theories that contradictory evidence was simply ignored. If one believes that stuttering is a learned behavior, then it should be expected to be continuously reinforced and grow. An important clinical implication of such models would be to recommend intervention as soon as possible to lessen the expected negative changes in the stuttering.

A significant important departure from the traditional model took place in 1971 with Van Riper's proposed developmental system. It recognized diversity in the path of stuttering according to four alternative tracks. His new system drew from information recorded longitudinally over several years in clinical files of 44 children. Note, however, that it was not derived by means of controlled scientific procedures.

Table 3.4: The Main Features of Van Riper's (1971) Four Developmental Tracks

	Features
Subtype Track I	Most cases of stuttering: 48% (21/44) Early onset (2.5–4 years) Gradual, episodic, previously fluent Starts with easy repetitions Normal speech rate, good articulation Lack of awareness of speech disruption Many cases recover Persistent cases progress to fast, irregular repetitions, then prolongations and tension; awareness, fear, and avoidance later on
Subtype Track II	Some cases of stuttering: 25% (11/44) Later onset than track I, as phrases and sentences emerge Gradual, chronic, not ever very fluent Part and whole-word repetitions, pauses, revisions Rapid rate (spurts), poor articulation, mumbled speech Lack of awareness of speech disruption Hesitations, revision, and false starts are added to hurried, irregular repetitions
Subtype Track III	A few cases of stuttering: 11% (5/44) Onset later like track II Sudden onset (often stressful event), chronic, previously fluent Blocks (laryngeal fixations, silent prolonged postures) Slow, careful rate, normal articulation Highly aware; some recover but many progress to complex and intense fears and avoidance patterns
Subtype Track IV	Rare cases of stuttering: 9% (4/44) Later onset (usually after 4 years of age) Sudden, episodic, previously fluent Unique patterns of speech disruption Initial whole words and phrases repeated for many units Normal rate, normal articulation Even if frequency increases, symptoms remain consistent Highly aware, but no avoidance No remissions

Note: Three of 44 cases did not fit any of the tracks.

Table 3.4 summarizes the main features of the four tracks. Although not specifically stated by Van Riper, Yairi and Ambrose (2005) observed that it is based on four variables or risk factors: (1) age at onset: early-late, (2) type of onset: gradual-sudden, (3) pattern of stuttering: repetitions-blocks-tension, and (4) concomitant speech-language problems. They noted, "For example, children exhibiting early and gradual onsets with repetitions as the dominant symptom (Track I) had better chances for recovery than those exhibiting sudden onsets, blocks, prolongations, and physical tension (Track III). Children with delayed speech (Track II) were also slower to improve than those with "otherwise normal speech" (p. 149). An important advantage of models that recognize developmental diversity according to risk factors is in allowing for differentiation in clinical decisions concerning intervention and counseling. For example, children in track IV may receive priority for treatment.

Natural Recovery

A most remarkable phenomenon of stuttering that occurs over time is its disappearance in a large percentage of the affected young children. The label *spontaneous recovery* has been the most commonly applied to this trend, implying that the recovery occurs without treatment. The term *natural recovery*, however, might be more suitable inasmuch as it has been argued that the observed recovery is not necessarily spontaneous but could be the consequence of external intervention, such as parental correction of the child's stuttering (e.g., Ingham, 1976; Ingham & Cordes, 1998). Whereas spontaneous recovery implies biological healing processes, natural recovery considers the possibility of environmental factors being responsible, at least in part, for the phenomenon. Of course, there is the all-important question as to who is "recovered." Recent investigators of this phenomenon who observed children who stuttered over several years listed several criteria, both objective and subjective, all indicating no stuttering for at least a year initially to be considered recovered and that no formal treatment should have been received by the child (Yairi & Ambrose, 1999a, 2005):

Criteria for Natural Recovery
- Clinician general judgment that the child had not exhibited stuttering
- Parental general judgment that the child had not exhibited stuttering
- Parental rating of stuttering severity as less than 1 on an 8-point scale (0 = normal; 1 = borderline; 8 = severe stuttering)
- Clinician rating of stuttering severity as less than 1
- SLD observed and reported as fewer than 3 per 100 syllables
- No stuttering present for a minimum of 12 months as judged both by parent and clinician
- Maintained no stuttering for 4 years to demonstrate stability of "recovered" status

Note that that information about the high percentage of natural recovery rests on two different types of evidence: indirect statistical inferences and information obtained through observations of children over time. The statistical inference uses the difference between the 5% figure of stuttering incidence and the 1% figure of its prevalence in the population (see explanation of these concepts in Chapter 2). The meaning of this comparison is that only 1 of 5 children who begin stuttering continues to do so. Put it differently: about 4 of 5 children who begin stuttering (80%) recover, presumably naturally. The second type of evidence come from either clinical observations or systematic research studies specifically intended to tap the level of recovery. Among the first calling attention to natural recovery was Johnson (1934). Based on his clinical observations, he estimated that natural recovery occurs in 30% to 40% of children who begin to stutter by age 8. Similarly, a 40% natural recovery by age 8 was estimated by Bryngelson (1938) based on inspection of 1,492 case files. These figures, as well as data reported in a good number of surveys, some of which are referred to later, were often based on a single person's impression and without specifying any criteria. (An interesting review of recovery can be found in Wingate, 1976. A summary table of reports is provided in Bloodstein & Bernstein Ratner, 2008, p. 86.)

Retrospective Evidence

Early systematic data on natural recovery were reported by investigators who employed retrospective methods. For example, information solicited about themselves from high school students and adults who stuttered in the past yielded nearly 79% recovery (Sheehan & Martyn, 1966). Or parents were asked about their children's stuttering history (e.g., Dickson, 1971; Glasner & Rosenthal, 1957). No further objective evidence, such as speech samples, was gathered, no criteria for stuttering or recovery were employed, and there was no verification of either the initial stuttering diagnosis or of remission. In the Glasner and Rosenthal (1957) study, parents' retrospective reports indicated that 54% of children who were said to have had stuttering history had recovered, 15% stuttered only occasionally, and only 31% continued to stutter habitually at the time of their study. Dickson (1971) also reported 54% recovery based on reports of parents of children in kindergarten through junior high school.

Longitudinal Indirect Evidence

Longitudinal investigations that followed children who stutter for several years provide considerably more valid recovery evidence than retrospective studies, although they have varied in methodological strength. A few suffer from the fact that their data were indirect. For example, Johnson (1955b) followed 46 preschool-aged children who stuttered for up to 5 years (mean = 30 months). Most had stuttered for less than a year at the first visit. Information on the children's status of stuttering was obtained several times during the follow-up period, but it was based on parents' reports not on direct observations of the children by the investigators or on objective tape-recorded speech samples. In this study, 72% evidenced complete recovery, and an additional 13% exhibited a decrease in stuttering severity. None received speech therapy during the course of the study. A few years later, Johnson et al. (1959) used a similar methodology with 118 stuttering children ages 2 to 7 at the time of the first interview, with a follow-up conducted 30 months later. Improvement was reported for 88% of the children, with 36% exhibiting complete recovery. It is noteworthy that only in 4% of the children did the stuttering severity increase, a finding that clearly negates the traditional view that stuttering *typically* grows in complexity and severity. We believe that the more advanced age of the children when entering this study yielded a lower percentage of full recovery because many children recover at younger ages.

Longitudinal Direct Evidence

Much more valid and reliable evidence has been generated by longitudinal studies that were based on direct monitoring of children's stuttering from near onset for a period of several years. These, too, have varied in methodological strength, such as how closely and how directly were children monitored, and how stuttering and recovery were specified and actually determined.

A critical parameter is the starting point of the longitudinal observations in relation to the time of stuttering onset. The longer the time gap, the more misleading the findings are likely to be because children who recover early, and there are many of them, are not accounted for. They are not included because (1) they do not stutter and investigators are not aware of them, and (2) if the investigators are informed about these already recovered children (e.g., by parents who already have a child who stutters in the study), there is no way of going back in time to capture the necessary direct data. Hence the reported percentage of natural recovery is in danger of being much is smaller than it is in reality. Illustrating this point is a study conducted in Germany that found 47% natural recovery (Fritzell, 1976). It is, however, hopelessly faulty because children were first observed between ages 7 and 9. As we know now, most recovery occurs before this age.

A very well-known longitudinal investigation conducted in England followed approximately a thousand children from birth to age 16 (Andrews & Harris, 1964). During this 16-year period, 43 children were identified to exhibit stuttering. Various professionals who visited the children's homes evaluated their speech periodically. Often, however, the examiners had to rely on parents' reports. Furthermore, the children's speech was never recorded for objective evaluation. Regardless, 79% of the children who stuttered recovered without treatment.

In this class of investigations we list additional five studies. High levels of natural recovery found in England were echoed in two small American longitudinal studies: 80% after 5-year follow-ups (Panelli, McFarlane, & Shipley, 1978) and 68% after only 2-year follow-ups (Ryan, 2001a). In these studies the children did not receive therapy. Three European studies were published more recently. In The Netherlands, investigators found 70% natural recovery among 23 children who stuttered and whose families were at high risk for stuttering because at least one parent stuttered (Kloth et al., 1995). The parents of children who exhibit persistent stuttering would also have a higher chance to persist in stuttering (Ambrose, Cox, & Yairi, 1997). Therefore the reported 70% recovery is probably a biased underestimate among the greater population of children who stutter. In Germany, 65 children were tracked for several years, beginning at age 5. After 3 years, 71% of the group had already recovered (Rommel, Hage, Kalehne, & Johannsen, 1999). It is quite likely that also in this study the 71% recovery is an underestimate, this time due to the late starting point of the follow-ups (age 5), a point highlighted earlier. Finally, in

Denmark, a longitudinal study of more than 50 preschool children yielded 71.6% recovery after 2 years. By the 5-year follow-up, recovery had climbed to 85%.

The Illinois Studies

Perhaps the largest and most intensive long-term longitudinal investigation of the development of childhood stuttering was conducted by Yairi and his colleagues at the University of Illinois. It obtained firsthand objective data in the form of audio- and video-recorded speech samples, as well as language, phonology, and many other data collected directly from the children and their parents. Another important advantage was that children were identified and initially recorded close to the stuttering onset. Therefore, it was possible to document cases of early natural recovery. The first study tracked 27 preschool children from approximately 6 months after onset, at 6-month intervals over 2 years. At that time, 67% exhibited complete recovery. Three years later, recovery reached to the 89% level (Yairi & Ambrose, 1992a). A second study included only 16 children but they were very young, 2 to 3 years of age, all exhibited moderate to severe stuttering, and they were first recorded within 12 weeks of stuttering onset (mean = 8 weeks), a very early starting point. For this group, the investigators focused only on the first 6 months following the initial testing. Within this very brief period, three children (19%) exhibited recovery according to the most stringent criteria. If just one less of the multiple criteria were considered, 38% had exhibited recovery. Of course, maintaining these achievements for a longer time was required to ascertain stable recovery (Yairi, Ambrose, & Niermann, 1993). The importance of this study lies in the demonstration of the strong trend for a quick, sharp decline in stuttering even within a few months past onset.

The largest Illinois study included 89 preschool children who stuttered who were 23 to 65 months old (mean = 38 months) at the first visit, all seen close to onset (Yairi & Ambrose, 1999a, 2005). As with the earlier studies, speech samples and other measures of stuttering were secured at 6-month intervals for the first 2 years. Beyond this period, data were secured at a yearly interval for years 3 and 4, and at the final visit several years later. Recovery from stuttering was determined using multiple criteria, including frequency of stuttering-like disfluencies in the recorded speech samples, clinician and parents' ratings of stuttering, and agreement among all. To avoid false classification of recovery, a failure to meet even a single criterion or if there was any doubt whatsoever was sufficient for classifying a child as persistent. The overall natural recovery rate at the end of the study was 79%, identical to the English findings (Andrews & Harris, 1964) and just under the Danish data (Månsson, 2000). It is of interest to note that Illinois investigators found that although reduction in stuttering may begin within a few months or even weeks after onset, the time period needed to reach complete natural recovery varies. Only 9% of the children fully recovered during the first year, an additional 22% during the second year, and so on. At the 4-year point, natural recovery occurred for 74% of the sample. It reached 79% within a year later. None of the recovered children received any formal speech therapy. Those children who persisted in stuttering did receive therapy. Yairi and Ambrose (2005) concluded that "given a child who has just begun stuttering, we can thus say that he/she has about a 65–80% chance of natural recovery by three to five years after onset, or a 20%

Table 3.5: Percentage of Natural Recovery from Stuttering in Longitudinal Studies

	N	Period of Sampling	Ages (Years)	Natural Recovery (%)
Johnson, 1955b	46	30 months	Preschoolers	72
Johnson et al., 1959	118	30 months	2–7	36
Ryan, 2001a	22	2 years	Preschool	68
Andrews & Harris, 1964	43	16 years	From birth	79
Yairi & Ambrose, 1992a	27	2 years	Preschool	89%
Yairi, Ambrose, & Niermann, 1993	16	First 6 months	2–3 years (from a few weeks after onset)	19% (3 measures) 38% (2 measures)
Yairi & Ambrose, 1999a	89	4–10 years	23–65 months	79%
Panelli, McFarlane, & Shipley, 1978;	15	Not specified. Possibly 2-12 years	Preschool	80%
Kloth et al., 1995	23	Up to 6 years	From close to onset	70%

chance of persistence" (p. 168). They cautioned, however, that the 70% to 80% recovery rate applies to children seen early in the course of their stuttering. Finally, on this note, natural recovery continues to occur throughout the years into adulthood although at much smaller percentages (Sheehan & Martyn, 1966; Wingate, 1964b, 1976). It appears that few people of senior ages stutter habitually. Table 3.5 summarizes the longitudinal studies cited.

A testimony for natural recovery is presented here from the same mother who described the onset of stuttering in her daughter, Denise (not a participant in our study). Her initial letter was cited earlier in the chapter. This follow-up account was written 2 years after onset.

I would like to let you know that Denise is doing fine now. Better than fine, actually. She is in kindergarten and is reading at a 3rd–4th grade level. She **never** stutters, and that nightmare has now, thankfully, become a thing of the past. When I reread the letter that I sent to you 2 years ago, it brought tears to my eyes. I was absolutely devastated at that time. It was heart wrenching. Denise was talking at an early age, and she has always been highly intelligent. To see her reduced to silence and tears overnight was more than I thought I could bear. Thank you so very much for your help and compassion. You will never know the comfort that you brought to me and my family during that time. I wrote to you out of sheer desperation. I honestly did not expect a response. (You did not know me or Denise, and you are probably very busy, etc.). Your letter back to me was my lifeline. I want to personally thank you again for your help.

I am so thankful that there are those of you in the field who are genuinely making inroads into this disability.

I do feel stuttering is a genuine disability. My baby was forced to stop communicating with us. I genuinely feel that stuttering is traumatic. The suddenness and the severity of it was staggering. Denise was 100% fine, and then WHAM! She was not experiencing any new routines (no new school, new friends, different home environment, etc.). Looking back, I can honestly say that I can see nothing that precipitated it in any way. I do not know what brought her out of it. We did our best to follow your suggestions. It was like her speech and her brain were at an impasse or something, and the signals were getting hopelessly stuck and circulated again and again along the same pathway. I am not sure what caused this, but I would be interested to hear your thoughts. I am still in awe of how severe it was. It was not an occasional word, but rather, OCCASIONALLY she would be able to speak a word WITHOUT stuttering. I am a registered cardiac nurse, and it reminds me of a certain cardiac condition where the impulse conduction for the heart gets "trapped" in a sense, and is constantly in a re-entry or circular loop. I don't know if that makes sense or not; in my mind it does (ha ha). But, that is what it reminded me of. She would literally look at me with these crazy wide eyes, like she were unable to stop speaking a particular word at times (not just stop the stuttering, but like she actually wanted to just stop speaking that particular word and her mouth just wouldn't stop). It frightened her. Usually, she would just stop talking, but there were times when I swear she couldn't stop speaking a particular word. Of course, she was so young, it would have been impossible for me to ask her this question and have her understand what I was asking (I also was afraid to draw attention to it). However, as a mother, I am confident that this was the case.

Denise is, in fact, a great communicator now. Her reading level is astounding, even to us. She finishes her grandfather's word find puzzle books, and we never see any signs of stuttering. In answer to your question, Denise did NOT receive speech therapy. We followed your recommendations and made sure that everyone else from her grandparents to her preschool teachers knew exactly what your recommendations were as well, so that we were all aboard the same train. She seemed to overcome the severe stuttering within a few months. She did, however, still stutter at times, especially when tired or not feeling well. Then, thankfully, one day it disappeared and never returned. It was such a bizarre thing.

I did not realize that your son also had an affliction of stuttering. I now know that you completely understand, not just from a clinical perspective, but from the perspective of a parent. I am so glad that your son recovered. As I mentioned before, she is doing well now. She excels in reading, spelling, and even math. At our first kindergarten conference a few weeks ago, her teacher told us that she was "very advanced." She also commented to us that Denise was doing so well, that she was, "far above all of her peers," and that "none of her peers are even close to being her intellectual equal." I don't say this to brag (although I am very proud of her), but rather to let you know, in case this somehow plays a factor.

Denise was also a very abstract thinker, which my father and others noticed at a very young age. For example, one day when she was maybe 15 or 16 months old, my husband and she were at the park. It was fall, and the sky was filled with birds

(continued)

flying south for the winter. My husband and her looked up at the sky, and Denise said, "Look Daddy . . . a 'V.'" She did not say, "Look Daddy! Birdies!" She said strange stuff like that all of the time. One day they were walking around the railroad ties that encircle the playground. She was 18 months old. She kept saying, "See Daddy! Octagon!" My husband was looking all around the playground trying to see where this supposed octagon was. After a short while, she became frustrated with him, because he kept saying, "Where baby? Where is the Octagon?" Finally, she pointed to the railroad ties and said, "See Daddy! Octagon!" As it turns out, the railroad ties that encircle the entire playground just happen to be in the shape of an octagon. However, the space is so large, that unless you could look down ON them from the sky, you'd never know it. But, she knew it just by walking on them while holding her Daddy's hand. These examples may mean nothing in relation to stuttering. If not, please forgive me for the rambling. However, in the off chance that they could, I thought that I would mention them.

Thank you again for all of your compassion, and your dedication to the field. My hope is that, one day, stuttering will be able to be treated so efficiently that no child has to suffer with it. I wish you the best of luck in your pursuits, and those of your students and colleagues. If, in your research, you find a link, please let me know, as I have heard that stuttering can be familial in nature. (Just in case stuttering rears its ugly head in our family again with another child, niece or nephew.)

Warm Regards.

An example, this one of stuttering development over a course shorter than one year, reflecting substantial improvement but not complete recovery, is seen in parental correspondence with us from far away. We present here 2 letters from a father—the first was received shortly after onset, the second about 10 months later.

Letter 1: Roy is now 3 years and 4 months old. Suddenly he began stuttering earlier in this month (November). It started over the course of a couple days, and within that time period he very quickly developed severe problems. He would get hung up on a word, repeating it several times. At first, he would repeat a word a few times. Then, it grew to several times, and eventually became a matter of repeating the word 10–15 times before he would either get through it or give up completely. This was a daily occurrence, over and over many times throughout the day. At the time he stuttered more than he spoke without stuttering. He clearly struggled with it, closing his eyes, tensing his body. As it became worse, he would just stop himself and say "Oh, I just can't talk anymore." For a 3-year-old, we thought that was a remarkable statement, that he was so very aware and conscious of the onset of his stutter, and aware that it didn't always used to be that way. I would rate his stutter at that time as moderate, based on my limited experience with this. Aside from my own mild stuttering issues as an adolescent, I know a good friend of my sister's who has a very severe stutter which completely prevents him from carrying on any sort of fluid conversation without constant interruptions. To me, that seems very severe, but there may be worse?

Stuttering continued to worsen from November through to the present (January). Within our nuclear family, we have grown accustomed to it and are very conscious not to add to any stress he might have been experiencing, in particular with regard to his own awareness of the stuttering. For example, we have not called attention to the stuttering, we let him work through it and wait patiently for him to complete his sentences without interruption. We spoke privately with our 2 daughters, ages 9 and 7, to remind them not to make fun of Roy and to be patient while he speaks without interrupting him. They are very concerned about him, too, knowing that his stuttering was unusual and came on suddenly.

Letter 2: Little Roy turned 4 years old approximately 2 months ago. Since writing to you, his stuttering has changed fairly dramatically. He still gets hung up on words, but doesn't repeat them 10–20 times and no longer completely shuts down in frustration (which was so sad to see him tearfully exclaiming things like "Oh, I give up, I just can't talk anymore," etc.). I would say that currently he has a mild stutter repeating a sentence 2–3 times until he gets it out. This happens often in conversation with him a couple dozen times daily. He doesn't seem to get hung up on individual words, rather he seems to get hung up on a concept or the subject matter in general to which he can often substitute words or phrases thus changing his tactic or approach to delivering his sentence. He has long pauses mid-sentence, as if to collect his thoughts, during which it seems he changes direction and alters what he was saying. He obviously has developed many compensatory mechanisms for it. Not being an expert in any way, I'm sure that I don't pick up on all the ways he has dealt with it, but here are a few examples: When he starts to get hung up, he substitutes another word, or immediately changes direction and attacks the concept from another angle. He often will still start a sentence over when he senses that he has made a speech mistake, and when that happens it is common for him to repeat the beginning of a sentence 2–4 times before he gets the concept out, if he doesn't take a new approach completely. He has also "adopted" or mimics a vocal throat tic from his older sister (8 years), which is sometimes interjected as a mild pause in his speech, which seems to be commensurate with moments when he is struggling to get through a word. He repeats phrases often, almost as if practicing them. Also, he hums and sings much of the day. I would say, however, that today most people, adults and kids alike, do not notice a significant deviation from whatever "normal" speech is when they hear Roy talk, but that if pointed out, they could see clearly that he is making conscious adjustments to his speech. We did not seek other professional help, other than my note to you, but it may have been very helpful if we had.

When his stuttering was at its worst, he was 3 years, 4 months old, and I talked to him about it and explained what it was. He seemed reassured. He seemed glad that somebody was talking to him about it. I was concerned that talking about it with him might make things worse if he was to feel ashamed, or, I wondered if I could increase the high level of anxiety it was already clearly causing him. He's a smart little kid, and

(continued)

I explained that I stuttered as an adolescent but it seemed to have gone away on its own. I also said that a lot of kids go through this when they're young and their brains are growing and learning so much. I said it would go away, knowing that it might not. He then went through a couple of months where it became clear he was really trying to work through it, perhaps merely coincidentally with our discussion of the issue, and sure enough, much of it went away or has since been masked by his compensatory responses.

At age 4, he still has a hard time forming certain sounds with his mouth, but I don't think that's particularly unusual for his age group and certainly not unusual compared to the speech progression of his 2 older sisters. For example, he has a hard time saying the "kr", "L", "th" sounds as in "Christmas" (kisst-mus), "lightning" (white-ning), and "then" (when) respectively. However, we have certainly noticed that Roy has a very good vocabulary for his age, and a remarkable ability to express even complex thoughts very clearly. He is, considering all things, a gifted little speaker. We also try to reduce his anxiety by not calling attention to his stuttering and let him work through it on his own without interrupting him, and I have never called attention to any of his compensatory strategies. He is not yet in school, but like our 2 other children, we will be looking to see if the classroom environment causes things to re-present, start up again, or get worse. We know that the classroom has typically been a very stressful place for the girls (now ages 8 and 10) and many of their tics and behaviors only appear in that environment. Interestingly, and sadly, the teacher(s) tend to handle them as disciplinary issues regardless of consultations in tic disorders . . .

Implications of Developmental Findings

Current information concerning the development of stuttering, natural recovery, and persistency has significant implications for theory, research, and clinical intervention. In the theoretical domain, it suggests the possibility that differences in etiological factors create at least two stuttering subtypes: those who persist and those who recover naturally. As we discuss in Chapter 7, recent research has provided supportive evidence of differences in the genetic makeup of these two subtypes. In the research domain, it would seem advisable that studies with young children be designed so as to distinguish between potentially recovering children and those destined to persist. For example, these subgroups should be differentiated in studies of the early language skills of children who stutter, or, in studying various characteristics of their parents. Taking natural recovery into consideration is especially important in studies that focus on the evaluation of therapies. Was a positive therapeutic outcome due to the treatment or, at least partially, to the strong likelihood for recovery? One way to answer this question would be to follow a nontreated group. Also, parent counseling and decisions concerning priority and timing for initiating treatment should be significantly influenced by the findings on natural recovery. For example, knowing that many children who begin stuttering recover on their own, should all of their parents be advised to seek help? Should clinicians be more selective when recommending who should receive therapy immediately and who may wait a while before rushing into unnecessary treatment? In other words, is it possible to predict the future development of early stuttering and use such information for clinical decisions and management?

Predictive Factors

Several attempts have been made to offer prediction criteria for future recovery or persistency. Pioneers in this area were Stromsta (1965), relying primarily on speech acoustic characteristics; Glyndon Riley, in his 1981 Stuttering Prediction Instrument for Young Children; and Cooper and Cooper (1985) in their list of prediction indicators covering a wide range of variables. These and other past formal and informal means of predicting persistency and recovery are covered in Chapter 13.

The most recent effort in this direction has been made by investigators at the Illinois Stuttering Research Program based on their longitudinal studies described earlier and summarized in Yairi and Ambrose (2005). They have shown that several biological factors provide various degrees of predictability. One of these is age. Children who persisted in stuttering tended to have somewhat later onsets than those who recovered, a trend supported by Buck, Lees, and Cook (2002). Gender is a stronger predictor. The 2:1 male-to-female ratio at the time of stuttering onset grew to 3.75:1 among children who a few years later persisted in stuttering. By comparison, the ratio among children who recovered was considerably smaller: 2.33:1. This means the rate of natural recovery for females is higher than for males. Furthermore, girls also recovered sooner than boys. On average, boys stuttered for 29.5 months prior to recovery as compared to only 24 months for girls. Perhaps the strongest predictor reported by the Illinois studies was the specific type of the child's family history of stuttering. Children who had a familial history of recovered stuttering had a 65% chance of following this pattern themselves. By contrast, children who had a familial history of persistent stuttering also had about a 65% chance of following their familial pattern. The investigators concluded that recovery and persistency are influenced by genetics (Ambrose, Cox, & Yairi, 1997). Hints of chromosomal differences between persistent and recovered stuttering also reinforce this conclusion (Suresh et al., 2006).

Another group of predictors was derived from speech factors. First, a strong predictor is the difference in the change in stuttering-like disfluencies (SLD) between the children who recover naturally and those who persist. As you can see in Figure 3.2, at the earliest stage of the disorder, there is no distinction in the amount of SLD exhibited by children in the two groups. By 7 to 12 months following onset, however, there are signs of divergence. From this point on, differences are clear and significant. Generally, the level of SLD decreases in those who recover, eventually reaching normalcy. For children whose stuttering persists, the mean SLD remains constant for

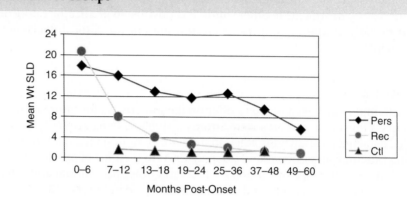

Figure 3.2: **Stuttering Frequency: Persistent, Recovered, and Control Groups**

Ctl = control; Per = persistent; Rec = recovered; SLD = stuttering-like disfluency.

a while but later also declines somewhat, although some of them increase their level of SLD. Hence the overall direction of SLD somewhere between 7 to 12 months post onset is important for predicting the future course of stuttering.

Also of interest are the findings that the levels of other disfluencies (more typical to normal fluency) were not different among persistent, recovered, and normally fluent children during the first 2 years after onset. This class is not an important component in the clinical evaluation, development, and prediction of stuttering, at least in young children. What counts are the up-and-down dynamics of SLD. Several additional speech disfluency features, such as type, length, and clustering, as well as secondary characteristics, are other potential predictors but appear to be weaker in power. The process of recovery seems to be associated not only with declining frequency of SLD but also with declining SLD length, fewer secondary characteristics (Throneburg & Yairi, 2001), and shorter disfluency clusters (Sawyer & Yairi, in press).

In regard to linguistic factors, it appears that, on average, near the onset of stuttering, these children's language skills are at or above age norms. The Illinois studies revealed the interesting finding that within 3 years post onset, the language performance of children who recovered naturally did not remain above average, whereas the language of children who persisted in stuttering tended to stay above average (Watkins, 2005; Watkins et al., 2000). At present, the predictive power of a child's language skills is not clear. Advanced language skills however, especially if they continue to develop at a fast rate, may constitute a risk factor for persistency. The predictive power of phonological skills is also limited. During the very early phase of stuttering, phonological skills distinguish between those who will eventually recover and persist, but by the second year of stuttering the difference between groups is greatly diminished and no longer statistically significant (Paden, 2005; Paden, Ambrose, & Yairi, 2002).

Summary

Onset

Improved scientific methods employed during the past 25 years have brought new light to the onset of stuttering. It appears that more than 60% of the children who stutter begin doing so prior to age 3, a figure that climbs to 85% by 4 years of age. The findings reinforce the notion that, by and large, stuttering is a disorder that begins in early childhood. These are earlier ages within a narrower range than has been previously assumed. The overlap of many stuttering onsets with the period of fast development of the speech mechanism, rapid acquisition of complex articulatory movement, and expansion of syntactic and other language faculties raises the specter of stuttering-articulation-phonology-language links. Onset of stuttering after age 4 may involve a different interaction of etiological factors.

Recent data on the symptomatology of very early stuttering dispel traditional views of the event of onset. Clinicians should be prepared for heterogeneity in what is observed and how it begins. They should be ready to encounter children whose onset was quite sudden. This is not parental imagination. They should also expect to witness early stuttering that is rather advanced in the wealth of its characteristics and, in some cases, is quite severe. Whereas repetitions of initial syllables and short words are almost universal, stuttering may begin with or without sound prolongations, blocks, accessory physical tensions, and with or without awareness and emotional reactions. Such early characteristics negate the diagnosogenic theory (discussed in Chapter 6) that suggests stuttering begins as normal disfluencies that turn into stuttering due to the reactions of overanxious parents. Clinicians should also keep in mind that because the onset of stuttering marks a definite change in the child's normally fluent speech, parents may be quite apprehensive about this development.

Development

As we have seen, great variability is also the hallmark of the development of stuttering after it has begun. Whereas some children present more severe and complex overt stuttering with the passage of time, accompanied with various emerging, often strong, emotional components, some children continue stuttering at a low level. Most importantly, the current solid evidence contradicts the traditional depiction of the disorder as always increasing in complexity and severity. The data clearly show that the most typical developmental trend of early stuttering is *downward*, decreasing in severity. Furthermore, in the majority of children who ever stutter, the process of amelioration leads to complete recovery without clinical intervention. Thus early childhood is not only the period when most stuttering begins; it is also the time when the disorder stops due to natural remission. The emerging information regarding predictive factors for recovery and persistency in stuttering is important to the understanding of stuttering in general and has major practical implications for research purposes, parent counseling, and treatment decisions.

STUDY QUESTIONS AND DISCUSSION TOPICS

1. What is the theoretical significance and what are practical implications of information concerning the onset of stuttering?

2. What major changes in information (e.g., in terms of age, gender, suddenness, severity, concomitant behaviors) about the onset of stuttering have resulted from recent pertinent studies?

3. What is meant by sequential developmental models of stuttering? What is the major premise of the various developmental schemes that have been offered? Which more recent research findings make that premise questionable?

4. What are the main findings concerning natural recovery in terms of timing, percentage, and other factors (e.g., age, gender, etc.)?

5. What are the implications of information concerning natural recovery for clinical decisions? For the identification of sample populations in research?

SUGGESTED READINGS

Ambrose, N. G., & Yairi, E. (1999). Normative disfluency data for early childhood stuttering. *Journal of Speech, Language, and Hearing Research, 42,* 895–909.

Ambrose, N. G., & Yairi, E. (2002). The Tudor Study: Data and ethics. *American Journal of Speech-Language Pathology, 11*(2), 190–203.

Månsson, H. (2000). Childhood stuttering: Incidence and development. *Journal of Fluency Disorders, 25,* 47–57.

Yairi, E., & Ambrose, N. (2005). *Early childhood stuttering* (Chapters 3, 4, and 5). Austin, TX: Pro Ed.

Chapter 4: Where Does It End? Advanced Characteristics, Rules, and Phenomena

LEARNER OBJECTIVES

Readers will be able to:

- Identify speech and physical behaviors associated with advanced stuttering.
- Understand research regarding the characteristics of people who stutter.
- Recognize the dynamics of stuttered speech as reflected in various phenomena and rules of stuttering.
- Develop appreciation of the emotional and cognitive aspects of advanced stuttering.

Advanced Stuttering

In Chapter 3, the characteristics of early childhood stuttering were described with just a few references to late occurring changes as depicted in Bloodstein's (1960b) developmental system. Although we commented that a good number of features seen in older individuals can also be observed in some young children, there are still marked disorder differences between children and adults who stutter. These include the proportions of certain disfluency types, the loci of stuttering, affective reactions, and others. Age and experience impact the stuttering disorder. For example, whereas 3-year-old children who stutter rarely experience negative reactions from others their age, many adults who stutter do experience such reactions. Also children's limited cognitive abilities and brief history of the disorder may limit their anticipation of stuttering events as compared with adults. As stuttering lingers on and becomes chronic, additional and more consistent features appear and/or old ones crystallize, to present a more complicated disorder. Furthermore, strong interactions among multiple systems can become firmly rooted beneath the surface of stuttering. Although Bleumel (1932) opined that incipient stuttering is a "pure" speech disturbance, we have alluded to stuttering as a complex disorder with multiple dimensions, especially when it persists over a longer period of time. This chapter presents the broad range of symptoms and dynamics that are encountered in advanced stuttering. Acknowledging its essence, however, stuttering is typically classified as a speech disorder (ASHA, 2008b). Therefore, in accounting for its advanced characteristics, we begin with the obvious attributes of advanced stuttering: speech features. These are rich in quantity and quality, and they include speech disfluency as well as other disruptions to suprasegmental properties.

Speech Disfluency

The interruption in the flow of speech, often referred to as speech disfluency, is the cardinal feature of stuttering. There is no stuttering without it. All the other characteristics frequently associated with the stuttering disorder, combined, would not be sufficient to amount to something that would merit the label "stuttering." As we explained in Chapter 1, however, the term *disfluency* and *stuttering* should not be equated. Disfluency has a wider meaning in that it covers all speech interruptions. Some of these are regarded as typically normal, whereas others are regarded as typically abnormal, mostly stuttering. The distinction is complicated in that not all disfluent events in the speech of people who stutter are necessarily stuttering; some are normal. Types of disfluencies usually regarded as stuttering, however, are sometimes present in the speech of normally fluent speakers.

The term *nonfluency*, later referred to as *disfluency*, was first used by Wendell Johnson in the mid-20th century. Because he was convinced that stuttering moments evolved from normal disfluencies, he used the term *nonfluencies* in his published works, for example, throughout the book *The Onset of Stuttering* (Johnson et al., 1959). Prior to that time, stutter events had been mainly called *spasms* (Johnson & Leutenegger, 1955; Van Riper, 1992). Johnson later adopted the term *disfluency* after Van Riper argued with him that it did not make sense to identify or count "non-somethings" (Van Riper, 1992, p. 83). In the 1960s, the term *disfluency* began to appear in publications by Johnson and his colleagues. For example, it is found in the title of the Iowa Speech Disfluency Test (Sander, 1961).

An important issue related to use of the term *disfluency* arises because research has shown that judgments of "stuttering" or "normal" are influenced by a host of factors. The label "stuttering moments" implies a value judgment by the listener. Various factors affect a listener's identification of a speech interruption as either normal or stuttering. Some are rooted in the objective properties of the speech segment in question, such as the specific type of disfluency. Sound prolongation, for example, is more apt to be perceived as stuttering than interjection (Young, 1961). Another property is the extent or duration of the segment. If the syllable *pa* in the word *patient* is repeated five times, it is much more likely to be judged as stuttering than if it is repeated only once or twice.

Other factors are rooted in more subjective influences, such as the listeners' background, life experience, and their cognitive set at a particular time. The same disfluent speech event may be judged differently by another listener or even by the same listener at different times or circumstances. In a well-known study, listeners were asked to mark down all stuttered interruptions in a speech sample. Other listeners were asked to mark down all normal speech interruptions. Significantly, the investigators found that a clear majority of events were counted either as normal or stuttered, depending on the instructions of what to listen for. When asked to listen for stuttering, more events were marked as such. When asked to listen for normal disfluency, more events were marked as such (Williams & Kent, 1958). Similarly, it is not surprising that a person who has family members who stutter may be more sensitive and inclined to judge speech interruptions as stuttering (Sander, 1968). Thus clinicians, older clients, and family members alike need to be aware that perceptions can be swayed by what the listener expects to hear. Unfortunately, the negative value judgment of "I hear stuttering" may have particularly grave consequences. As we alluded to in Chapter 3, according to one theory, if the normal-abnormal distinction of speech interruptions is blurred, and if a listener, say a particularly concerned parent who perceives a little child's speech interruptions as abnormal and erroneously labels them as "stuttering," the distressed reactions could push it over the edge and give rise to the impression of a stuttering disorder (Johnson et al., 1959).

In contrast to value-laden judgments, identification of speech disruptions according to descriptive disfluency types does not involve labeling them as "stuttering," "normal," "desirable," or "undesirable." Typical disfluency classes simply describe the speech behaviors (e.g., *syllable repetition* or *sound prolongation*). The listener is focused on objective dimensions. It then becomes possible to address questions about which disfluent speech classes are more typical in the speech of people who stutter and which are more typical of normally fluent speakers. The answer is therefore a matter of statistical probability, not subjective judgment (Bloodstein, 1970; Yairi & Ambrose, 2005).

Types of Disfluency

Clinicians and researchers have not yet agreed on a particular taxonomy of disfluency classification. This fact was illustrated when Kully and Boberg (1988) sent the same set of 10 speech samples (8 from stutterers, 2 from nonstutterers) to clinicians at various locations in the United States, Canada, Australia, and Great Britain. Across the nine respondents who returned their analyses, there were pronounced discrepancies in the stuttering, disfluency, and syllable counts. Although we challenge their conclusions that ignore these authors' own data,[1] the study highlights potential problems regarding communication among professionals because of the wide variety of procedural systems that different clinics use for such measures.

Disfluency classification systems began to appear in the literature in the late 1930s when several students of Wendell Johnson (e.g., Branscom, 1942; Davis, 1939) investigated speech interruptions in preschool-age children. Due to the technical limitations of audio recording in that period, their archaic repertoire included only

---

[1] Kully and Boberg (1988) emphasized the disagreement among clinics in identifying stuttering and disfluencies. The data in their Table 2 reveal that the average agreement between the two clinics that counted "percent disfluency" was 81.7%, a respectable level that was considerably better than agreement among clinics that counted "percent stuttering."

three types: syllable repetition, word repetition, and phrase repetition. Since then, a number of classification systems have been offered, but they mostly represent variations of the eight-type disfluency system employed by Johnson et al. (1959). For example, Campbell and Hill (1987) included 11 types. To cover speech interruptions found in advanced stuttering, as well as in normally fluent speakers, we opted to list and briefly describe the following disfluency types.

Types of Speech Disfluency

I. *Part-word repetitions.* Repetitions of sounds or syllables. No distinction is made between these two. For example, "a-ai," "f-five," "ba-baby," "mo-mo-mommy." Various speech sounds may be repeated including vowels and consonants of different types.

II. *Single-syllable whole-word repetitions.* For example, "but-but," "and-and." Here, and in all other repetitions of speech segments, it is important to distinguish disfluency from what is not. Some repetitions are intended for emphasis or for any reason (e.g., play in children). For example, a word repeated for emphasis, as in "very, very nice," is not counted as a disfluency.

III. *Multiple-syllable word repetitions.* Repetition of longer words, such as "Because–because." Similar exceptions for emphasis apply.

IV. *Phrase repetitions.* Repetition of any segment longer than one word, even a word plus a sound or syllable of the next word. "I was–I was going," and "Once up–once upon," are examples of this type of disfluency.

V. *Prolonged sounds.* These are audible elongations of vowels as in "a>>>>>ai like to go," or elongations of consonants, such as in "M>>>>>>y name is." Or "S>>>>ometimes." Prolongations may be voiced or voiceless.

VI. *Blocks and broken words.* The articulators (tongue, lips) or the vocal cords are held in fixed positions, either at the beginning of a word, such as in "C———cake," or in the middle of a word as in "The ta———able is set." Typically, the blocks are silent or accompanied with minimally audible sound. They are *within-word* phenomena.

VII. *Tense pause.* These are unusual breaks that occur *between* words, associated with tense sounds, such as escaping air (e.g., I like to———go home").

VIII. *Interjections.* Those are extraneous sounds such as "um, uh, er, and hmmm." Interjection, too, may be repeated such as in "um-um." Words and phrases such as "like," "well," or "you know" are not considered disfluencies.

IX. *Revisions and incomplete utterance.* A revision is when an utterance is modified but the general content remains the same (e.g., "I like–I want this ball"). An incomplete (abandoned) utterance occurs when there is an apparent change of thought in the middle of the utterance (e.g., "The baby is–let's do that").

The physiological correlates of disfluencies vary. Obviously, repetitions involve movement and positioning that are integral to the production of the specific sound except that they are unnecessarily repeated. Examples include approximation of the lips (Mo-Mo-Mommy), elevation of the back of the tongue (ka-ka-kite), movement of the whole tongue and jaw (I-I-I), tip of the tongue (Da-Da-Daddy), and others. Often, however, these movements involve observable and/or audible tension. When the repeated sounds are voiced, more tension in the larynx may be associated.

Some disfluencies may involve abnormal articulatory positioning. Those labeled as tense pauses, for example, are associated with *blockages* or *blocks* of the vocal tract to the point that no air can pass through and no sound, or only barely audible sound, is emitted. Such silent blocks may occur at one of several levels: larynx, tongue, or lips, or sometimes at multiple levels. In K——kite, the initial movement of the back of tongue against the hard palate is legitimate, but stays there in tight contact much too long. This is also referred to as *articulatory fixation*. When the vocal folds are tightly fixed, they are either in the abducted or adducted position—a *laryngeal fixation*. The specific disfluency examples given in the category of sound prolongations also involve *articulatory fixation*. The initial approximation of the articulators may be basically right, but they stay fixed in place for too long. In a prolongation, however, the fixation does not completely block the airflow, allowing for voiced prolongation such as M>>>>an or Z>>>>>ebra, or for a voiceless prolongation such S>>>>nake. Van Riper (1982) stated, "These blocking and closures are some of the most important phenomena in the multifaceted disorder of advanced stuttering. The stutterer senses such closure very vividly. For a moment he feels impotent, out of control" (p. 122).

Over the years, the various disfluency types have been combined, renamed, or removed altogether. In 1968, Williams, Silverman, and Kools combined sound prolongations, blocks, and broken words into a single category labeled *disrhythmic phonation*. Also *revision* and *incomplete phrase* were merged. In 1981, Yairi separated word repetition into two different types: *monosyllabic word repetition* and *multisyllabic word repetition*. Campbell and Hill (1987) divided part word repetition into *sound and syllable repetition* and added *hesitation*, and Ambrose and Yairi (1999) combined *multisyllabic word repetition with phrase repetition* into a single type and eliminated *tense pause*, which had low identification reliability.

Major Disfluency Classes

Significantly, scholars in the field have realized that disfluencies differ in the degree to which they are prevalent in the speech of people who stutter and normally fluent speakers, as well as in the extent to which they are perceived as stuttering or normal. Consequently, several attempts for grouping the various disfluency types to reflect such differences have been made. For example, Conture (1982, 2001) distinguished between *within-word disfluency* (including sound repetition, syllable repetition, and prolongation), which he explains are more likely to be "stuttering" and what he referred to as *between-word disfluency* (all other types), which are more likely to be "normal disfluency." Campbell and Hill (1987) distinguish between *more typical* and *less typical* disfluency. They describe their classification system as a continuum of disfluent speech behaviors. On one end of the continuum are the typical disfluencies of hesitations, interjections, revisions, and phrase repetitions; on the opposite end are the atypical disfluencies of sound repetitions, prolongations, blocks, and other signs of increased tension. In the middle are the "crossover" behaviors that could be either typical or atypical, depending on such features as numbers of repetitions per instance, or tension level. These disfluencies include part-word and one-syllable word repetitions. We find this classification problematic because the terminology employed uses normal (*typical*) as the reference within a framework of a continuum. It implies that stuttering is merely a change in degree of what normal speakers do, not something unique to the disorder. In our opinion, although there is some similarity in format (e.g., repetitions), the nature of the production of stuttering is different (Throneburg & Yairi, 2001).

The classification proposed by the Illinois Stuttering Research Program (Ambrose & Yairi, 1999; Yairi & Ambrose, 1992a) also consists of two disfluency classes, *stuttering-like disfluency* (SLD) and *other disfluency* (OD), and each includes three types. These are listed next.

The Illinois Disfluency Classification System

Stuttering-Like Disfluency	Other Disfluency
Part-Word Repetition	Interjection
Single-Syllable Word Repetition	Multisyllable Word and Phrase Repetition
Disrhythmic Phonation	Revision/Abandoned Utterance

By using the terms *Stuttering-like* and *Other*, the authors underscore that certain disfluencies are neither exclusively stuttering nor exclusively normal. The distinction between the two classes is accomplished by implying the greater probability of their occurrence in the respective group of speakers. Indeed, speech of children and adults who stutter contains a high proportion of disfluency types referred to as SLD. Also, it appears that the proportion of disrhythmic phonation (sound prolongations, blocks, and broken words) within the SLD is increased from early to advanced stuttering (Bloodstein, 1960b). Good-to-high interjudge reliability (between different judges) for SLD, reflecting agreement on the specific type and location of each disfluent event, has been reported in several studies as 0.86 and 0.89 or even higher (e.g., Ambrose & Yairi, 1999; Gregg & Yairi, 2007; Throneburg & Yairi, 2001; and others).

All in all, the three disfluency classifications (Conture, 2001; Gregory & Hill, 1999; Yairi & Ambrose, 2005) are in close agreement about the central characteristics of stuttering. They also recognize that a distinction between what is stuttering and what is normal can sometimes be difficult. Hence a small percentage of errors can be expected (Conture, 2001). Also, identification of a particular type of disfluency is sometimes challenging. For example, differentiating a repeated interjected "uh uh" from a repeated article "a, a," or making a judgment of how to categorize a sound that is prolonged as it is being pulsed in a repetitive manner. Is it a prolongation or repetition?

Dimensions of Disfluency

Frequency

The frequency of occurrence of each of the disfluency types and their total count has been its most commonly examined and reported dimension and is typically reported in terms of (1) the number of disfluencies per 100 syllables or 100 words, or (2) percent syllables or words that contain disfluency. (Methods for quantifying disfluency and stuttering are discussed in detail in Chapter 10.) Keep in mind, however, that even in advanced stages of the disorder, most of the speech of people who stutter is fluent. Bloodstein (1944) reported that, on average, only 10% of the words emitted by adults who stutter contain disfluencies regarded as stuttering.

It is equally important to realize that figures for the average, or mean, frequency of occurrence are likely to be misleading due to large fluctuations often observed within each individual who stutters from situation to situation and day to day. Perhaps the most remarkable variations are seen in several conditions that have been widely recognized to have an almost universal effect of temporarily reducing, or completely eliminating, the occurrence of stuttering. These include speaking alone, speaking to animals or babies, in the presence of high-level noise, singing, talking in rhythm (as paced by a metronome), talking in unison, and whispering, Some of these, especially noise, have been richly investigated and documented and are discussed further later in the chapter. Other factors, however, seem to have the influence of increasing stuttering, for example, time pressure (Guitar, Schaefer, Donahue-Kilburg, & Bond 1992; Stunden, 1965), the level of meaningful information in a message (Eisenson & Horowitz, 1945; Wingate, 1975), language complexity (Jayaram, 1984; Wells, 1979), and the size of audience (Young, 1985). Many other conditions are highly individualized. Some people increase the frequency of stuttering when speaking to specific persons, opposite sex, people in authority, or specific physical environments, and so on. One of us had experienced more stuttering when lecturing in a particular classroom. Bloodstein and Bernstein Ratner (2008) concluded that "What we know about the way stuttering varies in frequency can be generalized by saying that it is affected by communicative pressures" (p. 262). In addition to frequency of occurrence, speech disfluencies can vary in their length (e.g., duration) and spatial distribution (e.g., clusters).

Duration

One measure of length is *duration*, the time elapsed from the beginning to the end of a disfluent event. This measure can be applied to all disfluency types (e.g., sound prolongation or syllable repetition, or across both of them combined). Clinicians experienced in working with people who stutter, especially schoolchildren and adults, are likely to have observed at least a few disfluencies lasting 30 s or more. These certainly impact listeners. Such long disfluencies, however, are not too common.

Several studies found that most disfluent events in the speech of adults who stutter are quite short with a mean length for individual participants ranging from 0.5 to 3.7 s, with a group median of 0.9 s (Bloodstein, 1995). In one study, only 25% of the 30 participants exhibited mean durations for stutter events longer than 1.4 s (Bloodstein, 1944). This is not much longer than the mean duration of all disfluency types for preschool children, about 1.1 s, reported by Yairi and Ambrose (2005). Not much change seems to have occurred over time in this respect. Beyond the mean, there is interest in looking at the extreme ends of the range. Johnson and Colley (1945) reported that the mean of the 10 shortest blocks was 0.41 s, whereas the mean of the 10 longest was 4.1 s. The narrowness of this range is surprising because so much speech usually occurs in 4 s, there is an impression that much more time must have passed.

Interestingly, listeners' perception of the length of disfluencies complements the speech production measures. Studies have found that sound prolongations lasting 1 s or longer are most apt to be perceived as stuttering (Lingwall & Bergstrand, 1979; Zebrowski & Conture, 1989). Some prolongations are judged as stuttering after only a half second (Kawai, Healey, & Carrell, 2007; Susca & Healey, 2001). Again this should not be surprising because normally a single syllable in connected speech is uttered in less than a fifth of a second.

Examination of the age effect on the duration properties of sound prolongations show only modest changes as stuttering advances. Mean prolongation durations near stuttering onset were approximately 632 ms (standard deviation [SD], 211 ms), whereas 36 months later, nearing school age and stuttering persistence, the mean was elevated to 824 ms (SD, 350 ms). Although both mean values were less than 1 s, their relative values indicate that as stuttering continues there is a higher chance of longer durations (Throneburg & Yairi, 2001). Further maturing in age, the typical mean length of prolongations in school-age children and adults is about 1 s for either age group. The only difference is in the range. Zebrowski (1994) reported that the high-end mean value was 1.063 s for elementary school children. This is much lower than the high-end mean of 3 or 4 s for adults (see Bloodstein, 1995).

Although repetitive disfluencies could also be measured for their duration in time, usually their evaluation is handled differently. Length of these disfluencies is typically determined by counting the number of iterations per disfluent event. For these disfluencies, such as part-word or whole-word repetitions, length may be measured by the number of extra iterations of the repeated sound, syllable, or word. This measure is referred to as *repetition units* (Ambrose & Yairi, 1995). For example, "a-and" has one extra production of the vowel segment, which is counted as one repetition unit. If a speaker utters two extra iterations (e.g., "a-a-and"), it is counted as two repetition units. Again, from the listener's perspective, the number of repetition units also has an impact on the perception of stuttering as well as its severity (Sander, 1963). Obviously, a person saying "but-but-but-but-but-but-but-but-but" is bound to attract more attention and have his stuttering regarded as more severe than a person who says only "but-but-but." Yairi and Lewis (1984) and Ambrose and Yairi (1995) found that the number of repetition units was the measure that best differentiated stuttering from normally fluent children.

Unfortunately, many studies of disfluency in people who stutter have focused only on the frequency of disfluent events, neglecting information about length. For

The length of repetition type disfluencies is measured by the number of extra iterations of a speech segment. The concept underlying the measurement of repeated units is not what people expect, however. The repeated units are not the segments said after its first utterance. Instead, the extra repetition units are the ones uttered *before* the sound or syllable is finally blended with the intended word. Hence the sound or syllable eventually spoken as the fluent word is not counted (e.g., "but" in "b-b-b-but"), whereas the extra sounds or syllables uttered before the fluent word are the repetition units that are being counted (e.g., "b-b-b-" in "b-b-b-but"). This concept helps prevent an error in counting. Examination of the extra sounds or syllables at the start makes it easier to find the three units of length.

example, several investigations by Onslow and associates (e.g., Onslow, Andrews, & Lincoln, 1994) reported the percentage of syllables stuttered but not the length or number of repetition units for those syllables. If only the number of disfluent instances is reported, then the sentence "I-I am go-going ho-ho-me now" and the sentence "I-I-I-I-I am go-go-go-go-going ho-ho-ho-ho-home now" yield the same count: three instances of repetition. But were these the same stuttering severity? Obviously not. Hence important information is lost not only in research studies but also in most clinical evaluation and progress reports.

Although our clinical experience has included samples of disfluencies containing more than 20 repetition units for a word or a syllable, these are the exceptions. Unfortunately, very little data on repetition units have been published for school-age children or adults who stutter. One article could be found with such data for school-age children (Zebrowski, 1994), but none was found for adults. Data for normally fluent preschool children have indicated that between 80% and 87% of their repetitions had only one repetition unit (a-and), with a mean of about 1.16 (Ambrose & Yairi, 1995; Branscom, Hughes, & Oxtoby, 1955). The mean for the stuttering children was between 1.53 and 1.70 (Ambrose & Yairi, 1995; Yairi & Lewis, 1984).

Normally fluent people typically repeat a segment only once. In an important contrast, people who stutter not only produce more frequent instances of such repetitions, the number of units per repetition is also greater. Similarly, as stuttering progresses, the average number of units per repetition may increase. Children in elementary school who stutter exhibited sound/syllable repetitions with an average of 2.45 units per instance (Zebrowski, 1994). By contrast, preschool children who stutter evidenced a lower average of 1.72 units per instance (Yairi & Lewis, 1984).

Clusters

Another feature of stuttered speech, discussed in Chapter 3, is the tendency of disfluent events to occur in clusters of two or more on the same word or adjacent words. As mentioned, young children who stutter produce more disfluency clusters than normally fluent children (Hubbard & Yairi, 1988; LaSalle & Conture, 1995; Sawyer & Yairi, 2010, in press). Limited information has been made available for advanced stuttering. Two investigations supported a tendency for clustering in adults (Fein, 1970; Still & Griggs, 1979), but a study of school-age children did not (Taylor & Taylor, 1967). The latter study, however, applied different definitions and analysis methods. The significance of clustering is that it may contribute to the perceptual impression of "stuttering" or suggest greater severity. Further research is needed to test these hypotheses about the significance of clustering in advanced stuttering.

Physical Concomitants

We made reference to the physical concomitants of stuttering in Chapters 1 and 3. *Secondary* or *accessory characteristics* are other common terms referring to the physical concomitants of stuttering. Recall that concomitants occur in association with the main speech events of stuttering. Various physical movements and postures accompany stuttering events. Some are easily observed; others are not. Some occur covertly in the speech musculature, whereas others occur overtly in various body parts.

It important to understand that movement and/or postures regarded as concomitants are not necessary for the production of the intended speech. For example, engaging in a laryngeal block, the mouth may be widely open and some jaw movement observed. These gestures would have nothing to do with the production of the intended /i/ vowel.

Another physiological component sometimes observed in advanced stuttering is *tremor*. We have seen tremor in several clients, especially in the lips or jaw. Tremor is typically defined as a rhythmic, involuntary, oscillating movement of a body part. Physiological tremor is a normal phenomenon that affects all people when they engage in a sustained effort of muscle contraction. The typical oscillation rate of tremor is from 8 to 10 Hz. In some situations (e.g., being anxious or very tired), tremors can become exaggerated. In the person who stutters, tremors appear to occur in the speech musculature when tension increases in antagonistic muscles. Research of tremor has shown evidence of oscillations in electromyography (EMG) activity ranging from 5 to 15 Hz in the upper lip, lower lip, or jaw structures of children and adults who stutter (Kelly, Smith, & Goffman, 1995; Smith, 1989). These findings could reflect instabilities in their speech motor systems.

Physiological concomitants of stuttering include many types and numerous variations. They often involve tense body movements, especially in the head and neck, taking place in association with disfluency events. They contribute to the effect of tense, struggled speech, the perception of stuttering, its severity, and the overall degree of abnormality. The number of variations of secondary characteristics is almost limitless among and within individuals who stutter. For example, one individual explained that listeners have no idea that his toes are curling inside his shoes during moments of stuttering. A list of the most common observable characteristics is provided next, some of which are cited in Johnson, Darley, and Spriesterbach (1963).

Physical Concomitants (Secondary or Accessory Characteristics)

Head jerks	Head turns (side; down)
Forehead tension	Nostrils flaring/constricted
Eyes closed; squinting	Eyes widely open
Facial contortions	Lips pressured
Jaw closed tightly	Teeth grinding
Jaw wide open	Rotational or sideways jaw movement
Tongue protrusion	Throat tightened
Body swaying	Hand and/or arm movements
Irregular exhalation (blowing) during speech	
Irregular inhalations (gasping) in the midst of speaking	

The occurrence of most of these secondary characteristics during stuttering events in the speech of individuals ages 14 to 23 was investigated and confirmed by means of a motion picture camera, followed with a fine frame-by-frame analysis of the films (Prins & Lohr, 1972). The study, however, was confined to the head and neck. One finding was that the number of areas within the head and neck region involved in stutter events had a significant weight on the severity factor.

As mentioned, physical concomitants are viewed as *accessory* and *secondary*. According to Van Riper, they are accessory because they are not "basic"; that is, they are not part of the central stuttering core of sound/syllable repetitions and prolongations. And "[T]hey are secondary because they occur late in the developmental sequence" (p. 122). Reflected in much of the literature is a strong assumption that those accessories are acquired "behaviors" that are reinforced via instrumental learning (Brutten & Shoemaker, 1967; Van Riper, 1971).

Originally, so the thinking goes, secondary behaviors were used by the person who stutters to help cope with, or get out of, stuttering blocks. At a critical moment, the behavior happened to coincide with relief from a speech block. Over time the behavior becomes deeply integrated with the complex stuttering block, making it more severe. The stutterer's false belief that the behavior provides relief from the block, however, overrides any recognition that it actually does the opposite. Some clinicians have included secondary characteristics as targets for treatment (e.g., directly attempting to eliminate them). Others take the approach that they will diminish on their own once stuttering is decreased (Webster, 1980a).

We take a skeptical view toward interpretation of secondary behaviors as reinforced secondary reactions. As we discussed in Chapter 3, these supposedly "secondary" characteristics have been observed in young children from early stages of their stuttering. The possibility that these movements constitute an integral part of the neuromuscular disturbance in stuttering has not been ruled out.

Other Speech Characteristics

Voice

As stuttering persists, the speaker tends to have difficulty regulating dimensions of voice and speaking rate in addition to the disfluency. Various vocal phenomena, such as monotone, sudden sharp shifts in the vocal pitch, occasional vocal fry,[2] and strained voice, are common symptoms of advanced stuttering (Bloodstein & Bernstein Ratner, 2008). We have also observed cessations of phonation and changes in resonance quality, for example, the voice becoming quite denasal during stuttering. Some of these, such as vocal fry, are not abnormal but occur more frequently than in typically normal speech. Such characteristics are usually related to problems with regulating tension. Tense muscles are stiff, and stiffness offers resistance to movement. Excess tension could account for the speaker's sensation that the voice or speech mechanism is "stuck." Pitch inflection, an uncontrolled rise in pitch on a voiced speech sound, is a possible acoustic outcome of excess tension in the voice.

Monotonous vocal pitch and a number of other changes in vocal quality may be used as avoidance by the speaker to guard against stuttering. Vocal fry and monotonous pitch further add to the decline in overall quality of communication by the person who stutters. It is more difficult for listeners to focus on what the person is saying when, in addition to stuttering, the voice is flat and rough. Clinicians should be attentive to these dimensions in their overall therapeutic approach.

Acoustic and physiological research has supported laryngeal involvement in stuttering. In the 1970s and 1980s, there were many studies of both vocal reaction time (VRT), the interval between presenting a stimulus to the subject and the beginning of a vocal response, as well as of voice onset time (VOT), the gap between the release of a consonant and the beginning of vocal fold vibration on the following voiced sound (e.g., Adams, 1987; Hilman & Gilbert, 1977). Although findings were inconsistent, Ward (2006) concluded that, overall, adults who stutter (1) tend to exhibit longer VRT and VOT, and (2) evidence less control (greater variability) in this respect than normally fluent speakers. Studies that investigated electrical activity in the larynx of people who stutter using EMG techniques, found a higher level of muscle tonus and simultaneous contraction of antagonistic opening and closing muscles during fluent speech (Freeman & Ushijima, 1978; Shapiro, 1980). Other investigators, however, reported that people who stutter reduced EMG activity during fluent speech (Smith, Denny, Shaffer, Kelly, & Hirano, 1996). Conture, McCall, and Brewer (1977) used a motion picture to observe the larynx and also reported abnormal positioning during stuttering. The significance of laryngeal control has long been recognized by clinicians, for example in programs where easy voice onset is an important technique (e.g., Webster, 1980a).

---

[2] Vocal fry, also known as glottal fry, refers to the low-pitched, creaky sound of air weakly bubbling up through the vocal folds. It has a pulsating sound like the effect of running a finger along the teeth of a comb.

Speaking Rate

The traditional measure of verbal output is referred to as *overall speaking rate*. It is a global indicator of the amount of speech (number of words or syllables), including pauses and disfluencies, that a person utters in a given time. The overall speaking rate is lower (slower) for people who stutter than for normally fluent speakers. This is understandable because repeating the word "and" five times instead of just saying it once, and having additional interruptions, takes a longer time. Research has confirmed this common impression. Moderate to moderately high negative correlations of −0.72 and −0.80 between frequency of stuttering and overall speaking rate were reported by investigators (e.g., Aron, 1967, and Bloodstein, 1944, respectively). Therefore, overall speaking rate can be clinically useful in the evaluation of stuttering as well as in monitoring therapeutic progress.

Early on, Bloodstein (1944) reported the mean overall speaking rate during reading for adults who stutter was 122.7 words per minute (wpm), substantially slower than the mean of 170 wpm for normally fluent speakers (Walker, 1988). The difference in the two means is an excellent reflection of the growing communication problem as stuttering persists. Of course, diversity of rate is found in both groups. For people who stutter, the range is particularly wide, extending from 42 to 191 wpm. A satisfactory range for oral reading usually extends from 150 to 180 wpm (Fairbanks, 1960). It can be logically inferred that the slower the rate, the more stuttering.

The slower than normal overall speaking rate of people who stutter has raised the question of whether their speech movement during fluent speech also differs from normal. To this end, another indicator, *articulatory rate*, is used to measure the speed of speech only after pauses and disfluent segments are disregarded. Some data along this line have been provided for adults but usually in the context of another topic of research (e.g., Logan, Roberts, Pretto, & Morey, 2002; Onslow, van Doorn, & Newman, 1992; Prins & Hubbard, 1990). Articulatory rates have been reported in terms of either syllables per second or phones per second. A reduction in the variability of articulatory rate has been suggested as an indicator of posttreatment improvement (Onslow et al., 1992). Instructions for measurement of articulatory and speaking rates are presented in Chapter 9. Durations of articulatory movements, measured kinematically, tend to be slower generally in adolescents and adults who stutter than in normally fluent speakers (Archibald & De Nil, 1999; Zimmerman, 1980c; Zimmerman & Hanley, 1983). This slowness, also seen in acoustic measures, appears to be present across all transitions between consonant and vowel segments (Prins & Hubbard, 1990). The clinical implication of slower fluent speech is counterintuitive. If the speech of people who stutter is already slower, why is it therapeutic to slow their speech further? Some ideas are presented in Chapters 6 and 7 that deal with theories of stuttering.

This paradox is not unique to stuttering remediation, however. Treatment of dysarthria, which is also slower than normal speech, is achieved with further slowing by the speaker.

Emotional Characteristics and Cognition

Emotional Reactions

One of the most commonly recognized characteristics of advanced stuttering is the complex emotionality that evolves over time (Bloodstein, 1960b; Bloodstein & Bernstein Ratner, 2008). These emotions may include fear, dread, anxiety, being trapped, panic, embarrassment, shame, humiliation, anger, resentment, and other unpleasant feelings. The type of emotions varies in time relative to the moment of stuttering. Thus fear, dread, and anxiety are experienced in anticipation of the stuttering, before the attempted speech; feelings of being trapped and panic are experienced during the stutter event; feelings of shame, humiliation, anger, or resentment appear after stuttering had occurred. Whereas many laypeople might believe that people stutter because they are emotional, it would appear to be just the opposite: People become emotional because they stutter. Research has confirmed that heightened emotional reactions are common in people who stutter. Both *state* and *trait* anxiety are greater among those who stutter than in the general population (Craig, 1990; Craig, Hancock, Tran, & Craig, 2003). State anxiety is an emotional tension triggered by specific situations, and trait anxiety is a relatively stable tendency to be emotionally tense in situations.

At what stage of the disorder does stuttering evoke these feelings? As indicated in Chapter 3, initially, young children do not react to stuttering with the wide range of emotions and intensity that older children and adults do. As emotional reactions develop, three factors are apt to influence the level and timing of a child's reactions: (1) the child's sensitivity to stuttering, (2) other's reactions to stuttering, and (3) the child's reactions to others. Thus emotions emerge after the speaker becomes aware of the stuttering (Bluemel, 1932), that it is unpleasant to him or her, that a simple, well-intended attempt to communicate can deteriorate by means of a stutter into a terrifying feeling of being trapped, and that it attracts an upsurge of unwanted listener reactions, be they real or imagined. Loathing of stuttering develops after the stuttering beast has made mountains out of molehills.

Awareness is a complicated construct, and more knowledge is needed regarding its developmental stages. The mind is primed at an early age to detect novel stimuli. Seven-month-old infants tend to stare longer at novel stimuli than habituated stimuli (Fagan, 1984). At 14 months, infants who are shown actions with no opportunity to imitate them display recall of those modeled actions 4 months later (Meltzoff, 1995). At $2\frac{1}{2}$ years of age, children can provide verbal descriptions of unique events they experienced 6 or more months in the past (Fivush, Gray, &

Fromhoff, 1987). Children must be older, however, before biographical memories endure. Older children and adults find that autobiographical memories prior to age 3 or 4 are forgotten (West & Bauer, 1999). One's biographical memories become reliable at about 7 years of age (Rubin, Wetzler, & Nebes, 1986). Research has shown that a child's awareness of stuttering markedly increases between the ages of 4 and 5 years (Ambrose & Yairi, 1994; Ezrati-Vinacour, Platzky, & Yairi, 2001). Hence it would appear that sometime between the ages of 5 and 7 years, specific experiences of stuttering begin to have a lasting impression in a person's biographical memory.

It is no wonder that as such experiences multiply, the person who stutters often wants to avoid speaking situations, hold back from talking, mask stuttering with other behaviors, avoid looking at listeners, fear and think the worst of listeners, use unusual voice characteristics or say things in circuitous ways. Individuals vary in their emotional responses to stuttering, as all people do toward their negative experiences. Individuals develop fears to specific situations, people, words, and even speech sounds. Answering the telephone, for example, creates a specific situational fear experienced by many people who stutter. An example of specific word fear is saying one's own name when introducing oneself. One of our clients, an economics major, had a specific fear of the sound /m/. Hence he stuttered on many words beginning with /m/, especially on "millions." Another client scheduled to make a brief presentation in front of a class could not sleep the whole night before and was unable to eat breakfast until after the presentation was over. Nonetheless, people who stutter share remarkable empathy with each other concerning the emotional impact of stuttering. Feelings of anxiety about speaking, guilt over not having better speech control, and self-doubts about the ability to handle communication situations are common themes in group therapy or self-help group meetings. Many eventually choose their profession and particular job driven by the avoidance of speaking demands.

Research evidence suggests that stuttering increases anxiety (Ezrati-Vinacour & Levin, 2004). The extent of negative reaction varies widely among people who stutter, ranging from little to no anxiety to the opposite extreme of social phobia. Studies of adolescents and adults who stutter found they report greater anxiety than the general population but less anxiety than others with social phobia or psychiatric disorders (Kraaimaat, Vanryckeghem, & Van Dam-Baggen, 2002; Mahr & Torosian, 1999). More severe stuttering tends to be associated with a greater state anxiety than mild stuttering (Ezrati-Vinacour & Levin, 2004). The emotional reactions associated with advanced stuttering may grow in some individuals to such an extent that they become more of a handicap than the overt stuttered speech. In such cases, perhaps the strongest characteristics of advanced stuttering is avoidance behavior that may seriously affect day-to-day life and may lead to some social withdrawal. We believe that the emotional reactions should be considered when therapy is planned.

Avoidance behavior is one of the most predominant characteristics of advanced stuttering. One example is holding back from responding to questions in class, even when a student knows an answer quite well, for fear of the humiliation of stuttering. Or if there is an expectation of being called on, that student is apt to make an excuse to leave the room for the same reason. One young woman explained that she drove across a large city to ask one quick question just to avoid stuttering on the phone. She later explained that it was that incident that led her to realize just how much she was letting stuttering control her life, and that she never wanted to let it push her that far again. In a study of 200 adults who stutter, 20% reported turning down a job or promotions because of their fear of stuttering (Klein & Hood, 2004).

Cognition

The cognitive impact of stuttering has received some limited attention in research. Although lower self-esteem and social anxiety might be expected among those who stutter, some studies have had surprisingly opposite results that showed self-esteem was similar or more positive than age- and gender-matched controls (Hearne, Packman, Onslow, & Quine, 2008). Alternatively, one study found that adults who stutter rate themselves significantly lower on self-efficacy (Bray, Kehle, Lawless, & Theodore, 2003). The negative attitudes of people who stutter toward speech and communication have been surveyed through a variety of attitude scales. DeNil and Brutten (1991) found that 70 children who stutter, 7 to 14 years of age, had significantly more negative attitudes about communication than their age- and gender-matched control children who did not stutter. They tended to believe that others do not like the way they talk and will be unkind or make fun of them for stuttering.

There are a number of attitudes described in the nonscientific stuttering literature, common to people with advanced stuttering. One example is the tendency to think of one's self as a *giant in chains*. That is, the person tends to believe "If only I didn't stutter, I would have been successful at that endeavor." Stuttering skews one's perspective on how much of life's struggles would still be there even without stuttering. The stuttering attracts the blame for social or vocational setbacks. Another common belief is the tendency of expecting and fearing that stuttering will occur. The phenomenon of *expectancy* is described later in this chapter. Another cognitive obstacle is the extent to which all kinds of stimuli (e.g., sounds or words, situations, one's own emotions—excitements, doubts, etc.) are experienced as threatening to the endeavor to communicate. In therapy, managing these cognitive responses can be as critically important to remediation as addressing the strategies for speaking.

Concomitant Disorders

As we discussed in Chapter 3, young children who stutter also tend to exhibit other disorders with greater frequency than is found in the population at large, especially disorders of phonology and language. The pool of data for school-age children is

Table 4.1: **Comparisons of the Prevalence of Various Disorders in People Who Stutter and in the Population at Large**

Disorder	PWS (%)	General Population (%)
Phonology	16	6
Language	10	7
Learning disabilities	7	7
Reading disabilities	6	6
Other disabilities	5	N/A

N/A = not applicable; PWS = people who stutter.

much larger than that for preschool-age children, and there has been little interest in this domain as far as advanced stuttering in adolescents and adults is concerned. Among the larger sources, a survey of 358 speech clinicians who treated 1,060 school-age children who stutter found that 44% had one concomitant disorder, and an additional 24% had two or more concomitant disorders, adding up to 68% of the group (Blood & Seider, 1981). The percentage of children who exhibited only one of each concomitant disorder, as compared to population expectancy data according to ASHA, is shown in Table 4.1.

These data were supported by another survey of 241 speech-language clinicians from 10 U.S. states who treated 467 children who stutter (Arndt & Healey, 2001). They reported that 44% had one or more verified speech/language problem/s to accompany stuttering. Three disorder subgroups, phonology only, language only, and phonology and language disorders, each constituted nearly 15% among the total group of children who stutter. The clients, however, ranged in age from 3 to 20 years, making it difficult to draw inferences specifically to advanced stuttering. In a more recent, more comprehensive, and considerably larger survey, 1,184 school SLPs in 46 U.S. states identified 2,628 children who stutter in kindergarten through 12th grade. In this large sample, nearly 65% had at least one concomitant disorder. The distribution according to disorders was as follows: articulation, 33.5%; phonology, 12.7%; language (expressive), 13.5%; and language (receptive), 12.1%. Among other disorders were learning disabilities, 11.4%; literacy disorders, 8.2%; attention deficits, 5.9%; auditory processing, 3.8%; neuropsychological, 2.9%; behavioral, 2.4%; and sensory, 2.1% (Blood et al., 2003). Males displayed the greater proportions of nearly all types of disorders.

Such research has been criticized for its potential inflation of estimates because children with multiple needs are more apt to be referred and identified for services (Nippold, 1990, 2004). Although no direct links between stuttering and these disorders have been demonstrated, and they may well be completely independent of stuttering, clinicians who provide therapy for stuttering should probe for the presence of concomitant disorders to ascertain whether or not there are complicating conditions and to determine the therapeutic approach.

What does it mean that older children who stutter tend to have multiple disorders more often than the prevalence in the general population? Perhaps other speech-language problems make a speaker more vulnerable to fluency breakdown and stuttering. In contrast, stuttering itself may create the risk for developing additional speech-language problems. Finally, both stuttering and other speech-language problems may be related to yet another common underlying etiology. Research has not yet determined which of these possible implications are correct. Answers are also needed regarding whether certain aspects of treatment for other speech-language disorders put a child at risk for stuttering.

One reason why little research has been pursued related to concomitant language disorders in adults is because there has been no apparent reason to suspect that they exhibit poor language skills. Nevertheless, the past few years have seen growing interests in the language processing of this age group. For example, Scott Trautman and Cairns (2003) found that under time pressure, adults who stutter may have poorer language organization. Kleinow and Smith (2000) found that the speech motor stability of adults who stutter decreased when the speaking materials were more complex. They concluded that "language formulation processes may affect speech production processes and that the speech motor systems of adults who stutter may be especially susceptible to the linguistic demands required to produce a more complex utterance" (p. 548). Most recently, Weber-Fox and Hampton (2008) concluded that whereas linguistic abilities are normal in adults who stutter, underlying brain activity mediating some aspects of language processing may function differently.

The Dynamics of Advanced Stuttering

Patterns of Occurrence

Among the most interesting phenomena of advanced stuttering are the patterns of stuttering occurrence relative to previous stutter events. As we will see, three patterns demonstrate its predictability. In other words, these patterns reveal certain rules that show that stuttering is not as random as it often appears to listeners. Knowledge of the rules of stuttering is sometimes clinically useful even today. Better understanding should contribute more to its future clinical management.

Adaptation

Johnson and Knott (1937) published the first scientific report of stuttering adaptation. They observed that when a passage is read aloud several consecutive times, stuttering declines with each rereading. This phenomenon is known as *adaptation*. Several characteristics of the adaptation pattern are fairly consistent. First, the greatest reduction of stuttering is evident on the second reading, followed by a more gradual decline that levels off after five readings (Johnson & Inness, 1939; Jones, 1955). The typical result is a 50% reduction in stuttering from the first to the fifth reading. Like most conditions that reduce stuttering, the decline is only temporary. After a sufficient period, the original level of stuttering returns. Some adaptation occurs even if a speaker keeps on talking without saying the same words. Speaking words that are always changing, however, yields much less, about a 10% to 20% reduction (e.g., Gray, 1965a, 1965b; Johnson & Inness, 1939; Van Riper & Hull, 1955).

What do the characteristics of adaptation reveal about the nature of stuttering? For example, all types of disfluency decline, not just the stuttering-like disruptions (Silverman & Williams, 1971). On the one hand, this could suggest that all types of disfluency are governed by a similar mechanism. On the other, it might mean that one type of disfluency (e.g., SLD) exerts an influence over the other types. During adaptation, stuttering severity (e.g., intensity and duration of the prolongations) usually decreases along with its frequency (Trotter, 1955). Reduction in severity could indicate that a speaker's emotional reactive responses are diminishing. Consider that when a speaker reads a passage for the first time, the prospect of encountering moments of stuttering may be threatening. If by the end of the first reading of the passage, the stuttering moments were less threatening than the speaker anticipated, then the tension of anticipation will be reduced on the second reading, along with reaction-related aspects of disfluent speech.

Not all people who stutter display the adaptation effect, and among those who do, the amount varies (Kroll & Hood, 1976; Moore, Flowers, & Cunko, 1981; Silverman & Williams, 1971). Perhaps for those who do not adapt, stuttering on the first reading is more threatening than they anticipated, and so their reactive responses are heightened for the next readings. Surprisingly, milder stutterers tend to show greater adaptation than more severe stutterers (Gray, 1965a, 1965b; Van Riper & Hull, 1955). This could be explained by the possibility that adaptation reduces the reactive components of stuttering that people who exhibit milder stuttering are already more successfully managing. Finally, adaptation can take place whether successive readings are separated by 20 min, 1 hr, or even 24 hr (Leutenegger, 1957). This fact means that clinicians and researchers must be careful about evaluating progress with the same reading passage pre- and posttreatment. Rather than improving, the client may merely be adapting. The adaptation effect can be used in certain circumstances for clinical purposes. One such situation is when the client is to present a paper in class or present a project to his or her company's executives. Rehearsing the materials several times out loud in conditions as similar as possible to the actual situation, immediately before the upcoming event, might well reduce the level of stuttering.

How has adaptation been explained? From a learning theory perspective, the adaptation curve seen in stuttering is similar to the extinction curve seen in experiments with animals where an acquired behavior is made to disappear when reinforcement is removed. This interpretation supports the view that stuttering is a learned behavior (Wischner, 1950). From a psychological-emotional perspective, it was suggested that once stuttering occurs, the fear of stuttering is reduced, resulting in less stuttering in the following readings (Sheehan, 1958). Another explanation (Eisenson, 1958; Max & Caruso, 1988) proposes that some form of motor-sensory rehearsal is responsible: An articulatory-vocal "set" becomes established as a speaker repeats spoken material.

Many have believed that the adaptation phenomenon holds great potential. Some have proposed that it has the capacity to serve as a predictor of progress in therapy. Others have suggested that it could represent a basis for stuttering subtypes. By studying the subgroups who respond differently under adaptation conditions, the nature of stuttering and appropriate clinical intervention may become clearer (Johnson et al., 1963; Lanyon, 1965; Newman, 1963; Van Riper & Hull, 1955).

Which speech motor-sensory feedback systems (i.e., articulation, phonation, audition) might be essential to the adaptation effect? It appears that phonation could be the most important because oral rehearsal results in greater adaptation than either lipped or whispered rehearsal (Brenner, Perkins, & Soderberg, 1972; Bruce & Adams, 1978; Moss, 1976; Robbins, 1971). If the speaker needed to rehearse the articulatory pattern alone, then lipped or whispered rehearsal should be just as effective as voiced rehearsal. Other evidence supports the conclusion that suprasegmental (vocal) rather than segmental (phonemic) elements are crucial. For example, although the same words are repeated, adaptation can be prevented if commas are relocated to alter the rhythm and phrasing of the passage (Wingate, 1972).

Consistency

Another observation of the stuttering dynamics during repeated oral readings is a pattern called the *consistency* effect. This is the tendency for words stuttered on the final readings to be those that had been stuttered initially. This phenomenon has been observed and reported in a number of studies over many years (Johnson & Knott, 1937; Williams, Silverman, & Kools, 1969; Wingate, 1986). Although stuttering frequency and severity decline due to adaptation, the words still stuttered in the last reading tend to be among those stuttered during the first one. The *consistency index* is calculated by dividing the number of words stuttered in the first reading that were also stuttered in the subsequent reading, by the number of words stuttered in the first reading. Johnson and Leutenegger (1955, p. 211) reported a mean consistency index for adults who stutter of 69.3% (SD, 14.9%). Again, the consistency effect shows that stuttering does not occur randomly but follows certain rules. Like adaptation, it has been interpreted in terms of learning theory, in that once a word has been associated with stuttering, it acquires the role of a stimulus to trigger stuttering on subsequent occasions (Johnson & Knott, 1937).

Adjacency

Stuttering is never eliminated completely by adaptation, and the remaining stuttering events appear to be strongly tied to the word locations. The mystifying power of these locations became the occasion for yet another phenomenon observed by Johnson and his colleagues (Johnson & Millsapps, 1937), the *adjacency* effect. The essence of this effect is that stuttering tends to occur at the same locations as before, even when previously stuttered words are removed from the reading passage being rehearsed. That is, stuttering tended to occur on the words adjacent to locations where stuttering had occurred before.

Expectancy

The previous three effects dealt with the patterns of stuttering events relative to their own occurrence. The phenomenon of *expectancy* is different in that it implies some impact of the person's cognition on the actual occurrence of stuttering. Specifically, expectancy refers to the ability of the person who stutters to scan ahead and predict with a good measure of accuracy, although not perfectly, what words or parts of words will be stuttered. This phenomenon was revealed when subjects were instructed to mark a passage according to places where they thought they would stutter. When an unmarked passage was later presented for them to read, a majority of locations had been predicted accurately. Expectancy is very commonly experienced by many people who stutter: They know when, sometimes how, they will stutter. Like other phenomena described earlier, expectancy suggests that anticipatory anxiety is important to stuttering. It produces danger signals that lead to apprehension that lead to physical tension in preparing to cope with the upcoming stuttering. As Johnson (1948) opined, it is this tension that actually causes the stuttering. Therefore, reducing the emotional threat of stuttering would appear to be a worthwhile therapy goal. But because client predictions of stuttering are incorrect on a fair proportion of instances, they may also benefit in therapy by gaining more realistic expectations of when stuttering is apt to occur. As we discuss in Chapter 11, the ability to anticipate stuttering has been used in therapy, training clients to begin changing expected stuttering behavior before it actually occurs.

Loci of Stuttering

It was stated earlier that the adaptation, consistency, and adjacency phenomena demonstrate that there are forces that influence the occurrence of stuttering in the stream of speech, some under certain conditions, some more generally. The elements of spoken language also offer a certain degree of power to predict when stuttering events occur in general communication situations. Early investigators examined the linguistic variables associated with the specific locations (loci) of stuttering events, hoping that, to the extent stuttering could be predicted, its governing rules might be better understood and the disorder better treated.

In 1945, Spencer Brown reported that the occurrence of the stuttering of adolescents and adults was not random but commonly associated with specific language structures. Analyzing speech samples, he observed that stuttering tended to occur on (1) content words (versus function words), including nouns, verbs, adjectives, adverbs; (2) long words (versus short words); (3) consonant-initial words (versus vowel-initial word locations); and (4) sentence-initial (versus final locations). The more factors congregate in a single word, the higher is its chance to be stuttered. These locations became known as "Brown's four factors" because they supposedly accounted for most stuttering instances. Unfortunately, this type of research is confounded by the proportions of occurrence of the factors and the extent to which they overlap. For example, most content words are longer words, and most content words are consonant-initial. Later researchers concluded that the effects of these factors were not independent of each other (Quarrington, 1965; Soderberg, 1967, 1971). Initial sentence position was primarily responsible for the locations (Brown, 1945; Wingate, 1988). Other types of locations have been shown to attract stuttering, including words conveying "prominent" or important information (Lanyon & Duprez, 1970), unfamiliar words (Hubbard & Prins, 1994), and stressed or accented syllables and words (Prins, Hubbard, & Krause, 1991; Wingate, 1984).

Stuttering loci observed in adults are not the same as those in children. Prior to age 8, the loci of stuttering are not as predictable and almost run in an opposite fashion. Children often stutter on function words, short words (most of their words are short), vowel-initial words, and familiar words (Bloodstein & Gantwerk, 1967; Bloodstein & Grossman, 1981; Natke, Sandrieser, van Ark, Pietrowsky, & Kalveram, 2004). Consider the child who says: "I I I I I want to go." The first word "I" fits all four of these categories. Research suggests that the shift in stuttering locations to the advanced pattern may begin as early as age 5, be mostly complete by age 12, but continue to progress into adulthood (Au-Yeung, Gomez, & Howell, 2003; Howell, Au-Yeung, & Sackin, 1999).

Table 4.2 provides a list of typical stuttering loci and whether they are common only in adults or in both children and adults. Examples of each of the loci are also given.

Table 4.2: **Examples of Typical Loci of Stuttering (Shown in Bold and Italics) for Adults and/or Children**

Stuttering Location	Utterance Example	Typical Age Group
On the first three words of the utterance	"***The Galapagos Islands*** offer a warm respite from the vicissitudes of life."	Both adults and children
On initial sounds or syllables of the words	***Th***e ***Ga***lapagos ***I***slands ***o***ffer a ***w***arm ***r***espite ***f***rom ***th***e ***vi***cissitudes ***of*** ***l***ife."	Both adults and children
On the content words (nouns/verbs/adjectives/adverbs)	The ***Galapagos Islands offer*** a ***warm respite*** from the ***vicissitudes*** of ***life***."	Adults, not children
On longer words (more sounds/letters)	The ***Galapagos Islands*** offer a warm ***respite*** from the ***vicissitudes*** of life."	Adults, not children
On consonant-initial words	***The Galapagos*** Islands offer a ***warm respite from*** the ***vicissitudes*** of ***life***."	Adults, not children
On unfamiliar words	The ***Galapagos*** Islands offer a warm respite from the ***vicissitudes*** of life."	Adults, not children
On the stressed syllables (after the first three words[3])	The Galapagos Islands ***of***fer a warm ***re***spite from the vi***cis***situdes of life."	Adults

---

[3] See Hubbard (1998).

In sum, the locations of advanced stuttering can be divided into word-based factors and utterance-based factors. Word-based factors include initial position, sound class (consonant), length (in phones, letters, or syllables), syllabic stress, word familiarity, propositionality, and phonological complexity. Utterance-based factors include initial position (first three words), grammatical class, length (in syllables, words), propositionality, clause type (verb phrase), clause boundaries, and initiation of phonologic words. The vulnerability of early word and utterance position as a common location of fluency breakdown has led some researchers to notice its uniqueness as the time when the highest demands are placed on speech planning systems, both linguistically and motorically. The loci phenomenon is discussed further in Chapter 7 in regard to theories of stuttering.

> The loci suggest a strong link between stuttering and language, although many of the locations are also typical of normal disfluencies (Silverman & Williams, 1967). Some researchers propose that stuttering locations reveal more about the nature of speech-language production itself rather than stuttering because other so-called speech errors (not disfluencies) also tend to occur at these same locations. Hence these loci may merely inform us where the pieces of speech-language structure can be fit together or taken apart. There remains much more to understand about why speech breaks apart, *when* it does, and *the way* it does (i.e., as SLD or other).

Conditions That Diminish Stuttering

One of the most mystifying, but fascinating characteristics of the disorder of stuttering is its amelioration, that is, its improvement, in an extensive array of diverse conditions. It has been supposed that if the common link among the various ameliorating conditions were found, it would unlock the nature of stuttering. Furthermore, it would provide important information concerning therapeutic methods. Unfortunately, researchers have not yet found that link. It is also unfortunate that the reduction in stuttering is usually only experienced while the condition is present; when removed, the stuttering usually resumes its previous level. This aspect, however, has barely been investigated.

For more than half a century, scholars of stuttering have been aware that many conditions may induce fluency. Bloodstein (1950) surveyed 204 people who stuttered, ages 16 to 44 years, regarding conditions that may reduce stuttering. The participants reported experiencing reduction of stuttering in a total of 115 conditions, ranging from speaking when mildly intoxicated to acting a part in a play. A selected set of such conditions and the corresponding percentage of respondents who experienced either marked reduction in, or no stuttering at all, are shown in Table 4.3.

Relevant to clinicians in particular, several of the ameliorating conditions have indeed been employed for purposes of treatment of stuttering (Bloodstein & Bernstein Ratner, 2008). Those conditions, some of which we describe in later

Table 4.3: **Number of Respondents and Percentages Who Reported Marked Stuttering Reduction in 20 Fluency-Inducing Conditions**

Fluency-Inducing Condition	N	Absent or Hardly Any Stuttering (%)
Reading aloud in unison with others reading same material	50	100.0
Singing*	46	100.0
Speaking to an animal	50	94.0
Speaking in time to a rhythmic swing of your arm	26	92.3
Speaking to an infant	37	91.9
Swearing in ordinary conversation	47	87.2
Speaking with no one else present	45	86.7
Lipped speech (Perkins, Rudas, Johnson, & Bell, 1976)	30	83.0
Reading aloud with no one else present	49	81.6
Imitating a foreign dialect	33	69.7
When very considerably intoxicated	25	64.0
Imitating another person's manner of speaking	36	63.9
Speaking in a sing-song manner	33	60.6
Speaking in a monotone	30	60.0
Speaking and writing simultaneously	28	57.1
Whispering	46	52.2
Acting a part in a play	112	43.8
Repeating sentences after someone else	37	40.5
Speaking more slowly than usual	44	38.6
Reciting from memory	44	27.3

*The frequency and regularity with which the observation of an immediate reduction in stuttering during singing has been reported led Wingate (1969) to conclude that it may be one "of the few universal facts about stuttering."

Based on information from A rating scale study of conditions under which stuttering is reduced or absent by O. Bloodstein. *Journal of Speech and Hearing Disorders, 15*, 29–36. Copyright 1950 by American Speech-Language-Hearing Association. All rights reserved.

chapters concerned with stuttering therapy, are listed in Table 4.4. Note that a good number of them are created by instrument-generated stimuli.

Although the previous Bloodstein survey provided interesting information from the subjective experiences of people who stutter, research that examines the effects of ameliorating conditions with firsthand laboratory observation is important. Moreover, instead of answering the question about what percentage of people experience reduction, direct observation addresses the question of how much stuttering is reduced in these conditions. A study by Andrews, Howie, Dozsa, and

Table 4.4: **Ameliorating Conditions of Stuttering Used for Therapeutic Intervention Purposes**

Ameliorating Condition

Delayed auditory feedback (usually 200–250 ms)

EMG biofeedback for less muscle activity (lip, larynx)

Metronome-timed speech

Masking noise

Reduced speaking rate

Voluntary stuttering, especially if repeated to gain control

Emotionally distracting/intense stimuli

Hypnotic suggestion

Monotone speech

Response contingent stimulation (shock, tone, light, words, time-out)

Repeating the same word/s over and over

Singsong speech

Guitar (1982) examined three adult men who stutter under 15 different fluency-inducing conditions. Seven of these conditions reduced stuttering by at least 90%: singing, chorus (unison) reading, shadowing, response contingent stimuli, slowing, syllable-timed speech, and prolonged speech under delayed auditory feedback (DAF). The results are summarized in Figure 4.1 in order of most to least amount of reduction of stuttering.

Two examples from scientific literature illustrate how research of this phenomenon can aid our understanding of the nature of stuttering. First, Stager, Jeffries, and Braun (2003) compared the brain activity patterns using PET (positron emission tomography) in adults who stutter with adults who do not stutter under two fluency-inducing conditions, singing and pacing speech. Results showed that the brain areas that were more active during the fluency-inducing conditions were the auditory association areas that process speech and voice, and motor regions related to control of the larynx and oral articulators. This was true for both participant groups. The activation, however, was more robust in the left hemisphere of those who stutter during the fluency-inducing conditions. The authors suggested that the patterns of brain activity may indicate that under the fluency-inducing conditions, speakers are self-monitoring speech production more closely (a primarily left hemisphere function). Because both groups showed similar patterns, it was proposed that the sensory-motor and cognitive demands of self-monitoring for the tasks, not the task itself (i.e., singing) were responsible for fluency.

A second example of research that applied knowledge of ameliorating conditions was conducted by Sparks, Grant, Millay, Walker-Batson, and Hynan (2002). The fluency

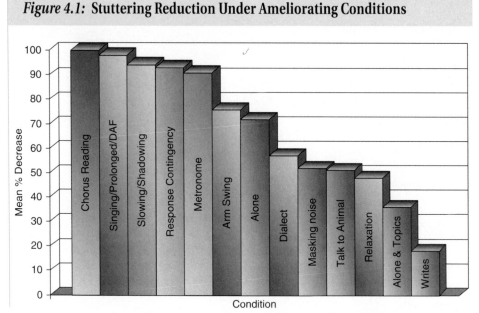

Figure 4.1: Stuttering Reduction Under Ameliorating Conditions

Based on information from Stuttering: Speech pattern characteristics under fluency-inducing conditions by G. Andrews, M. Dozsa, and B. Guitar. *Journal of Speech and Hearing Research, 25,* 208–216. Copyright 1982 by American Speech-Language-Hearing Association. All rights reserved.

of four adolescent speakers, two with mild and two with severe stuttering, was studied under slow and fast speaking rates with DAF or without DAF as a control condition. Fluency for the speakers with mild stuttering was the same for the two conditions; for speakers with severe stuttering it decreased by 90% for the two DAF speaking conditions as compared with no DAF. It appears that the severity of stuttering could be an important indicator of whether a speaker will respond to a fluency-inducing condition. Those with more severe stuttering may be more likely to benefit. The findings raise the possibility that the fluency-inducing effect of DAF is not necessarily its tendency to slow speech down.

As mentioned earlier, situations of communicative pressure tend to trigger more frequent or worse episodes of stuttering (Bloodstein & Bernstein Ratner, 2008). Such situations include having to say one's name, telephone calls, repairing miscommunications, or responding to "What did you say?", large audiences or groups, authority figures, prolonged anticipation time prior to a talking turn, and words or sounds believed to be difficult. Each speaker, however, may perceive communicative pressure in different ways. Some have difficulty speaking with the opposite sex and others with the same sex. Many have difficulty speaking to large groups and do much better one on one, but others have trouble with face-to-face individual encounters and do much better in front of large groups. Detailed information on how an individual person who stutters responds could enhance the planning and execution of therapy, for example, in planning desensitization programs (see Chapter 10).

Summary

As stuttering progresses into later childhood and beyond, the fully developed characteristics of advanced stuttering become more evident. This can be seen across the various domains of the disorder. A variety of disfluency types, frequency levels, and event durations are possible, influenced by anticipatory reactions. Generally speaking, as the proportion of sound prolongations and blocks in the total disfluency tend to increase, disfluencies are more apt to occur in the form of clusters where more than one disfluency type are together at the same location. A wide array of physical behaviors associated with the stuttered speech becomes more visible, adding to the complexity and apparent abnormality of the disorder. Suprasegmental characteristics of voice quality, prosody, and speaking rate are also influenced by stuttering. A critical aspect of advanced stuttering is the tremendous growth in the emotional reactions that people who stutter develop, primarily negative emotions that lead to avoidance of speech and possible social withdrawal.

Several predictable phenomena can be observed, such as adaptation, consistency, and adjacency. These may have some clinical implications. Unlike early stuttering, the stuttering loci in more advanced stages tend to be associated with language characteristics of longer, less familiar content words. The role of language in the occurrence of advanced stuttering is not well understood. Investigating the potential stuttering to language link may shed much light on the disorder. Also, stuttering can be greatly decreased, albeit temporarily, under various unique conditions, a number of which can be incorporated in treatment. All these phenomena indicate that stuttering is governed by certain rules still waiting to be understood.

STUDY QUESTIONS AND DISCUSSION TOPICS

1. What are the main changes that occur in the speech characteristics of advanced as compared to early stuttering?

2. What are the main developments in the emotional and social domains?

3. What considerations should enter into the selection and application of a disfluency classification system and why?

4. Does anxiety cause some stuttering and/or does stuttering cause some anxiety, and what evidence exists to support either? What is the difference between state and trait anxiety?

5. What are possible reasons why the loci of stuttering shift from their typical patterns in early childhood to their different pattern in older childhood and after?

6. Do you think that the various ameliorating conditions of stuttering are apt to share one common underlying cause, or are they more likely to produce their effects for a variety of different reasons? Why?

SUGGESTED READINGS

Andrews, G., Howie, P., Dozsa, M., & Guitar, B. (1982). Stuttering: Speech pattern characteristics under fluency-inducing conditions. *Journal of Speech and Hearing Research*, *25*, 208–216.

Bloodstein, O., & Bernstein Ratner, N. B. (2008). *A handbook on stuttering*. Clifton Park, NY: Delmar. See Chapters 10 and 11, which discuss stuttering as a response.

Perkins, W., Rudas, J., Johnson, L., & Bell, J. (1976). Stuttering: Discoordination of phonation with articulation and respiration. *Journal of Speech and Hearing Research*, *19*, 509–522.

Wingate, M. E. (1976). *Stuttering: Theory and treatment*. New York: Irvington. Chapter 8.

Chapter 5: Why Do People Stutter? Evaluating Theories and Models

LEARNER OBJECTIVES

Readers of this chapter will understand:

- The nature of scientific theory.
- Why stuttering theories have been numerous and diverse.
- Criteria that may be applied to evaluate the credibility of theories and models of stuttering.
- The potential role of subtyping in the characterization of stuttering.

Theories and Models

Having presented in Part I of this book some answers to the general questions of what is stuttering and who stutters, we now turn our attention to the question of how stuttering has been explained, that is, theories of stuttering. We begin with the more elementary question of what makes a good theory in general and then address the specific considerations of what makes a good theory of stuttering. First, the necessary components for generating testable theories and models of phenomena are identified. Next, problems as well as possible solutions pertinent to theorizing and modeling stuttering are generated. Subsequent chapters then provide an overview of specific theories and models of stuttering.

In common use, the word *theory* denotes an opinion, conjecture, or specula-tion. In other words, the term is often applied to an unsubstantiated guess or a per-sonal hunch about a phenomenon of interest. In the scientific arena, however, the meaning is different. A scientific theory is a proposed explanation, framework, or model of a natural or social phenomenon or set of phenomena. It is proposed in relation to scientific data and should have the potential to be tested experimentally. It should enable prediction of future occurrences of, or changes in, the phenome-non under certain conditions. Scientific theories are tentative and may be modified based on the acquisition of new information. Whereas the term *theory* is occasion-ally stretched to refer to a theoretical speculation that is currently unverifiable, the criterion of a scientific theory is its testability or refutability.

At times, the term *model* is used in the context of a theoretical proposition. A model goes further in that it represents an ideal prototype of the major parts of a complex phenomenon or a system, and it is especially helpful in explaining the underlying *dynamics* of the system; it makes assumptions about how it works. Most of you probably have seen diagrams presenting models of an atom or models closer to home showing the components of speech communication between a speaker and a listener. The terms *theory* and *model* are often used interchangeably; however, the terms have slightly different meanings. Whereas a theory is a conceptual system of understanding for the purpose of explaining and/or predicting a phenomenon or phenomena, a model is a representation of the phenomenon in terms of a set of variables and the relationships among them. Some theories take the form of a model or include a model as a component, but other theories do not. When a *theory* takes the form of a *model*, the two terms may be used interchangeably as referents.

Although the literature is rich with references to "theories" of stuttering, and, to a lesser degree, "models" of stuttering, it is also true that each proposed explanation tends to be limited to one or a few aspects of the disorder, such as the decline in the frequency of stuttering under noise, larger incidence of stuttering in boys than in girls, the decline in stuttering in repeated readings of same material, and many others. It is doubtful, therefore, that most would, or should, be regarded as "theories of stuttering" according to the common scientific meaning of the term. At best, some are merely *theoretical notions*, whereas others are speculations or guesses. Similarly, few, if any, actual models of stuttering exist because most fail to go beyond hypothetical explanations of the disorder. Still, there are many proposed so-called theories of stuttering and, in turn, many organizational schemes or classifications of those theories. How can the student of stuttering begin to understand the nature of these various theories and their contribution to our knowledge of this complicated communication disorder? Following, we suggest a possible approach to this endeavor.

Much of our knowledge of phenomena is dealt with on two levels: theoretical and practical. Musical knowledge illustrates this point. The music theory, among other things, describes the elements, such as notes and keys, and the relationships among them, such as scales, intervals, or chords. On the practical side, the elements and relationships permit musical compositions to be created, played, or sung. The aim of our theoretical knowledge of stuttering is to describe the relevant elements and the interrelationships of those elements. Theoretical knowledge, in turn, will facilitate our practical management of stuttering: its prevention, assessment, and treatment.

How to Analyze a Stuttering Theory

Prior to the examination of any theory, it is essential to determine what it tries to explain. As discussed in Chapter 1, the term *stuttering* may be constrained in referring only to moments (events) of speech disruption. Or it may be used in a more inclusive fashion with reference to the human condition of a speech disorder, including all of its associated aspects and effects. It follows, then, that the student should first ask whether the theory under study is supposed to explain stuttering events or stuttering as a disorder. Similarly, it should be determined whether an isolated aspect or a subset of stuttering phenomena is being explained, as opposed to a comprehensive account for stuttering.

After determining what a particular theory attempts to explain, the nature of its content should be examined. Such analyses reveal that the field of speech pathology has borrowed ideas and knowledge from the disciplines of medicine, psychology, and education. Accordingly, some organically based, psychologically based, or learning-based theories of the stuttering disorder have been developed. There are several ways to categorize theories of stuttering. Bloodstein's (1995) etiological schema included classifications of theories into the following types: breakdown, repressed need, and anticipatory struggle. These three broad contextual categories provide one framework for thinking about stuttering theories, but other perspectives exist. Guitar (1998) describes theories in terms of factors that appear to contribute to stuttering. The organically based theories are covered in the context of *constitutional* factors, and the psychological and learning-based theories are explained on the bases of *developmental and environmental* factors. He also offered other possibilities, including motor-based, psycholinguistic-based, or social-based theories. The chapters covering the specific theories of stuttering in this text, both as a disorder and as abnormal speech events, classify them broadly according to psychological and biological theories.

Science, Superstition, and Stories About Stuttering

Historically, human notions of the cause and correction of stuttering have varied widely. In a historical account of speech disorders, Klingbell (1939) noted that several centuries B.C., Hippocrates, "The Father of Medicine," thought that stuttering may be due to chronic diarrhea that he observed in people who stutter, the treatment of which resulted in ulcers. One story from ancient Greece proposes that Demosthenes, the statesman, improved his stuttering by the exercise of speaking with pebbles in his mouth. Among many others, Klingbell also lists De Chauliac (A.D. 1300–1380), who ascribed stuttering "to convulsions, ulcers, or other or other affections of the tongue, to paralysis, or to moisture of the nerves or muscles." Several surgical interventions were performed on the tongues of people who stuttered beginning in 1840 by the German surgeon Deiffenbach and later by others because it was believed that anatomical defects cause stuttering.

According to Klingbell (1939), prosthetic devices were also developed and patented in the 1800s. For example, in 1838, Itard, a French physician, constructed ivory or gold forks placed in the cavity of the alveolar arch of the lower jaw for the purpose of supporting the supposedly weak tongue. Other constructed devices to be worn over the tongue to add to its weight and supposedly improve stuttering. In contrast, in the early 1900s, people who stutter were given lessons in elocution, reflecting the belief that stuttering is caused by insufficient practice with skills of word usage and pronunciation (Wingate, 1997). It is still true today that, in some cultures, religious ceremonies are conducted to cast out the evil spirits that are thought to cause stuttering (St. Louis,

1986). Although it is understandable why ancient peoples or the contemporary general population may have many diverse ideas and experience confusion over the cause of stuttering, it has also been true that scientists have expressed vastly divergent perspectives on this disorder.

The long unresolved search for the cause of stuttering frequently has been compared to the story of the blind men and the elephant (Johnson, 1958):

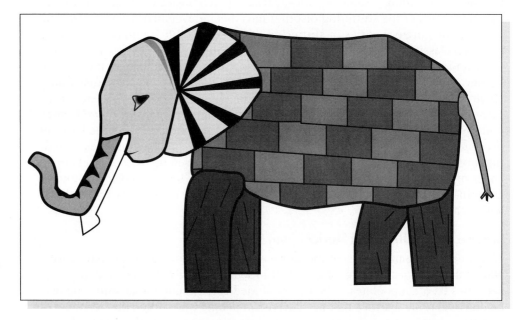

A fable from India tells of six blind men who had never met an elephant before visiting the Rajah's palace. The first blind man touched its body and announced, "An elephant is like a wall." The second grasped its ear, and corrected: "An elephant is like a fan." The third man wrapped his arms around a leg, and declared: "The elephant is like a tree." The fourth felt the trunk and countered, "The elephant is more like a snake." The fifth was poked by a tusk, and warned: "The elephant is like a spear!" And the sixth held the tail, and concluded: "The elephant is like a rope." An argument developed as each man insisted on his on own perspective. When the Rajah heard them, he instructed: "The elephant is bigger than each part you have touched. Only by putting all your parts together will you understand what the elephant is really like."

Unfortunately, this is exactly the kind of problem that has plagued the development of stuttering theory over the years. Although many causal theories have been proposed, often they have been limited to one, or a select few, of the various facets of stuttering. To date, no one has quite managed to blend the elements of truth of the various theories into a single, clear, testable, and, therefore, satisfactory system of explanation. A story could be told about stuttering that parallels the story of the six blind men and the elephant, only the story would be about six researchers who sought to explain stuttering. In this story, each researcher observed a different stuttering phenomenon (or phenomena) and applied the results, reaching a different conclusion about its cause. The first researcher, after observing that people do not stutter when they sing, concluded that stuttering must be a problem of vocal dysfunction. A second researcher, who observed that people do not stutter when speaking in time to a metronome beat, asserted that stuttering must be a problem of speech rhythm. Yet a third researcher, who experimented with the control of speech fluency using delayed auditory feedback, reasoned that stuttering must be caused by a disorder of the auditory system. A fourth researcher, noting enhanced fluency when people speak in a monotone, decided that stuttering must be caused by deficient skill with suprasegmentals such as inflection and intonation. The fifth researcher, who observed that in a stuttering block, the speaker stops air from flowing, proposed that stuttering must be a problem of respiration. Finally, the sixth researcher, who found that unison speech is nearly always fluent, argued that stuttering arises from psychological reactions invoked only when talking to other people (i.e., difficulty with communicating meaningful, propositional speech).

> In an exchange of commentaries in 1990, diverse views regarding stuttering were expressed. Bloodstein opined that it is not worth being concerned over precise definitions of stutter events or observer agreement of judgments because the essence of stuttering should be recognized as "a tense and fragmented way of speaking" (Bloodstein, 1990, p. 393). Ingham asserted that we need more sophisticated observational measures for stutter events to establish a data-based understanding of the disorder. Smith said an all-encompassing framework is needed—one that does not take an either/or stance on the question of biological versus behavioral but allows for the contribution of both, among other factors. Finally, Perkins insisted on concern with what most distresses the person who stutters—the sense of a loss of control.

If the story actually ended there, the problem might be manageable, but stuttering researchers and clinicians have not limited their perspectives to only six conclusions. Rather, we are faced with a plethora of old, new, and recycled observations and related conclusions about stuttering, each from another point of view. Because researchers struggle with the multiple and inconsistent findings related to stuttering, conflicts regarding interpretation abound. The essential nature of stuttering has been highly controversial. An example of controversy between two opposing views is as follows: "I can find no evidence that the person who stutters is physically different from anyone else, therefore stuttering must be psychological," whereas the opposite stance may be asserted: "I can find no convincing evidence that people who stutter are psychologically different from anyone else, therefore stuttering must be physical." Such examples suggest that how we think about stuttering influences our theoretical position. Like the matter of whether the cup is half empty or half full, notions about causality and the nature of stuttering may be different depending on whether, for example, we consider the onset of stuttering to represent the acquisition of new disfluency symptoms or the loss of an already existing fluency. Similarly, because stuttering itself leads to frequent consternation for those who stutter, conflicts among researchers have been frequent as well. The literature in stuttering is sprinkled with frequent exchanges in the form of letters to the editor representing the struggle with resolution of differences and communication of diverse perspectives. One example is the series of commentary papers (letters) published by Bloodstein (1990), Ingham (1990), Smith (1990), and Perkins (1990b) revealing controversy about the nature of stuttering, its perceptual definition, and the conditions for validating when it has occurred.

The Need for an Integrated Framework

Because ideas about stuttering have been so numerous and difficult to reconcile, many scholars have appreciated the proposal that "workers in the area of stuttering should adopt a multifactorial, nonlinear, and dynamic framework" for the disorder (Smith & Kelly, 1997, p. 205). By multifactorial, it is meant that many variables contribute to the occurrence of stuttering. By nonlinear and dynamic, it is meant that even slight differences may upset the balance of interactions among processes within the complex speech/language production system, yielding disproportionately large disruptions of speech in the form of stuttering. Within the context of a multifactorial model, a wider variety of diverse facts and associated phenomena can be explained. Another potential advantage of multifactorial models is that they may aid in the discovery of how different combinations of variables lead to specific profiles of the stuttering disorder. In this respect, the concept of stuttering subtypes or several different profiles for stuttering is relevant. We discuss the topic of subtypes later in this chapter.

Modeling the complex interaction of multiple etiological factors in stuttering raises issues and challenges. To illustrate, consider Figure 5.1, in which components

Figure 5.1: **Hypothetical Example of a Multifactorial (Multiple Components) Model of Stuttering**

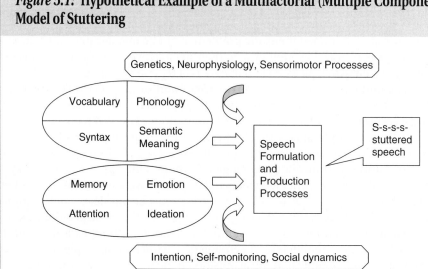

that may influence stuttering are presented in a flowchart. The uppermost section represents the various underlying physical constitution factors. The ovals represent language abilities at the top, psychological factors in the middle, and interpersonal and relational dynamics at the bottom. Additional and/or alternative factors could be shown in such a model. The flowchart could also be augmented by including feedback loops, interactions among factors, and by emphasizing the relative influence of various aspects (e.g., by means of size of the font). The specific details of this multifactorial dynamic model would need to be worked out, but the purpose at this point is to grasp the concept for this type of theoretical proposal.

Criteria for Strong Theories and Models

Recall that a theory is a scientific framework that accounts for a set of facts or observed phenomena. Scientific theories are based on evidence and lead to predictions about future occurrences that may be observed and tested. Thus when various models and theories of stuttering are presented in the chapters that follow, what criteria should be applied in evaluating their strength? We suggest the following nine criteria:

> *Validity.* To be valid, the theory must fit observed phenomena. If a researcher proposed that stuttering is caused by inaccurate articulation, someone might challenge the theory with data revealing a substantial proportion of people who stutter who do not make articulation errors. As conflicting facts or observations are uncovered, they undermine the validity of a theory. Although most scientific theories are challenged by some exceptions to their rules, those that face too many lose credibility. Hence scientists must maintain openness to new ideas. When a prevailing theory has become popular, people tend to ignore inconsistent evidence; instead, they doubt the unexpected findings. Consensus of opinion does not validate a theory and is not a substitute for hard data. A theory must always be reexamined in light of the factual evidence.
>
> *Exhaustiveness.* Theories are most useful when they provide a comprehensive explanation that speaks to all the related observations and phenomena. When only one or a limited number of associated phenomena are explained, it is less than satisfying. If a theory only explains why stuttering tends to occur at the beginnings of utterances, but not its variability across situations, it does not account for all the phenomena. It has failed the test of being exhaustive. Rarely is a theory completely exhaustive; nonetheless, a strong theory of stuttering would account for its variability related to a host of factors and conditions.
>
> *Elegance.* This criterion refers to theory simplicity. A theory is elegant when it explains a large number of observations in the most succinct way. When a theory is elegant, specific observations are satisfactorily replaced by a comprehensive generalization.

Parsimony. This is the capability of using the smallest number of variables or components to account for the greatest number of facts. When there are numerous phenomena to explain, as is the case with stuttering, with its many ameliorating conditions, varying symptoms, and so on, it is particularly challenging to develop a parsimonious theory. Can a comprehensive, multifactorial model of stuttering also be parsimonious? Which components of stuttering theory are necessary? For example, if a theory were developed that included psychosocial, psycholinguistic, and psychoemotional dynamics, one should consider whether the psychosocial and psychoemotional factors are independent or overlap in some way. The necessity of each component of a theoretical model must be tested and based on experimentation.

Exclusivity. Overlap of content or concepts within a theory means the factors are not exclusive. Such overlap contributes to confusion and complication. Similarly, across theories, if overlap is present, then researchers must be careful not to consider the ideas to be anything new. For example, one model of stuttering may suggest that emotional reactions are a cause of its progression, and another may attribute its escalation specifically to anxiety. When the second theory is proposed, it could be criticized for not being sufficiently exclusive from the original proposal because anxiety could be viewed as a part of emotional reactions. A new theory is more credible when it contributes concepts that are actually distinct from others.

Testability. As mentioned previously, it is very important for a theory to be testable. If there is no way to disprove the hypotheses generated by the theory, then the theory has no basis in observable facts. Without observable facts to support the theory, it is no better than myth.

Let's say that numerous reports revealed that stuttering continues to occur regardless of variations in the speaking conditions. Someone may generate the idea that stuttering happens in the presence of mystery element Q. According to the scholar who proposed this new theory, element Q has unknown properties except that in its presence, stuttering occurs. Such a theory must be discouraged because there is no way to test it. The theory cannot be proved or disproved until some concrete properties of Q are actually described. It should be clear, therefore, that a theory is not sufficiently credible unless it can be tested.

Prediction. Much of a theory's strength is its usefulness in forecasting future observations under specified conditions; in other words, it needs to be predictive. If certain factors are present, would stuttering consistently occur? If certain factors are not present, can stuttering be prevented?

Consistency. It is important for the various components of a theory to agree with each other. Within any proposed theory, there is the possibility of contradictory content. For example, if a theory suggests a motoric cause for stuttering but proposes that motor deficits are not involved, it is unsatisfying as much as it contradicts itself. When components of a theory work together

Table 5.1: Criteria for Evaluating the Credibility of a Theory or Model

Valid	The model fits the observed phenomena.
Exhaustive	The model explains all associated phenomena.
Elegant	The model is succinct (explains multiple observations with a larger generalization).
Parsimonious	The model uses the smallest number of components to explain the most facts.
Exclusive	The model does not overlap with other explanations.
Testable	The model and its components can be tested and proved or disproved.
Predictive	The model makes predictions about future observations.
Consistent	The model's components do not contradict each other (internal consistency).
Flexible	The model can be expanded or changed with new information.

well, without contradicting each other, the theory is more credible because it is internally consistent.

Flexibility. A theory is an ever-changing, expanding system of understanding. It must be able to accommodate change as new observations and discoveries are made. The issue of whether a theory can be readily modified and refined to accommodate new knowledge describes its property of being dynamic or flexible.

Table 5.1 summarizes the nine criteria just presented and discussed.

Testing Theories and Models

Having reviewed criteria for a strong theory, what issues need to be considered and what problems are encountered in application? History suggests stuttering has been the topic of more research in the field of communication disorders than any other area. So why is it taking so long to develop a strong theory of stuttering?

Potential difficulties arise in regard to *observation*. Scientific theories should be supported at least by observed evidence. It is quite difficult to evaluate the causal nature of particular variables in relation to stuttering. It requires careful consideration of their properties, their timing, and the nature of their association to stuttering. As we alluded to in Chapter 3, it is extremely difficult for scientists to observe the very first stuttering episode of a 3-year-old to support their theory that parental reaction to normal disfluency has been the cause of stuttering. Those holding to the theory may count on the fact that it is almost impossible to prove them wrong. Furthermore, to test theories, research must include experimental (dynamic) support and not merely circumstantial evidence. For example, based on observed circumstantial evidence of a number of people who stutter, one might propose that stuttering can be caused by attempts to speak on inspiratory airflow. Dynamic evidence should be obtained, however, by experiments designed to manipulate the variable of inspiratory airflow to observe the resultant effect on stuttering. Only if stuttering was observed to respond to the direct manipulation of the variable could we conclude the relationship is potentially causal rather than circumstantial. Association between two or more phenomena or factors is insufficient for demonstrating causal relations. Of course, sometimes the contribution of variables is not simply a matter of "yes" or "no." A factor may contribute to better fluency without directly causing it. Certain variables may improve (e.g., noise) or exacerbate (e.g., fatigue) stuttering, even if they are not directly responsible for it. This is why the separation of circumstantial from dynamic evidence is essential.

Still another issue that poses a challenge to theorizing is the *precision* of the observations made of the phenomena under study. Those seeking to explain stuttering must observe stuttering. If a scientist mistakes another form of nonfluent speech, for example, cluttering, for stuttering and then formulates a theory or model based on the results, conclusions may be drawn that are not pertinent to actual stuttering. If scientists do not carefully isolate and define the essential speech characteristics of stuttering, to distinguish it from other forms of speech breakdown, erroneous conclusions are likely to result, leading to faulty theories and models.

Several more difficulties arise when scientists attempt to draw causal inferences from observations of any given phenomenon. One is that of co-occurrence. Let's return to the inspiratory airflow hypothesis. Suppose that nearly every time someone stutters, there is evidence of an attempt to speak on inspiration. One possibility is that the inspiratory airflow has a causal connection to the stuttering. It could also be the case, however, that both the inspiratory airflow and the stuttering are separate results of the same underlying, yet unknown, abnormality. Also, factors deemed responsible for a given phenomenon must have unique roles in relation to it. For example, fatigue might be a proposed component in a model of stuttering, but if fatigue leads to the interruption of many kinds of human abilities besides speech fluency, a case may be made that this factor does not play a critical, unique role.

Another issue central to theories concerning living organisms (i.e., humans) is the element of *time and age*. What is meant here is that variables causally related to the phenomenon may not be identical, and/or may not occur in the same proportions or hold the same importance, across its life stages. For example, a plant grows underground without light for a while, but later, after it appears above ground, light aids substantially, or may even be necessary, to its growth. That is, the effect of light varies in relation to the stage of the plant's life. The same is apt to be true with respect to stuttering; that is, variables responsible for the onset of stuttering in early childhood may be different (in type and/or degree) from those maintaining it later, as a person ages. For example, anxiety, so common in older children and adults, is seldom an apparent factor at the earliest stage of stuttering in preschool children.

In general, testing theories of stuttering has been remarkably challenging due to (1) inherent difficulties of observing its onset, an important aspect of several theories, (2) its changing characteristics during aging, (3) the inconsistent occurrence of stuttering-related speech events from moment to moment and from situation to situation, (4) technical limitations in testing theories (e.g., what can animal research offer?), and (5) ethical problems for setting up scientific experiments (e.g., conditions that may induce a person to stutter), and (6) a highly likely possibility that stuttering results from a multiplicity of factors. Further, the relevance of factors may differ depending on the age, development, and experiences of the individual, as well as the number, type, and amount of specific factors.

> A theory is a set of interrelated concepts, principles, and definitions that present a systematic view of a phenomenon, specifying relationships among the relevant variables for purposes of description, explanation, and prediction (Kerlinger, 1986). What must take place in order to arrive at a sound theory? Scientists need to agree on a framework specifying the exogenous (e.g., environmental) and endogenous (e.g., genetic) variables to be studied. Measurement issues must be resolved. Hypotheses must be generated and tested to reveal the systematic relationships among the variables. Confounding factors or control variables must be isolated. Finally, skillful experimentation and multiple observations must be undertaken to refine the range and boundaries of relationships among the variables.

Are There Stuttering Subtypes?

With few exceptions, every entity in the universe can find its place within a system of classification. Systems of classification usually take the form of taxonomies with a hierarchy of divisions and subdivisions. The scientific classification of plants, for example, is based on a hierarchy moving from broad to specific cases according to phylum, class, order, genus, and species. The taxonomic system applied has an important role in the organization and enhancement of knowledge about any particular entity. It is the basis by which we understand which things are similar and which things are different. The question of subtypes is the matter of whether there are subdivisions to be made among people who stutter and/or what form of classification system to apply.

Although certain features of stuttering are relatively consistent, such as the age at onset of the disorder and the presence of certain core speech disfluencies, there are large differences in many aspects of the disorder across people who stutter, including variations in expression of symptoms and their severity. As discussed in Chapter 1, in addition to symptom diversity, in many ways the disorder of stuttering is interwoven with linguistic, phonetic, cognitive, social, emotional, physiological domains, as well as others. Additionally, it has been explained as emerging from a wide range of possible etiologies. A hint of possible taxonomic development for stuttering disorders is evident in literature. For example, a basic division of stuttering disorders has been noted according to age at stuttering onset. Stuttering with an onset in childhood (prior to adolescence) is considered *developmental*, whereas adult onset stuttering is considered to be *acquired*. Within the developmental stuttering framework are two types of divisions—*classic stuttering* and *cluttering*—distinguished mainly by symptomatology. Within the acquired stuttering framework, there also have been two types of cases—*neurogenic* stuttering and *psychogenic* stuttering—distinguished primarily on the basis of etiology.

With these multiple related domains and etiological classes in mind, is it possible that stuttering is not a single disorder? That is, might different combinations of several or all of the factors just cited create variations that are substantial enough to make clinically meaningful differences? After all, similarly sounding hoarse voices can be a symptom of vastly different disorders: vocal fold cancer, vocal fold infection, or vocal fold paralysis. Alternatively, is it possible that stuttering is a single disorder but contains subtypes of overt variations, such as seen in cleft palate speech that may result from unilateral cleft, bilateral cleft, and other types of clefts? The fact is that for a long time stuttering has been generally considered to be a unitary disorder without an acceptable subclassification system. St. Onge and Calvert's (1964) remark that stuttering has been viewed as a "pathognomonic monolith" (p. 160) nicely summarizes this perspective. The two scholars, however, questioned this view by posing these questions: "What are we studying when we study stuttering? Whatever it is, is it one, several, or many?" (p. 160) and went on to imply that stuttering is not a unitary disorder.

An altogether different view has stipulated that stuttering, at least its overt speech features, is not even a unique disorder but a *quantitative* deviation along the continuum of normal speech disfluency. In other words, stutterers simply do more of the same of what normally fluent speakers do (Bloodstein, 1970). We disagree with Bloodstein and posit that stuttering is a unique disorder, qualitatively different from other disfluent speech. Still the question of whether it composes discrete subtypes deserves attention. The implications to the development of theory and related research are obvious. If subtypes exist, do they differ in their etiological components or the relative contributions of other factors? Does the nature of the disorder vary significantly among its subtypes? Do they follow different developmental courses, such as natural recovery or chronic stuttering? Not less important is the question of whether subtypes respond differentially to various treatments.

Van Riper (1982) noted that that the concept of stuttering subtypes is traceable to at least the 16th century when it was proposed that stuttering is caused by either brain hyperexcitability or by emotionality. New subtype classifications of stuttering have surfaced throughout the modern history of speech pathology as reflected in the writings of Froeschels (1943) and the more current work of Riley and Riley (2000). In a recent review of the literature, Yairi (2007) suggested that many of the systems offered can be grouped into seven categories based on their frame of reference. These are listed next with an example of a classification under each category:

I. *Etiology*: Brill's (1923) classification based on personality problems (e.g., depressive, psychoneurotic, psychopathic) and stuttering.
II. *Prominent stuttering characteristics*: Froeschels (1943) classification of Clonic and Tonic stuttering.
III. *Reaction to drugs*: Alm's (2004b) classification of Type 1 and Type 2 stutterers who, respectively, decrease or increased stuttering in response to dopamine.
IV. *Biological characteristics*: Hinkle's (1971) classification of right ear preference (RE), left ear preference (LE), and no preference (NE), reflecting hemispheric brain dominance, and are also associated with a different stuttering pattern.

V. *Concomitant disorders*: J. Riley's (1971) distinction between stuttering children exhibiting language deficits and those exhibiting inferior motor skills.

VI. *Developmental course*: Van Riper's (1971) four distinguished developmental courses of stuttering.

VII. *Statistically generated models* (multifactorial): Prins and Lohr's (1972) Types I—syllable repetitions/sound prolongations, and Type II—secondary physical movements, word substitutions.

Although ideas have been generated, little research has been conducted that is specifically concerned with stuttering subtype differentiation (e.g., Berlin, 1954; Feinberg, Griffin, & Levey, 2000; Schwartz & Conture, 1988). More typically, researchers have focused on a single dimension of stuttering (e.g., disfluency behaviors, motor skills, language abilities, personality, brain hemispheric lateralization, and others), thereby overlooking the multifaceted nature of the problem. These studies were also restricted in scope (e.g., small numbers), lacked adequate experimental controls, and were not situated within a clear theoretical framework. Perhaps due to these limitations they have not succeeded in generating strong evidence for straightforward typologies. So far, the scientific activities in this area have not translated meaningfully into the practical levels of either clinical management or the design of studies. None of the proposed classification systems for stuttering as a disorder has been adopted by a significant number of professionals. In spite of more sophisticated recent research (see reviews by Seery, Watkins, Mangelsdorf, & Shigeto, 2007, and Yairi, 2007), it would appear that the inclination to investigate and treat stuttering as a single disorder has generally prevailed. The point most related to this chapter is that if subtypes of stuttering need to be recognized, then our theories and models of stuttering need to be sufficiently dynamic to accommodate the requisite divisions and subdivisions.

Summary

Many diverse ideas about the cause of stuttering have been proposed. The so-called theories of stuttering have been based on etiologic models borrowed from the fields of medicine, psychology, and education, and they represent potential classifications of theories. There have been many controversies over the cause of stuttering. The numerous and diverse observations of stuttering and associated phenomena have led to varied opinions about the nature of the disorder. Multifactorial theories and model and subtype profiling based on multiple dimensions may lead to more satisfying models of stuttering.

Theories of stuttering must meet a number of evaluation criteria to be considered credible; that is, each must fit observed phenomena, make predictions about future observations, and be testable. An acceptable theory must explain all of the associated phenomena in the most succinct way. Its components must not contradict each other nor overlap with other possible explanations. Finally, it must have the potential to be expanded and/or changed with the acquisition of new information. Research will add credence to a theory when it reveals dynamic rather than merely circumstantial evidence. Stuttering is not apt to be explained by simple principles overgeneralized across the heterogeneous population of people who stutter. There is reason to believe that the etiology of stuttering may be different from the factors that precipitate its onset and that govern its progression.

Satisfying taxonomies of stuttering disorders and stuttering events have yet to be developed. It is also not yet clear whether stuttering is better understood as a condition varying along a continuum (dimensional) or as a condition characterized by heterogeneous subtypes. Subtypes may eventually be identified through profiling of multiple etiologic source factors or through more sophisticated models of the systems underlying speech fluency. In the chapters that follow, we examine possible etiologic source factors and attempt to expand our understanding of systems that contribute to fluency and stuttering.

As briefly discussed earlier, theories of stuttering have been grouped in several ways. For the tutorial purposes of this textbook, the question of why people stutter is handled by breaking it down into several subquestions: Is stuttering motor-physiological? Is stuttering psycho-emotional? Is stuttering cognitive-linguistic? Is stuttering developed or learned? Is stuttering genetic? Is stuttering multidimensional? As we explore each of these potential etiologies, it will be important to understand that the answers to these questions are not mutually exclusive. Moreover, it is worth remembering that the various source factors may be differentially relevant for separate subtypes of stuttering disorders.

STUDY QUESTIONS AND DISCUSSION TOPICS

1. What is the difference between a theory and a model?
2. What difficulties are encountered in attempting to provide observational data in support of a theory of stuttering?
3. Generate a *theory* statement related to stuttering, and answer these questions:
   a. Is your theory related to the stuttering event or the disorder?
   b. Is your theory about an isolated aspect or a comprehensive explanation?
   c. How well does your theory meet the criteria of being valid, exhaustive, exclusive, predictive, consistent, parsimonious, elegant, testable, and dynamic?
4. Ask a few people from outside the field of communicative disorders whether they believe stuttering is a biologically or psychologically based disorder, and to explain why they think that way. Were you surprised by what they think? Why? Did they use facts as a basis for the belief? Are there facts that you know about stuttering that were not considered in their beliefs?
5. Based on what you know about stuttering, do you think the disorder may be better characterized in terms of subtypes? Why or why not?

SUGGESTED READINGS

Packman, A., & Attanasio, J. (2004). *Theoretical issues in stuttering*. New York: Psychology Press.

Perkins, W. (1999). *Stuttering and science*. San Diego, CA: Singular.

Wingate, M. (1997). *Stuttering: A short history of a curious disorder*. Westport, CT: Bergin & Garvey.

Chapter 6: Is Stuttering Psychological? Psychoemotional, Psychobehavioral, and Psycholinguistic Theories

LEARNER OBJECTIVES

Readers will be able to understand and critically evaluate:

- Theories of the psychoemotional contributions to stuttering.
- Theories of the psychobehaviorial contributions to stuttering.
- Theories of the psycholinguistic contributions to stuttering.

Is Stuttering Psychological?

Many speech-language clinicians, including ourselves, have been asked by people in social situations, or by clients and/or their family members in clinical settings, whether stuttering is "psychological." The typical underlying meaning of the question is whether stuttering is caused by "nerves" or psychological issues. Repeated experience has taught us that most laypeople raising this question already think so; their questions merely seek confirmation of their own beliefs. Furthermore, a study based on personal interviews of adolescents who stutter regarding their "theory" of stuttering found that they, too, adhere to psychological factors as probable causes (Fraiser, 1955).

Usually these presumptions treat the concept of "psychological" with a limited perspective confined to the psychoemotional, if not psychopathological, domain. The extent of various psychological dimensions, however, and their potential contributions to stuttering is, in fact, much broader. We recognize three major classes of psychological theories of stuttering: psychoemotional, psychobehavioral, and psycholinguistic. Psychoemotional theories propose that stuttering is based in some psychological maladjustment. Psychobehavioral theories attribute stuttering to learning or conditioning processes. Psycholinguistic theories explain stuttering in terms of cognitive systems underlying the production of speech and language. In the following sections, we explore the essence of these theoretical orientations, related research, their contributions to the understanding of stuttering, and their clinical implications.

Psychoemotional Theories

Psychoemotional theories propose that psychological traumas or emotional disturbances or personality characteristics are the original cause of stuttering. Early written accounts of these psychologically based models of the genesis of stuttering emerged in the 1920s, and investigations of stuttering as a psychopathological disorder reached a peak around the 1950s (see Goodstein, 1958, and Sheehan, 1958, for comprehensive reviews). The early psychoemotional theories of stuttering (e.g., Brill, 1923; Coriat, 1928, 1943b) were influenced by the basic premises of psychoanalytic theory, originally offered by Sigmund Freud (1899, 1901). One such assumption was that behaviors and actions can be triggered by earlier traumas to the psyche. The *psyche* was, in essence, the human soul or self, placed in central charge of thoughts and actions. Freud conceived of the psyche as having three parts: the id, the ego, and the superego. The *id* consists of unconscious instinctual drives, the *ego* engages in conscious decisions, and the *superego* is the moral conscience judging the goodness or badness of thoughts and actions. For example, if the ego experiences a threat or trauma, and the id is inclined toward self-protection through violence, the ego may notice violent thoughts surfacing into consciousness. The superego may judge violent thoughts and actions as unacceptable, and so in turn, the ego may refuse to deal with them, pushing the impulses back deeper into the id's unconscious motivations (i.e., *repressing* them). Thus reactions to trauma within the psyche may be repressed but rise to the surface of ego consciousness as compulsive thoughts or actions, still basically violent but having a more acceptable form. So stuttering, for example, might stem from a violent impulse that was repressed and converted into a more acceptable form.

Freud proposed that conflicts of a sexual nature are at the heart of nearly all psychoneuroses, which are mental disturbances characterized by disordered thoughts and actions expressed in socially acceptable forms. For example, repressed unconscious sexual desires of the id might be turned into anxiety or physical symptoms because these are more acceptable socially. A number of Freud's followers (and the authors of this text) disagree with the idea that all psychoneuroses are primarily rooted in psychosexual conflicts. This idea, however, had a strong influence on several early stuttering theories, and some elements of these theories contributed to later psychoemotional theories of stuttering.

Because stuttering begins in childhood, the early theories were based on Freud's model of child psychosexual development. Freud maintained a child's psyche is developed in response to the id's sexual energy or drive, referred to as *libido*. The libido takes on a different character at various stages and/or ages of early childhood. The three psychosexual stages and corresponding ages were the *oral* stage (0 to 18 months); *anal* stage (18 months to 3.5 years), and *phallic-oedipal* stage (3 to 6 years). The following examples of stuttering theories propose psychoneuroses that vary in relation to the particular stage of its development.

During the oral stage, the libido is concentrated in the lips and mouth. Sucking is the child's main source of pleasure. Emotional disturbances may arise, for example, if the mother is resentful about nursing or when weaning takes place. Some children may not like it. Generally, psychoemotional fixation at this stage is seen when there is a continued need for oral gratification. Eventually this will result in a personality characterized by dependency and passivity throughout life if not adequately resolved.

Coriat (1928) opined that stuttering primarily represents a fixation at the oral stage. He explained it was a symptom of an unhealthy solution to the unconscious conflict between a wish for infantile suckling, which is socially unacceptable, and the need for a more appropriate behavior. Summing it up in his own words, Coriat stated that "in the speech of stammerers the illusion of nursing is maintained and the oral gratification continued by this illusory substitution for the maternal nipple, the stammerer thus retaining his mother into adult life" (quoted by Hahn, 1956, p. 29). The symbolic nature of the outward symptom—stuttering, strange as it might be seen—is demonstrated by this example.

During the anal stage, libido is concentrated in gratification of the anus as the child becomes focused on fecal elimination and retention. Children are often fascinated with their own feces; some may even try to put them in their mouth. Toilet training is the backdrop for ensuing psychoemotional issues. Parental interference and pressure can create emotional disturbances at this stage eventually leading to problems with self-control and compulsiveness, but also underlying anger and aggressiveness. At this age, however, expressions of infantile anger and aggressiveness are no longer socially acceptable.

Fenichel (1945) regarded stuttering as a psychoneurosis originating at the anal stage of psychosexual development. Conflicts stemming from ungratified urges toward the retention and expulsion of feces are resolved in an unhealthy manner when the child displaces its expression upward to another sphincter, the mouth. This is another case of stuttering serving as a symbolic symptom. It is an acceptable form of "smearing" listeners with aggressiveness and hostility. Because stuttering is socially tolerated, even if painful to the child, the expression of true feelings goes unpunished. Bear in mind that these dynamics are buried deep within the unconscious psyche. The person who stutters is not aware of it. The constant neurotic anxiety experienced is general and nonspecific because the source remains known.

The common theme of the early psychoemotional theories depicts stuttering as a deep-seated neurosis involving a conversion reaction. The unconscious mind converts its hidden, objectionable urges into an openly acceptable form, even if unpleasant, expressing them as stuttering. Early proponents often debated about whether the stutterer's unmet psychosexual impulses in infancy were oral or anal in nature (Carp, 1962; Glauber, 1958; Lowinger, 1952; Moskowitz, 1941). Counterintuitively, anal, rather than oral, fixation was the most frequently supported basis for stuttering (Bloodstein, 1995; Dickson, 1954, 1971; Fisher, 1970). These theories were the first among several implicating parent-child interactions in stuttering etiology.

More recent psychoanalytic theories of stuttering were presented in the middle of the 20th century (e.g., Barbara, 1954; Glauber, 1958; Travis, 1957). Sheehan (1953) proposed that stuttering was a symptom of repressed needs, inhibited aggressions, or other "unspeakable feelings" (an expression used later by Travis, 1971) leading to simultaneous urges to speak and to hold back from speaking. Noting strong rejection of stuttering children by their fathers, Clark and Snyder (1955) contended that stuttering reflects basic disturbances in the child-father relationship, including fear of authority figures and lack of well-defined masculine identification. Similarly centered on parental influence, Murphy and Fitzsimmons (1960) viewed stuttering as a tension-reducing symptom emanating from parents' overprotective attitudes. Travis (1957, 1971) explained that the person who stutters is caught in the conflict between repressed urges to suck, eat, evacuate, and explore sexual pleasures, and the parentally induced inhibition of these forbidden needs. The person resents, even hates, these impositions, must abide by them, and has guilt feelings for even harboring such drives. These must be repressed. At the same time, there are mixed feelings of love and guilt toward the parents. Such conflicts are unconsciously resolved through a symbolic symptom: stuttering. It allows the person to express the forbidden impulses and simultaneously punish the guilt without showing these urges to others.

Logically, psychoemotionally oriented theories that depict stuttering as a psychoneurosis also advocate psychoanalysis as the therapy of choice. This technique aims at bringing the unconscious closer to conscious to allow the client better insight into the real problems, and thus be able to deal with them in a more healthy manner. Several programs based in this approach are discussed in Chapter 10. The main criticism of the previous theories, however, is that they were largely based on circumstantial evidence. The supporting observations tended to be strongly influenced by a biased perspective. In the next section, some of the research related to psychoemotional disturbances in people who stutter is discussed.

Related Research

The early theories generated interest in whether people who stutter possessed personality characteristics similar to other groups with psychoemotional disturbances. Investigators, intent to put the hypothesis of similarity between stutterers and people with abnormal psychology to the test, conducted studies that compared people who stutter with psychiatric populations using a variety of methodologies and subjects across age ranges. Goodstein (1958), for example, compared adults who stutter with psychiatric patients. He concluded that the stutterers were not maladjusted by comparison, but found that they were more anxious, tense, and socially withdrawn than the third group, normal subjects. He cautioned, however, that it was impossible to know whether such attributes represented factors influencing the etiological development of stuttering or problems that emerged as a consequence of social reactions to stuttering. Sheehan (1958) similarly opined that the absence of a definite personality pattern among those who stutter made them different from other populations with emotional disorders, such as hysterical aphonia or depression. Nevertheless, he entertained the possibility that different personality dynamics among participants who stutter may have been obscured in typical group studies. He went further to support the concept of stuttering subtypes, stating that "it might follow that there are several different kinds of stutterers, psychologically speaking" (p. 24).

Nearly a quarter of a century later, Sermas and Cox (1982) assessed measures of abnormal personality among three groups: patients who stutter, patients with brain dysfunction (BD), and patients with personality disorders without brain dysfunction (NBD). To their credit, they employed multiple sources of data: psychiatric interviews, projective tests, and personality tests. The stuttering group scored significantly higher than the other two (BD and NBD) groups only on the interpersonal sensitivity subscale of one test. This subscale taps feelings of personal inadequacy, inferiority, and negative expectations during interpersonal interactions. The psychiatric interviews revealed that almost half of the stuttering group displayed noteworthy obsessive-compulsive tendencies, and 25% had experienced some depression. None of the stutterers, however, showed formal neurotic symptoms. Also, there was an insignificant trend for the stutterers to score higher than the other two groups on the measure of obsessive-compulsiveness. The interpretation of this investigation is limited by the absence of a control group of nonstuttering nonpsychiatric participants, the small sample size of 19 per group, and the participants' wide age range, from 16 to 48 years. Nonetheless, it would appear that although people who stutter are adversely affected by stuttering psychologically, they are not, as a group, evidencing any consistent form of personality disturbance.

What results of research could lead to acceptance of the commonly held belief that stuttering is rooted in psychoemotional causes? The potential evidence could take several forms. First, the onset of stuttering could frequently coincide with psychologically agitating events. Second, a sudden rather than gradual onset might be seen as more consistent with the premise of a psychologically agitating event. Third, natural recovery from stuttering would be found to co-occur in association with conditions that improve psychological adjustment. Fourth, if psychological (i.e., mental-emotional) states, such as anxiousness, nervousness, or fears, were at the root of stuttering, then age of stuttering onset would be distributed fairly evenly across the lifespan because people at any age can be vulnerable to such states. Fifth, apparently the most important, if certain personality characteristics or signs of emotional maladjustments were consistently noted among those who stutter, it would lend credence to an association between those psychological factors and stuttering.

What, then, do we know about these possibilities? Answering point by point to the above, stuttering onset coincides with emotionally stressful events in approximately 40% of the cases, but these vary in nature and are not typically traumatic. Similarly, onset tends to be sudden in about 40% of cases (Yairi & Ambrose, 2005). There is lack of support, however, for an association between chronological age and the onset of stuttering: Onset is sharply skewed to the early childhood period (see Chapter 3). Next, although psychological factors are sometimes important to the amelioration of stuttering among older children and adults undergoing treatment, research has not thus far revealed a noticeable role for these factors in the massive natural recovery experienced by preschool children. Finally, there have been mixed research results with respect to stuttering and personality links, but the bulk of the evidence has not revealed a specific stuttering personality profile or indication of psychological maladjustment (Bloodstein, 1995; Bloodstein & Bernstein Ratner, 2008).

Thus the evidence for a psychoemotional problem as the main cause for the onset of childhood stuttering is largely unsupported by research. If this is the case, why should we be interested in psychological theories of stuttering? Several answers come to mind. First, psychological dynamics could be one of several contributing factors responsible for the onset of stuttering in a subset of cases. Second, although psychological factors may not account for stuttering onset, they could contribute to the maintenance and progression of stuttering. Third, even if emotional states and personality traits are insufficient to predict cases of stuttering consistently, such factors may help to explain the timing of occurrence of speech events regarded as stuttering. Fourth, some people who stutter also exhibit emotional problems that, although not the cause of stuttering, complicate the problem and interfere with therapy. The individual's personality and temperament characteristics are also factors that influence the client's responses to therapy, for example, willingness to enter speaking situations with strangers. It is not surprising, therefore, that psychological theories and factors continue to attract interest, and exert influence on stuttering research and intervention. The review of additional research related to these questions appears in the next sections on factors of personality, anxiety, and temperament.

Personality Factors in Stuttering

Even if the evidence does not uphold theories of stuttering as an expression of psychopathology, another factor possibly contributing to stuttering etiology is personality structure. Goodstein (1958) published a review of a large number of personality studies of children who stutter. These investigations employed many kinds of instruments: formal tests of observation, personality inventories completed by parents, and free (word) association tasks. Regardless of methodology, results generally yielded no significant differences between groups of children who stutter and their nonstuttering peers. In the same publication, Goodstein also detailed findings and summarized results of approximately 40 personality studies of adults who stutter. Assessment tools used in these investigations included projective techniques, clinical interview, paper-and-pencil tests, and a variety of other inventories such as the Minnesota Multiphasic Personality Inventory (Walnut, 1954). A similar conclusion was drawn that no particular personality pattern of people who stutter could be identified based on the research. People who stutter appeared to represent the broad range of individual personalities that characterized people who do not stutter.

Also published in 1958, Sheehan reviewed 17 investigations with adults, school-age children, and preschool children who stutter in which projective techniques (e.g., Rorschach ink blots, Thematic Apperception Test pictures) or scales of aspiration levels were used. About half of these studies reported no significant differences between controls and individuals who stutter at various ages on multiple variables, such as morality, aggression, impulsivity, and obsessive-compulsive tendency. A few of these studies, however, suggested that those who stutter have greater tendencies for obsessions, compulsions, aggression, and ego defensiveness. Contradictory findings were also reported regarding levels of aspiration. Highlighting the inconsistent results of research, Sheehan, like Goldstein (1958), concluded there was very little to show that those who stutter, as a group, were different from anyone else. As mentioned earlier, however, the tendencies toward certain personality characteristics among adults who stutter could represent the impact of stuttering on the person rather than the cause of the stuttering.

Anxiety

There are two main areas of research relating anxiety and stuttering. One explores the potential influence of anxiety on stuttering events and their frequency. The second examines the tendency for people who stutter to experience anxiety.

Although it is not known to what extent increased response latencies set the stage for increased stuttering, the hypothesis appears tenable. Weber and Smith (1990) noted that the timing of elevated autonomic nervous system arousal was strongly associated with stutter events in people who stutter, and concluded that emotional factors may affect stuttering moments. In contrast, Gray and England (1972) found that the correspondence between stuttering frequency and anxiety was marginal in their 15 adults who received deconditioning treatment. Wingate (1975) observed that although 9 of 10 young adults who stutter claimed high predictionabilities for upcoming stuttering, their stuttering moments often did not occur on expected word locations. He raised doubts about the extent to which emotional responses trigger stutter events. He did not appear to consider the possibility, however, that these speakers may have just as much trouble predicting their emotional fluctuations as they do their stuttering. These results do not disprove a connection between anxious emotion and stuttering moments, only that a speaker's predictions of both may not be as strong as they believe.

Blood, Wertz, Blood, Bennett, and Simpson (1997) found that 75% of their 12 adults who stutter reported increased disfluency and stuttering on days with increased stress. By contrast, Toomey and Sidman (1970) found that although all four adults who stutter reported having anxiety in their threat-of-electrical shock situation, two increased and two decreased stuttering during the condition. Caruso, Chodzko-Zajko, Bidinger, and Sommers (1994) observed increased speech latency (longer reaction time) by those who stutter in a condition of cognitive stress, specifically speed pressure during a Stroop task (naming the color in which a word is presented, whereas the word itself spells a different color).

Regarding the second major research area related to stuttering and anxiety, a number of recent studies have noted significant differences in anxiety level/type between adults who stutter and normally fluent controls. Greiner, Fitzgerald, Cooke, and Djurdjic (1985) reported that adults who stuttered scored significantly higher than normally fluent controls on their measure of anxiety, the Willoughby Personality

Schedule (WPS, WPS-R). They suggested that those who stutter may have word-specific anxiety, situation-specific anxiety, and/or general anxiety. Later, Fitzgerald, Djurdjic, and Maguin (1992) used the same instrument (WPS-R) with a group of Yugoslavian adults who stutter and essentially replicated the findings of the Greiner et al. (1985) investigation. Specifically, stutterers scored higher on social isolation and social sensitivity, and lower on social confidence compared to control subjects.

Craig (1990) administered Spielberger's State-Trait Anxiety Inventory measure, called the STAI (Spielberger et al., 1983), to a large group of 102 adults who stutter before and after behavioral therapy for stuttering. Anxiety levels were also compared with a control group. Those who stuttered scored significantly higher on *state anxiety* in demanding speech situations, but they also scored higher than the controls on chronic, or *trait*, anxiety. Following treatment, the anxiety levels of those who stutter were in the normal range, although their scores remained higher than those of the controls. In a more recent investigation, Craig, Hancock, Tran, and Craig (2003) explored the associations between stuttering and anxiety in 63 people who stutter, age 15 or older, identified through a random telephone survey concerned with the incidence of stuttering. Using the STAI inventory, the stuttering group was found to have significantly higher anxiety scores than a nonstuttering control group. Thus more specific research supports the impression that people who stutter tend to experience significant state anxiety as a result of stuttering. Additionally, recent research findings concerning chronic trait anxiety in adults who stutter raises the possibility that personality is a predisposing factor for stuttering persistence.

Temperament

Several experts have proposed that one relatively stable dimension of personality, temperament, may contribute to the etiology of stuttering. Temperament refers to an "individual's sensitivity and responsivity to environmental demands" (Caprara & Cervone, 2000, p. 87). Individual temperament differences explain why people respond differently to the same stimulus conditions. Research suggests that temperament traits can be identified within the first year of life and, generally, remain stable throughout the lifespan (Caprara & Cervone, 2000).

Guitar (2006) suggested that a sensitive (i.e., reactive) temperament may predispose a child to stutter. Similarly, Perkins (1992b) suggested that children at risk for persistent stuttering were apt to be those who are more easily intimidated. Some evidence supports these hypotheses. For example, Riley and Riley (2000) found increased sensitivity (reactivity) and higher self-expectations among 50 school-age children who stutter, and Oyler (1996) concluded that school-age children who stutter were significantly more vulnerable and sensitive than children who do not stutter.

As mentioned in earlier chapters, some differences in temperament characteristics have been noted between preschool-age as well as school-age children who stutter and normally fluent children. The children who stutter were more reactive and more irregular in physiological functions, had less regulation of emotion and attention, were less apt to habituate to environment or adapt to changes in routine, and were less distractible when engaged in a task (Anderson et al., 2003; Karrass et al.,

2006; Schwenk, Conture, & Walden, 2007). Significantly less adaptability in children who stutter has been reported in several other studies as well (Embrechts, Ebben, Franke, & van de Poel, 2000; Howell et al., 2004). Findings in the opposite direction (i.e., being more adaptable), however, were reported in other investigations (e.g., Lewis & Golberg, 1997; Williams, 2006).

Although it is unclear whether tendencies toward greater sensitivity and reactivity and lower adaptability in children who stutter represent factors contributing to the etiology of stuttering at onset, it appears that personality differences are evident in children who have stuttered for a while. But these traits may not be specifically related to stuttering. Hauner, Shriberg, Kwiatkowski, and Allen (2005) reviewed temperament literature for children with a variety of communication disorders and concluded that children with speech and language disorders displayed significantly greater "sensitivity, anxiety, distractibility, neuroticism, withdrawal, and difficulty in adaptability" (p. 637) when compared to typically speaking peers. Hence children who stutter may merely show personality tendencies typical of children with a variety of communication disorders, not specifically linked to stuttering.

> Psychoemotional dimensions of stuttering may originate from several planes. As a primary cause, stuttering could be the overt symptom of an underlying psychoneurosis. From this vantage point, the disorder is energized by an unconscious conflict arising between, or among, opposing needs or motives of the psyche. From another angle, psychoemotional factors, such as extremely sensitivity temperament traits or anxiety tendencies, may serve in the role as secondary causes, by predisposing the speaker either to start stuttering or to persist in stuttering. Finally, seen from the flip side, people who stutter may be prone to develop psychoemotional disturbances as a result of stuttering.

Summary of Psychoemotional Theories

The popular long-standing laypersons' belief that stuttering is caused by emotional problems has also found expression in experts' theories, or theoretical notions, about this possible etiology of stuttering. The early theories in the modern era of speech pathology (the first third of the 20th century) were strongly influenced by Sigmund Freud's psychoanalytic theory of the human psyche with its strong emphasis on deep-seated, unconscious emotional problems and conflicts, which are outwardly expressed in physical symptoms such as stuttering. The stuttering, although unpleasant, serves as symbolic expression of the inner needs. Theories along this line were influenced by later variations of the psychoanalysis framework, and they continued to appear for several decades. For the most part, however, research studies have *not* offered sufficient evidence to support these theories. Research has failed to show that those who stutter are characterized by abnormal psychology, nor has it sufficiently described how such psychopathological factors would contribute to the disorder.

In many of the related studies, psychoemotional characteristics were inconsistent across subjects and across studies. When differences were found in emotional-social behavior (e.g., greater withdrawal from social activity), these can easily be seen as a normal reaction of the person who stutters to the difficulties presented by his or her speech problem. Recent studies, however, have provided reasonable evidence for greater levels of trait anxiety in people who stutter as well as hints of possible greater sensitivity in terms of temperament. It is interesting to note here that the diagnosogenic theory of stuttering (discussed in the next section), which is framed primarily within learning perspectives, emphasizes the child's sensitivity to listeners' reactions as an important factor in the onset of stuttering. Perhaps Sheehan's notions of subtypes of stutterers is worth renewed consideration because there may be a subgroup of people who stutter who have at-risk personalities. Further research is needed to examine whether psychoemotional factors (e.g., hypersensitivity) might have a role in the persistence of stuttering.

Psychobehavioral Theories

The basic concept underlying the psychobehavioral theories is that stuttering is a learned behavior, that is, an acquired rather than constitutionally based disorder. This learning may take place in a variety of ways. It may progress slowly as in the formation of a habit, consistent with a gradual onset of stuttering. Gradual learning might suggest that some form of reinforcement is shaping the behavioral response. Or stuttering could be acquired through a very brief motor problem-solving learning process, consistent with a sudden onset of stuttering. Indeed, as discussed in Chapter 3, both gradual and sudden onsets of stuttering have been reported in the literature.

The foundations for psychobehavioral theory were established by Pavlov (1927) in his work concerning classical conditioning, and by B. F. Skinner's (1953) research on operant conditioning. These two modes of behavioral conditioning are quite different. Classical conditioning involves a learning process in which more features in the environment (i.e., stimuli) can elicit the *same* response through a process of association. In the famous example, Pavlov's dog responded at first with saliva when food was presented but later also salivated to the ringing of a bell, after its sound had been paired with food. Next, additional stimuli that were paired with the bell or other already conditioned stimuli also triggered the same response—salivation. In other words, classical conditioning is a process of response generalization in which the subject makes the same response to an ever-growing number of stimuli that occur *before* the behavioral response. In contrast, operant conditioning is aimed at changing the response (behavior), based on events that occur *after* it has occurred. This process can result in a narrowing down (rather than generalization) of the desired response as it is modified by the impact of what follows it (e.g., reinforcement, punishment, or other consequences). For example, a professor pacing the classroom while lecturing may be conditioned to gradually reduced pacing, and finally position himself in a particular spot as a result of the students showing great interest when he happens to be in that spot and their lack of interest when he moves away.

The interest in the application of behavioral principles to stuttering resulted in a host of new theoretical perspectives, some of which are reviewed here, that incorporated one or both of these two types of conditioned learning processes. These, in turn, prompted new research, especially of operant conditions that bring the stuttering response under stimulus control (Flanagan, Goldiamond, & Azrin, 1958; James, 1981; Martin & Siegel, 1966). For an extensive review of the experimental literature related to the effects of response contingent stimulation on stuttering, see Prins and Hubbard (1988). This group of theories has had significant impact on stuttering therapy as evidenced in a number of clinical programs that employ conditioning procedures (e.g., Brutten & Shoemaker, 1966; Costello, 1980; Ryan, 1971).

Stuttering as a Reactive Avoidance Behavior

One of the earliest theories of stuttering to suggest that a child's speech behavior could be modified by its environmental consequences was developed by Wendel Johnson at the University of Iowa. Although his ideas were not based in behavior modification principles, and he placed a heavy emphasis on emotional reactions to disfluent speech, the theory is being categorized as *psychobehavioral* because it purports that stuttering is a learned response. This well-known view saw its early hints beginning in 1942 when Johnson concluded from his original study of stuttering onset that what parents described as their young child's "first stuttering" was quite similar to what parents of nonstuttering children observed as their child's normal disfluent speech.[1] Johnson's views saw further development when a few years later he elaborated on the early findings, concluding that "Stuttering, as a clinical problem, as a definite disorder, was found to occur not before being diagnosed but after being diagnosed. In order to emphasize these findings, I have coined the term **diagnosogenic**; stuttering is a diagnosogenic disorder in the sense that the diagnosis of stuttering is one of the causes of the disorder" (Johnson, 1944a, p. 33). Following additional studies based primarily on parent interviews and some speech samples recorded a while after the time of onset (see Chapter 3), his later publications (Johnson et al., 1959) proposed what came to be popularly known as the *diagnosogenic* or *semantogenic* theory concerning the etiology of stuttering. *Diagnosogenic* means that the diagnosis causes the disorder. *Semantogenic* means that the mere labeling of the problem is powerful enough to create the problem.

Relying on data that showed most, if not all, young children exhibit speech disfluency as they develop speaking skills (e.g., Davis, 1939), Johnson felt that stuttering began when overanxious parents erroneously labeled these normal disfluencies as "stuttering." In his own words, "stuttering begins not in the speaker's mouth, but in the listener's ear" (1955a, p. 11). His research findings indicated that the parents of stuttering children tended to be pedantic, perfectionistic, demanding, anxious, and overprotective. Commensurately, they held such unrealistically high child development standards and expectations that they tended to be more disappointed in their child's

---

[1] The study was described in detail by Johnson (1955b).

performance. In particular, these parents appeared to be overanxious about speech, and they were quick to react negatively to the child's normal disfluencies. Responding to the parents' lead, the child reacted unfavorably to his or her own normal disfluencies, becoming anxious. By actively attempting to avoid these unapproved disfluencies, tension built up that led to a worsening of the disfluency. The child's continued failings invited even stronger parental reactions, leading to further effort on his or her part to avoid disfluencies, resulting in further tension that eventually spiraled what began as normal disfluency into a real stuttering problem. This view is also reflected in Johnson et al.'s (1948) definition of stuttering as "an anticipatory apprehensive hypertonic avoidance reaction" (p. 206). He conceptualized it to be nothing other than what a speaker does trying not to stutter.

The diagnosogenic theory maintained dominance in the field well into the 1970s, and some scientists and clinicians may still adhere to it. It was attractive in its simplicity and based on premises that are almost impossible to prove wrong. Can anyone prove that the very first disfluencies labeled by parents as "stuttering" were really "normal"? As we discuss in later chapters, it had a profound influence on the treatment of stuttering. For young children, treatment became largely indirect, keeping the child out of therapy so as to not call attention to his or her speech. Instead, therapy focused on parent counseling, advising them regarding better parent-child interaction. Parents were to reduce communicative pressure, be patient listeners, and accept stuttering without reacting. For adults, an important implication of the theory was a reorientation of the person's perspective on the problem, encouraging him or her to view self as a speaker rather than a "stutterer," with particular emphasis on the use of descriptive language when thinking and talking about stuttering. In other words, assuming responsibility for the behaviors that bring about the stuttering allows the person to change and improve (Johnson, 1961a).

With time, the idea that stuttering is caused by listeners' reactions to normal disfluency began to lose ground as contradictory evidence accumulated. Table 6.1 lists the evidence Johnson believed to support his theory as well as our counterevidence that contributed to its fall.

The learning-oriented diagnosogenic theory exerted strong and lasting influences but was not firmly linked to learning theory principles. Theoretical as well as clinical questions were left open. For example, why and how does stuttering continue or become reinforced in spite of being so painful? Why is the stuttering block eventually released? Therefore, other investigators stepped in to present stuttering within a more formal behavioral conditioning framework. Among the first attempting to correct this deficiency was Wischner (1950), who proposed that stuttering involves a learned anxiety reaction system. This theory is discussed next.

Stuttering as a Conditioned Anxiety Response

In 1950, Wischner incorporated principles from the conditioning models of both Pavlov (1927) and Hull (1943) to construct his theory. He pointed out that the stuttering

Table 6.1: **Supporting and Counterevidence for Johnson's Diagnosogenic Theory**

Supporting Evidence*	Counterevidence
1. Speech data for some stuttering children in the study and their matched nonstuttering controls revealed certain *overlap* in the overall frequency of disfluency.	1. Disfluencies of nonstuttering children are *far less frequent* than what Johnson thought, especially in certain critical types of disfluency (Ambrose & Yairi, 1999; Yairi, 1981, 1983).
2. Parents' descriptions of early stuttering were similar to descriptions of disfluent speech of control children.	2. Many parents have reported that they perceived abnormal speech in their child from the first day of stuttering (Yairi, 1983).
3. Parents overwhelmingly depicted a gradual onset with uneventful circumstances.	3. Sudden onsets of stuttering have been found to comprise nearly 40% of all cases (Yairi & Ambrose, 1992b, 2005).
4. Johnson's speech data showed that every disfluency type found in the speech of the stuttering children was also present in the speech of control children.	4. Critical types of disfluencies near the onset of stuttering are substantially different from normal not only in frequency, but in type, proportions, length, and speed (Ambrose & Yairi, 1999; Throneburg & Yairi, 1994; Yairi & Hall, 1993; Yairi & Lewis, 1984). In fact, Johnson et al.'s (1959) own disfluency data do not support the assertions he made (see McDearmon, 1968).
5. Data for normally speaking preschool children revealed that disfluency is a normal phenomenon (Branscom, Hughes, & Oxtoby, 1955; Davis, 1939).	5. Disfluency in normally fluent children is a normal phenomenon but limited (Yairi, 1981).
6. Parents reported no statistically significant differences between children who stutter and normally fluent controls in many aspects of health and development.	6. Evidence for a strong *genetic component* to stuttering has been growing from several directions, including identification of several chromosomes as likely sites for genes underlying stuttering (Ambrose et al., 1997; Suresh et al., 2006).
7. Children who stutter are often sensitive to negative listener reactions to their disfluent or stuttered speech and seek to avoid reprisal.	7. Experimental studies and surveys revealed that parents' calling attention to their child's stuttering with instructions such as "slow down" and "take a breath and start over" may have contributed to his or her improvement (Martin, Kuhl, & Haroldson, 1972; Wingate, 1976). Although the child may have been destined developmentally to recover, parental instructions did not hinder recovery.
8. Reports indicated there were societal/cultural variations in stuttering prevalence related to the extent of community emphasis on speaking skills. The Shoshone Indians, for example, were reported to have no word for stuttering and no cases of it (Snidecor, 1947). By not labeling or calling any attention to disfluencies, Johnson thought their tribe had successfully prevented stuttering altogether.	8. Revisiting the societal/cultural factor it was discovered Native Americans do have a word for stuttering and did know of individuals who stuttered (Zimmermann, Liljeblad, Frank, & Cleeland, 1983). It appears that stuttering is found universally.
9. Data showed that listeners might vary greatly in their perceptual judgments of speech as normal or stuttered (Tuthill, 1946; Williams & Kent, 1958).	9. Studies showed that negative verbal responses, mild electrical shock, loud sounds, and other aversive stimuli, administered as the immediate consequence of stuttering moments, often result in substantial declines in stuttering (Costello & Ingham, 1984; Prins & Hubbard, 1988).

*Items without a reference are based on Johnson et al., 1959.

adaptation curve (see Chapter 4) is similar to a behavioral extinction curve obtained in animal experiments and that stuttering increases as the anticipation periods prior to talking gets longer. Equating anticipation with anxiety, stuttering was seen to be similar to other behaviors evoked by the avoidance of unpleasant (noxious) stimuli. This is commonly seen in experiments with guinea pigs trapped in a cage, running around frantically to avoid electric shock that is terminated when a certain lever is pressed or floor grid is found.

Imagine learning to walk the tightrope at the same time you are performing in the circus. The rope is high above the ground, without nets to catch you. All the eyes of the spectators are glued to your every movement, scrutinizing every bobble. The combination of the fear of falling and the lack of confidence in performing cause the tension to build inside you. All your effort is concentrated on trying to maintain your balance, but your extreme level of tension and mounting anxiety causes you to lose balance over and over again. Each time you feel yourself start to fall, you jerk yourself around in a haphazard array of arm and leg movements until you finally regain your composure and prepare to move forward again. You manage to stay on the high wire until you reach the safety of the opposite platform, but your journey there has been filled with a chaotic display of flailing limbs and unusual postures. Perhaps this experience parallels the nature of stuttering as an anxiety response.

Wischner asserted that expressions of parental disapproval of the child's normal disfluency constitute noxious stimuli that create anxiety. The anxiety (anticipation) concerning further painful parental reactions to disfluencies motivates the child to avoid them by changing his or her disfluent speaking behavior. Typically, these attempts end up with mounting tension to the point where real stuttering ensues. Soon, in a classical Pavlovian manner, other stimuli, such as words, situations, and certain people, are conditioned to become anxiety-provoking stimuli that cause stuttering. Stuttering persists in spite of being painful due to the principle that learning takes place as a result of drive reduction (Hull, 1943). Stuttering is self-reinforcing because the anxiety that builds up prior to talking is greatly relieved when the stuttering finally occurs and is completed. The reinforcing power of the sharp fall in anxiety *immediately* after a stuttering event is greater than the adverse social reactions that follow. The physical behaviors (secondary characteristics) are also reinforced because the person who stutters is convinced that they actually helped "get the word out." Eventually, these tensions and movements become integrated into the stuttering pattern.

One weakness of Wischner's theory is that many young children do not appear anxious at the time of stuttering onset. Additionally, many children present sudden onset, which does not support the notion of a gradual learning of behavior. The theory has, however, logical clinical implications. Although extinction of responses set up by avoidance conditioning is difficult, it is still possible if an animal in a cage ignores the danger signal and the expected negative consequence does not materialize.

Accordingly, stuttering should diminish if speech disfluency is experienced in the absence of noxious stimuli so that the anxiety is deconfirmed. By inference, remediation for adults is possible through behavioral modification, particularly through the process of *desensitization* that lowers anxiety and sensitivity to listeners' reactions. Practicing easy voluntary disfluencies that do not invite negative reactions should be helpful. For young children, Wischner's ideas, like Johnson's, imply that parents must be counseled to accept the child's stuttering and stop reacting to it.

The Conflict Theory of Stuttering

Although Wischner's theory strengthened the view that stuttering is an acquired behavior shaped from normal disfluency, additional aspects, such as the initial trigger (is it normal disfluency?) and the nature of dynamics underlying the moment of stuttering leave room for additional contributions. Sheehan's (1953) conflict theory varies from Johnson's and Wischner's ideas in two respects. First, the underlying cause of stuttering is proposed to stem from different fears, such as fears of specific words or speaking situations, as well as unconscious fears of exposing the ego to the threat of failure, and others. These fears stimulate conflict between any of several pairs of opposing drives, such as the drive to speak and the drive to avoid stuttering, the drive for expression of self versus the drive to avoid exposing one's self, between conscious speech control versus automatic processes, and others. Convolutedly, then, subconscious psychoemotional elements are injected into this primarily psychobehavioral theory.

Second, regarding the dynamics that trigger moments of stuttering, Sheehan used studies of approach-avoidance conflict in animals as the model. In this experimental paradigm, a hunger drive motivates the animal to move toward the food, but when the food is approached, an electric shock is delivered and the animal retreats to avoid pain. Going back and forth, the animal eventually freezes in one place, where the strengths of the opposing drives are equal. This is comparable to the person who stutters who finds himself or herself in a conflict between the urge to speak and drive to avoid speaking and stuttering, regardless of the source of the fear and conflict. Freezing occurs when approach and avoidance drives reach an equilibrium. This is analogous to the stuttering block. Repetition and prolongation would represent oscillating and stopping at the point where the two-drive gradients cross. Stuttering is learned and persists because it is being self-reinforced through reduction in anxiety during the block when the approach drive finally prevails and the word is uttered.

Later, Sheehan (1970) posited that the central problem with stuttering is a self-role conflict. Because the person who stutters speaks fluently at times, he possesses two roles: the stutterer and the fluent speaker. He or she constantly attempts to embrace the fluent role by hiding/minimizing the stuttering in social contacts, hoping to "pass" as a normal speaker. The guilt feelings about the pretense mount to tension, resulting in stuttered speech. Although Sheehan's ideas account well for variations in stuttering frequency with situational factors, such as audience size and identity of the listener, it fails to be exhaustive with respect to explaining why singing, which also involves expression of emotion and specific words, is not also stuttered.

Sheehan's theory has had influential clinical implications. Accordingly, treatment should be primarily a matter of gaining mastery over fear, decreasing the tendencies for avoidance while increasing the approach drive. He strongly advocated that the person who stutters should actively accept, rather than hide, the role of the stutterer, by bringing stuttering out into the open. The inclination to hide stuttering strengthens the avoidance drive and the related psychoemotional conflicts that are expressed in stuttering moments. Clients should openly talk about their stuttering, even allow for some stuttering on purpose. By being open about stuttering, tension is reduced and stuttering is decreased.

Stuttering as an Operant Behavior

A further significant theoretical development is seen in Shames and Sherrick's (1963) application of a strict operant conditioning frame of reference to stuttering. It is similar to the Johnson and the Wischner notions in that stuttering is said to emerge from normal disfluency. The principal difference from these two, as well as from Sheehan's ideas, lies in their reliance only on observable behaviors and their consequences. There is no allowance for intermediating emotions, such as anxiety or guilt feelings, that are prominent in the previous models.

Accordingly, normal disfluencies, probably of physiological origins, are modified by complex interactions among four modes of behavioral learning: positive reinforcement, negative reinforcement, punishment, and extinction (nonreinforcement) as they impact speech. Positive reinforcement is said to have taken place when introduction of a stimulus increases a response. Removal of positively reinforcing stimuli reduces the likelihood of the response (extinction). Punishment is said to have taken place when presentation of a stimulus decreases a response. Removal of punishing stimuli increases the likelihood of the response (negative reinforcement). Table 6.2 summarizes the four modes, or principles, of operant learning for purposes of behavior modification (conditioning).

For most children, disfluency is diminished through either extinction, being ignored by parents and others, or through verbal punishment, (e.g., "Stop it."). In a smaller number of cases, children's disfluency may draw positive reinforcement, such as listeners' attention. Listeners may be truly interested in what the child says or tune in because the disfluent speech draws attention. Subsequently, the disfluencies are emitted in increasing numbers. Some children may become normal speakers

Table 6.2: Description of Various Forms of Behavioral Modification

Term	Stimulus Manipulation	Behavioral Outcome
Positive reinforcement	**Presented** after behavior	Increase
Punishment	**Presented** after behavior	Decrease
Extinction	**Withheld** after behavior	Decrease
Negative reinforcement	**Withheld/removed** after behavior	Increase

who exhibit a good number of normal disfluencies. In a few children, however, it might be that primarily syllable and single-syllable word repetitions are reinforced. As explained in Chapter 1, when these disfluency types increase in number, they are likely to be perceived as stuttering, drawing more attention and being further reinforced.

Stuttering persists when environmental consequences continue to reinforce it through multiple complex types and schedules of reinforcement, both positive and negative, punishing and extinguishing. Random reinforcement is particularly effective in shaping behavior that is difficult to extinguish. Also, once established, stuttering provides the child with secondary gains, such as being excused from being called on to recite in class. These add to the mix of reinforcements that shape the behavioral response.

Regarding remediation, Shames and Sherrick (1963) supported behavior modification techniques that employ reinforcement of desired fluent speech and extinction, as well as nonreinforcement of stuttering. In fact, several operant conditioning therapy programs have been developed (e.g., Costello, 1980; Ryan, 1971). Some operant conditioning principles can be seen in many therapy programs. Although this model of stuttering is powerful in terms of explaining various dynamics of stuttering, especially the triggering of stuttering by neutral stimulus cues, it, too, fails the criterion of being exhaustive in explaining various ameliorating conditions. The precise stimulus-response factors critical to stuttering dynamics have never been uncovered. Also, the model does not explain why stuttering only rarely begins at ages other than childhood.

Two-Factor Theory of Stuttering

An interesting contribution to stuttering theory as an outgrowth of behavioral learning was made by Brutten and Shoemaker (1967), who posited that both classical and operant (instrumental) conditioning play major roles in the disorder. This double-pronged approach was motivated by studies that showed conflicting behaviors: Whereas some stuttering behaviors increased when penalized, others decreased. That stuttering could decrease under stimuli regarded as unpleasant negated a widely accepted assumption at the time that predicted it to increase. It also created a challenge concerning the choice of conditioning techniques for therapy. To consolidate the behavior variability and the contradictions, Brutten and Shoemaker suggested that stuttering comprises at least two distinct behavioral phenomena: (1) core stuttering features (prolongations and repetitions) that result from anxiety acquired through classical conditioning, and (2) secondary stuttering characteristics learned via instrumental conditioning. These two processes comprise their "two-factor theory."

Stuttering begins when the child undergoes strong emotional experiences (anxiety) that naturally result in motor instability, including speech fluency disintegration. This assumption appears reasonable given that many people experience difficulty performing even simple motor tasks, such as sticking a key in the car door lock, when upset or frightened. Next, strong anxiety is paired (conditioned) with many stimuli and situations (e.g., different people), all becoming capable of triggering anxiety that induces stuttering-type fluency failures. A parallel instrumental learning takes place when the person who stutters attempts to cope with in-progress stutter events (to get the word out) or prevent anticipated stuttering. These attempts involve secondary characteristics, such as swaying of the head or arms. When successful, they are strongly reinforced as well.

The theory fails to be exhaustive, like its predecessors. It is not clear why some individuals develop a stuttering problem related to experiencing negative emotion whereas other individuals do not. It does not explain why stuttering is a disorder primarily of early childhood. Its premises conflict with evidence that the "classically conditioned" disfluency types can be decreased when time-out periods are delivered as their consequence (James, 1981; Martin & Haroldson, 1971). Moreover, other phenomena, such as the consistency of stuttering loci (see Chapter 4) with respect to language, suggests that other factors besides negative emotion and conditioned associations contribute to fluency failure.

This theory, like the conflict theory of stuttering, has supported therapeutic techniques, such as systematic desensitization, that are detailed in Chapter 10. The fears and anxieties that prompted initial disintegration of fluency must be lessened through therapy that addresses emotions and attitudes. Desensitization approaches are implicated. Finally, the stuttering behavior itself must be decreased through extinction (removal of reinforcers) and positive reinforcement of desired behaviors.

The Anticipatory-Struggle Hypothesis

Yet another angle within the learning domain of stuttering theory is encountered in Bloodstein's (1987, 1997) *anticipatory-struggle hypothesis*. The theory suggests that for some children, the complex, automatic, serially ordered motor activity required for speech appears overwhelming, causing them to initiate it with excessive tension and fragmentation—stuttering. They are thus prone to experience failure and frustration when speech develops. Any kind of difficulty or pressure involving speech during childhood might lead to stuttering. For example, phonological and articulation problems could cause frustration when a child attempts to communicate but is not always understood. Out of that frustration, the child soon believes that speaking is difficult and learns to struggle when stuttering is anticipated. The implication for remediation is that if people who stutter could forget that they stutter, they would have "no further difficulty with speech" (Bloodstein, 1997, p. 170). Similarly, parents can best support recovery in their children by preventing the belief that talking is difficult.

As supporting evidence, Bloodstein (1997) pointed to research that has shown stuttering can be eliminated for short periods by the power of suggestion, highlighting the impact of an individual's beliefs about stuttering on its perpetuation. Also, stuttering is governed by self-fulfilling prophecies, for example, words, sounds, or letters stuttered once and noticed by the speaker, are more likely to be stuttered again. Similarly, the longer a person must wait before talking, the speaker's anticipation grows stronger and stuttering becomes more likely.

Like the previous theories, the *anticipatory-struggle hypothesis* fails to account exhaustively for ameliorating conditions (e.g., rhythm and singing). It is also not clear how its concepts should be tested. Even if it were determined that "speech is hard" for children, why do they develop a debilitating belief about speech difficulty instead of displaying symptoms (as some children do) of more frequent phonological, semantic, or syntactic errors without stuttering? Although the hypothesis aptly describes the nature of stuttering in its advanced form, it is less clear that it fits stuttering close to onset. Children are less accurate than adults at predicting their stuttering; about half predict less than 50% (Avari & Bloodstein, 1974). In our experience, many young children do not display either anxiety or tension when stuttering begins. Also, a number of adults have reported feeling perfectly relaxed yet still stuttering. The model further does not fully explain why or how there is a shift from a "speech is difficult" belief into an overwhelming experience of a "block" that entirely prevents speech from happening.

The Demands-Capacities Model

Included in the context of psychobehavioral theory is the *demands-capacities model* of stuttering (Adams, 1990; Starkweather & Gottwald, 1990). Although some researchers have also considered it a multifactorial model, it is primarily a theory of behavioral responses or capacities in relation to stimulus demands. In simple terms, stuttering arises when a child attempts speech performance beyond his or her abilities. Adequate capacities, especially in four domains (cognitive, linguistic, motor, emotional maturity) are needed to withstand corresponding environmental demands and still produce fluent speech. No deficits are implied in this model; if the conditions exist in which demands (e.g., expectation to use new and complex language structures) exceed capacities, fluency can be expected to fail.

> Tremendous multitasking may be needed by the stay-at-home mother of a toddler. Within the same 10 minutes, Mom may need to juggle activities of preparing a cake for a social event, cleaning the dishes, adding softener to the laundry load, keeping the baby out of the garbage can, answering the phone, and so on. As the number of demands increases, and she reaches the limits of her capacities to give each task the time and attention it requires, there is a greater likelihood of a mishap (e.g., an egg dropped on the floor). Mom's weakened performance is not due to any inadequacy on her part. The multiple demands simply overloaded her attentional capacities. In a similar manner, the demands-capacities model proposes that various demands of communication (e.g., figuring out which words to say, selecting the desired intonation, time pressure to say it quickly, etc.) can overwhelm the child's speech system—and disfluent events occur as the result.

As evidence for the *demands-capacities model*, nearly all speakers find that speech fluency tends to break down in highly demanding situations, such as speaking publicly, conveying complicated concepts, reciting tongue twisters, and feeling threatened for accountability. With respect to children who stutter, this model accommodates well the research findings that many who persist remain above average in language skills

(Watkins & Yairi, 1997; Watkins, 2005). Cyclical patterns of stuttering during the early developmental period also can be explained by this model. If the rate of various developing capacities does not keep pace to meet the demands, greater disfluency ensues. As capacities meet or surpass demands, fluent speech is recovered once again.

In terms of the limitations, the theory does not fit the facts on all accounts because there are occasions when some children stutter in what appear to be low-demand situations. On the flip side, this model does not explain why sometimes high-demand situations do not result in moments of stuttering. For example, some people who stutter can be very fluent when speaking to large audiences. With respect to intervention, the theory stresses the importance of addressing any imbalances among demands and capacities, and especially working with parents to alter environmental demands on children's speech performance (Starkweather & Givens-Ackerman, 1997).

Summary of Psychobehavioral Theories

Psychobehavioral theories view stuttering not as what a person is, or what is wrong with him or her, but as a behavior that can be acquired by means of various and complex processes under various conditions. The review of a range of theories has demonstrated this point. In principle, the learning point of view assumes that just about everyone may acquire stuttering given the proper circumstances. Once acquired, many stimuli may trigger stuttered speech that may be reinforced and modified by its consequences, either internal (e.g., anxiety reduction) or external (listener's reactions). Very different in orientation from the psychoemotional theories, psychobehavioral theories offer considerable insight into the dynamics of stuttering moments, but the reasons for initial onset are often obscure. These theories are concerned with observable phenomena, however, and therefore lend themselves more readily to scientific experimentation. From a clinical viewpoint, they have supported several therapy programs, and are by nature optimistic because, supposedly, whatever is learned can be unlearned.

Psycholinguistic Theories

Psycholinguistics is the study of the psychological processes (*psycho-*) underlying language use (*-linguistic*). A speaker can sometimes be disfluent in the process of correcting an error in selection of word stress. For example, after uttering a syllable repetition of "re-re-re-relative," a non-stuttering speaker was retrospectively aware that during the "re-re-re" the word "related" (with 2nd syllable stress) was just under the surface, ready to come out by mistake, until finally the intended stress pattern for "relative" (1st syllable stress) was ready and produced for the intended word. This is an example of a disfluency resulting from a failed psycholinguistic process. A number of researchers have proposed that the occurrence of some stuttered speech may result from subtle aberrancies or deficiencies in the underlying psychological processes responsible for transforming word selections into integrated patterns of suprasegmental (voice inflection) and segmental (phonemic) speech gestures. Theories that explain stuttering in terms of these dynamics are considered *psycholinguistic* theories.

We must clarify what the psycholinguistic domain *is* in contrast to what it *is not*. Psycholinguistic processes are primarily responsible for the retrieval and assembly of language elements. A "disorder of phonology" or "a disorder of language" does not necessarily imply a disorder of retrieval and assembly. A *disorder of phonology* or of *language* implies impaired knowledge of the elements and/or rules governing the use of phonemes, or of words to convey meaning. A child may adopt an erroneous set of phonemes (deficient in number or lacking features in his or her language) or apply unusual rules for their combination. Still, the child may have no trouble using that set of deficient phonemes in the way they intend, although it is difficult for listners to understand. Likewise, a child may lack vocabulary (lexical) items or generate unique words or word combinations that are erroneous in the target language but still select and order these words as intended and in a timely fashion. Psycholinguistic theories of stuttering do *not* propose that people who stutter are lacking in their knowledge of the phonology or vocabulary of their language. In contrast, they propose that the processes or systems responsible for the retrieval and integration of those elements are failing to operate smoothly.

A psycholinguistic theory might assert that stuttering is a "disorder of phonological *encoding*." Encoding refers to the subconscious cognitive activity of generating the elements of the code. Therefore a *phonological encoding disorder* refers to an impairment of a system or process responsible for the timely and precise retrieval of phonological elements, primarily phonemes. As an analogy, imagine a manufacturing plant. The parts (phonemes) are available in their storage area, and even the procedures (phonological rules) for putting the parts together are established, but the manufacturer's mechanical systems for the assembly of the parts into a product are weak and/or breaking down. This results in a faulty product. Similarly, a *disorder of lexical (word) encoding* indicates that the speaker, even if he or she has an ample vocabulary (lexicon) and well-developed morphosyntactic knowledge, has a problem, or weak mechanism, within the systems responsible to retrieve and assemble those words into an utterance. The distinction between systems responsible for psycholinguistic processing versus those responsible for knowledge of the linguistic elements is an important one because they may break down independently. A speaker can have problems with the cognitive systems that handle the assembly of the language regardless of sufficient knowledge related to the phoneme or word elements and rules for combining those elements for the language itself.

Psycholinguistic Processes Resulting in Fluent Speech

Before examining psycholinguistic theories of stuttering, it is important to consider a model of the processes underlying normally fluent speech production. Based on experimental research, Levelt (1989) proposed that the processes for generating fluent speech consist of three major phases: conceptualization, formulation, and articulation. Each phase receives the by-product of the previous phase in sequential order. During conceptualization, the speaker conceives the message. In formulation,

Figure 6.1: Model of Psycholinguistic Processes Underlying Speech

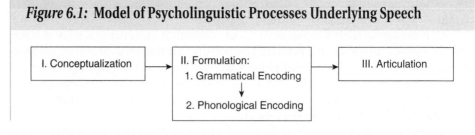

its grammatical and phonological representations are generated. Finally, in the articulation phase, the representations are transformed into motor programs that reach the peripheral speech musculature, which acts to achieve the desired acoustic outcomes of speech. Figure 6.1 shows the phases in sequence.

The assembly of speech is handled during the formulation phase, which is further divided into two sequential subphases: grammatical encoding and phonological encoding. In grammatical encoding, the underlying semantic and syntactic representation is prepared; in phonological encoding, the syllable and sound (phoneme) specifications are made. Finally, when the idea, word selection, and structural form have been retrieved, then the movements of speech (i.e., articulation) can be generated and produced. If the speaker needs to hold up the initiation of articulation, for example, while chewing and swallowing food, then the retrieved thoughts and word forms can be held temporarily in a short-term memory storage (referred to as the buffer) until the vocal tract structures are available.

The psycholinguistic processes of speech production mostly take place without conscious awareness on the part of the speaker (Levelt, 1989). Retrieval of words, grammatical structures, intonational patterns, and phonemic elements are achieved with operations that are fully "automatic." The speaker does not have to devote attentional resources to these activities; therefore they occur in parallel without mutual interference. Even more importantly, they operate simultaneously with the actual act of speaking. Simultaneous psycholinguistic processes make it possible for articulation to follow conceptualization almost immediately. The implication of simultaneous speech-encoding processes that do not need conscious attention is that the latter parts of an utterance can be planned while the earlier parts are being articulated (Howell, 2002; Kempen & Huijbers, 1983; Levelt, 1989). The fact that early products of speech planning usually are immediately delivered while subsequent sections are being prepared is referred to as a "staged and feedforward" process (Levelt, Roelofs, & Meyer, 1999).

The nature of psycholinguistic processes is illustrated by "tip of the tongue" and "slip of the tongue" phenomena, common to all speakers. When a speaker has an idea (perhaps envisioning the flowers in the garden) but cannot find the right descriptive word, then the conceptualization stage was accomplished, but formulation failed. If the wrong grammatical form is selected, the result may be a *semantic* slip of the tongue, such as the error of saying "pansies" instead of "violets." Although conceptualization was accurate (envisioning the violets), the word-generating (formulation) process has failed at the grammatical encoding level. Similarly, phonological encoding can break down when a speaker knows the word he or she wants to say (grammatical content was retrieved) but has trouble finding the sound and syllable sequences for it. Partially successful phonological encoding may retrieve the initial sound (e.g., 'v') but not the rest of the sounds in the word. The speaker senses the word is near and expresses, "It is on the tip of my tongue." If phonological encoding fails, however, the error could result in a "slip of the tongue," such as saying "violence" for "violets."

Psycholinguistic Factors in Stuttering

What do simultaneous word retrieval processes mean for stuttering? It has long been noted that when someone stutters on a particular word, it might not be the word being uttered that is the problem at all. It may be another word that is being retrieved simultaneously that has not even been uttered yet. Or the words being stuttered may also hold clues to underlying processes related to stuttering. Might the locations of stuttering within and/or between words in connected speech tell us something about its nature? There are still many questions to answer regarding the relationship of stuttering to psycholinguistic processes. Why do people who stutter typically become held up after the utterance of word fragments? When and how is the word assembly process breaking down? Several researchers have offered possible theories.

The Covert-Repair Hypothesis

One theoretical perspective that received considerable attention during the past two decades is the *covert-repair hypothesis*. This model explains stuttering as an outcome of hyperactive self-monitoring of inner speech (Postma & Kolk, 1993; Postma, Kolk, & Povel, 1991). An error in the centrally devised speech plan (e.g., in the phonetic plan) is detected subconsciously and because the speaker's system attempts correction before it reaches the surface, he or she stutters. Restated in another way, disfluencies occur when the speaker is late repairing errors in the phonological system that arise during their formulation. The term *covert* refers to things hidden or unseen, and the term *repair* refers to the speaker's attempt to correct the original formulation and replan the intended speech. An underlying assumption of the theory is that people who stutter may have some form of deficit with the capacity for phonological encoding. At typical rates of speech, their process of generating the phonological elements does not keep up well. Alternatively, perhaps their tendency to talk too fast makes it difficult to correct errors in a timely fashion, leading to disfluencies (and the need for slower speech). Some supportive evidence takes several forms. First, stuttering appears to be a moment in which speech is held back. Second, most fluency breakdown appears to occur at points of transition between sounds within words. Third, people who stutter have been observed to be slower with silent reading (i.e., a "covert" process). The implication of this hypothesis for stuttering intervention is that people who stutter should take more time (slow down) to initiate and do talking; they may benefit by practice of speech sound combinations.

The counterevidence for this theory has been noted in two ways. First, research (Postma & Kolk, 1992) shows that people who stutter do not make more speech errors than those who do not stutter, and second, a subgroup of children who stutter have no difficulty with complicated phonological sequences (Seery, Watkins, Ambrose, & Throneburg, 2006). Also, phonologically difficult words, or words that followed them, did not draw more instances of stuttering than other words (Howell & Au-Yeung, 1995; Throneburg, Yairi, & Paden, 1994). Additional research related to the phonological proficiency of children who stutter did not find problems (Bernstein Ratner, 1997a; Louko, Edwards, & Conture, 1990; Nippold, 2001).

The Fault Line Hypothesis

Wingate hypothesized that stuttering is a defect in the language production system, an indication of a lack of synchrony in the assembly of linguistic elements. He explained that stuttering occurs at the "fault line" of phonological formulation where initial consonant and vowel are joined. These elements are "unitized" by the generation of syllable stress. Thus stuttering represents a failure to merge the prosodic and phonologic aspects of speech (Perkins, Kent, & Curlee, 1991; Wingate, 1988). Wingate reasoned that because the specific sounds that are the loci of repetitions or hesitations are usually recognizable and appropriately articulated, that the difficulty is not with the production of those sounds but with moving past the sound to the production of the next phonetic element. He conceptualized stuttering as a "phonetic transition defect" (1988, p. 11) in which the speaker has trouble connecting the speech elements rather than with producing the elements themselves. Although these ideas sound as if they suggest motoric bases, Wingate (1988) insisted that the fault line for stuttering originated at a central rather than a peripheral level of speech production processes.

Wingate observed that the common element describing the loci of most stutter events is that they occur on stressed syllables. The linguistic factors associated with the loci of stuttering as described by Brown (1945) (word length, initial sounds, content words, and initial words, etc.) were explained by Wingate as all sharing the common element of linguistic stress. He reasoned that the execution of stress is primarily a phonatory function requiring laryngeal adjustments for pitch and loudness. This inference, combined with the view of stuttering as transition defect, led Wingate to conclude that the data showed a general difficulty for stutterers to produce stressed vowels, with the implication that the central processing difficulty leads to a failure to make the neurophysiological adjustments necessary for speech.

Even if stuttering occurs predominantly on stressed syllables, the fact remains that not all stressed syllables are stuttered. In some languages, such as Hebrew, the stress occurs on the last syllable of most words. In addition, in a variety of speaking conditions, stressed syllables are not stuttered at all (e.g., talking to one's self, etc.). Thus it would appear there is more to stuttering than a phonatory transition defect for the execution of stressed syllables. It is also not clear that stressed syllables are the primary locus of stuttering in young children, and the course of stuttering development was not addressed directly by Wingate's theory. The correspondence of stuttering and early prosodic development warrants further research. Before children develop contrastive word stress in their multiword utterances, there appears to be a tendency to give each word emphasis (no contrast). Use of intonational contrasts appears to develop separately from durational contrasts (Snow, 1994; Patel & Brayton, 2009). Investigations are needed to explore whether stuttering onset (or significant increase in disfluent speech) coincides with some form of transition between stages of prosodic development.

The clinical implications of Wingate's model are similar to those of the previous psycholinguistic hypothesis. That is, people who stutter may benefit by speaking slower to allow the additional time needed for their linguistic assembly processes. Because stressed syllables are particularly vulnerable to stuttering, these locations may especially need a slower, easier approach. Finally, given the speaker's difficulty with phonatory transitions, another clinical target would be the management of voicing for speech.

The Neuropsycholinguistic Theory

The essence of Perkins, Kent, and Curlee's (1991) proposal is that stuttering results when the syllable framework is not ready at the same time as the speech sounds (segments). They assert that fluency is interrupted by asynchronies between the arrival of syllable frames and segmental fillers, and that time pressure to continue the attempt to speak ultimately precipitates the stutter event. Basic to their neuropsycholinguistic theory of stuttering is the understanding that speech is planned hierarchically as well as sequentially. Sequentially, speech sounds must be ordered within words, and words must be ordered within sentences. Hierarchically, however, the onset initial sound (onset) and final vowel-consonant ending unit (coda) must be inserted within the syllables, and syllables must be inserted within the intonational phrase. When the various components of the speech plan, both sequential and hierarchical, are being generated, they must all be ready at the necessary time for speech to move forward smoothly. If the syllable frames are ready, and the onset retrieved, a speaker may initiate talking under time pressure even if the coda or pattern of the rest of the intonational phrase has not been resolved. When the rest of the pattern is not forthcoming, the asynchrony in the delivery of the syllable components for production is evidenced as stuttering. Stuttering is the speaker's time- and place-holding activity until all of the speech components are properly arranged and ready for final execution.

Although this hypothesis offers a suitably complex account for why speech breaks down in the form of disfluency, it does not offer any further insight into why children are prone to this breakdown rather than adults. Moreover, it has offered little insight into why the conditions such as singing, delayed auditory feedback (DAF), choral reading (unison), and so on, facilitate the synchronization of these components. This theory, like the others, offers a model to explain why those who stutter should approach speech more slowly, but otherwise does not offer straightforward therapeutic applications.

The way freight trains are loaded may help to illustrate the concepts of syllable frames and sound fillers central to the neuropsycholinguistic theory of stuttering. As train cars are moved along the track, the freight must be loaded into each car. Each car must wait for its freight before it can move forward and let the next car be filled. In speech, each syllable is like a train car that must be loaded with the sound segments, like the freight. If the freight (sounds) arrive before the train car (syllable) arrives, then the freight (sounds) may spill out (repeat?). Alternatively, if the train cars (syllables) move forward, but the freight (sounds) are not ready, then the position of the car may be fixed (prolonged?) waiting for the sounds to arrive.

Related Research

Stuttering Loci

In Chapter 4 we explained that the loci of stuttering coincide with specific elements and structures of spoken language. The more factors may congregate in a single word (e.g., unfamiliar, longer, content word, etc.), the higher its chance to be stuttered. These loci have led to the question of whether there are significant links between stuttering and language. Are these loci special for stuttering? Evidence suggests that stuttering locations may merely reflect the nature of underlying psycholinguistic processes in general, rather than the specific nature of stuttering. Research shows that these loci are vulnerable locations of disruption for all speakers, stuttering or not. For example, the initial sounds of words often attract stutter events, but these same locations also attract slips of the tongue by all speakers. When speech sound transpositions occur, they are most often on the initial sounds of words (MacKay, 1970). For example, a common speech error could take the form "root fest" for "foot rest" switching the initial sounds of the words. It would be highly unusual, however, for a speaker to switch the final sounds of the words to produce the error: "foost ret."

Conditions of Psycholinguistic Interference

The multilevel parallel system of speech planning and production raises questions as to how each subsystem can be protected from interfering influences by other parts of the system. Bosshardt (2002) examined the effect of concurrent psycholinguistic processing activities on the speech of adults who stuttered and normally fluent individuals. The experiment consisted of the primary task of repeating words continuously and secondary tasks, either silent reading or word memorization, to be accomplished simultaneously. In addition, two conditions related to phonemic content were compared. In one condition the phonemic content of words was simi-lar between the primary and secondary tasks. In the second condition, the phonemic content was dissimilar. Speech fluency analysis revealed that those who stutter were significantly more disfluent when similar words were read or memorized concur-rently with the word repetition task than when dissimilar words were involved. By contrast, there was no significant difference in disfluency between these stimulus conditions for those who do not stutter. Bosshardt concluded that people who stutter are more sensitive to interference from concurrent cognitive processing tasks compared to people who do not stutter and that their phonological and articulatory systems are not efficiently protected from interference by attention-demanding processes. Thus, when a person who stutters encounters challenging phonological patterns, the weight of these demands would be expected to interfere with speech fluency. This raises the question of whether the phonological systems of individuals who stutter are more error prone than for people who do not stutter.

Stuttering and Phonologic Complexity

Throneburg, Yairi, and Paden (1994) studied children who stuttered at ages 29 to 59 months, selected to represent four conditions: severe stuttering/good phonology, severe stuttering/poor phonology, mild stuttering/good phonology, and mild stuttering/poor phonology. Words were classified according to seven possible types of phonological difficulty: consonant clusters, multiple syllables, late-developing sounds, and the four possible combinations of these three. Words that were not phonologically difficult (i.e., none of those just listed) constituted an eighth category.

A conversational speech sample with approximately 1,000 words was recorded for each child near stuttering onset, and the frequencies of words in the eight categories were analyzed. Also, stuttered words were identified, and the proportion of these in each of the eight categories was determined. Results showed that the largest proportion of stuttered words (about 50%) used by each of the four groups of children were "not phonologically difficult." That is, they fit none of the seven categories of phonological difficulty. The proportion of stuttered words among each of the seven categories of difficulty was small, and no category was more prevalent than any of the rest for any of the four participant groups. The investigators concluded that phonological difficulty was not associated with the locations of stuttering in young children. More specifically, the phonologic difficulty (complexity) of a word does not predict the occurrence of fluency breakdown regardless of a child's stuttering severity or phonologic ability. An almost identical conclusion was reached by Howell and Au-Yeung (1995).

Although phonologic ability level does not appear to predict the coincidence of stutter events with phonologically difficult words, the Throneburg et al. (1994) investigation did not address whether stuttering tends to coincide with phonological errors irrespective of word difficulty. A later investigation by Wolk, Blomgren, and Smith (2000) analyzed the frequency of simultaneous disfluency and phonological errors in 4- to 5-year-olds, with coexisting stuttering and phonological disorders. Analysis of their speech samples revealed that overall, the occurrence of stuttering was not more frequent on syllables with phonological errors than on syllables without phonological errors. There was, however, a significantly higher stuttering frequency on word-initial consonant clusters with phonological errors than on word-initial consonant clusters without phonological errors. These results suggest most stuttering is not associated with phonological production demands, but some stuttering is.

Priming of Linguistic Structures

Priming studies are another means of exploring whether stuttering is a symptom of failed phonological encoding processes. In an auditory priming paradigm, the participant is presented with an auditory stimulus, such as a word that sounds like the name of the picture they will see, prior to being shown the picture to be named. The experimenter can then examine whether primed conditions yield faster or slower response latencies and thereby assess the function of psycholinguistic processes.

Using this paradigm, Byrd, Conture, and Ohde (2007) compared picture-naming performance between young children who stutter and normally fluent children. Three auditory priming conditions were created to test neutral, holistic, and incremental phonological encoding processes. For example, if the target word was "book," a neutral prime might have sounded like "d," a holistic prime would have sounded like "ook," and an incremental prime would have sounded like "b." The children's speech reaction times (response latencies) were measured from the onset of picture presentation to the onset of participant response. The investigators observed that as children who do not stutter grew older from 3 to 5 years of age, there was a shift from being significantly faster in the holistic priming condition to being significantly faster in the incremental priming condition. By contrast, the majority of both 3- and 5-year-old children who stutter exhibited faster reaction times in the holistic than the incremental condition. It was inferred that children who stutter tend to be delayed in making the developmental shift in phonological encoding from holistic to incremental processing, and that such a delay may contribute to their difficulties generating fluent speech.

Summary of Psycholinguistic Theories

In contrast to psychoemotional and psychobehavioral theories, psycholinguistic theories of stuttering have nothing to do with environmental factors and emotional responses. Unlike motoric perspectives of stuttering (see Chapter 7) that emphasize dynamics of speech execution, psycholinguistic viewpoints shift the focus to central cognitive processes involved in the planning of speech. Psycholinguistic theories provide us with insight into the nature of disfluent speech, but they generally do not offer the breadth of explanation necessary to understand the full picture of stuttering etiology and onset. They also have fallen short of accounting for all the phenomena related to stuttering (e.g., ameliorating conditions). They do help to account for the various loci of stuttering and illuminate the associations of speech and language assembly processes and stuttering.

Summary

Is it possible that psychoemotional, psychobehavioral, and psycholingistic factors all contribute to stuttering? The answer is undoubtedly positive. Although research evidence does not support the notion that stuttering originates from some form of psychoemotional disturbance, it remains possible that temperament has a role in the persistence of stuttering and the person's handling of the problems it presents. Additionally, stuttering and anxiety are related; however, more evidence suggests that stuttering leads to anxiety rather than the other way around. Regarding psychobehavioral contributions, research has demonstrated that the frequency of stuttering can be manipulated by delivery of contingent reinforcements. This fact alone is not sufficient to prove that stuttering is a learned behavior, but it does imply that environment serves an important role in the triggering of stuttering moments. Both classes of theories have had substantial influence on the clinical management of stuttering. Familiarity with them enhances clinicians' insight into their therapeutic regimens. Psycholinguistic theories of stuttering support the hypothesis that speech fluency may be interrupted by psycholinguistic processes that govern the assembly of sounds and words into connected speech, but future research is needed to reveal the exact nature of their role in the occurrence of stuttering.

STUDY QUESTIONS AND DISCUSSION TOPICS

1. Paradoxically, stuttering has been described as both tension-provoking and tension-reducing. Compare and contrast the psychoemotional versus psychobehavioral views of this paradox.

2. Provide a psychobehavioral explanation for the acquisition of secondary behaviors of stuttering.

3. Describe the tendency for a person to stutter on his or her own name from a classical conditioning perspective. Is this psychobehavioral view sufficient, or might psychoemotional factors play a role in this tendency? Explain.

4. How would the persistence versus recovery of stuttering be explained in terms of operant conditioning? Is this view of stuttering progression sufficient? If not, what facts regarding recovery and persistence of stuttering are *not* explained by psychobehavioral dynamics?

5. A child is heard to stutter on the initial word "Mommy" of a multiword utterance. Is it appropriate to conclude that the word "Mommy" is difficult for the child to say? Why or why not? Offer an explanation for this location of fluency breakdown based on psycholinguistic processes underlying speech production.

SUGGESTED READINGS

Bernstein Ratner, N. (1997). Stuttering: A psycholinguistic perspective. In R. Curlee & G. Siegel (Eds.), *Nature and treatment of stuttering* (2nd ed., pp. 99–127). Boston: Allyn & Bacon.

Costello, J. (1980). Operant conditioning and the treatment of stuttering. In W. H. Perkins (Ed.), Strategies in stuttering therapy. In J. L. Northern (Series Ed.),

Seminars in speech, language and hearing. New York: Thieme-Stratton.

Ezrati-Vinacour, R., & Levin, I. (2004). The relationship between anxiety and stuttering: A multidimensional approach. *Journal of Fluency Disorders, 29*(2), 135–148.

Fisher, M. (1970). Stuttering: a psychoanalytic view. *Journal of Contemporary Psychotherapy, 2,* 124–127.

Chapter 7: Is Stuttering Biological? Neurological, Motor, and Genetics Perspectives

LEARNER OBJECTIVES

Readers will become familiar with:

- Evidence related to genetic theories of stuttering.
- Theories of stuttering as a symptom of brain dysfunction.
- Theories of stuttering as a symptom of motor dysfunction.
- Multidimensional theories and models of stuttering.

Introduction

During the 18th century, it was suggested that an abnormally large tongue causes stuttering by interfering with its mobility and proper positioning. This is a prime example of a belief in an anatomical basis for stuttering. Another idea circulating many years ago was that the tongue of a person who stutters is too weak, incapable of moving sufficiently fast or far enough in the oral cavity. This is an example of a belief in an abnormal function, or physiological basis, for stuttering. Might stuttering have biological bases, such as physical and/or physiological abnormalities (e.g., a thick tongue or a shallow breathing pattern)? Is stuttering the symptom of an underlying neurophysiological impairment? Is stuttering caused by a structural abnormality? Is there a genetic basis for it? These are the types of questions that have led to a variety of what could be called *organic* theories of stuttering. Scientists have speculated that stuttering could be the result of a variety of physically based limitations, such as inadequate neural structure and organization, deficient capacities to regulate speech timing, weak sensorimotor integration for speech targets, and impaired self-monitoring processes. Again, could stuttering be related to any or all of these issues?

It seems reasonable to hypothesize that at least some cases of stuttering may have a neurophysiological basis. Neurophysiology refers to the function of the nervous system. Perhaps the most apparent signs are the hypertonicity associated with stuttered speech (often affecting the entire body), some uncontrolled movements, respiratory irregularities such as gasping, and tremors associated with stuttering events (see Chapter 4 for a review of secondary characteristics). Observing these, West (1958) wrote that "if a specialist in convulsive disorders, without any previous experience with, or knowledge of stuttering, came upon a stutterer, he might at once label the disorder a seizure. Such a specialist would compare stuttering with the spasms that sweep through the muscles of the head, neck, and upper extremities when the athetotic person attempts to speak, or with the seizures mechanism of a mildly epileptic" (p. 175). In fact, West hypothesized that "Stuttering is primarily an epileptic disorder that manifests itself in dyssynergies of neuromotor mechanism for oral language" (p. 197).

A second phenomenon that prompts the idea of a neurophysiological component to stuttering is the variety of stuttering symptoms witnessed as a result of neurological damage secondary to strokes, head injuries, and so on (e.g., Rosenbeck et al., 1978). In a number of these patients, the stuttering symptoms ceased with natural recovery or after medical treatment for the neurological lesions. Third, the vulnerability for stuttering of certain groups, such as males, identical twins, and families with stuttering histories, suggests a genetic component to stuttering (Kidd, Kidd, & Records, 1978; Yairi, Ambrose, & Cox, 1996). Fourth, the remarkable way in which stuttering subsides under conditions of altered phonation (e.g., unison singing, whispering) or alterations in auditory feedback (e.g., loud noise, delayed auditory feedback [DAF]) suggests that underlying neurobiological systems play a role. Finally, when the stuttering of some individuals is particularly chronic and unyielding, even to conditions that often ameliorate stuttering, such symptomatology is more consistent with what could be expected from a physically based disorder.

An important question in regard to the preceding is "What evidence would be needed to establish a physically based stuttering disorder?" In Chapter 5, we pointed out several challenges to be addressed by research in order to identify potential physical bases for stuttering. It was suggested that evidence should be found in children who stutter close to the onset of stuttering. If research only examines evidence in adult populations, the physical conditions could have developed secondary to stuttering, perhaps as a response to the disorder over many years. These conditions may not be the cause but rather the result of stuttering. Also, organically oriented theories must account for why the stuttering symptoms generally are not constant but so highly variable.

Another question is relevant to clinical implications: What would it mean to intervention approaches if stuttering was caused by some deficiency in the individual's physical constitution? One obvious conclusion would be that our interventions and expectations of clients' progress must be altered accordingly. On one hand, psychological and behavioral approaches to modification would have to be understood as compensatory rather than remedial measures. On the other hand, efforts to discover/develop medical treatments (drugs, electrical stimulation, surgeries, etc.) would probably receive greater attention.

Genetic Perspectives

Although the idea of multiple etiologies of stuttering has been frequently expressed in the literature, so far not a single cause of developmental stuttering has been unequivocally identified. One thing we know with increasing certainty, whatever the cause of stuttering, it is in large part genetically transmitted. This may be structural brain features, functional brain features, motor abnormality, personality or temperament characteristics, or others. But which one (or ones) is still unknown. Furthermore, a particular characteristic that increases the susceptibility for stuttering may not, by itself, cause the stuttering. But, when it co-occurs with certain other characteristics, stuttering may be expressed. It is possible, then, that something is inherited that only under certain conditions causes stuttering. It is interesting to note that quite frequently a child with a nonstuttering parent inherits stuttering from a grandfather who stutters. Is it possible that the parent carries certain traits conducive to stuttering that are not overtly expressed in this individual? (See discussion and data by Subramanian & Yairi, 2006.)

To be sure, genetics may be relevant to various theories of stuttering so that some time in the future we will know what is being transmitted and, thus, a particular theory will receive strong support, even confirmation. Nevertheless, the body of data that supports genetic transmission of stuttering, and the models that depict the kind of transmission, should not be construed as a theory of stuttering because it does not attempt to suggest the cause of stuttering, the dynamics of stuttered speech, or rules that govern stuttering. Evidence for genetic factors to stuttering from different types of data is briefly described next.

Familial Incidence

For many years, clinicians working with children and adults who stutter have noticed that the disorder runs in families. One of the authors (Yairi) has had an extensive familial history of stuttering on the paternal side, including his father, two uncles, one aunt, a cousin, a brother, a son, and a nephew. A letter from a father of a child who began stuttering reflects this common situation. It also suggests the possibility that, at times, stuttering may be linked with other inherited conditions and disorders.

I have read several articles you've authored and beg your indulgence on behalf of my 3 1/2 year old son. He suddenly began stuttering a few weeks ago. . . . There is a strong history of both motor and vocal tics in my family. I have 3 children. My oldest daughter, 9, was diagnosed with Tourette's syndrome[1] at age 6. She still has excessive eye-blinking (more like eye squinching). My second daughter, now 7, has a throat-clearing tic and some obvious OCD[2]-type behaviors and sensitivity issues, mostly related to food and eating. And, of course, I am writing you regarding my youngest, our son, who has recently developed a severe stutter.

Moving up the family tree, I have 4 siblings and we ALL have various motor and vocal tics, though none of us were ever diagnosed with Tourette's, Autism, ADHD, ADD, OCD, etc. However, we're all aware that we're "different." We're all functioning,

(continued)

---

[1] It is regarded as a genetically inherited disorder with onset in childhood, characterized by the presence of multiple motor tics. These include facial movements, eye blinking, throat clearing, and/or sniffing. Tics of the vocal folds result in uncontrolled random phonation. Some exhibit tics as well as characteristics of other conditions, such as obsessions, compulsions.

[2] OCD refers to Obsessive-Compulsive Disorder.

well-adjusted adults (for the most part), and most would say, I think, that we're "normal"; but we know better. I, too, struggled with a stutter as an adolescent, but seem to have developed sufficient compensatory mechanisms to have buried the issue—until my son started stuttering! Now, my own stuttering seems to be returning—and I'm 45.

Still further up the tree, my father was diagnosed, at age 7, with Sydenham's Chorea in 19XX. He had a neck and eye twitch, which he recalls as being stress-related. A year off from school seemed to have "cured" him, though he still displays several vocal tics. Tourette's Syndrome didn't come to be called such until the 1970s, I believe. Dad is now 70 and recently retired after a successful business career. He had 2 brothers, at least one of which had many motor and vocal tics—deep knee-bends, throat-clearing, and foot-shaking. . . . That individual, my late uncle, had 2 daughters (now middle-aged) who freely engage in laughter with me and my siblings, all being first cousins, about how strange it is that we all have such strikingly similar behaviors, especially that we did not all grow up together. We'd all be open to participating in a 3-generation genetic study. The genetics are remarkable to all of us, especially from my wife's perspective [because she] sees most of this much more clearly than even we do. . . .

Clinicians' observations have been substantiated in a good number of studies. One of the first surveys found that 46% of the probands who stuttered (in the genetic literature, the person whose relatives are surveyed is referred to as the *proband*) had a family history of stuttering compared with only 18% in probands who did not stutter (Bryngelson & Rutherford, 1937). A review of 28 studies concluded that the majority of them yielded familial stuttering in 30% to 60% of those who stutter as compared with under 10% for families of normally fluent controls (Yairi, Ambrose, & Cox, 1996). In their own research, these investigators found 71% of stuttering children had stuttering histories in their immediate (parents and siblings) or extended family. Most of them, 43%, had stuttering in their immediate family only, and 28% had at least one parent with such history. This type of information, however, is insufficient to reach conclusions about the genetic nature of stuttering because it failed to take into account size of family and the specific familial class of the relatives who stuttered. For example, a person may report one stuttering relative in a family of only 4 members, whereas another person reports one relative who stutters in a family of 16. Or one person may report a father who stutters, whereas another person reports a second cousin who stutters. Still, the information provided a strong motive for better research approaches.

Twin Studies

Twin research compares the similarity, referred to as the *concordance*, of the two members of a pair of identical twins in relation to a particular trait, say stuttering. Identical twins develop from a single fertilized egg (which is why they are also called maternal or monozygotic twins) and, therefore, share 100% of their genes. Hence close similarity for the trait is expected. The level of similarity for the same trait is then compared to that of nonidentical (fraternal or dizygotic) twins, who develop from two fertilized eggs and therefore share only 50% of their genes like any non-twin siblings.

Clearly, the approach highlights the relative role of the genetic versus the environmental effects underlying the trait or behavior under study. Specific to our topic, the question is if one member of a twin pair stutters, does the second member stutter too? The answer tends to be positive. In spite of the different methods employed for ascertaining probands and family members who stutter, several investigations reported a much higher concordance for stuttering in monozygotic than in dizygotic twins (Andrews, Morris-Yates, Howie, & Martin, 1991; Felsenfeld, Kirk, Zhu, Statham, Neale, & Martin, 2000; Godai, 1976; Howie, 1981). In the Howie study, for example, in two thirds of identical twin pairs in whom stuttering was found, both members stuttered. If stuttering was purely genetic, all pairs with one stutterer would have concordance. But in a third of identical twin pairs in which stuttering occurred in one member, the other member was not affected. Hence the findings have strengthened the evidence for genetic components to stuttering but also indicated environmental influences.

Family Aggregation

Unlike surveys of the percentage of people who stutter having familial history of stuttering, aggregation studies analyze the detailed distribution patterns of stuttering in the familial pedigrees (trees), accounting as well for gender, family size, and degree of relatedness (e.g., first degree = siblings; second degree = cousins). The most important feature of these studies is that statistical methods, such as *segregation analysis*, allow investigators to determine the most likely mode of genetic transmission by matching the familial distributions of stuttering against several possible genetic models. These are listed here:

- No genetic components
- Multifactorial polygenic (MFP; environmental factors + many genes)
- Single major locus (SML; one or a few main genes are involved)
- Mixed (both MFP and SML components)

Investigators Kay and Garside carried out the first aggregation study in the United Kingdom, which was published by Andrews and Harris (1964). They concluded that the data for stuttering had the best fit with a model that depicted a disorder controlled by a primary gene with contributions from other genes (SML). Their data, however, also allowed for the possibility of a purely polygenic inheritance (MFP). Over the next several decades, other researchers have proposed and tested genetic models to explain the transmission of stuttering as a family trait. A large-scale investigation of possible genetic factors in stuttering was conducted at Yale University (i.e., Kidd, 1977, 1980; Kidd, Heimbuch, & Records, 1981; Kidd, Kidd, & Records, 1978). They concluded that the data could fit any of three models: multifactorial polygenic, single major locus, and mixed (Cox, Kramer, & Kidd, 1984; Kidd, 1980).

Two more recent reports came from the University of Illinois Stuttering Research Program where all families were identified through young children shortly after stuttering onset. Their samples provided a considerably more complete representation of the population of people who stutter. This team was the first to report statistically significant evidence for both a single major locus and a polygenic transmission of stuttering (Ambrose, Yairi, & Cox, 1993). The finding is particularly encouraging because it should be easier to isolate one or a few primary genes than to identify many genes.

A few years later, the Illinois team conducted an investigation that was primarily aimed at comparing the genetic bases of two subpopulations: children who recovered spontaneously from stuttering and those who developed persistent (chronic) stuttering. They concluded that the developmental pathways of persistence and natural recovery were related to differences in genetic factors. Specifically, that both forms of stuttering share a common major gene, but persistent stuttering involves more complex genetic factors because it involves additional genes (Ambrose, Cox, & Yairi, 1997).

> Regardless of the research progress concerned with *how* stuttering is propagated, it is still unclear *what* is being transmitted genetically that contributes to the cause of stuttering. The "what" could be related to personality trait/s, speech motor skills, sensory feedback characteristics, neural timing properties, or other constitutionally based abilities or features impacting fluency. Because a combination of factors may interact to cause susceptibility, even nonstuttering family members can transmit genetic characteristics that could lead to the disorder. The good news is that if a major gene is involved, there is a high chance to eventually locate it.

Biological Genetics

In view of accumulated findings from behavioral/statistical research, recent years have seen a major shift to genotyping research. Typically, the first phase in such research is known as *linkage analysis*, which uses body tissues, such as blood, to identify chromosomes, and the general region within each one of them, where genes underlying stuttering are located.

These studies have yielded positive initial findings (Riaz et al., 2005; Shugart et al., 2004; Wittke-Thompson et al., 2007). The largest genotyping study was conducted by the Illinois Stuttering Research Program, which extracted DNA from blood samples of 585 individuals. Their findings suggested that genes from three different combinations of chromosomes: numbers 2 and 9; 7 and 12; 7 and 18) may result in stuttering. Additionally, there were sex differences in respect to specific chromosomes, showing the strongest linkage signal on chromosome 13 for males and 21 for females (Suresh et al., 2006). At this point, however, no specific genes underlying stuttering have been isolated on any of the chromosomes.

Summary of Genetic Perspectives

A growing body of evidence supports the existence of a genetic basis for stuttering. The incidence of stuttering among family members of those who stutter is significantly higher than among family members of those who do not. It is more likely for both members of an identical twin pair to stutter compared to both members of a fraternal twin pair. Family aggregation studies indicate there might be a single major locus for the genes underlying stuttering, and that a polygenic transmission could also be responsible. Finally, biologically based genotyping studies are revealing the specific chromosomes with the greatest linkage signal for stuttering. It is still not known what exactly is being transmitted, whether genetic differences are primarily affecting aspects of motor, linguistic, temperamental, or other factors in speech development. Research is needed to reveal which factors are the major players and whether there are subtypes influenced by different sets of factors.

> Current knowledge about genetics and stuttering is useful for diagnosis, prognosis, treatment, and counseling. For example, if a child who begins to stutter has a family history of persistent stuttering, it raises a red flag of a higher risk that he or she will follow that familial pattern of persistent stuttering. Alternatively, if the child has a family history of recovered stuttering, there is a much better chance for natural recovery. Inasmuch as there are several genetic pathways leading to stuttering, the prospect for improved future identification of subtypes is reinforced.

Theories of Brain Dysfunction

One reasonable hypothesis about the genes underlying stuttering is that they seed an atypical development of brain structure and function. Several points of evidence lend support to this idea. First, as indicated earlier, individuals with brain damage often exhibit fluency problems. Although overall their disfluent speech characteristics are different from those exhibited by people who stutter (Yairi, Gintautas, & Avent, 1981), some patients reveal remarkable similarity to developmental stuttering. Second, a growing number of studies report brain structure differences between people who stutter and normally fluent people (Chang, Erickson, Ambrose, Hasegawa-Johnson, & Ludlow, 2008; Foundas et al., 2003). Third, other biophysiological differences in adults who stutter, such as atypical cerebral blood flow during speech and stuttering, have been documented (Watson & Freeman, 1997). Fourth, brain activation patterns in adults who stutter are different from normal (Beal, Gracco, Lafaille, & De Nil, 2007; Brown, Ingham, Ingham, Laird, & Fox, 2005). Fifth, reduced stuttering as a result of therapy is associated with changes in patterns of brain activity (De Nil, Kroll, Kapur, & Houle, 2000; De Nil, Kroll, Lafaille, & Houle, 2003). It is not surprising, then, that theories proposing brain-related causes of stuttering would attract interest. Several are briefly reviewed here.

Cerebral Hemispheric Dominance

One of the earliest published theories of stuttering proposed that it arises from an improper balance of control between the two cerebral hemispheres. A pioneer of 20th-century stuttering research, Lee Travis (1931), proposed that stuttering is caused by a lack of hemispheric dominance, more commonly referred to as the *cerebral dominance theory*. The theory rests on the nature of hemispheric innervations as relay centers of neural signals to the opposite (contralateral) side of the body.

To accomplish simultaneous movement of both sides of the body working together toward a common goal (e.g., oral postures for speech), it is assumed that each brain hemisphere must participate in a carefully orchestrated set of neural signals. If the hemispheres operated independently, then there would be no predicting whether their signals to musculature on opposite sides would be coordinated. For example, both left and right *masseters*, muscles on opposite sides of the face, must be activated concurrently to move the jaw up and down. Similarly, both sides of the tongue, a single muscle structure, must be active together for changing position from one vowel gesture to the next, across syllables.

The cerebral dominance theory assumes that to accomplish simultaneous movement, one brain hemisphere must take the lead in establishing the movement pattern while the other hemisphere follows to match it. The theory suggests that the brains of people who stutter lack the necessary dominance. Hence stuttering arises from a conflict over which cerebral hemisphere should take the lead. As the hemispheres attempt to resolve the confusion, the result is an asynchrony (mistiming) of neural impulses from both sides to the speech musculature, and, in turn, a disruption to the fluent execution of speech. In other words, the theory proposes that overt stuttering events are the result of neurological blocks.

In its time, the cerebral dominance theory gained strength based on a combination of facts. For one, hemispheric functions exert contralateral control, being responsible for muscles on the opposite side of the body. Second, the notion of cerebral dominance and body-side preferences for various motor activities was recognized. And third, it was known that oral language expression in right-handed people, the majority of the population, arises mainly from left-hemisphere regions (Wernicke's and Broca's areas).

To explain the lack of cerebral dominance for speech in people who stutter, it was suggested that they were naturally left-handed with a right hemisphere dominance for speech. Their handedness, however, had been changed, perhaps through adult pressure to do so. The shift from left- to right-handedness led to an underused, weakened right hemisphere that was losing its dominance for the person's speech. The result: lack of cerebral dominance with confusion and conflict over which hemisphere should take the lead. Stuttering presumably occurs as the hemispheres struggled over which side should dominate control for the act of speech.

The cerebral dominance theory attracted considerable attention and influenced widespread public thinking about stuttering. Many parents and schoolteachers were blamed for stuttering because they had shifted a child's handedness for writing, causing hemispheric conflict. Even at the time of writing this textbook, an elderly man who stuttered told one of us he was still inclined to believe what he had been told as a child: He stuttered because his writing handedness had been switched in elementary school.

Early support for the theory came from several directions. For example, in a survey conducted by one of Travis's students, a majority of 13 children trained to change handedness developed stuttering within 1 year (Fagan, 1931). Several studies measured electrical activity in the speech musculature using *electromyography* (EMG). For example, one EMG investigation revealed that the action potentials from right and left masseter muscles, responsible for lower jaw movement, were unequal during stuttering, unlike those measured in normally fluent speakers (Travis, 1934). Morely (1937) reported similar findings. although a substantial proportion of the electromyographic (EMG) abnormalities of speakers who stutter were during their fluent speech, and not only during stuttering. Several investigators used an *electroencephalograph* (EEG) to record the cortical electrical activity of people who stutter. They found that the alpha brain waves during fluent speech were somewhat larger and slower than those of normal speakers during fluent speech (Travis & Knott, 1936; Travis & Malamud, 1937).

From the mid-1940s to the beginning of the 1970s, the cerebral dominance theory lost ground in good part because research concerned with brainwaves (e.g., Rheinberger, Karlin, & Berman, 1943; Scarbrough, 1943) and bilateral speech muscle function (Williams, 1955) failed to support it. The latter investigator employed EMG to study the masseter muscle and found that the same anomalous activity observed in people who stutter was also seen in normal controls when they faked stuttering. In other words, it was the specific jaw movement involved in stuttering that caused the abnormal signals, not necessarily abnormal muscle activity causing the stuttering (Williams, 1955).

The theory also weakened when new evidence surfaced regarding handedness. Research revealed that the majority of left-handers, 60% to 70%, were left-hemisphere dominant for speech, not right dominant as previously assumed. Also, rather than being an "all or none" phenomenon, handedness was shown to be a continuum of varying degrees of ambidexterity across the human population, with the more adept hand varying across different skills (Daniels, 1940). Research had also shown that shifting handedness for writing in 23 children did not cause stuttering (Ojemann, 1931).

The cerebral dominance theory had several logical clinical consequences. For a while, some clinicians began retraining people who stutter in shifting from their right to the left hand, aiming to return them to the supposedly original handedness. It was believed that the increased left-hand usage would also strengthen their right cerebral hemisphere to the point of retaking its dominance and restoring fluency

(Williams, 1955). With the hope that cerebral dominance might be influenced and improve speech, both Wendell Johnson and Charles Van Riper participated in the act of constraining their right forearms (and hands) in plaster casts for a year. Neither, however, found this process afforded any relief for their speech (Travis, 1978a). A much greater influence spawned by this theory is seen in the advocacy of procedures that encourage the stutterer to remain "objective" during stuttering. Inasmuch as the cause is organic in nature, went the logic, the best the client can do is accept the stuttering and reduce emotional reaction to minimize further aggravation of the neurological-based affliction (Bryngelson, 1931).

Interestingly, Travis abandoned his brain-related theory of stuttering for a period, shifting his attention to psychoanalytical perspectives on stuttering (Travis, 1957). Some research activity concerned with brain function and structure of people who stutter continued at low levels for about 25 years before a new surge of interest emerged in the 1970s. Lee Travis (1978b) himself contributed to promoting this renewed trend when he published two articles where he asserted he had never disavowed the cerebral dominance theory. He summarized relevant research related to the Wada test,[3] auditory evoked potentials, and dichotic listening studies in people who stutter, proposing that the resultant differences still supported a problem with interhemispheric functions.

Excessive Right Hemisphere Activity

Later brain research continued to generate interest in the possible role of hemispheric activity in stuttering. Based on studies that used *positron emission tomography* (PET), an imaging technique that produces a three-dimensional map of the functional processes in the body region being scanned, the idea emerged that rather than a lack of cerebral dominance, the overactivation of the right hemisphere during speech leads to stuttering. Recall that normally, brain activity during speech is greatest in Broca's and Wernicke's speech-language centers in the left hemisphere. Two studies that employed the technique revealed different brain activity patterns for stutterers in both oral and silent reading conditions compared to baseline levels. The focal area of excess activation was the right frontal motor cortex, right behind the central sulcus (De Nil, Kroll, Kapur, & Houle, 2000; Kroll, De Nil, Kapur, & Houle, 1997). Consequently, they proposed that people who stutter may have innate, or early acquired, differences in brain activation patterns, namely excessive right hemisphere activity. The researchers stressed the importance of early intervention for stuttering when the brain's plasticity is greatest, so that activation patterns may be changed. Additional support for increased right-sided brain activation in adults who stutter was reported by Preibisch et al. (2003). Again, in both speech and non-speech tasks, greater right hemisphere activation was demonstrated by participants who stuttered.

---

[3] In the Wada test, sodium amobarbital is injected into one of the internal carotid arteries to shut down temporarily the function of the one associated cerebral hemisphere for several minutes. This is done to evaluate the functions of the opposite hemisphere. The patient is asked to talk, respond to questions, engage in memory tasks, and so on. The test was named after Juhn Wada, the Japanese-Canadian neurologist who invented it.

Despite these robust results, the theory for the role of excessive right hemisphere activation has been challenged by others who offer alternate explanations. Because these studies were conducted only with adults, it was argued that excessive right hemisphere activation could be the result, rather than the cause, of stuttering or other developmental domains (Buchel et al., 2004). Moreover, it could be that the right hemisphere activation arises primarily as a reflection of stuttering movements and might be noted even if nonstuttering speakers voluntarily imitated stuttering. It has also been pointed out that right hemisphere activity could represent compensation for other brain differences that cause stuttering (Fox et al., 2000; Ludlow, 2000). Alm (2004b) explained that if the basal ganglia were not providing adequate timing information to the supplementary motor area, then SMA activation with increased right-side dominance would show up as compensatory processes during stuttering. This explanation is consistent with findings by Fox et al. (1996) and Ingham, Fox, Ingham, and Zamarripa (2000). Other recent research also revealed additional brain areas involved with stuttering, not necessarily situated in the right hemisphere (Fox et al., 2000; Ludlow & Loucks, 2003).

Further Evidence of Brain Differences

Scientists have been making great strides toward a better understanding of the brain. As our knowledge of the neurological underpinnings for fluent speech expands, it serves as a foundation for revealing the brain regions and processes potentially responsible for stuttering. The neurological basis for action is particularly relevant to fluency because speech is composed of movements. A sequenced chain of commands begins with the anterior frontal region of the cortex (where action is planned), and projects through the cingulate, supplementary motor area, and premotor area, and then to the primary motor area. This hierarchical activation pattern is enhanced by tandem connections of these areas with other cortical areas so parallel activations can take place as well. For example, action may be influenced by sensory feedback, as well as being enhanced by information from other brain areas. Figure 7.1 and Table 7.1 illustrate the brain regions used for these functions.

Although currently there is no formal theory of how brain structure and function cause and sustain the disorder of stuttering, a growing body of scientific data indicate there are brain differences between people who stutter and normally fluent speakers. These can be organized into three areas. The next two are covered in this section: brain structure and brain physiology. The third area, auditory processing of perceptual stimuli, is discussed in the next section.

Brain Structure

Brain-imaging research has yielded data that indicate possibilities of structural (anatomical) differences between adults who stutter and normally fluent controls. Among the most interesting studies were those conducted by Foundas, Bollich, Corey, Hurley, and Heilman (2001) and by Foundas et al. (2004) reporting a rather atypical right-left asymmetry for the stutterers, with the left planum temporale, the

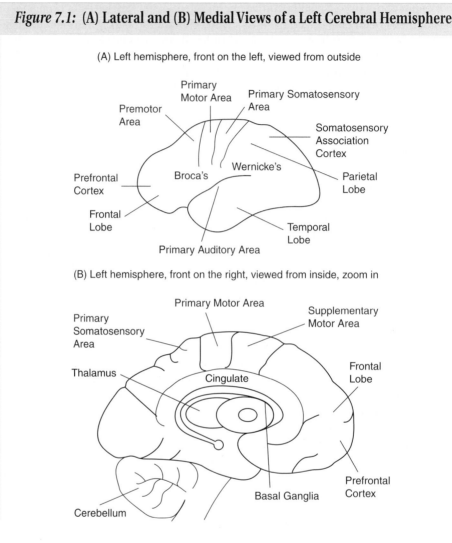

Figure 7.1: **(A) Lateral and (B) Medial Views of a Left Cerebral Hemisphere**

(A) Left hemisphere, front on the left, viewed from outside

Primary Motor Area

Premotor Area

Primary Somatosensory Area

Somatosensory Association Cortex

Prefrontal Cortex

Broca's

Wernicke's

Parietal Lobe

Frontal Lobe

Temporal Lobe

Primary Auditory Area

(B) Left hemisphere, front on the right, viewed from inside, zoom in

Primary Motor Area

Supplementary Motor Area

Primary Somatosensory Area

Thalamus

Cingulate

Frontal Lobe

Basal Ganglia

Prefrontal Cortex

Cerebellum

center of the Wernicke's area, a critically important cortical center for language processing, tending to be smaller than the right. By contrast, in the normally fluent controls, the left planum temporale was larger than the right. Also they noticed a larger number of gyri (the convolutions seen on the surface of the cortex) in the brains of stutterers. These observations led to the hypothesis that perhaps auditory processing of language is different in people who stutter. Complementary findings included an increased volume of white matter in the right hemisphere (Jancke, Hanggi, & Steinmetz, 2004) and reduced white matter integrity in the left hemisphere (Sommer, Koch, Paulus, Weiller, & Buchel, 2002).

Table 7.1: **Summary of the Brain Regions and Their Functions for Producing Movements**

Speech Function	Brain Region
1. Decisions are made about the type and characteristics of actions to be taken (e.g., lift tongue blade to touch alveolar ridge)	Parietal lobes and prefrontal motor areas
2. Anticipatory planning and initiation of movement based on past experience (e.g., start contracting muscles to raise tongue)	Primary motor area and supplementary motor area
3. Integration of sensory and spatial information used to guide movements (e.g., tongue is short distance from center)	Posterior parietal cortex and premotor area
4. Specifications for the sequence and duration (timing) of movements: Activities of each body part are coordinated with precision (e.g., open lips and raise tongue, then exhale air)	Cerebellum
5. Movements are inhibited until time for their delivery (e.g., wait to breathe until tongue is ready)	Basal ganglia indirectly involved with the thalamus

Brain Physiology

In the section on Travis's cerebral dominance theory, we mentioned studies of brain activity using EEG. More recent research has employed several modern technologies, among them *magnetic resonance imagery* (MRI), which provides clear images of and *contrast* between different soft tissues such as neural (e.g., brain), and various types of muscles. You will find that many modern studies of stuttering employ MRI. Still, several brain studies conducted by F. Freeman and colleagues employed other techniques, including electrophysiologic (QTE) and metabolic regional cerebral blood flow (rCBF) as measures of brain function. These investigators reported a tendency toward longer laryngeal reaction times (LRT) in a subgroup of people who stutter with below normal right-left asymmetry of blood flow in certain regions of the temporal lobe (Watson et al., 1992). Longer LRTs implied that people who stutter did not initiate voiced sound, such as that used for speech, as quickly as others. In another study, adults who stuttered and also exhibited language deficiencies had significant blood flow asymmetry (left < right) in certain regions of the temporal and frontal lobes compared to those without language deficits (Watson et al., 1994).

The only brain-imaging study of children who stutter found to date was conducted at the University of Illinois Stuttering Research Program with 9- to 12-year-olds. The investigators reported that risk for childhood stuttering in general was associated with deficiencies in left hemisphere gray matter volume. Children who persisted in stuttering also had reduced white matter integrity in the left hemisphere speech area (Chang et al., 2008, p. 1133). Because this result was unlike previous findings of anatomical increases in the right hemisphere for adults who stutter, Chang and colleagues proposed that whereas the left hemisphere may reveal differences in stuttering children, right hemisphere differences may reflect the lifetime influences of stuttering by adults.

More recently, brain blood flow measures obtained by means of PET were applied to males and females who stutter (Ingham et al., 2004). Differences were found, although, interestingly, not in brain regions correlated with variations in stuttering. All in all, the findings just described support the notion of brain differences between people who stutter and normally fluent speakers. They also indicate that (1) stuttering subgroups might be identified by the relative magnitude of blood flow abnormality in the brain, and (2) gender differences in susceptibility and recovery may be related to brain differences between males and females who stutter (Yairi & Ambrose, 2005).

Summary of Brain-Related Theories

There have been several significant theoretical points of view regarding stuttering as a function of abnormal brain activity. These have hypothesized that stuttering occurs secondary to a lack of cerebral dominance, or excessive right hemisphere activation, or from a hypersensitive brainstem reflex response. Some quasi-supportive evidence has contributed to ongoing speculations and additional inquiries about the role of the cerebral hemispheres and supportive neural structures in stuttering. Research has also suggested that there may be differences in people who stutter with respect to brain anatomy, such as various deficiencies in white and/or gray matter, and with respect to brain physiology, for example as evidenced in blood flow.

Theories of Auditory Processing

Another direction, prompted in part by brain research, explains stuttering as a disorder of auditory processing. Studies have reported reduced brain activity in the temporal region known to be responsible for auditory functions during stuttering (Fox et al., 2000; Watkins, Smith, Davis, & Howell, 2008). Such observations add to the concern with whether people who stutter process auditory stimuli in the same way as those who do not stutter.

The Role of Audition

It is well recognized that normal speech development relies heavily on the close relation between speech control and audition. That is, adequate sensory-to-motor integration processes between hearing and speech are essential to its production. For example, deaf children do not develop normally sounding speech because they lack auditory feedback about their speech output. A potential connection between hearing acuity and stuttering is supported by the very low incidence of the disorder in the deaf population (Montgomery & Fitch, 1988). Other evidence for the interactive relation between audition and speech is the *Lombard sign* (also known as the *Lombard effect*), observed when people automatically raise their voices by a predictable amount when speaking in noise (Harlen & Tranel, 1971). Therefore, it is of special interest to note, as seen in Chapter 4, that when people who stutter speak in the presence of a sufficiently high noise level, their stuttering is substantially reduced (Wingate, 1976). Similarly, amelioration of stuttering is seen when people who stutter hear their own speech through a DAF instrument (Perkins, 1973b; Sparks et al., 2002; Wingate, 1970) or other form of altered auditory feedback, such as frequency-shifted auditory feedback (Stuart et al., 2004). In contrast, it has been shown that DAF can induce disfluencies in normally fluent people (e.g., Jones & Striemer, 2007; Lee, 1950; Van Borsel, Sunaert, & Engelen, 2005). Finally, several scholars have suggested classifications of people who stutter based on their dichotic listening, which is an indirect method of probing auditory processing (see review by Yairi, 2007).

Explanations of the Stuttering-Audition Link

In what ways has the stuttering-audition link been explained? Several theoretical notions have been proposed in this regard. In the first experiment of noise effects on stuttering, Shane (1955) proposed a psychological explanation. Adhering to the Johnsonian ideas that stuttering results from people's anxiety about their own stuttered speech, Shane postulated that because people talking in noise cannot hear their own speech, they cannot be critical of it, become apprehensive, and stutter. Another plausible explanation is based on motoric rather than psychoemotional factors. A person's manner of speaking changes in conditions of altered auditory stimulation. For example, a person tends to speak more loudly and sustain vocalization longer in masking noise (Cherry & Sayers, 1956). Another change in speaking manner was noted by Wingate (1976), who cites more than 25 articles reporting that DAF results in slower speech. The combination of changes in articulation and vocalization, summed up as an alteration in prosodic pattern, could be the mechanism responsible for fluency when auditory stimulation is altered, as concluded by Wingate (1976).

The relation between stuttering and audition was heavily researched by Cherry, Sayers, and Marland (1955) and Cherry and Sayers (1956). These investigators conducted a series of experiments on the effect of loud sounds on stuttering using tonal and noise stimuli in selective frequency bands, all delivered either via air or bone conduction. They concluded that the largest reduction in stuttering, to nearly elimination, occurred under low-frequency, bone-conducted noise. Additionally, they had people who stutter use *shadowing* speech, attempting to follow that person's speech in very close time proximity, almost simultaneously. This too was very effective in reducing stuttering. Considering all these findings, the investigators proposed a third theory: Stuttering is a perceptual defect. According to them, it seemed reasonable to hypothesize that people who stutter suffer from a defective auditory feedback loop that interferes with accurate speech motor activity, causing disfluent speech. By overriding the reliance on one's own feedback, for example by means of noise or by having the person rely on external feedback (shadowing), stuttering can be averted. As we discuss in Chapter 12, miniature instruments that generate masking noise or deliver DAF or other altered auditory feedback signals to the ears have been employed in the treatment of stuttering.

Harrington (1988) developed a more specific version of the idea that stuttering is a perceptual disorder involving auditory feedback. He hypothesized that people who stutter experience a defect in the timing of auditory feedback. The lagging auditory feedback causes the speaker to expect to hear sound earlier than the system feeds it back. The speaker therefore waits (prolongs) or repeats the speech segment in an effort to correct the mismatch of information about speech timing. Observations that stuttering is frequently ameliorated in conditions of DAF or under loud noise were taken as supportive evidence. Also, people who stutter appear to need more time to speak fluently, as if they are permitting their auditory system sufficient time to feed back the sound of speech.

Summary of Auditory-Related Theories

Evidence from multiple sources suggests a special relation between audition and stuttering, particularly as evidenced in the effect of noise and DAF on diminishing overt stuttering. One limitation of these theories is that they do not account for the fact people sometimes begin stuttering, as seen in their facial and oral tension and apparent attempt to speak, before they have uttered any vocal sound. How, then, can stuttering occur if there is no sound fed back through the defective auditory system? Additional questions were raised when research demonstrated reduction in stuttering when noise was presented only during nonphonated periods of speech (Sutton & Chase, 1961) or in only one ear when self-hearing is still preserved in the other ear (Yairi, 1976). It is also a fact that not all individuals who stutter respond with more fluency in the conditions of either noise or delayed auditory feedback. It would appear, therefore, that if the auditory defect theory holds, it may only be relevant for a subgroup of individuals who stutter. Although the stuttering-audition link is still misunderstood, it has already been exploited for therapeutic purposes.

Theories of Motor Dysfunction

Earlier in this chapter, we pointed out that various ideas about motor factors contributing to stuttering have been entertained for hundreds of years. During the first third of the 20th century, when stuttering became the subject of systematic research, motor abilities of people who stutter began to be researched in controlled laboratory studies. Among early investigators, West and Nusbaum (1929) compared people who stutter (PWS) and people who do not stutter (PWNS) on their speed of jaw and facial muscle contraction. The slowness exhibited by the PWS in the action of these muscles was interpreted to be a cause, or related to the cause, of stuttering. The investigators stated that slowness suggests a neuromuscular imbalance that may result in stuttering. Other investigators, who looked at breathing, found general malfunctioning of the breathing mechanism during stuttering (Fletcher, 1914; Fossler, 1930; Travis, 1927). Cross (1936) investigated a large range of motor skills and reported that although PWS were not inferior to PWNS in unimanual (use of a single hand) tasks, they were significantly inferior to them in bimanual tasks.

One of the challenges to the study of potential motor sources of stuttering is determining the most pertinent questions to address. What kind of a breakdown and in what system(s) is evidenced as stuttering? Is stuttering but one symptom of a general, extensive motor disorder that might have additional, apparently unrelated symptoms? Does the underlying problem, whatever it is, exist during nonstuttered speech? In nonspeech systems? On a broad level, three types of movement-related systems could play a role in breakdown of speech fluency: sensory perceptions, motor actions, and executive (central) decisions. In combination, these three systems aid the speaker's control of motor speech.

The diagram in Figure 7.2 can be used to illustrate these three systems. Regarding movement decisions, there must be instructions from brain centers to the speech structures as to (1) whether to move, (2) when to move, (3) where to move, (4) what distance to move, and (5) what speed to move. With respect to actual movement or action, the structures (e.g., the tongue) must both respond to command and achieve the target parameters. Sensory perceptions (feedback) are essential for generating instructions for the movement in progress because they are the source of information about the structures' position (e.g., spatial location of the tongue), size/weight (e.g., how heavy is the tongue?), activity (e.g., is the tongue moving already?), contact (e.g., is the tongue touching something?), and elastic properties (e.g., is the tongue resistant/stiff?). Research could be conducted to reveal which of these dimensions are most important where stuttering is concerned.

Figure 7.2: **Three Systems Involved in the Regulation of Movement**

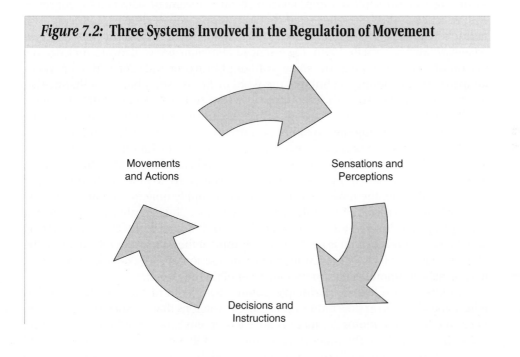

Movements and Actions

Sensations and Perceptions

Decisions and Instructions

Speech, among other physical movements, is potentially controlled or regulated with a combination of feed forward and feedback processes. Feedback occurs when the person receives information about the outcome of movement *after* it has occurred (e.g., was the intended sound spoken?). In feed forward, the parameters of movement are established *before* the action, and no attention is given to tracking or checking on the result of the movement that takes place (as is often the case when swearing or yelling). Feed forward processes are considered *open loop* because they consist only of the instructions and the actions. Sensory information is used prior to the initial decision for action but is not consulted while action is in progress. Feedback processes, by contrast, are *closed loop* in that during the action, sensory information is consulted and used to adjust and refine the movement.

Motor Learning Theories of Stuttering

A model of motor learning "may prove to be a valuable theoretical framework to interpret changes in stuttering" (Caruso & Max, 1997, p. 213). Motor learning theory deals with the science of how skilled actions are developed, how practice and its associated variables influence permanent changes in performance, and how trial-and-error processes are involved in learning. Because speech is a motor act, we can expect its acquisition and refinement to be governed by motor learning principles. A number of these principles can be examined relative to the facts and phenomena of stuttering. One principle of motor learning is that movement skills can be improved with practice. It has been suggested that adaptation, the decline of stuttering with multiple readings of the same passage, may reflect the benefit of practice or *motor rehearsal* (Max & Caruso, 1998). Experienced clinicians are well aware that when a person who stutters repeats the same word or phrase over and over, with no particular instruction regarding technique, the word or phrase soon becomes fluent. This has been demonstrated in the laboratory as well (Brutten & Dancer, 1980). In motor learning terms, *massed* practice (e.g., saying each word over multiple times) can be as effective at improving speech motor performance as *distributed* practice (e.g., saying the whole passage or paragraph over multiple times) (Schmidt & Lee, 2005). The greatest challenge to the application of the motor rehearsal hypothesis to stuttering, however, is that the fluency gains do not readily generalize to new conditions or spoken material. Here, the motor learning appears to apply only to the particular passage or item rehearsed, often only for a limited time. Thus another motor learning principle, *generalization* after rehearsal, does not hold up in the case of stuttering and fluency. More research is needed to determine if the gains from rehearsal can be effectively generalized. For example, the manipulation of the schedule of rehearsal may reveal conditions that improve carryover of fluent speech.

Another motor learning principle potentially related to speech fluency is that rehearsing an action in slow motion generalizes to actions that are sped up. There is no need to relearn the motor act just because a different rate is used (Schmidt & Lee, 2005). In theory, then, the practice of a slow rate of fluent speech in therapy should carry over to conditions where a faster rate is used. In reality, however, speakers who stutter must be careful not to attempt rates beyond their capacity to sustain the desired fluent speech movement. Another motor principle is Fitts's law of speed-accuracy trade-off (Schmidt & Lee, 2005). The precision of a motor act will deteriorate if the attempted rate is *too* fast. Fitts's law reminds us that there is an inverse relationship between the difficulty of a movement and the speed with which it can be performed.

Dynamics of motor learning may eventually be important to our understanding of stuttering. Consider the child who discovers a button to push, and does it over and over again, just exploring it. Perhaps there are young children who, by chance, find and explore the means of triggering stuttering, exploring it over and over again without being able to help themselves from it. Impulse control and the refined regulation of action take some time to develop. In the meantime, the child may often trigger stuttering, making it an unintentionally practiced habit. These motor learning principles and possibilities lead us to consider a few concepts of stuttering that possibly qualify as motor theories. These are briefly discussed next.

Brainstem Reflexes: A Disorder of Movement

Kinematics, the study of how things move, has been applied quite extensively in stuttering research. In 1980, Zimmermann conducted a series of kinematic investigations using cinefluorography, a method of producing x-ray motion images. The images were used to measure movements of oral and facial structures involved in speech, such as the lower jaw and tongue, of people who stutter. Zimmermann's (1980b) research found that adults who stutter produced oral movements during fluent speech, such as transitions between consonants and vowels, steady state portions of vowels, or when building up movement speed, slower than normally fluent speakers do. He interpreted the findings to suggest that stuttering should be considered a disorder of movement triggered by brainstem reflex responses. Zimmermann conjectured that stuttering was due to a speaker's reduced tolerance for oral speech movement that deviates from the typical range in both space and time. When movements either overshoot or undershoot the speaker's intended targets, they trigger conflicting afferent (sensory) and efferent (motor) brainstem reflexes to correct the movement. The resultant struggle between the original movement and the reflex corrective response could be abnormal oscillatory movements (repetitions), frozen postures (silent blocks or voiced prolongations), or something else that constitutes stuttering (Zimmermann, 1980c). These ideas ignored the possibility that slow movements could be a result, rather than the cause, of stuttering. A particularly interesting observation during stuttered speech, was that just prior to terminating stuttering blocks, adults often repositioned their oral structures, lowering the jaw and changing the lip and/or tongue shape. The clinical implication of this theory was that people who stutter need to speak more slowly so as to move the articulators within the allowable range of space and time in order to avoid triggering brainstem reflex interference. It also implied they should learn to assume new articulatory postures (e.g., lowering the jaw) to release blocks.

The Zimmermann theory was based, in part, on his data that revealed problems with lower jaw movement. Since that time, investigators have paid particular attention to the jaw, gaining insights about its movement associated with stuttering. For example, one team of investigators found that although both PWS and PWNS employed the same control strategies for the jaw when speaking fluently, the stutterers' opening and closing jaw movement were more restricted as well as slower to build up speed (Jäncke, Bauer, Kaiser, & Kalveram, 1997). More recent research of the jaw uncovered significantly greater target errors and spatial variability in PWS than in PWNS, but there were no differences in the velocities and durations of movements (Loucks, De Nil, & Sasisekaran, 2007). The researchers suggested that the jaw-phonatory discoordination of their stuttering participants indicated either an oral proprioceptive or a motor control deficit. One of the challenges to these conclusions is that they fail to explain why such limitations seem not to be imposed during singing, choral speech, rhythmic metronome speech, and so on, that, in general, tend to be fluent.

Sensorimotor Dysfunction

Earlier in this chapter we stated that although stuttering appears to have a genetic base, it is uncertain what is being genetically transmitted. Later, we reviewed studies that found differences in brain activity in both the motor and somatosensory regions of the cerebral cortex for people who stutter. Hence one of the possibilities is that a person who stutters inherits a sensorimotor system that is insufficient to support fluent speech. Some evidence for this general frame of reference is seen in studies that reported people who stutter had slower sensorimotor response times, for example, vocal or manual responses to visual or auditory stimuli (Cross & Cooke, 1979; Till, Goldsmith, & Reich, 1981). If the sensorimotor systems of people who stutter do not offer timely or otherwise reliable feedback related to the speech musculature, fluency breakdown might occur. This, in essence, is the context of the sensorimotor model of stuttering as reflected in the DIVA (Directions into Velocities of Articulators) model of stuttering.

The DIVA model was developed by Max and colleagues at Haskins Laboratories (Max, Guenther, Gracco, Ghosh, & Wallace, 2004). These researchers hypothesized that people who stutter have trouble acquiring or activating the internal schemes necessary to integrate feed forward and feedback forms of speech motor control. The imbalance arises from inaccurate feed forward programming for speech movements during early childhood, which, in turn, creates an excessive need for dependence on sensory feedback to regulate speech motor activity. The preponderance of feed forward errors, in turn, makes it difficult for the child to engage in a stable and complete mapping process for speech movement targets. Reliable internal maps are necessary so that sensorimotor systems can appropriately guide the speech structures. Uncertain targets may lead to groping, prolonged, or repetitive movements while the structures find their bearing.

A role for motor programming factors underlying stuttering is supported by the hyperactivation of right hemisphere motor and premotor areas, as well as the left cerebellar areas in people who stutter (De Nil et al., 2000; Fox et al., 2000). A tendency for deficient auditory sensory feedback is supported by findings that the auditory cortex tends to be underactive during speech and stuttering (Fox et al., 2000). Also relevant is the research of Sommer et al. (2002) who found that adults who stutter had abnormal white matter pathways for the orofacial area in the primary sensorimotor cortex of the left hemisphere.

Evidence of Motor Differences

Regardless of etiology, it is clear that stuttering manifests itself as a breakdown in the execution of speech movements. Motor involvement is apparent from the observable physical tensions and abnormal articulatory actions and postures during the disfluent speech events at the heart of the disorder. The secondary characteristics add to the general impression of motor involvement. Some of the ways that people who stutter differ in motor system function, however, are detected only through instruments that provide data about the abnormal patterns of activation of muscle groups in the lip, jaw, tongue, or larynx during stuttering. The past several decades of stuttering research have seen a wealth of studies that employed acoustic, kinematic, electromyographic, and other methodologies to derive these data. Measures have included reaction time, various kinematic and temporal parameters of speech, spatial dimensions of articulation, dynamics of articulatory, phonatory, and respiratory aspects of speech production, and activation and tension of various oral, laryngeal, and other muscles of speech. Both static and relative dimensions of a variety of these motor-related parameters have been examined, often in the context of fluent speech.

> Research has provided evidence of atypical or abnormal movement patterns in the *fluent* speech of people who stutter. This could indicate that their physical systems carry the seeds of stuttering moments constantly, just under the surface. The physical system is thus vulnerable to produce the stutter, whereas other factors (e.g., environment, emotion, attention, etc.) play a role in precipitating it. The finding of atypical physiological dynamics beneath the surface of fluent speech in people who stutter would lend support to the view that stuttering is not just a more severe form of normal disfluency. The physiological vulnerability to stutter is something that normally fluent people presumably do not have.

Further examples of research findings concerning the different anatomical areas and functions involved in speech production—respiration, phonation, and articulation—are presented next.

Oral Motor and Articulatory Differences

Clearly, people who stutter often have higher levels of EMG activity (tension) during speech compared to nonstuttering controls. Such tension can be particularly great during stuttering moments (Freeman & Ushijima, 1978; Shapiro, 1980). Levels of EMG, however, do not necessarily correlate with stuttering severity (McClean & Runyan, 2000). Fluent speech presumably depends on carefully orchestrated activation of the various muscle groups. Activations could fail by either being inappropriately timed (out of sequence) or inappropriately strengthened (for the level of force). Another possible miscalculation leading to stuttering would be an inappropriate "balance" of interaction between jaw and lip/tongue activation. With a similar hypothesis in mind, it was reported that EMG data obtained from people who stutter frequently reversed the normal sequence of lip muscle activation, particularly when they stuttered (Guitar, Guitar, Neilson, O'Dwyer, & Andrews, 1988). The authors suggested that there could be problems of activation mistiming underlying stuttering, or that these sequencing patterns could represent an anticipatory hypertension secondary to stuttering.

Another form of evidence for a motor deficit in people who stutter arises from measures of their fluent speech that is slower than it is in normally fluent controls (Zimmermann, 1980a). Although this tendency is evident in preschool children who stutter (Meyers & Freeman, 1985), it is not clear what the tendency toward slowness indicates. It could suggest the speakers are proceeding with caution when they speak, analogous to traversing a minefield where stuttering moments are the landmines that could be triggered. Another explanation is the possibility of weak kinesthetic and/or proprioceptive capacities that do not support the certainty of a faster pace. Some research has suggested evidence for the latter (Archibald & De Nil, 1999). If an orofacial control problem arises during the early stages of speech acquisition, it might prompt stuttering (McClean & Runyan, 2000). Alternatively, stuttering itself could upset the parallel maturation of the neural system. Kelly, Smith, and Goffman (1995) conducted EMG research with children who stutter and who do not stutter at three age levels: preschool, school age, and adolescence. When the three oldest children stuttered, their muscles exhibited tremorlike oscillations in the 5- to 15-Hz range in the upper lip, lower lip, or jaw. By contrast, the younger children who stutter and their controls exhibited peak activity mainly in the 1- to 4-Hz range. It was proposed that as children who stutter continue to experience stuttering symptoms while their neural systems mature, they may tend to develop tremorlike instabilities in their speech movements.

If persons who stutter do have underlying instabilities that interfere with regulating the force of their movements, this could be evident in greater motor variability even during their fluent speech. In fact, several studies have revealed that people who stutter display greater variability of speech movements during fluency (Zimmermann, 1980a). Other studies, however, have revealed no significant differences in the variability of kinematic speech measures between adults who do and do not stutter (Max, Caruso, & Gracco, 2003). At least one study found evidence of higher motor stability in people who stutter, which might suggest either reduced variability in movement or more rigidity (Smith, Goffman, Zelaznik, Ying, & McGillem, 1995). Of particular interest in this regard is a study that demonstrated the effect of language complexity on the speech motor system of people who stutter. The investigators applied an index of motor stability (STI) to study lower lip movement while manipulating utterance length and complexity. Overall, people who stutter had significantly higher STI scores than control subjects. Only for the stutterers, however, did the scores increase significantly between the baseline speech material and the condition that employed increased length and complexity of speech (Kleinow & Smith, 2000).

Finally, little research of this type has been done with preschool children closer to the onset of stuttering because kinematic data are difficult to collect from participants who cannot sit still for very long. Acoustic data are easier to obtain for young children and are cautiously interpreted as an indirect representation of articulatory movement. For example, one study looked at articulatory speaking rate (Hall, Amir, & Yairi,

1999), and another focused on changes in the second formant (F2) transition in fluent speech because variations along the time and frequency domains usually reflect tongue movement (Subramanian, Yairi, & Amir, 2003). Overall, however, both studies revealed little differences from normally fluent peers.

Vocal Physiology Differences

There is a long history to the idea that the larynx is responsible for, or at least an important contributor to, stuttering. This can be seen in the early 19th-century idea relating stuttering to a spasm of the larynx (e.g., Arnott, 1828). Bryngelson (1932) reported reduced pitch range in adults who stutter. With time, such guesses were replaced by better, scientifically based evidence of laryngeal motor mismanagement by people who stutter. In the early research, acoustic laryngeal data predominated because it was noninvasive and relatively easily obtained. Measuring voice onset time (VOT), the time elapsed between the release of a stop-plosive consonant and the beginning of vocal fold vibration for the following voiced sound, was a popular target. Results across studies have been inconsistent, however, with some reporting longer VOT for PWS (e.g., Agnello & Wingate, 1972), whereas others reported no differences from PWNS (Jancke, 1994). Others revealed that PWS exhibited slowness of voice onset time, laryngeal reaction times (LRT), and poorer timing of performance on DDK tasks as compared to PWNS. Nevertheless, no differences were found in other physical systems, such as reaction times for manual button pressing, and non-speech vocal activity such as inspiratory phonation and expiratory throat clearing (Till, Goldsmith, & Reich, 1981; Watson & Alfonso, 1987).

Investigators who used EMG techniques reported no systematic relation between LRT and stuttering severity (Watson et al., 1992). These results suggested that if people who stutter do have motor system insufficiencies, they primarily affect the phonatory behavior rather than the whole body's physical capacities. More recently, Max and Gracco (2005) compared the coordination of oral and laryngeal movements of stuttering and nonstuttering adults. Both kinematic and acoustic techniques were employed to measure the correlation between the gap in the stop consonant /p/ in fluent utterances and the voice onset time (VOT) of the following sound. No significant kinematic differences were found. The participants who stutter, however, had longer durations for the consonant gaps and the VOT, as well as greater variability. Overall, the data reflect a mixed picture in which the fluent speech production of PWS is somewhat slower than that of PWNS but the overall pattern of speech movements is not disrupted.

Research of laryngeal behavior during stuttering events has revealed abnormal timing of intralaryngeal muscle contraction. Video photography of the larynx showed that many stutter events involved simultaneous contractions of antagonistic vocal fold abductor and adductor muscles (Conture, McCall, & Brewer, 1977). At about the same time, EMG techniques showed that stutter events were associated with greater levels of laryngeal muscle activity and "disruption of normal reciprocity between abductor and adductor muscle groups" (Freeman & Ushijima, 1978, p. 538). These findings were complemented by video photography research of the larynx during stuttering events. The vocal folds were more likely to be inappropriately adducted and less variable in their movement during sound prolongation than during sound/syllable repetition. The type of sound (voiceless versus voiced) and the type of stuttering (sound prolongation versus sound/syllable repetition) interactively influenced the vocal fold movement and the overall position of the larynx in the throat (Conture, Schwartz, & Brewer, 1985).

In contrast to the often cited excessive force observed during stuttering, Smith, Denny, Shaffer, Kelly, and Hirano (1996) found evidence of insufficient force when they studied the larynx of adults who stutter. Their measures of intrinsic laryngeal muscles revealed that "compared to periods of fluent speech, intervals of disfluent speech are not typically characterized by higher levels of activity" (p. 329). The adults they studied displayed a lower operating range of muscle activity during conversational speech, leading to the conclusion that adults who stutter do not routinely evidence excessive levels of intrinsic laryngeal muscle activity. Thus, if people who stutter do have problems regulating the degree of muscular force behind their speech movements, this could be evidenced in insufficient, not only excessive, levels of force. One might expect insufficient force to be accompanied by reduced variability of movement, and a certain extent of motor variability is necessary to facilitate effective motor learning (Schmidt & Lee, 2005).

Again there are only a few studies with preschool children related to vocal fold function, and they have reported acoustic measures. For example, no differences in fundamental frequency between the stuttering and normally fluent groups were reported by Healey and Bernstein (1991), but significant differences were found in shimmer (cycle-to-cycle amplitude perturbations), although not in jitter (cycle-to-cycle frequency perturbations) during fluent speech (Hall & Yairi, 1992).

Respiratory Physiology

Some of the secondary behaviors of stuttering include irregular breathing, gasping, and a fast rate of speech. These observations lead researchers to wonder if aspects of breath management are disordered in people who stutter. Early investigators found general malfunctioning of the breathing mechanism during stuttering (Fletcher, 1914; Fossler, 1930; Travis, 1927). Recent research by Raczek and Adamczyk (2004) also yielded evidence that breathing during stuttering tends to be less effective. They observed that during stuttering, carbon dioxide (CO_2) concentrations were one-fifth lower than during fluent speech. In the 1950s, CO_2 treatments were applied to people who stutter with mixed but mainly ineffective results (Ingham, 1984; Kent, 1961). These CO_2 treatments were applied, however, because they were the popular therapy for psychiatric and psychoneurotic disorders, not because stuttering was believed to be a form of respiratory system dysfunction.

In a study of respiration during fluent speech, people who stutter tended to display substantially higher or lower lung volumes than controls who do not stutter (Johnston et al., 1993). If people who stutter must adjust their lung volumes to reach atypical levels in order to sustain fluent speech, it may be very difficult for them to retain such changes for longer periods of time. This could account for why their periods of fluent speech are highly variable and prone to relapse. Poor timing of breath patterns in adults who stutter have been observed by others (Williams & Brutten,

1994). This, too, could be a symptom of difficulty sustaining lung volume levels. Finally, still other research has shown that atypical respiratory control affects both nonspeech and speech conditions performed by people who stutter. They appear to have more difficulty in tasks that require fast-paced, precisely timed, or highly rhythmic breathing (Denny & Smith, 2000).

Summary of Motor-Related Theories

Motor abilities of people who stutter have been suspected as the cause of stuttering for a long time. Early laboratory studies focused on a wide range of gross motor skills, such as unimanual and bimanual skills, respiratory function, speed of jaw movement, and EMG data from articulatory muscles. The motor breakdown of speech fluency could arise from one of the three major systems involved in movement: sensory perception, motor action, or central decision/instruction. Motor learning theories, brainstem reflex models, and sensorimotor dysfunction have also been proposed to explain stuttering. Modern research has targeted the major components of the speech production system, looking both at stuttered and fluent speech for possible seeds of the stuttering disorder. Abnormal functions of the articulatory, phonatory, and respiratory systems have been observed in people who stutter, particularly during their stuttering. Speech is a complicated motor act, and much more research is needed to understand the related factors underlying stuttering and fluency.

Summary

Various characteristics of stuttering and of the population of people who stutter make it reasonable to hypothesize that the disorder has neurophysiological bases. Robust evidence for strong genetic components to stuttering reinforces this view. Nevertheless, what is being genetically transmitted remains unknown. Several theories, or theoretical notions, stemming from the neurophysiological orientation present a wide range of concepts, such as lack of cerebral dominance, excessive right hemisphere activity, abnormal auditory processing, deficient brainstem reflexes, motor learning, or sensorimotor integration. Regardless of the particular theory, a growing body of positive findings has emerged concerning differences in brain structures and processes between people who stutter and people who do not stutter. Much of it, however, has been acquired from adults who stuttered for years, leaving open the question if these deviations were present at the onset of stuttering or are just by-products of a prolonged disorder. Therefore, much more brain research with increasing focus on young children soon after stuttering onset is warranted.

Proceeding down to the periphery and the speech production musculature, differences in motor activity during stuttering have been found in nearly every region of the vocal tract (lips, jaw, vocal folds, and respiration) but no particular dysfunction is common to all people who stutter. During fluent speech, differences in muscle activation sequencing and slower rate of movements appear to suggest seeds of stuttering. Models of motor learning and testing whether related principles are consistent with stuttering phenomena could be helpful to understanding the nature of stuttering and fluent speech change.

Already a decade ago, one speech scientist asserted that when relevant research with adults is examined, on balance it would appear to suggest that the speech production processes of those who stutter are somewhat different from those of normally fluent individuals (Kent, 2000). Such conclusions, however, would be considerably more qualified in regard to young children who stutter for whom limited research has shown small differences, if at all, from normally fluent peers (see reviews by Conture, 1991, and Yairi & Ambrose, 2005). Perhaps these children do not exhibit pervasive speech motor deficits but may exhibit different thresholds for perturbation. Here too, an alternative explanation is that the reported dysfunctions in adults may represent compensations or anticipations for the possibility of stuttering. If a theory of motor dysfunction underlying stuttering is to be validated, considerably more research is needed to uncover the nature of the dysfunction. We conclude that the current state of the art research in genetics, brain anatomy, brain and motor physiology, and motor dysfunctions of people who stutter reveals signs of a generally unstable/unreliable neuromotor system for speech. Many questions, however, remain unanswered.

STUDY QUESTIONS AND DISCUSSION TOPICS

1. What observations about stuttering would seem to make it reasonable to hypothesize that stuttering may have a neurophysiological basis?
2. Why study the fluent speech of people who stutter?
3. What kinds of evidence have supported genetic components to stuttering? Explain.
4. What kinds of evidence have supported brain structure and function as factors underlying stuttering?
5. What evidence has supported a relationship between stuttering and audition?
6. Explain Zimmermann's theory of stuttering as a motor disorder.
7. Explain how it can be that stuttering is associated with so many different dimensions of the physical and neurophysiological system.
8. How would treatment for stuttering differ if research were to reveal that the specific cause of stuttering was:
   a. a genetic defect?
   b. a brain abnormality?
   c. an auditory processing dysfunction?
   d. a motor system deviance?
   e. a respiratory system dysfunction?

SUGGESTED READINGS

Caruso, A., Max, L., & McClowry, M. T. (1999). Perspectives on stuttering as a motor speech disorder. In A. Caruso & E. Strand (Eds.), *Clinical management of motor speech disorders in children*. New York: Thieme.

De Nil, L. F. (1997). Stuttering: A neurophysiological perspective. In N. Bernstein Ratner & C. Healey (Eds.), *Current perspectives in stuttering: Nature and treatment*. Hillsdale, NJ: Erlbaum.

Watkins, K., Smith, S., Davis, S., & Howell, P. (2008). Structural and functional abnormalities of the motor system in developmental stuttering. *Brain, 131*, 50–59.

Yairi, E., & Ambrose, N. (2005). *Early childhood stuttering*. Austin, TX: Pro-Ed. Chapter 9, "Genetics," pp. 285–312.

Chapter 8: Stuttering Therapy: Issues, Directions, Research, Ethics

LEARNER OBJECTIVES

Readers will be able to:

- Analyze issues related to the therapy-theory connection.
- Distinguish potential long-term goals of stuttering treatment.
- Examine and categorize various treatment approaches.
- Become familiar with issues of evidence-based practice, clinical efficacy, and clinical research related to stuttering.
- Reflect on clinician qualities that enhance clinician-client rapport.
- Contemplate issues concerned with clinical ethics.

Introduction

The earlier parts of this book dealt with the definition of stuttering, its nature as event and as disorder, prevalence, onset and progression, variations and unique phenomena, the characteristics of advanced stuttering, and the various theories about stuttering. Whereas this knowledge is interesting in itself, it fulfills a greater purpose when integrated and applied to decisions concerning treatment. The realm of knowledge related to the clinical management of stuttering encompasses a host of aspects all of its own. The literature, however, reveals that often this enterprise has had little connection to the breadth of the knowledge previously described. Prior to reviewing the relevant clinical literature, several questions are worth considering: Is it important for treatment to be theory-based? What are the possible aims of treatment? How do we make order out of the variety of treatment approaches to be considered? What are the objectives of evidence-based practice? How can we meet the challenges associated with clinical efficacy research? What qualities are desired in clinicians? What are the essential ethical considerations? This chapter deals with these issues as underpinnings to the general topic of the clinical aspects of stuttering.

Theoretical Considerations

We propose that treatment of stuttering should emanate logically from theory, formal or informal, about the cause and factors that influence stuttering (Guitar, 2006; Yairi & Ambrose, 2005). Because it is likely that multiple factors contribute to the disorder, varying across clients, clinicians may need multiple techniques to individualize treatment appropriately. A sensible clinician can be expected to practice intervention approaches consistent with either a known theory or his or her own set of beliefs and associated rationales. In either case, an evidence-supported theory and rationale are ideal.

Despite the importance of theoretical foundations, history suggests that a number of therapies, some of which are currently practiced, originated from layperson or clinician hunches. A few were later recognized for their beneficial effects and received experimental support. A classic example is the technique of rate control. For many generations, parents and friends have implored people who stutter to talk slower. In his youth, one of us had been so advised by relatives and neighbors. At the time, no particular rationale was provided. The approach originated from "gut-level" instincts. By now, many clinicians incorporate different versions of slow speech practice into their therapeutic regimens; furthermore, the method has been backed by both theoretical rationale and research data (Curlee & Perkins, 1973; Onslow, Costa, Andrews, Harrison, & Packman, 1996).

Conditions found to ameliorate stuttering (see Chapter 4) have been adapted for formal therapy. For example, long ago it was noticed that when people who stutter talk in noisy environments, their stuttering may be substantially reduced as long as the noise continues. Although this phenomenon is not understood, it has been adopted in treatment regimens incorporating portable miniature noise making instruments such as the Edinburgh Masker (Dewar, Dewar, Austin, & Brash, 1979). The therapeutic rationale is simply based on the obvious reason that it works, not because of any theory about the cause and nature of stuttering.

As Van Riper (1973) commented, there have been a number of therapies grounded only in the principle that if the treatment works, it does not matter much why. This is known as the *pragmatic* approach to therapy, sometimes combining procedures into an *eclectic* program representing different philosophies and methods. The effectiveness of some pragmatic stuttering therapies has been supported by research, for example, the noise application program (MacCulloch, Eaton, & Long, 1970) and the Lidcombe program, which targets speech disfluencies in children who stutter (Onslow, Packman, & Harrison, 2003). Admittedly, then, in spite of our advocacy, therapy-theory links are not always essential for clinical success. If certain procedures are found to yield reliable positive outcomes independent of any theory, or without a complete understanding of why they work, it makes sense that they should be used providing there is research evidence to support the effectiveness of the applied practice.

Still, we have several reservations about the preceding statement. Although picking and choosing procedures from diverse approaches may yield more efficacious therapies that fit both the client and the clinician, there is a downside. For example, a single clinician cannot be an expert in every method. Perhaps more importantly, if clinicians do not understand or cannot explain why their treatment works, it is difficult, if not impossible, to provide clients with a rationale. This handicap interferes in therapy because the rationale, as presented to the client, can greatly influence the therapeutic process. Yairi and Ambrose (2005) stated,

> When identical procedures are presented to the client with different rationales, it results in different understanding, responses, and learning. When a person who stutters is told to speak slowly so that (a) he can better attend to and analyze what he does in speaking, or (b) he can better cope with neurological spasms, or (c) he can better control his hostile reaction to the listener, very different learning takes place. (p. 409)

Without a theoretical framework, it is difficult to determine what needs to be done if the therapy fails.

The preceding examples of pragmatic therapies for stuttering notwithstanding, there is ample evidence that from early on, discernible links between clinicians' theories of stuttering and the prescribed treatment were the rule rather than the exception (see reviews by Klingbell, 1939; Sheehan, 1970; Wingate, 1997). Centuries ago, when the cause of stuttering was believed to reside in the tongue, caused by either its oversized or weak musculature (Brosch & Pirsig, 2001), treatment was prescribed accordingly: Size was reduced by removing pieces from the tongue; weak movement was enhanced with hot spices, supporting prosthetic devices that elevated it, and so on. Obviously if the theory itself is not well founded, a strong theory-therapy link is not enough to yield the best treatment approach.

Other interesting illustrations abound. For example, when Oto, in the 19th century, regarded stuttering as a problem of transitions between speech sounds, he recommended phonetic drills and a conscious effort to integrate articulatory transitions as the logical treatment (see Sheehan, 1970, p. 40). Similarly, relegating the cause of stuttering to muscular spasms of the larynx, several clinicians, for example, Ssikorski (1891), Sandow (1898), and Makuen (1941), offered vocal exercises as well as maneuvers for repositioning certain laryngeal muscles to prevent spasm. When stuttering was explained as an outward symptom of deep-seated conflicts, it was treated by the application of psychotherapy (e.g., Brill, 1923).

These examples also remind us that the theory-therapy link is only as good as the theory itself. Furthermore, theories may have negative influences on whether intervention is viewed as beneficial. In the extreme case, certain religions object to all treatments, leaving the remedy entirely in God's hands. Another example is the far-reaching influence of the diagnosogenic theory of stuttering (see Chapter 6). Because of the theory's claim that calling attention to the child's disfluency causes and sustains stuttering, direct stuttering therapy was often withheld from young children for more than three decades, especially in the United States. The theory, which has lost much of its credibility over the years, also inflicted undue pain on many parents by assigning the cause of stuttering to their behavior.

In spite of the qualifications just described, we adhere to our proposition that the theory-therapy link is advantageous. A theory-driven therapy provides clinicians with a frame of reference. If clinicians believe stuttering is a symptom of a psychological problem, then they should not be applying an oral motor treatment. A theory also provides the rationale for the therapeutic approach, an understanding of why specific procedures are applied, and a logical basis for sensible alternatives when progress fails to occur, rather than yielding a haphazard trial and error strategy. Theories, however, need to be tested in order to be refined or modified and thus give rise to better methods of treatment.

Unfortunately, the field suffers from large gaps between the stuttering therapies and the stuttering theories, mainly because of the narrowness of the theories. For example, the covert repair hypothesis (Postma & Kolk, 1993) proposes that disfluencies result from problems in premotor phonological encoding in which the speaker attempts to correct speech errors before they are uttered. The theory seems to provide a rationale for therapies that emphasize slower speaking rate. It does not, however, offer any guidance for intervening with the client's psychological attitudes, an important domain within the grand scope of the disorder of stuttering.

> The therapies for stuttering have only been as comprehensive as the theories supporting them. Theories of stuttering thus far have been limited in scope. For example, the psychoanalytic theory was narrowly focused on the emotional etiology of stuttering and on psychoanalysis as its treatment. It neglects the potential impact of stuttering on a person's behavioral reactions and how these can be handled. It has nothing to say about the speech aspects of stuttering and what can be done about changing them.

There is also the phenomenon of therapies that originate from a certain theoretical position and then spread out, incorporating procedures that are not rooted in the theory. For example, a clinician may counsel parents against calling attention to stuttering, based on Johnson's diagnosogenic theory. She may also advise that parents model slow speech and use simple language. In this case, a theoretical connection for the latter advice does not exist and the experimental evidence to support the procedure is scant. If a clinician believes persistent stuttering is ultimately genetic, then why is success being expected from a behavioral reinforcement approach to treatment? Perhaps the weak theory/therapy connection in stuttering during the past 25 years reflects the absence of a strong theory accepted by scientists and understood by the public (Siegel, 1998).

The Objectives of Therapy

Knowing that the vast majority of people who stutter begin by age 4 (Yairi & Ambrose, 2005) and certainly by age 6 (Andrews, 1984), preschool children present with a brief history and little experience with the disorder. By contrast, it can be assumed that the great majority of afflicted school-age children have been stuttering for a good number of years and that adults have stuttered for many years. Naturally, the longer their stuttering history, the greater is their experience with the disorder. Having missed the best opportunity for natural recovery, on one hand, and having formed strong associated emotional reactions and habits of dealing with stuttering, on the other, the question arises as to what are the realistic goals of treatment for them? Are the same goals applicable to school-age and preschool-age children alike? With respect to the latter question, increased knowledge in the future concerning stuttering subtypes may lead to differential treatments. At the present time, however, and recognizing some distinction should be made between preschool and older ages of people who stutter, from our perspective there is substantial commonality among all age groups in respect to the general therapeutic aims.

The three major alternatives to consider in setting up long-term therapeutic goals for people who stutter are increased fluency, reduced stuttering, and improved emotional adjustment.

Increased Fluency

Naturally Fluent Speech

Naturally fluent speech is produced by speakers who feel, think, and behave like normally speaking individuals when they talk. In essence, the aim is a complete cure. This can be a realistic goal for preschool children. Indeed, as discussed at length in Chapter 4, most of them experience natural recovery. Also many who received therapy do well either due to therapy or to the combination of natural recovery forces and therapy. This goal appears to be similar to Guitar's (2006) therapeutic outcome labeled *spontaneous fluency*.

When applied to older children and adults, achieving complete cure in both the fluency and the psychological domains of speaking by means of any of the current therapies typically has been viewed as unrealistic. Clinicians tend to believe in the potential for improvement, even substantial, but up to a point (Manning, 2001; Sheehan, 1980). The main reason for being guarded has been the limited long-term success of therapy. Also, it may have been influenced by organic theories of stuttering that intuitively imply constraints on the power of speech therapy to alter physiological or biochemical structures and processes. There are indications, however, that speech therapy can alter the brainwaves of people who stutter (e.g., Boberg, Yeudall, Schopflocher, & Bo-Lassen, 1983; De Nil, Kroll, & Houle, 2001). It also remains possible that with the advent of new medical treatments, such as gene therapies, stem cell implants, and so on, full cure may, in time, become a realistic goal for a growing number of clients.

Deliberately Fluent Speech

Deliberately fluent speech is produced by the speaker who exercises a conscious mental and/or behavioral monitoring of speech that normally fluent speakers usually do not use. Clearly, this subcategory presents quite a different goal from the first one listed. It is similar to what Guitar (2006) called *controlled fluency* as a therapeutic outcome. This goal presents a paradox for some individuals who stutter because one abnormality may have substituted for another that still makes the person uncomfortable. Also, the required self-monitoring is tremendously difficult, attempting to attend to one's own speech production while simultaneously tracking the development of the intended message. This multitasking demand might even result in triggering some disfluent or stuttered speech, the opposite of the intended outcome.

Reduced Stuttering

The goal is to lessen the abnormality of overt stuttering, and, as a by-product, to also decrease its frequency. This objective appears close to what Van Riper (1973) labeled as "fluent stuttering" and to what Guitar (2006) refers to as "acceptable stuttering." Note, however, that what is acceptable, and to whom, is a wide-open question. The goal may also be described as "managed stuttering."

Fluent, or so-called acceptable, stuttering occurs when the movements involved in the production of discontinuities in the speech stream are managed deliberately by the speaker. This can perhaps be likened to a person with spasmodic extremities attempting to "smooth out" the uncontrollable movement. It is a counterintuitive concept in that most, if not all, of those who stutter seek therapy to get rid of their stuttering, not keep it going.

Improved Cognitive-Emotional Adjustment

The goal is to change emotional and social behavior related to speaking without directly addressing speech itself. Such changes, however, are expected to yield the by-product of diminished stuttering. This broad goal of indirect influence on stuttering may be reached in diverse ways. It may reflect elements of Travis's (1931) concept of mental hygiene, Bryngelson's (1931) ideas of an objective attitude, Sheehan's (1970) role acceptance, and others. In this sense, one could refer to this goal as a form of "attitude control."

General Therapeutic Approaches

What has been done and what can be done to achieve the three optional stuttering treatment objectives presented earlier? A review of the clinical literature on this topic reveals numerous therapies, reflecting extremely diverse subjective factors with respect to clinicians' theoretical positions, personal beliefs about stuttering, professional backgrounds, or preferred eclectic strategies. Cultural values and religious beliefs also have had some effects (Leith, 1986). There are also more objective factors, such as the multidimensional nature of the disorder, that influence the focus and character of the therapy. At times, these factors overlap. It is to be expected that psychologists, by virtue of their professional training, gear their therapies to the emotional aspect of stuttering, which, in some cases, is a very significant component of the disorder. In a similar vein, speech clinicians would tend to focus on the overt speech characteristics, whereas physicians show more interest in body function and medication.

> A naive observer of therapy, not knowing for what problem it is provided, may witness that one client soaks his feet in a pail of cold water, a second client is hypnotized, and a third one receives a shot in the rear end. Such an observer will be amused to learn that all three were being treated for stuttering. In fact, it has not been uncommon that a single client received several, if not many, extremely diverse therapies. One of us presented an incomplete list of 16 different therapies, including the three mentioned earlier, that he had received (see Yairi & Ambrose, 2005, p. 402). Also Johnson (1946) listed a good number of therapies that were applied to him.

Unfortunately, it is not only the layperson who is at risk of becoming confused about stuttering therapy. Students and professionals in speech-language pathology too are exposed to the same risk. Hence prior to answering the question of how to accommodate any of the broad treatment aims presented here, it is wise to lessen the confusion by organizing the numerous therapies into a small number of categories based on their commonalities.

There are several reasonable classifications for types of therapy. Examples include therapies to change speech directly versus therapies to change speech indirectly; aided therapy, such as using delayed auditory feedback (DAF) or electromyography (EMG) instruments, versus unaided therapy, such as stuttering modification or fluency reinforcement; therapies for treating the parents versus therapies where parents are the agents of treatment; therapies focused on broad permanent change of the disorder, such as psychotherapy, versus therapies focused narrowly on immediate change of the events, such as stuttering modification techniques. Therapies might also be classified according to how the stuttering problem is conceptualized. For example, some approaches related to psychotherapy, emotions, and attitudes address stuttering in terms of the "loss of control" definition that Perkins (1990a) defends, whereas other approaches address stuttering in terms of speech behaviors to be modified by means of techniques such as those developed by Onslow, Packman, & Harrison (2003) or Ingham (1999). Notice the overlap because some therapies can be described within more than one classification system.

Traditionally, stuttering therapies have been informally distinguished according to two categories: anti-anxiety and anti-stuttering (Williams, 1968). This oversimplified classification fails to consider fundamental differences among approaches, excludes a number of important therapies, and does not accommodate more recent developments. Yairi and Ambrose (2005) offered a more representative nine-category classification of stuttering therapies based on the common theme of the specific clinical techniques that have been employed. In writing this book, the set of possible long-term treatment objectives provides the framework for a modified scheme that includes 12 general therapeutic approaches for stuttering:

I. Focus on Improved Adjustment
  1. Resolving psyche and personality disturbances
  2. Promoting calmness and relaxation

   3. Modifying emotional reactions
   4. Modifying cognitive sets
II. Focus on Reduced Stuttering
   5. Modifying or replacing stutter events
   6. Decreasing stutter events
III. Focus on Increased Fluency
   A. Achieving Deliberately Fluent Speech
      7. Fluency shaping
      8. Fluency reinforcement
   B. Achieving Naturally Fluent Speech
      9. Instrument-based therapies
      10. Pharmaceutical treatments
      11. Strengthening supporting skills (e.g., oral motor, phonology, language)
      12. Environmental management

Having outlined the general therapeutic options, it should be made clear that each represents a number of underlying specific techniques that have been employed to achieve it. For example, personality problems (approach 1) have been resolved by different psychotherapies, and relaxation can be realized by practicing certain movements, through meditation, and others. Fluency shaping (approach 7) can be achieved through very slow (stretched) speech or by applying easier voice initiations. Hence the clinician is faced with the challenge of developing a therapy program by choosing among numerous possibilities. She or he may opt to pursue one approach by means of a single technique or several techniques, or prefer to pursue therapy through multiple approaches, which, of course, imply also several techniques. As a matter of fact, clinicians have combined and/or integrated stuttering modification with psychologically oriented approaches such as anxiety reduction (Van Riper, 1973) and anxiety reduction with stuttering modification and fluency-generating approaches (Guitar, 2006). Also note that approaches to stuttering therapies have seen considerable alternations in popularity among professionals. Whereas resolving personality problems as the main approach peaked during the first half of the 20th century, at present it is out of favor. The use of various fluency-enhancing techniques, for example, slow speech, was employed over a long period of time, lost its popularity during the middle two quarters of the 20th century, and has seen a considerable surge since the late 1970s. Finally, some approaches have targeted specific age groups more than others. For example, instrument-based therapies (approach 9) have been applied primarily with adults, whereas environmental management (approach 12) has been applied primarily with preschool children. The major clinical techniques and programs developed within each of these major approaches are described and discussed in subsequent chapters.

Clinical Applications

Developing Appropriate Long- and Short-Term Objectives

A number of considerations must be made when setting the clinical goals and objectives for persons who stutter. Although these are not largely different from those appropriate for individuals with speech sound disorders, a few are particularly worth noting: Which goals and objectives will make the most impact on the speaker's effectiveness as a communicator? Which steps will the client be most ready and able to undertake? Are there changes that if made in one area will promote change in other areas? Are the conditions and expectations commensurate with the individual's lifestyle and cultural background, communication needs, and/or developmental stage? What will offer the most relief for his or her experiences of communicative stress?

Goal setting with adolescents or adults is best accomplished together with the clients so they are encouraged to feel a sense of ownership of the process. Similarly, the parents of young children should be involved in the treatment planning for their child. When developing therapy objectives, clinicians should be clear and completely define all the components according to the formula: Treatment objective = Who + will do what + to what degree of accuracy + under what conditions. Sometimes even seasoned clinicians overlook the defining conditions and write imprecise or insufficient goals, such as "John will perform his fluency targets with 95% accuracy." Such a statement may seem sufficient at first, but in fact, there is no way to tell when the client has satisfactorily met this objective. It lacks specific information, such as the nature of conditions on John's performance (independently? after imitating? given an indirect model?) or the speaking context (on sentences? in spontaneous conversation? during oral reading?) or location (therapy room or classroom?), or even the time frame (in one session? across two consecutive sessions?). Finally, a major problem with such an objective is that the measurement basis has not been specified. Compare the relative stability of a 95% achievement if the client has performed only 20 utterances as compared to 100 utterances. An example of an objective that specifies the particular task, conditions, and measures needed is "*John will independently apply a slow, easy speech initiation strategy on 100 utterances with 95% accuracy during spontaneous conversation with his peers across two consecutive group sessions in the therapy room.*"

Individual Versus Group Therapy Sessions

Therapy can be delivered in a variety of formats, including individual, group, and, recently, also via the Internet (electronic therapy). So far, the individual format has been dominant in stuttering therapy. It is obvious that an individual format where clients have the therapist's full attention during the session affords the most flexibility for zeroing in on the client's needs. It takes the one-on-one contact for the clinician to have a firsthand understanding of the problem and to get to know the client, his strengths and weaknesses, and together, to formulate goals. Additionally, many adolescent and some adult clients who stutter initially are not comfortable sharing feelings, discussing stuttering, or practicing speaking skills in the presence of other clients. Group therapy in additional to individual therapy, however, can be a particularly valuable component of the overall treatment approach, especially with others who stutter who are approximately the same age. Advantages of group therapy are discussed in Chapter 9. Sometimes, it may be the only format available. Regardless, the clinician has to make a decision about the format or formats of the program.

Implementing Treatment

Several of the intervention principles that apply broadly in the practice of speech pathology are appropriate for fluency intervention. For example, a long-term goal should be broken down into a progressive sequence of intermediate, short-term, down to session-specific objectives. Unrealistic goals can easily lead to a strong sense of failure even if considerable improvement has been achieved. Some procedural considerations that tend to be shared in common across approaches to communication disorders treatment, to be considered in stuttering and fluency intervention, are described next.

Increased Awareness and Self-Monitoring

With any speech target, it is important for the client to have a clear awareness of the nature of that target. In fluency therapy, for example, the target may be self-knowledge of the overt features of the disorder, a fluency-enhancing strategy, or avoidance behavior. Generous amounts of modeling and instructional support are important when teaching new target skills (Landers & Landers, 1973). The modeling and feedback are gradually faded out as the client demonstrates consistent success independently. Clinician feedback is best when it offers specific descriptions of performance (e.g., "your lips touched together gently that time") and should be applied more often than vague general praise (e.g., "good job"). In motor learning terms (Schmidt & Lee, 2005), knowledge of performance (i.e., what movement pattern occurred) is more instructive than knowledge of results (i.e., whether outcome was successful or not). Adolescent and adult clients need to develop habits of ongoing self-evaluation and self-monitoring, both of the old and newly learned behaviors, to ensure an enduring result. That is, clients need to be able to serve as their own clinician. For this to happen, the client needs plenty of practice in self-evaluation and self-monitoring in the presence of the clinician where the impressions can be compared/contrasted with the clinician's. Finn (2003c) has reviewed in detail the value of self-regulation in fluency therapy.

Conditions of Practice

In nearly every learning experience, especially for changing speech processes, some component of practice is needed. Although the old adage asserts that "practice makes perfect," the new wisdom warns that "practice makes permanent." So it is important before encouraging repeated practice to ensure the client is performing the target behavior in just the desired way. Because it is relatively easy to achieve fluent speech in the confines of the clinical setting, it gives a misleading impression that only a minimal amount of practice of new skills should be required. In fact, however, the speaking approach needs to be practiced over and over, multiple times and in multiple conditions. Manning (2006) highlights the thousands of hours of practice and perseverance essential to becoming a competent performer (e.g., a dancer), to remind us that the time needed to develop proficient speech skills may require no less. If many hours of practice will be necessary, then the client should spend time talking for the largest percentage of their therapy sessions.

The motor learning literature reveals some conditions of practice to enhance learning. Motor practice is most effective when the conditions are varied rather than consistent. For example, one treatment implication may be that rather than practice of the same set of words every clinical session, words sets used for speech practice should be varied continuously. Similarly, instead of the same tone of voice applied consistently in practice, the speaker needs to practice techniques in conditions of varied intonation patterns and stress emphasis. Finally, if the motor learning principles are applicable to speech fluency learning, then 8 hours of practice in 2 days may not be as beneficial as 2 hours of practice on each of 8 days (Schmidt & Lee, 2005). Still, recent research has raised some questions concerning the effect of practice on people who stutter, showing that after practice, instead of decreasing reaction times and increasing accuracy like those who do not stutter, people who stutter continued to demonstrate slower reaction times and decreased accuracy in a color recognition naming task (Smits-Bandstra & De Nil, 2009). Further studies are needed of the nature of these apparent speech learning constraints. Under what conditions do people who stutter make improvements in speech performance? Would greater numbers of practice trials afford speech performance gains? If this finding suggests an underlying area of speech performance deficiency where little gain is possible, then what compensatory or adaptive strategies will contribute to speaker success?

It is important to understand, however, that extensive practice in stuttering therapy has some unique perspectives compared with practice in other speech disorders, say correcting articulation of speech sounds. Where speech production is concerned, the person with articulation disorders practices to develop fine motor skills, such as tongue placement. In learning how to modify a stuttering block, clients learn the motor adjustment required to reduce tension and get out of the block, but they often can do this in a relatively short time. The extensive practice with modifying hundreds and thousands of blocks is necessary not so much for developing fine motor skills but to change the clients' beliefs and confidence in what he or she can do. People who stutter often feel they have no control over stuttering. Extensive practice in modifying blocks changes this entrenched psychology. In other aspects of stuttering therapy, practice does not involve motor skills whatsoever. For example, clients learn to identify various features of their overt stuttering by observing themselves in the mirror or listening to their recorded speech. Again, the intention of extensive practice goes beyond the client's ability to identify all the features. Its other, not less important, objective is to increase clients' realization that some aspects of stuttering are their own doing.

Generalization and Transfer

Generalization to many situations, conditions, and people is an essential component of most procedures in stuttering therapy. Even if the client can apply the target strategies in the clinic session, how well can the client apply the strategies in other circumstances? It was just mentioned that speech practice should take place in a variety of conditions for better learning. A certain amount of practice across situations, conditions, and people should be incorporated into therapy to facilitate transfer of learning. Incorporating others—family, teachers, and friends—both for motivational support and for practice in variable conditions can be important. Some clinical tools of transfer include use of situation hierarchies, event or daily log notations, employing self-regulating habits, and role play. For example, after achieving adequate skills modifying stuttering blocks in the therapy room, clients can practice their skills speaking to other people brought into the therapy room, then in speaking to other people in the clinic, then in easy situations out of the clinic, and so on. Finn (2003a) highlights the use of everyday, real-life elements in speech therapy and emphasizes that clients must gain a sense of self-efficacy, that is, the belief that they have capacities and skills to enable them to generalize and maintain achievements.

Skill Maintenance and Prevention of Relapse

With adolescent and adult clients, there is almost a certainty of some experiences of relapse following therapy. Thus it is important to prepare the client for this expectation and help them achieve a readiness to meet that experience before it occurs and gain confidence in being able to recover from speech fluency failures. Some experts have even suggested not dismissing a client until at least one major relapse has been addressed together (Manning, 2001). Another option may be to simulate or role-play such an experience for practice and adjustment of attitudes. Adoption of realistic expectations is important for the prevention of relapse. When too much of a premium is placed on the experience of relatively continuous fluency, the client is apt to be more at risk for problems later on.

Blood (1995) recommends that relapse management include client instruction for how to "approach, understand, and solve problems" (p. 171). He developed a game for adolescents to change their cognition about speech systematically, used as a supplement to changing speech motor skills. In the game, called POWER², the players move their pieces along a game board and draw cards to answer questions about a variety of situations (e.g., not being able to say a word to order your food). The players are sometimes required to respond in a way that is constructive and proactive, and, at other times, in a way that is reactive and less productive. By engaging in these opposite types of responses, the players gain a better awareness of their nature and what is preferable. Topics and activities in the game raise issues of (1) permission to stutter or not, (2) ownership (of the speaking difficulty), (3) well-being and social support, (4) self-esteem and self-talk,[1] (5) resilience (bouncing back after stuttering moments), and (6) responsibility (handling life and processes of change). Rather than assuming that attitudes will change if speech improves, the idea is to empower the speaker with attitudes and problem-solving approaches that will help him or her be prepared for the bumps in the road ahead. Many clinicians also follow systematic maintenance programs whereby periodic contact with the client, either in person or via telephone, continues after dismissal from the regular therapy. This is typically done with decreasing frequency.

Evidence-Based Practice

During the past 20 years, the concept of evidence-based practice (EBP) has come to occupy greater centrality in speech-language pathology, including stuttering (Bernstein Ratner, 2005). This is the current trend among other health professions, especially those concerned with behavioral health management. In its strictest

---

[1] Self-talk, and its application in therapy, are addressed in Chapter 10.

meaning, EBP is a philosophy that holds that therapy must be supported by research findings that provide positive evidence that it is effective. Framed more broadly, evidence-based treatment is a clinical decision-making process that integrates (a) the best scientific evidence with (b) the individual clinician's expertise (Sackett, Rosenberg, Gray, Haynes, & Richardson, 1996). Taking this definition, the question of which one of the two components assumes primacy in driving treatment decisions has been the subject of debates in various health fields (Watts-Jackim, 2004), including the area of stuttering. This is seen in the conflicting views expressed by J. Ingham (2003), arguing for the centrality of research evidence, and Yaruss and Quesal (2002), who give considerable weight to clinicians' experience and judgment.

The "research-first" choice seems to be the obvious answer for two reasons. First, it is difficult to trust the clinicians' subjective impressions of what works. Suspicion must be upheld because in too many cases, clinicians' instincts have been wrong. The stuttering literature is filled with a host of unfounded clinician advice to parents of preschool children just beginning to stutter, such as "ignore the child's stuttering, be a good listener, use short, simple language, and have the child go to bed early." These suggestions, and other advice, have remained popular, although their clinical merit has barely ever, if at all, been tested. Furthermore, there have been studies that negated some advice, showing, for example, that calling attention to stuttering in young children may in some cases actually reduce it (Martin, Kuhl, & Haroldson, 1972; Wingate, 1976). Other scholars concluded that the premise underlying clinicians' admonition for parents to reduce the length and complexity of their utterances when conversing with their children has no experimental support. In fact, they cautioned about potential long-term harmful effects of such advice to the child's language development (Miles & Bernstein Ratner, 2001).

> There are virtually no data on the effects of being a good listener, style of toilet training, early bedtime, and so on, on children's stuttering. Similarly, although research has revealed that parents of children who stutter tend to be overprotective, the direct effect of increase or decrease in overprotectiveness on stuttering has not yet been demonstrated (Yairi & Ambrose, 2005). Although none of these forms of advice have been shown to work, they are still being disseminated in parent counseling. Ingham and Cordes (1998) stated that a range of popular treatments persists even in the face of evidence showing them to be ineffective. In other words, the sole justification for the therapy is the clinician's "feeling" that it works. We doubt that such practices would be met with much tolerance in medicine.

The second argument of the "Research First" proponents is that although limited knowledge about treatment effectiveness necessitated reliance on clinician preferences in earlier times, that status has changed. They posit that the current body of information allows differentiation among more effective, less effective, not effective, and harmful treatments (Sackett, Rosenberg, Gray, Haynes, & Richardson, 2000).

Those who favor the "Clinician Judgment" position, however, could raise the following reservations: (1) for some disorders, available treatment effectiveness data are limited, (2) research has been plagued by various methodological weaknesses, (3) critical measurements have often been overlooked, (4) interpretations of the data vary greatly, and (5) the evidence might not always be particularly meaningful. (See Lilienfeld, 2003, for an interesting discussion of these issues.)

An argument can be made that all of these negating points apply, to some degree, to stuttering. Undoubtedly, progress has been made as evaluated in several reviews of the clinical research literature (Andrews, Guitar, & Howie, 1980; Andrews et al., 1983; Bothe, 2004; Cordes, 1998), but the current database leaves much to be desired in terms of quantity and quality. A strong supporter of evidence-based treatment opined that "One legitimate limitation to our ability to rely on research evidence to guide our treatment is the dearth of published treatment efficacy studies" and that "Stuttering treatment researchers have not conducted definitive randomized clinical trials" (J. Ingham, 2003, p. 202). Less than two decades ago, only six studies with a total of 14 participants were identified as dedicated to clinical effectiveness of therapy for preschool-age children who stutter (Yairi, 1993). Undoubtedly, more information for this age group has become available since then, markedly due to the contributions of Onslow and his colleagues in Australia in developing the Lidcombe program (see Onslow, Packman, & Harrison, 2003). Still, less experimental progress has been achieved for treatment of school-age children and adults who stutter during the same period, and little comparative treatment research has been carried out.

Those favoring the "Clinician Judgment First" will also point out that a guideline published by the American Speech-Language-Hearing Association (ASHA) states that criteria for determining treatment of stuttering based entirely on empirical evidence would be "too restrictive" and that common practice should also be considered (ASHA, 1995, p. 26). Indeed, a strictly evidence-based treatment approach has its limitations. Some therapies for stuttering do not lend themselves well to be researched and proven effective because they focus on less defined variables (e.g., attitudes, and their exact procedures are difficult to repeat with consistency). Many past studies measured effectiveness primarily in terms of number and length of stuttered events but overlooked measures of more covert aspects (e.g., emotional reactions and interpersonal functioning; Blood & Conture, 1998). And there is always the factor of the client's preference, the particulars of each case, and the clinician's degree of comfort. Finn (2003c) stated that "An evidence based-framework can be described as an empirically-driven, measurement-based, *client-sensitive* approach for selecting treatments" (p. 209). ASHA advises that the best research evidence must be considered in relation to the "individual's preferences, environment, culture, and values regarding health and well-being" (ASHA, 1997; 2007b). This means that clinical decisions require discernment on the part of clinicians who must sometimes work in support of a client's opinions and circumstances, and at other times work to effect change in a client's opinions and circumstances.

Another very important question is tied to restrictiveness: Does a given evidence-based program allow the clinician any flexibility and creativity? Suppose a clinical center in a hospital adopts a single therapy program for adults and a single program for children who stutter. Must a clinician practice the same approved protocol in each case? Must a clinician follow all 20 steps in the ELU therapy (Costello, 1983)? If not, how many steps can be omitted? At what point do the changes amount to a deviation from the approved research-based treatment? And what about tested programs that do not yield meaningful results to the client, for example, the person who cares more about overcoming fears of speaking in social events than about being 100% fluent? These are serious questions to consider.

A Case Study

The challenges associated with EBP are illustrated with a practical case applying a five-step process outlined by Sackett et al. (2000). A 7-year-old African American boy is referred for stuttering treatment. The first step is to develop a clinical question (e.g., will advising parents and teachers to speak more slowly to the child provide a supportive environmental factor toward his smooth speech?). The skill of generating the clinical question will vary greatly across clinicians, their knowledge, experience, values, and judgments.

The second step, finding the best relevant information, may uncover several studies pertinent to the clinical question (e.g., Guitar & Marchinkowski, 2001; Stephenson-Opsal & Bernstein-Ratner, 1988; Zebrowski, Weiss, Savelkoul, & Hammer, 1996). This step involves challenging decisions about how many and which search engines to use, what keywords to search on, and when the search has been sufficient.

Step 3 raises the issue of how to engage in critical examination of the studies that are found. This is one important reason for including research methods courses in the university curriculum of speech-language pathology programs. The studies should be examined for their background, rationale, participants, procedures and conditions (controlled factors), measures, reliability, results, and implications. A clinician may note that the articles mainly found that children who stutter benefit from slower speaking rates by their parents. But what if the gender and stuttering symptoms of her client did not match any of the children in the studies under scrutiny? What if there are no studies to be found with children of the same age and culture? Are the results still applicable to her client? Even if generalizing results is a sensible option, is it justified in this case? An adult's model of slow speech may enhance child fluency but not necessarily by slowing the speech of the child (Stephenson-Opsal & Bernstein Ratner, 1988). Perhaps more critical factors may be operating. For example, Bernstein Ratner (2004) explained that longer turn-taking latencies may be the effective outcome of instructing parents to slow their speech, and that the increased latency of adult responses might be the factor that enhances fluency as suggested by Newman and Smit (1989). Based on the set of articles identified in step 2, the clinician may conclude that she needs to advise adults to slow their speech around the child. She would explain that the slow-paced environmental condition is beneficial to fluency even though the child is not apt to mirror this speech rate. However, if the additional review article is found (Bernstein Ratner, 2004), the clinician may conclude that she should advise parents to wait before responding to their child, increasing the latency of conversational turn-taking.

With the fourth step, application, the clinician would instruct the adults who speak with the child according to her findings, duplicating the type of instructions given in the research studies. In the fifth step, evaluation, the effect of the procedure on the child's fluency is determined. Finally, if the outcome does not indicate a substantial effect, the clinician will have to determine whether her instructions were insufficient or whether the evidence does not apply for the specific client. In our opinion, this five-step process, although challenging, is nonetheless valuable.

Clinical Research

What kind clinical research has been done to provide the sought-after scientific evidence for stuttering therapy? In this respect, a significant distinction exists between clinical *outcomes* and clinical *efficacy* research. The first addresses only whether significant change occurred posttreatment, but the latter is concerned with proving that the specific treatment, not something else, is responsible for the change. Treatment efficacy can be considered in terms of two main components: effects and efficiency. An examination of treatment *effects* (i.e., outcomes) is concerned with whether change has occurred, the nature of that change, and client satisfaction with the change. An examination of treatment *efficiency* considers whether the change was cost effective, whether all parts of the treatment were necessary, and whether another treatment could have worked faster. *Efficacy* ultimately is concerned with how well the treatment achieves both effects and efficiency (Dowden, Stone-Goldman, & Olswang, 2006; Olswang, 1998).

Evaluating Efficacy

Efficacy research requires rigorous design. Typically, studies are conducted in laboratories or other controlled settings and employ randomized trials, careful selection of participants, well-trained clinicians, blind data analysis, and so on. One problem is that frequently there is no clear indication for whether such laboratory conditions and levels of reported success can be transferred to treatment conducted in typical work environments that all too often are impossible to control. This leads to effectiveness-focused research that seeks to explore the extent to which the intervention, when deployed in the field, yields the intended results, and factors that interfere with, or increase, the therapeutic results (Moscicki, 1993; Stuart, Treat, & Wade, 2000).

Clinical efficacy research in stuttering can be directed to answer many questions. Example for *adults*: Does a particular therapeutic approach (e.g., psychotherapy; noise application) result in a long-term cure or decrease in stuttering? Which therapeutic approach (e.g., stuttering management versus fluency management) yields better and/or faster results? Is therapy oriented toward the emotional aspects of stuttering as effective as therapy oriented to the speech aspect? What is the optimal number and frequency of therapy sessions? Example for young *children*: Are early predictions of chances to exhibit natural recovery accurate? Does early intervention result in a higher percent of complete cure than natural recovery without clinical intervention? Is indirect intervention (parent counseling) as effective as direct therapy with the child? The implications of some of these clinical questions to understanding the nature of stuttering are quite obvious.

Group Studies

The most common clinical research design employs group comparisons in which a certain treatment is administered to participants, with or without a control group, over a certain period. Pre- and posttreatment measurements are made of the behavior under investigation, as well as single or multiple follow-up measures. The strongest efficacy studies are randomized controlled clinical trials characterized by several features. First, they involve a test treatment (therapy) delivered to one group, another treatment or treatments delivered to other groups, and/or a control group receiving no treatment. Second, the clients are assigned into each group randomly. Third, subjects are selected with careful epidemiological, ethnic/culture, and other factors that might impact the results. For example, testing the effect of new stuttering therapy with children between ages 2 and 4 is likely to be problematic because of the high rate of natural recovery in this age group. Fourth, data analysis is performed at a different site than the treatment center and by independent investigators who are blind to the purpose of the study.

You should keep in mind that because efficacy research examines the effect of treatment on organismic variables (e.g., speech), it may be closely tied to theoretical issues and can further our scientific knowledge of the disorder under investigation (Olswang, 1993). For example, comparing preschool-age children receiving therapy soon after stuttering onset with children who do not receive treatment should generate important information about developmental processes of early stuttering, such as natural recovery (e.g., if the latter group improved without treatment). Similarly, when modified parental behaviors are the experimental variable in a treatment study, we can test hypotheses regarding the role of environmental factors in precipitating stuttering.

Although recent years have seen a growing number of studies concerned with the evaluation of therapies for stuttering, for the most part, they do not constitute randomized clinical trials. In a study that compared the effectiveness of the ISTAR Comprehensive Stuttering Program as employed in the Netherlands and in Canada, the number of participants was small, 22 and 16 respectively; no control groups were employed in either site, hence no random assignment of subjects was possible (Langevin, Huinck, Kully, Peters, Lomheim, & Tellers, 2006). There have been, however, a few exceptions. Among them is the Franken, Kielstra-Van der Schalk, and Boelens (2005) study comparing two therapy programs for children using a randomized design, and the Jones et al. (2005) investigation that included 54 children randomly assigned either to receive the Lidcombe program of intervention or to a nontreatment control group. On the whole, however, other procedures essential to unbiased clinical trials in stuttering have not been commonly adopted. Such procedures include careful control of subject selection, for example, history of persistent or recovered stuttering in the family, administration of treatment in several clinics, blind analyses of data, and others.

Single-Subject Studies

A rather popular means for conducting clinical research in various behavioral/emotional disorders, also in the area of stuttering, has been single-subject studies. These are used to observe changes occurring in an individual as a result of a treatment or treatments. Whereas typical studies compare groups of subjects, this type of research compares treatment effects on one or several individuals, each examined alone. The terms *single-subject study* simply indicates that each participant serves as her or his own control. This is accomplished by looking at the person's performance while alternating between treatment and nontreatment phases of the study. For example, the first phase includes eight consecutive sessions (4 weeks) of no treatment followed by a second eight-session phase in which punishment is administered upon stuttering, followed by a third phase during which reinforcement is administered upon stuttering, followed by a fourth phase of no treatment once again. Such alternating cycles may repeat several times. Thus, whereas typical studies allow for one or just a few observational sessions in which the target behavior is measured, the single-subject design is advantageous in allowing repeated multiple observations of stuttering. McMillan (2004) points out that this feature also minimizes the effect of normal variations.

Several clinical studies in stuttering have employed single-subject design. For example, Martin, Kuhl, and Haroldson (1972) demonstrated the effect of response contingencies with two preschool-age children: one stuttered severely (37% of syllables) and the other moderately (10% of syllables). During the base rate phase (about 3 to 5 sessions), the child talked with the puppeteer examiner. In the treatment phase (10 to 32 sessions), a 10-second time-out immediately followed every moment of stuttering. The time-out consisted of the puppet stage sound and lights being turned off. In the final extinction phase (about 10 sessions), the time-out treatment was no longer administered. In both children, stuttering frequency dropped down to below 1% and remained at that level after the time-out treatment had been removed. Follow-up visits approximately 1 year posttreatment revealed continued levels below 1% by each child.

Although single-subject experiments do not supply evidence that is as strong as group experiments with respect to generalization of results, they nonetheless play an important role in demonstrating the specific conditions that may affect clinical outcomes. When characteristics or symptoms of single-case subjects (e.g., age, severity level, disfluent behaviors, etc.) match the client being served, similar stages or considerations in treatment may be applicable.

Issues Regarding Efficacy Research

Aside from the logistic difficulties in pursuing clinical efficacy research, several funda-mental questions are yet to be resolved, such as how effective therapy should be evidenced. If in terms of overt stuttering, what parameters should be reported: fre-quency, duration, severity, clustering of disfluencies, speech naturalness? What other aspects of the disorder should be investigated: for example, changes in attitudes and social adjustment regardless of overt stuttering? Can they serve as sufficient evidence of therapeutic success? (see Thomas & Howell, 2001). Should clients' self-assessment be taken as evidence or only external observations? (see Quesal, Yaruss, & Molt, 2004; Rustin, Boterill, & Kelman, 1996).

Another question is what level of change should be taken as evidence of success-ful treatment. When stuttering frequency is the measure, should the absolute or percentage change be regarded as a significant indicator of success? Specifically, is a reduction in three stutter events, say from 10 to 7 per 100 words, sufficient evidence supporting the technique employed? If yes, would a reduction in three stutter events from 20 to 17 per 100 words be viewed as sufficient evidence? Or should a specific percentage change, say 30%, be set as minimally acceptable? In that case, someone initially exhibiting 6 stutter events per 100 words would have to drop by only 2 events, to settle at 4 events per 100 words. But is a reduction in 2 events perceptible enough to be meaningful?

A third relevant issue is the amount of treatment and its distribution. Should we stipulate the number of sessions or the overall duration of the program as standard? And, of course, there is the well-known tendency for relapse in adults who stutter, estimated by several investigators as approximately 70% (e.g., Craig, 1998). For how long should follow-ups continue in order to declare success?

In addition to seeking out clinical research literature, clinicians will want to test the efficacy of their own treatments. In a schools setting there are ample opportuni-ties for small breaks that give the clinician a chance to observe whether treatment has been having a beneficial impact when compared to the "no treatment" periods, or whether treatment effects are maintained and generalized in the posttreatment variable conditions. The clinician must wrestle with the various questions and decide what criteria are indicative of individual client success with therapy.

The Client-Clinician Relationship

The roles that the speech clinician will serve during stuttering intervention are many and diverse: counselor, coach, educational resource, and comrade model. The clinician must shift readily among modes of interaction to meet the client's needs. More impor-tant than these roles, however, are the personal qualities the clinician brings to the therapeutic relationship. Certain qualities facilitate the rapport, trust, and openness necessary to the therapeutic progress. Without sufficient trust, clients may not report attitudes and feelings honestly, resulting in misleading data and progress assessment.

The famous clinical psychologist Carl Rogers (1957) asserted that professionals who intend to practice a person-centered approach to facilitating therapeutic change must display qualities of empathy, self-congruence, and unconditional positive regard. Although there are other desired qualities, we believe these three form an important foundation for the client-clinician relationship in the context of stuttering intervention. Clinicians, and those preparing themselves to become clinicians, who lack experience with people who stutter may find it particularly challenging to display these qualities and facilitate therapeutic change for their clients. These can be developed in several ways, as discussed next.

Empathy

Empathy is about understanding the nature of the problem the client faces. It has been said that only someone who stutters can understand what a person who stutters experiences. Some people go so far as to assert that unless the clinician is a person who stutters, her or his therapy will not be effective. Although it may be true that clinicians who do not have a stuttering history may never fully comprehend the stuttering experience of their clients, several steps can be taken to improve that empathy:

1. Simulating various forms of stuttering in speaking situations with strangers, friends, in public places, on the telephone, and so on, to experience the range of accompanying feelings and listener responses. Feelings experienced prior to, during, and after stuttering, as well as listeners' responses should be examined. Placing oneself in others' shoes facilitates empathy.
2. Participation in stuttering support groups. This affords the opportunity to encounter a greater number of people who stutter, and so become familiar with their feelings about speaking, stuttering, speech therapy, and clinicians. Among other experiences, it can be an eye-opener to sometimes encounter negative opinions about therapy and the reasons for such animosity. These experiences seed ideas for doing things differently in therapy.
3. Reading newsletters and other publications of support groups keeps ongoing familiarity with what children and adults who stutter are saying about their speech problem. Examples of sources are listed in Table 8.1.

Similarly, watching video commentaries prepared by people who stutter (e.g., *Transcending Stuttering*, etc.) and participation in online groups (e.g., STUTT-L, visit: www.mnsu.edu/comdis/kuster/stuttlfaq.html), provide the experience of dialogue about stuttering.

Self-Congruence

Self-congruence is about being authentic and genuine. People with self-congruence do not hide or disguise feelings but own and admit them. They are less apt to play a role rather than being themselves. Self-congruence by professionals enhances the trust of their clients because the clinician is objective and open to perceiving the real selves of others. It creates an atmosphere in which the client can perceive himself or herself more clearly, the negative as well as positive aspects, without experiencing them as a threat. Clinicians can enhance their self-congruence by adopting an objective awareness of their thoughts and feelings through regularly recording self-observations and selecting

Table 8.1: Support Groups

Group	National Association of Young People Who Stutter	National Stuttering Association	Stuttering Foundation of America
Newsletter title	*Friends*	*Letting Go* (newsletter for adults) *Stutter Buddies* (newsletter for children)	*The Stuttering Foundation Newsletter*
Address	145 Hayrick Lane Commack, NY 11725-1520	119 W. 40th Street 14th Floor New York, NY 10018	3100 Walnut Grove Road, Suite 603 P.O. Box 11749 Memphis, TN 38111-0749
Web site	www.friendswhostutter.org	www.nsastutter.org	www.stutteringhelp.org

an entrenched habit for changing or elimination, studying objectively the difficult process of change over the course of several weeks or months.

Unconditional Positive Regard

Psychological health is encouraged when people sense they are completely acceptable as they are. The clinician's warmth and high regard toward the client must not be preconditions. To this end, the clinician should be desensitized to stuttering and be comfortable when it occurs. The client must be fully respect-worthy and acceptable, with or without stuttering. It is not that stuttering must be seen as desirable, only that whether or not stuttering behaviors are observed, the clinician regards the client with full respect and high regard.

Strategies for developing a desensitized attitude toward stuttering by a clinician are similar to what they might be for a client (e.g., watching a videotape of severe stuttering, remaining comfortable and focused on what the speaker has to say). The following self-questions serve as guidance: What attitudes make it difficult to remain comfortable? Is it difficult not to be distracted by stuttering? Was it the stuttering itself or pragmatic behaviors that most interfered with communication?

Listener respect for the speaker who stutters should also be given attention. By intentionally studying the behaviors of listeners for how they do and do not show their respect for speakers, clinicians may identify ways to improve their own listening behaviors. Examples may be reducing tendencies to hurry the speaker by their own fast speaking behaviors, using appropriate and comfortable eye contact, and so on.

Clinicians may also need to examine their own attitudes toward themselves, especially in regard to things disliked. Being overly self-critical can be addressed through the practice of letting go of severe judgments, becoming more gentle toward oneself. The point is that the more gently we respond to our own shortcomings, the more gently we are apt to respond to others. This gentleness should not be confused with permissiveness or a relaxed attitude toward self-discipline. Beginning clinicians should be encouraged to self-evaluate their recordings of therapy sessions and minimize the amount of time they spend talking. How can the client accomplish enough practice if the clinician tends to talk 10 times as often (Costello, 1977) in the therapy session?

The client-clinician relationship is especially important to the process of therapeutic change for people who stutter. The qualities just discussed will serve to enhance this relationship. Several authors have addressed this issue with special reference to stuttering in ways that may further enrich your understanding (e.g., Manning, 2001; Shapiro, 1999; Van Riper, 1975).

Ethics

According to the *Internet Encyclopedia of Philosophy* (Fieser, 2006), "The field of ethics, also called moral philosophy, involves systematizing, defending, and recommending concepts of right and wrong behavior" (www.iep.utm.edu/e/ethics.htm). The practice of speech pathology involves various encounters between clinicians and clients that are embedded in moral context. Clinical ethics issues include patient rights, confidentiality, truth-telling, informed consent, disclosure of optional treatment, recommendations for treatment, advice, and more. We assume that general courses and textbooks on speech pathology address the domain of clinical ethics in our field, including the ASHA code of ethics. Therefore, only issues with special relevance to stuttering are covered here. A good way to demonstrate the magnitude and seriousness of ethics in stuttering therapy is through listing questions as we have done here. These are categorized according to whether they tend to arise with treatment of adults versus children.

Questions Concerning Ethics

Questions Concerning Adults

1. Is it sound practice to base diagnosis primarily on the judgment of a person who states that he or she stutters?
2. Should I use only strict evidence-based therapies?
3. Is it ethical to tell a client that the goal for therapy is the achievement of normal speech?
4. Is it ethical to instruct a client to stutter on purpose in the clinic or at home as part of the therapy?
5. Is it ethical to instruct a client to stutter on purpose talking to strangers in the street, store clerks, and so on?
6. Is it ethical to use mild electrical shock to punish stuttering?
7. Is it ethical to stop people in the street and stutter to them on purpose just to practice?
8. Is it ethical to substitute one abnormal speech (stuttering) with another (e.g., rhythmic speech)?
9. Is it ethical to recommend purchase of an expensive fluency-aiding instrument rather than providing speech therapy?

Questions Concerning Children

1. Is it ethical to postpone therapy for a preschool-age child immediately after onset, just because of the high chances for natural recovery?

2. Is it ethical to recommend therapy for a preschool-age child immediately after onset, knowing the high chances for natural recovery?
3. Is it ethical to counsel parents to not correct their child's stuttering? To correct it?
4. Is it ethical to counsel parents of a child who stutters to talk to him or her in a simple language?
5. Is it ethical to tell parents that perhaps their behavior caused the child's stuttering?
6. Is it ethical to tell parents that perhaps some of their behavior aggravates the child's stuttering?
7. Is it ethical to train children to be assertive when others make fun of them?

As scientific advances are being made in genetics, drugs, brain imaging, and other areas, more questions arise. Genetics raises several concerns, especially privacy issues. A genetic analysis could bring uninvited results, significant to the individual, as well as current or future children. What should be done with such information? Sometimes obtaining genetic information requires participation from other family members who may be unwilling to cooperate. Is there a proper ethical principle to persuade their participation? A rather sensitive issue is counseling. Suppose an infant is at high risk for stuttering even before the onset of speech. Should parents be counseled? If so, how and when should counseling be offered? Who should provide the counseling? Another thorny issue pertains to the use of pharmaceutical agents. Suppose a pharmacological treatment for stuttering has been developed but with some risk that disfluency will persist. Some parents would want their child to take the drug, even though stuttering is not a life-threatening condition. How do parents weigh the risks versus the benefits, especially for the one who has never stuttered? We will not provide any opinions. Indeed, these are serious questions that clinicians should be prepared to answer as they formulate their own personal code of ethics in conjunction with the professionally accepted principles.

Summary

Prior to an examination of various forms of treatment for stuttering, it is important to consider several broad issues that impact clinical decisions. Clinical intervention is ideally based in a theoretical rationale. The absence of strong comprehensive theories of stuttering poses a substantial challenge to this endeavour. Yet successful eclectic therapy programs should be recognized and considered with all other factors. Three major potential aims of stuttering treatment were identified. These center on producing fluent speech, reducing stuttering, and improving social-emotional adjustment. The 12 general approaches to stuttering treatment, aimed at achieving these goals, were classified into four areas of focus: psychological factors, stutter events, fluency, and environment. A separate but all-important issue is the qualifications and qualities of good clinicians. The therapeutic nature of the client-clinician relationship can be enhanced by qualities of empathy, self-congruence, and unconditional positive regard.

The pursuit of evidence-based practice has both its merits and its hazards. Whereas the merits of evidence-based treatment are obvious, it may also present considerable rigidity in practical implementation. Similarly, the field must face multiple challenges before we can answer all our questions about clinical efficacy. Scientists and clinicians have procedures to aid their progress in these areas, but considerable care must be taken in the handling of data and its interpretation. Unfortunately, the limited well-controlled clinical research pertaining to the treatment of stuttering conducted to date, whether employing group or single-subject design, has left many common clinical practices untested. Finally, clinical practice must be conducted within commonly accepted rules of ethics by the society at large and the profession of speech pathology. Ethical questions of special relevance to stuttering were brought to the forefront.

STUDY QUESTIONS AND DISCUSSION TOPICS

1. What is the reasoning behind the advocacy of a therapy-theory link?
2. Do certain forms of evidence-based rationale provide a sufficient basis for treatment even in the absence of a definitive theory of stuttering? Give examples in support of your opinion.
3. What are the three major long-term therapy objectives for stuttering? Explain/discuss the differences among the goals stated.
4. Although the three major treatment goals, fluent speech, reduced stuttering, and improved adjustment, can each be targeted in isolation, these areas also may interact. In your opinion, could progress in each of the areas influence progress in the other two areas? Why?
5. The chapter presented 12 treatment approaches classified into three classes. What are the classes?

Elaborate on the uniqueness of each. Explain the differences.
6. If you were charged to categorize these 12 treatment approaches, what classification system would you develop and why? What features would you base your system on?
7. Make a list of the challenges that clinical efficacy research must address in the field of stuttering. Which challenges pose the most serious threats to our progress with treatment knowledge and why?
8. What is your opinion regarding the significance of each of the clinician qualities suggested in this chapter? Do you think they are important? Suggest at least two additional qualities.
9. What would your answers be to the questions listed in the section on ethics?

SUGGESTED READINGS

American Speech-Language-Hearing Association. (2003). *Code of ethics*. Retrieved May 1, 2008, from www.asha.org/docs/pdf/ET2003-00166.pdf

Guitar, B. (2004). *Stuttering: An integration of contemporary therapies* (Publication No. 16). Memphis, TN: Stuttering Foundation of America.

Olswang, L. (1998). Treatment efficacy research. In C. Frattali (Ed.), *Measuring outcomes in speech-language pathology* (pp. 134–150). New York: Thieme.

Packman, A., & Attanasio, J. (2004). Theories and treatment. In *Theoretical issues in stuttering* (pp. 143–156). New York: Psychology Press.

Van Riper, C. (1975). The stutterer's clinician. In J. Eisenson (Ed.), *Stuttering, a second symposium* (pp. 453–492). New York: Harper & Row.

Yairi, E. (2006). The Tudor Study and Wendell Johnson. In R. Goldfarb (Ed.), *Ethics: A case study from fluency*. San Diego, CA: Plural Publishing.

Chapter 9: Assessment of Adults and School-Age Children

LEARNER OBJECTIVES

Readers of this chapter will understand:

- The purposes and rationale for the initial evaluation of stuttering and its components.
- Appropriate stuttering evaluation procedures.
- Specific procedures for speech recording and the various methods of disfluency analyses and measures available.
- How stuttering severity is evaluated.
- Administration and scoring of different available scales/checklists/assessment protocols for stuttering.
- How to interpret comprehensive evaluation data, make recommendations for therapy based on assessment results, and prepare professional clinical reports.

General Considerations

Assessment of Stuttering

There is wisdom in the maxim attributed to Charles Kettering that "a problem well-stated is a problem half-solved." The goal of assessment is to be able to artic- ulate an understanding of the nature of a presenting disorder and associated com- munication difficulties, so that appropriate treatment objectives and activities may be pursued. One end result of an assessment is a *diagnosis*, which refers to the identification of a specific condition usually not apparent at the beginning. For example, in medicine, when a patient complains about abdominal pain, the underlying problem must be isolated from the range of possible ailments, such as food poisoning, ulcers, ruptured appendix, cancer, and so on. This is not the case with advanced stuttering, where just about all those who seek professional help state the correct diagnosis, *stuttering*, when they first contact the clinician. Given this reality, with some qualifications to be addressed next, the main assessment task is that of characterization and quantification of the client's stuttering and related factors, not the diagnosis of something not readily apparent (Yairi & Ambrose, 2005).

Differentiation

As stated, a classic diagnostic objective is the differentiation of the client's problem from other possible clinical entities. For a long time, stuttering has been viewed as a single disorder. Delineation and application of meaningful clinical subtypes began to be examined more closely only recently. It has been suggested that stuttering subtype distinctions could be based on etiological factors, gender, personality characteristics, specific stuttering characteristics, language abilities, concomitant disorders, and others (Seery et al., 2007; Yairi, 2007). Although an acceptable subtype system for stuttering is not currently available, a few distinctions can be made. For example, diagnoses may differentiate psychogenic versus neurogenic stuttering or developmental versus acquired disorders (Seery, 2005). Therefore, clinicians engaged in assessment should be aware of the fine details of fluency disorders and be prepared to differentiate possible subtypes of stuttering, as well as stuttering from other fluency disorders, such as language-based disfluency. Although false diagnoses of stuttering in school-age children and adults are not common, there can be times when teachers, parents, and pediatricians refer children to speech-language clinicians because they diagnosed the problem as stuttering when the problem is another form of fluency issue or not even fluency. The clinician needs to listen closely to the client's concerns, carefully observe structure and function of the speech and hearing mechanism, appraise normal and abnormal communication characteristics, and recognize the barriers that prevent the client from speaking freely. More about assessment of fluency disorders other than stuttering is covered in Chapter 15.

The general components of a stuttering assessment are not substantially different from those applied in the evaluation of other communicative disorders. They include the gathering of background and case history information, observing speech production in controlled speaking contexts, assessing the severity of the overt stuttered speech as well as that of the overall disorder, and discerning factors contributing to the communication difficulties. Where assessment of stuttering differs, however, is the relatively large variability in the disorder and the special concern given to evaluating the client's emotional reactions associated with the speaking difficulties, as well as his or her attitudes about speaking. This difference reflects the often large emotional component of advanced stuttering. As we explained in Chapter 4, this component can be more of a problem than the core overt stuttering by itself.

Multidimensionality

One reason why it is especially important to expand the evaluation beyond the speech domain is the multidimensionality of the stuttering disorder. Consistent with ASHA's knowledge competency standards for the assessment of communication disorders, speech-language clinicians must be prepared to consider the "etiologies, characteristics, anatomical/physiological, acoustic, psychological, developmental, and linguistic and cultural correlates" (ASHA Standards, 2008b) of fluency disorders. In the case of stuttering, although assessment of these correlates do not typically lead to the identification of the direct etiology of the disorder, it does help to reveal how individual abilities and characteristics in these correlates (domains) contribute to the complex picture of what triggers stutter events and why the disorder persists.

Several commercial instruments are available to guide the clinician through a comprehensive fluency assessment. One example is the *Overall Assessment of the Speaker's Experience of Stuttering* (OASES) developed by Scott Yaruss (see Yaruss & Quesal, 2006). With this protocol, the clinician analyzes information about the total stuttering disorder, including (1) the client's broad views of stuttering, (2) affective, behavioral, and cognitive reactions to stuttering, (3) functional communication difficulties, and (4) the impact of stuttering on the quality of life. Speech is addressed in section (3) related to communication difficulties. Another instrument, developed by Charles Healey and colleagues, the *CALMS*, addresses five key components believed to be central to maintaining stuttering: Cognitive, Affective, Linguistic, Motor, and Social factors (Healey, Scott Trautman, & Susca, 2004). The model is intended to highlight the individual differences among those who stutter as well as relative strengths and weaknesses among the five CALMS components.

Variability

One of the hallmarks of stuttering is its variability. Rarely does a person who stutters produce all the possible stuttering behaviors, yet some who stutter may not even demonstrate the usual features (Barr, 1940). Stutter events vary both across and within individuals who stutter. Within the same individual, the severity and types of stutter events can vary considerably at different times and in different situations. As described in Chapter 4, certain situational contexts (e.g., talking with an infant, saying typically automatic phrases) can be ameliorating conditions, whereas others can be aggravating conditions (e.g., saying one's name, talking on the telephone). Although there are trends of stuttering variability that are similar across clients, such as the contexts just mentioned, responses to speaking conditions are different across individuals. For example, one client may seldom stutter during interpersonal conversation but have severe stuttering events during oral reading or talking over the telephone. Another client may rarely stutter in oral reading but exhibit severe stuttering during conversation. Hence it is desirable to obtain speech samples in a variety of conditions so that the range of variability and the influence of different contexts for a particular client are appreciated by the clinician.

Special Considerations for School-Age Children

For the sake of minimizing unnecessary repetition, this chapter addresses the initial evaluation of both adults and schoolchildren. Although there are several important procedural modifications necessitated by age differences, the commonalities, such as the kind of information sought or the specific procedures of analyzing speech samples, prevail. Thus when the clinician applies the information presented here, the procedures should be adapted flexibly to suit adults, high school students, or children in elementary school.

Typically, an initial evaluation conducted with adults involves only the client who provides the history background, fills out questionnaires, and offers a relatively mature level of self-awareness of emotions and attitudes. Most high school students are able to function similarly but may lack information pertaining to their history. They should be able to respond to most of the case history questions listed later in the chapter. It is obvious, however, that a question about the person's wife or children's reactions to stuttering should be skipped or reworded to fit the particular individual's circumstances. For many children, asking about parents' and siblings' reactions would be more appropriate. The presence of one or both parents is welcome and may be helpful, but it is not essential for the narrow purpose of the evaluation. Relevant missing information may be secured at a later time.

By contrast, a full evaluation of a third grader would greatly benefit from a parent's participation. Many of the case history questions can be answered only by the parent, not only regarding the stuttering history but regarding emotional reactions, social impact, and so on. It is wise to interview the parent alone before talking with the child. Again, a good number of questions from the list can be presented but with altered wording to suit the child's age, apparent behavior, maturity, and intellectual aptitude. It is also important to examine the complete profile of the child's communication abilities (i.e., articulation and language testing), as well as the academic impact of stuttering. In addition to parents, the clinician may need to interview several persons important to the client, such as teachers and professionals who have evaluated or treated the child for stuttering or other communication disorders. In the table of case history questions, presented later, the last section contains extra questions that may be especially relevant for school-age children. The *CAT-R* and *SEA Scale* are additional tools designed specifically for this age group. As mentioned, procedures for recording and analyzing speech samples are similar to those used with adults. Some children, however, are less verbal or cannot read well enough, requiring more flexibility in obtaining sufficient speech samples, using passages appropriate to the child's ability level. Finding topics of special interest to the child can be particularly important to enhancing the client's motivation and receptivity.

Assessment Objectives

Based on the previous discussion points, a set of evaluation objectives could be proposed for the adult/adolescent/school-age child fluency assessment. Specifically those aims are to:

1. Establish rapport with the client.
2. Obtain background and case history information.
3. Describe the client's speech characteristics.
4. Understand the client's home, social, and work environment.
5. Identify conditions and variables affecting the client's speech.
6. Understand the impact of the communication disorder on the individual's life.
7. Provide information about the nature of fluency/stuttering and its treatment.
8. Recommend a plan of action for the client.

Background and Case History

The purpose of the case history portion of a clinical evaluation is to provide an organized record of all the relevant information concerning the client's condition, problem, or disorder that might be useful in its treatment and related counseling. This may encompass a detailed account of factors ranging from the initial onset and development, to the current status of the stuttering. In the case of children, the history includes such details as the home environment and family background (e.g., genetic factors, family dynamics, and attitudes), parental and/or caregiver legal rights over the client, and whether stuttering varies predictably in any conditions (e.g., emotional responses, certain settings/people, time of day). Also very important information is the nature and effects of present or past treatment. Although not all of the data collected may eventually prove useful, the case history provides clinicians with an overall picture of the problem at hand, sometimes with critical information as to what direction to pursue in treatment or which ones to avoid.

The initial contact with the client and the circumstances surrounding the referral for services are important foundations for the entire assessment and remediation process. During the first moments of interaction with the client, the clinician begins to establish the rapport and trust that will open the lines of communication between them. In Chapter 8 we elaborated on the clinician's qualities that underlie an ideal client-clinician relationship, so critical for successful therapeutic processes. For now, let it just be said that clinicians need to express genuine interest in their clients as people, and have the strength of courage and understanding to journey along with their client on the ups and downs of their path to improved speech.

The circumstances of referral could make a major difference in the trajectory of the treatment process. If a client is self-referred, has individually reached a point of courage and resolve to enter into the treatment process, then foundations for change have already been established. In contrast, if an employer, professor, or family member has urged the client to seek help, and the client is undertaking the therapy mainly to please others, then the process could be already jeopardized. In the latter case, the clinician will need to devote time to educating both the client and those who referred him or her about the nature of treatment, and the critical matter of the client's independent motivation and readiness to undertake the arduous process of change.

Table 9.1 lists a set of potential case history questions to be included during the initial interview with the client. The question *"What do you do when you stutter?"* is particularly important because it begins the process of examining the stuttering as a behavior on the part of the client. It also reveals the client's understanding of stuttering and whether there is readiness to discuss it in terms of his or her own initiated speech movements and consequent emotional reactions, or just how much it is ascribed to a mysterious extraneous force or impulse that arises out of nowhere, over which the client has no control (Williams, 1957). Later on, in therapy, the clinician will strive to have the client develop a point of view of stuttering in which his or her own doing is a big part of the disorder. Finally, even if the client is able to discuss stuttering in terms of self-initiated behaviors, there can be a certain amount of mismatch between the characterization of stuttering events and reactions described by the client and what the clinician observes. In some cases, the clinician will need to observe much more in order to develop an understanding of what the client is experiencing. In other cases, the clinician will need to guide the client toward an improved level of self-awareness to promote therapeutic change.

Table 9.1: Case History Topic Areas and Potential Interview Questions

I. Stuttering History	a. Do you remember, or have you been told about when you began stuttering?
	b. From how far back do you remember stuttering?
	c. Are you aware of any factors/events surrounding the time of onset? Do you think any of these was the cause of the stuttering?
	d. How has stuttering progressed over time? Has it been up and down? Only gone up? Only down? About the same all the time?
	e. Have there ever been time periods, for example, several weeks, when you hardly stuttered at all?
	f. Have there been other relatives who stutter? Who? When? Did any of them stop stuttering? Who? When?
II. Treatment History	a. Who referred you to us?
	b. Have you received any treatment? When? Where?
	c. How long did each treatment last? Frequency of sessions?
	d. What were the therapy approaches?
	e. What were the results for each treatment?
	f. What technique has helped you the most? And the least?
	g. What led you to seek help at the time(s) you did?
	h. What led to your interest in therapy right now?
III. Current Speech Description	a. Currently, what are your main problems related to your speech?
	b. How would you describe your speech and your stuttering?
	c. What do you do when you stutter? (Show me)
	d. What is the severity range of your stuttering—is it mild, moderate, or severe? What is the most common severity? In what situations?
	e. Do you know when you are going to stutter?
	f. Describe what you experience/feel/think just *before* you stutter.
	g. What do you experience/feel/think *during* stuttering?
	h. How do you react/feel *after* you have stuttered?
	i. What kinds of things do you do to cope with stuttering moments? (Clinicians should probe for avoidance/postponement methods and speech modifications.)
IV. Environmental Variables Affecting Speech	a. What increases your stuttering? (e.g., places, situations, friends, other people, sounds, words)
	b. What decreases your stuttering? When is speech easier for you?
	c. When do you stutter the most? The least?
	d. How much talking do you do each day? In what settings?
	e. With whom do you usually talk (family, friends, colleagues, superiors, strangers)?
	f. How do others respond to your stuttering (friends, teachers, strangers)?
	g. What are your plans related to school? Are you attending school now? If not, when did you last attend school? Has your school situation been comfortable regarding your speech?
	h. What are your plans related to work? Are you working now? Part or full time? Where? If not, when did you last work? Where? Is your work situation comfortable in regard to your speech?

Table 9.1: **Continued**

V. Impact of Stuttering on Quality of Life	a. Does stuttering affect your relationships with family? With whom? How? (If married, with spouse and/or children? If young, with parents and/or siblings?) b. Does stuttering affect your social life? How? c. Do you ever talk about stuttering? If so, with whom? d. Has stuttering affected your school achievements? e. Has stuttering affected your choice (or plans) of career or job/vocation? f. Does stuttering affect you in any way we haven't mentioned? g. If you didn't stutter, how do you think life would change?
VI. Other Relevant Case History	a. Have you ever had any other speech or language difficulty? b. Any difficulty reading or writing? c. Is English your first and only language? d. Have you tended to move a lot or live mostly in one location? Has moving been associated with changes in the stuttering? How? e. Are you currently taking medication that could affect speech? If so, what medication? For what health condition? Does this health condition affect your speech in general? The stuttering? How? f. Have you ever had difficulty hearing? When was your last hearing test?
VII. Client's Perspective	a. Do your feelings and mood affect your speech? How? b. How would you describe yourself as a person? For example, easygoing, serious, ambitious, good-humored, energetic/calm? persistent/easily gives up? self-confident or unsure? enjoys people? afraid of new situations? c. During this interview, has your speech/stuttering been typical? Better or worse than usual? How? d. What do you know about stuttering? e. What do you believe causes stuttering? f. How important is your speech therapy goal? (Relative to other goals?) g. What do you hope/expect to gain from speech therapy? h. What do you think you will need to do to change your speech? i. Are you ready to make those changes? j. Do you have any questions?
VIII. Identifying Information	a. Who referred you? b. Check spelling of name, correct birthdate, current address, phones, and so on. Where/how do you wish to be contacted? c. Are there others (doctor, family, caseworkers) with whom you would like for us to share information regarding your speech services? (fill out proper consent forms) d. Do you wish for a copy of our evaluation report to be sent to your home? And/or reviewed with you, in person?
IX. Additional Questions for School-Age Children	**For interviewing children:** a. Do you go to school? What grade are you in? b. What subjects do you like most? Least? c. Are you in any after-school activities? Sports? Music? Hobbies? d. What do you like to do best? Why? e. Tell me about some things you do well. f. Do you like talking? How much talking do you do each day? Where? With whom? g. Do you participate in class discussions? Answer questions? h. Do other children make fun of your stuttering? i. Are your teachers understanding of your stuttering problem?

(continued)

Table 9.1: **Continued**

For interviewing parents:
a. Does stuttering affect how {child name} does in school?
b. Does {child name} stutter the same at school and at home?
c. Aside from speech, does {child name} struggle with any other areas (for example, in school or with developing other skills)?
d. Is a typical day for {child name} fairly calm or busy? How/Why?
e. Are there frequent big family gatherings?
f. Does he or she play with neighborhood children? Do they get along? Has teasing been an issue? How has it been handled?
g. Does {child name} prefer to play alone? or with others? Has stuttering appeared to affect play or socializing?
h. Does stuttering affect your family or you in any way(s) we haven't mentioned?
i. How important do you think speech is to {child name}?

Another important question centers on the client's attitudes and expectations. Is the client expecting that the clinician will impart a treatment, for example, sets of prescribed exercises, a powerful electrical stimulation, hypnosis, or all sorts of other treatments that should do the job of removing the stuttering? Or does the client understand that she or he will have to work diligently toward a process of multiple changes, keep practicing new speaking behaviors, altered emotional reactions and social interaction, and move out of his or her comfort zones to accomplish the various therapy objectives? If the client expects the former, then the clinician will need to devote time to educate the client about the nature of speech therapy for stuttering, the essential approach, and the work to be done to accomplish change. That is, therapy is not about "fixing" stuttering for the client but is aimed to provide the client with skills and abilities that will have to be practiced to deal effectively with stuttering and improve communication. Clients ought to realize that stuttering therapy often requires doing the very things that they least like to do, for example, speak on the telephone, talk to strangers, make oral presentations to groups, and so on.

Each individual will have his or her own painful memories and strong emotions related to stuttering that may need to be released. The clinician is to be ready to listen closely to the expressed feelings, appreciate the client's perspective, and offer the reassurance that it is safe to expose those feelings and experiences in the clinician's presence. The clinician's acceptance of the client's feelings and experiences, just as they are, is apt to go far in promoting progress. Because the client may need to enhance skills of self-comfort in the wake of emotional distress, the clinician can note and validate such skills of self-understanding as the client may already evidence.

Observations and Examinations: Speech

Speech Sample Context

In as much as disfluent speech is the cardinal feature of stuttering, it is only logical to expect that analyses of speech samples would typically play a central role in the assessment of the disorder. They are the means by which fluency, disfluency, and associated factors are observed and quantified for the sake of diagnosis and treatment decisions. Due to the variability of stuttering across situations, at least two, ideally three, separate speech sample contexts are recommended for an in-depth evaluation (Costello & Ingham, 1984; Gregory, 2003). With adolescents and adults, those usually consist of a spontaneous speech sample, such as conversation or monologue, oral reading, and another speaking context with individual relevance (e.g., classroom, group discussion, phone call, etc.).

A conversation and monologue are different in that there is frequent turn-taking during conversation. In contrast, a relatively continuous stream of speech is delivered during a monologue. If the clinician speaks as little as possible to encourage a monologue, the collection of a large sample can be accomplished more quickly than if there is an exchange of conversational speaking turns. Hence a monologue is a more efficient means to reach the goal of quickly obtaining a large speech sample for type/frequency analysis of disfluencies. A monologue, however, is not the most common form of daily speaking context; if a primarily valid and representative sample of speech is desired, conversation may be a better choice. Conversation, with its many shifting topics and potential interruptions, may also exert more pressure on the client, thus providing more examples of stuttering events.

To elicit a spontaneous monologue, the examiner prompts with requests such as "Tell me about your hobbies/interests." or "Tell me about the work you do." A standard monologue elicitation procedure known as the *Job Task* (Johnson, 1961a) is conducted by asking the client to talk for 3 minutes about a current job or vocation, future jobs or those held in the past, or current school classes and other activities to prepare for employment. In addition to describing the vocation, the client should say why she or he chose the job, as well as anything else about it that she or he would like to discuss. The client is given a minute or so to prepare before starting. If the client stops talking too soon, the clinician prompts with additional questions to elicit more talking. For a monologue sample, the clinician should note whether any adaptation occurs with continued talking, that is, some speakers tend to become more fluent as they keep talking. Such adaptation may suggest a milder or more readily modified form of stuttering.

Sometimes, for efficiency, a clinician might choose to record the initial interview as a form of conversational speech sample. If this context is selected, considerations should be given to whether the sample is representative of daily conversations. The topics discussed in the initial interview could elicit either more mild or more severe forms of stuttering than are typically encountered. Therefore, depending on the particular objectives of the fluency assessment, the clinician might want to select the speech sample context with consideration of the balance of priorities between efficiency and representative validity. It is important to obtain information about the client's level of education and reading ability prior to selection of the reading passage. This will prevent the uncomfortable experience of asking a client to read material that is either way beyond or way below his or her abilities. Perhaps the most important factor in deciding the sample context is whether the clinician will compare the client's disfluency in terms of type and frequency or any other measure of stuttering, only to other speech samples generated by the client (relational assessment), or to published reference data (normative assessment). If the latter is the goal, a valid comparison depends on selection of a sample context that reasonably matches the one/s used to generate the normative data set.

Speech Sample Size

How long should a speech sample be to obtain valid and reliable data for analysis? Unfortunately, this is not an easy question to answer because, so far, only two studies have compared disfluency data obtained from different sample sizes: one with adults who stutter and one with adults who do not stutter. Both reported nonsignificant differences for the number of disfluencies more typical of stuttering among speech samples ranging from 300 to 1800 syllables (Logan & Haj Tas, 2007; Roberts, Meltzer, & Wilding, 2009). Some sources suggest a modest 200 syllables for each situation or speaking mode: conversation and oral reading (Riley, 1994), or 300 to 400 words (Shapiro, 1999). Others recommended an amount of speaking time, such as 3 minutes (Johnson, Darley, & Spriesterbach, 1963; Ward, 2006). And several sources addressing evaluation do not specify speech sample size (Manning, 2001; Wingate, 1976). Initial information directly relevant to the effect of speech sample size was provided by Sawyer and Yairi (2006) based on samples of speech from preschool children. They reported that longer samples, upward of 1200 syllables, were necessary to capture all the relevant disfluent speech behaviors. It is unjustified at the present, however, to generalize this finding to adolescents and adults.

One of us (CS) requires at least 300 words or syllables for the adult spontaneous speech sample, conversation, or monologue. She reasons that if the measure will be per 100 units, then 300 represents three times the sampling unit basis. When evaluating baseline measures, at least three data points are required to establish a trend (Barlow, Hayes, & Nelson, 1984). In contrast, a minimum standard of 600 syllables was advocated by Yairi and Ambrose (2005). They argue that the larger sample size is necessary to sample certain disfluency types adequately, for example, disrhythmic phonations or repetitions of four or more units (e.g., Bu-bu-bu-bu-but), which generally occur at a much lower frequency, especially in mild to moderate stuttering, than other disfluencies but yet are very important contributors to the overall impression of stuttering and its severity. They opined that "it is advisable to have at least three tokens for any given type of disfluency. Just one could be random, two are insufficient to identify a pattern or obtain a mean, but three indicate that the behavior is more than a fluke, presenting some semblance of pattern or typicality" (p. 106). Again, although their comments were made in regard to young children, it may be even more critical for older children who may have found ways to suppress their stuttering-like disfluencies and be at risk for underdetection of their speech problem.

As explained, the issue of sample size is important for the purpose of counting the frequency of specific disfluency types. This, however, is not the case if the clinician is interested only in assigning an overall rating of stuttering severity. When stuttering appears to be severe, a short sample can suffice. The milder the stuttering, the longer the sample size necessary to rate severity with confidence.

For the oral reading context, longer samples are usually not necessary to find out whether this condition differs from spontaneous speech samples. Although the per 100 unit basis will be applied in measurements, a paragraph of oral reading is often enough to reveal the severity of stuttering in that context. If the examiner is looking for adaptation or wants to establish a baseline frequency measure, then a passage of least 200 syllables would offer more representative data. Also, time may be the more appropriate standard of sample size length. If a client displays considerable struggle, with blocks lasting many seconds long, then measuring the number of fluent words or syllables spoken in 3 minutes is apt to be more meaningful than the number of disfluencies or stutter events per 100 words.

Measures of Stuttering or Disfluency

A variety of systems of analysis have been employed to measure and report the amount of stuttering in speech samples. Although they appear similar, important differences exist among systems. For example, the frequency of stuttering per 100 words is quite different from the percentage of stuttered words. Both measures are based on the clinician's subjective perception that some instances of stuttering occurred. The first measure, however, provides more accurate information in that it allows for counting more than one stuttering event on the same word (e.g., A-a-ari-zo-zo-zo-na has two events). The second measure allows for counting only one stuttering instance per word. Thus A-a-ari-zo-zo-zo-na is counted as only one stuttered word. In this case, the first method reports twice as much stuttering for the same amount of speech. These measures of perceived stuttering events, however, do not provide information about the kind of stuttering that took place. They only reveal the total number of the events. A third measure, the objectively counted frequency of various disfluency types per 100 syllables or words, yields much more information on the specific characteristics of the client's speech. It not only reveals how many interruptions are contained in the speech, but it provides specific descriptions of them, discriminating among repetitions, sound prolongations, interjections, and other types or forms. This is meaningful information to have.

In 1988, Kully and Boberg sent an identical set of speech samples to multiple clinical sites to be analyzed for stuttering frequency, and they discovered that the approaches and event counts differed substantially across sites. Although their specific procedures and findings have been seriously questioned (Ryan, 1997; Yairi, 1997[1]), such disagreement can be understood given the fact that there are many ways

---

[1] Yairi (1997, p. 54) stated that "Although Kully and Boberg (1988) emphasized the disagreement among clinics in identifying stuttering and disfluencies, an inspection of their Table 2 reveals that the average agreement between the two clinics which counted "percent disfluency" was 81.7%, a respectable level that was considerably better than agreement among clinics which counted 'percent stuttering.'"

in which stuttering has been quantified. The major differences among metrics of stuttering come from two parameters. First is the target/s of interest, that is, what is being measured. Second is the sampling units or period over which measurements are made. The target may be any of the following: (1) perceived stuttering events (also referred to as "moments," or "instances," of stuttering), (2) descriptive disfluency types, or (3) perceptually fluent speech. The sampling units can consist of syllables, words, or time intervals (see discussions by Yairi, 1997, and Yairi & Ambrose, 2005).

> Another train car analogy (see Chapter 6) may help illustrate the different ways speech samples may be analyzed. The general question is: How much cargo is there? One way to find an answer is to look in each train car for whether it contains boxes of cargo, count the cars with cargo in them, and divide by the total number of train cars to arrive at the percentage of train cars with cargo. This method is like measuring % syllables (or words) stuttered. Another way to find an answer is to count all the boxes of cargo in the entire train, then divide by the total number of train cars. This calculation yields the number of cargo boxes per train car. By multiplying that number by 100, the number (frequency) of cargo boxes per 100 train cars is estimated. This latter method is like measuring the frequency of stuttering (or disfluencies) per 100 syllables (or words). The information yielded by the two ways of obtaining measures is different.

Depending on the combinations of target (e.g., disfluencies, stutter events) and sampling units (e.g., syllables, words, time intervals), different measurement methods may be applied. In one method, all disfluent instances are counted and their frequency relative to the overall number of sampling units is calculated. This method results in the frequency of disfluencies per 100 syllables or words. In contrast, each sampling unit (e.g., each syllable) can be examined for whether the target feature (e.g., stuttering) is present. For example, among the 274 syllables sampled, how many are perceived as stuttered? This method yields the measure of percentage syllables stuttered. If preferred, each word, rather than each syllable, is analyzed. Table 9.2 shows the formulas for several types of speech behavior analyses.

Table 9.2: **The Target Behaviors, Sampling Units, and Formulas for the Various Measures of Stuttering from Speech Sample**

Type of Measure	Target Feature	Sampling Unit	Formula
Disfluency frequency per 100 syllables or words	Descriptive disfluencies according to type	Syllables or words	$\dfrac{\text{No. disfluencies} \times 100}{\text{No. syllables or No. words}}$
Percentage of words stuttered	Perceived stuttering	Words	$\dfrac{\text{No. stuttered words} \times 100}{\text{No. words}}$
Fluency frequency index	Perceived fluency	Words	$\dfrac{\text{No. fluent words} \times 100}{\text{No. words}}$
Frequency of stuttered intervals	Perceived stuttering	5-s intervals (or shorter) of speech	$\dfrac{\text{No. stuttered intervals} \times 100}{\text{No. intervals}}$

To derive the first measure in the table, the number of disfluencies in the entire sample is divided by the number of syllables in the sample. The outcome is then multiplied by 100. Alternatively, multiply the number of disfluencies in the sample by 100, and then divide by the number of syllables. A clinician who specializes in stuttering will want to shift flexibly among these methods, depending on the assessment needs. If a clinician wants to obtain a severity rating using the *Stuttering Severity Instrument* (SSI-4) by Riley (2009), then the percentage of syllables stuttered metric would be applied. If, however, there is an interest to obtain an analysis of the specific types of disfluent characteristics displayed by the client, then a calculation of disfluencies per 100 words (or syllables) could be used. Both of these methods of analysis are based on the clinician's review of previously recorded audiovisual speech samples and are referred to as *offline* analysis. Alternatively, if during a clinical session, a reliable *online*[2] method of stuttering data collection is desired, judgments of whether 5-s time intervals in the sample contain stuttering might be helpful (Cordes & Ingham, 1994, 1999). Another measure that may be useful to assess progress in stuttering treatment is the fluency frequency index (FFI), based on the number of fluent words per total words (Shapiro, 1999). Of course, this is not a direct measure of the stuttering per se. It provides information about the amount of speech not affected by the disorder and may help focus the client's attention on fluent rather than disfluent speech. In sum, there is no universally adopted system of speech sample analysis for purposes of evaluation of stuttering and fluency. Clinicians may opt to employ a single method with which they feel comfortable or train themselves in several methods that they are capable of using as the need arises.

Several additional methods have been proposed for measuring fluent, also called *stutter-free*, periods of speech. Costello and Ingham (1984) offered the following two measures, among several more: the average *duration* of the three longest nonstuttered intervals measured in seconds and/or minutes, and the average *length* of the three longest nonstuttered intervals measured in numbers of syllables. An alternative to measuring fluent time periods is the measurement of disfluent time. Starkweather, Gottwald, and Halfond (1990) suggested the percent time disfluent (PTD) measure. PTD is derived by summing up the duration of all disfluencies in a sample, then calculating its percentage of the total duration of the sample. In a later publication, Starkweather and Givens-Ackerman (1997) referred to this same measure as the percentage of discontinuous speech time (PDST). Sometimes measures like these, or disfluent or fluent time periods, are particularly useful for showing progress with treatment.

Speech Recordings and Transcription

Audiovisually recorded samples are more desirable than audio samples alone because visual information is there to aid the interpretation of an event. For example, a silent pause may represent a type of disfluency, such as a static oral posture, or it could simply be a moment when the client stopped talking to think about at something. An audio recorded sample, however, may be a useful backup if the video technology fails.

---

[2] Note that the term *online* here is synonymous with "live" and must not be confused with the common but entirely different meaning for the term *online* of being connected to the Internet.

The audio recording system should be checked in advance for sound clarity and unwanted noise. The gain control switch should be turned off in recorders that have this feature to avoid variations in loudness and loss of some speech, especially at the beginning of utterances. Another decision regarding *video* recordings has to do with what view of the client to frame (e.g., full face, full body, upper body, etc.). Because it is of interest to capture potential secondary behaviors that can involve arm movements as well as upper body posturing, it is desirable to obtain a video image that includes the upper body from the waist to the head, at a distance close enough to reveal oral postures and facial expressions.

Once a speech sample is recorded, the next step is making a written transcription of it to facilitate detailed analyses. For this task, it is usually best to start by transcribing only the client's words in an utterance without noting the disfluencies. The next step, analysis, is made easier when each spoken utterance is distinguished in the transcript by starting it on the next line. Knowledge of the context of the words beforehand aids in resolving challenging questions, such as whether an utterance was a word "a" or an interjection "uh." In our practice, we review (listen to) the recorded speech sample as many times as necessary to ensure the most valid and reliable transcript as the basis for the analysis.

Procedures for Speech Sample Analysis

After all the words in the speech sample have been determined, the examiner can then listen again to the utterances, marking the location of the specific target according to the clinician's preferred measure or the particular need. It is also helpful to add in the transcript any comments or behavioral observations that could aid interpretation later (e.g., "started to speak before examiner finished" or "coughed and scratched his head"). Notes about secondary behaviors (e.g., "looks away," "gasped," "head jerk," "lip tension," etc.) are also useful to include where applicable in the transcript. Braces can be used to set these apart from the spoken words.

If *percentage of stuttered words* is the desired measure, each word perceived with confidence as stuttered is marked. As explained earlier, the stuttered words are then counted and their percentage in the total number of words in the speech sample is calculated. In a 369-word sample containing 23 stuttered words, the percentage of words stuttered is $23/369 \times 100 = 6.23\%$.

If *percentage of stuttered syllables*[3] is the desired measure, the procedure is very similar. Each syllable perceived as stuttered is marked, the total number of syllables in the sample is counted, and the percentage of stuttered syllables is calculated. In a speech sample of 443 syllables containing 65 stuttered syllables, the familiar math involved is as follows: $65/443 \times 100 = 14.67\%$.

When specific disfluency analysis is desired, the clinician indicates on the transcript each of several disfluency types (e.g., syllable repetition, interjection, sound

---

[3] In published literature, the terms "percent syllables stuttered," "percent stuttered syllables," "percentage of stuttered syllables," and "percentage of syllables stuttered" are all synonymous, as are the parallel terms where "words" is used in place of "syllables."

prolongation), using a simple marking code. This can be aided by applying a different-colored highlighter for each type of disfluency where it occurs.

After the transcript is completely marked, the occurrence of each type in the sample is counted and its frequency per 100 syllables is calculated and tabulated. Then, the total frequency per 100 syllable of *all* types combined is derived. The clinician may also wish to derive subtotals of these disfluency types grouped as Stuttering-Like Disfluency (SLD) and Other Disfluency (OD), or other desired categories. A display of this type of analysis in a 566-word speech sample, in which a total of 147 disfluencies (25.97 per 100 words) were identified, is illustrated here:

Disfluency Type	Per 100 words
Part-word repetitions (45)	7.95
Whole-word repetitions (19)	3.36
Disrhythmic phonation (33)	5.83
SLD Subtotal (97)	**17.14**
Phrase repetitions (12)	2.12
Interjections (34)	6.01
Revisions (4)	0.71
OD Subtotal (50)	**8.83**
Disfluency Total (147)	**25.97**

Selection of Sampling Units

Prior to the analysis, the examiner must decide what sampling unit to apply, usually words or syllables. Several considerations will be needed. First, if comparisons will be made to published data sets, then the same constituents, words or syllables, must be applied in the analysis. If a direct match is not possible, adult sample estimates may be made by converting the word count to a syllable count (or vice versa), applying a 1.5:1 syllables-to-words ratio. By contrast, samples from young children, typically users of more monosyllabic words in their speech, would be converted with a smaller ratio of approximately 1.15:1 (Yaruss, 2000).

The following example illustrates the conversion of a syllable metric to a word metric. Suppose a 600-syllable speech sample was collected with 60 disfluencies. The frequency of disfluency is 10 per 100 syllables. If the clinician wants to compare this value to the norm, which is about 7 disfluencies per 100 words for adult spontaneous speech, then a conversion is needed. By applying the ratio of 1.5 syllables per word, the number of words is estimated by dividing 600 syllables by 1.5, yielding 400 words. The disfluency frequency can then be recalculated based on 60 disfluencies per 400 words, which would be 15 per 100 words. The result turns out to be considerably higher than the normative standard.

Second, there may be practical factors in the choice of unit applied. If the word or syllable information is already available to the examiner (e.g., a reading paragraph), time can be saved and allotted instead to the analysis process. Third, there may be an interest in the nature of the disfluent speech relative to language or speech planning. Conceptually, the number of words would better reflect the amount of language produced, whereas the number of syllables better reflects the amount of speech produced. The more multisyllabic words used by a speaker, the less the word count reflects the speech motor demands of the utterances. Syllable counts are apt to capture such demands more closely. Finally, the total counts of either words or syllables tend to be more accurate when smaller sections of the speech sample are summed first. For example, next to each line in the transcript, the examiner would record the count of words or syllables, then for each section or page subtotals are derived, and finally the subtotals are added to arrive at the grand total of words or syllables.

Rules for Syllable or Word Counts

An essential rule for counting words or syllables in the speech samples of people who stutter is that the count should be based on the number of words or syllables that would have been spoken had there been no disfluent speech. For example, "bu-bu-bu-but" counts as one spoken syllable. Additionally, standard rules for what should, and should not, be counted as a word or syllable have been offered (Brown, 1973; Guitar, 2006; Retherford, 2000). We suggest the following conventions, adapted from those sources:

1. Repeated, interjected word or phrase segments are not included in the counts.

    e.g., "The ba-ba-ba-baby is uh uh crying." has 6 syllables, 4 words.

2. Words that precede or follow revisions *are* included in the word count.

    e.g., "The infant—the baby is—has been crying." has 11 syllables, 8 words

3. The following are considered to be one word:
    a. Expressions like "Oh boy" (2 syllables).
    b. Acronyms like "MTV"
    c. Proper names like "Mary Kay"
    d. Catenative forms such as "gonna" or "hafta"
    e. Ritualized reduplications such as "bye-bye" or "so-so"

Although some clinicians may prefer to exclude unfinished or abandoned words, we usually include any partial words that are still intelligible, counting only the portion that was actually uttered (e.g., "bana-" and "stra-" would be 2 syllables + 1 syllable = 3 syllables).

Additional rules ensure that word or syllable counts are not artificially inflated with a preponderance of utterance types that are either atypical, exceedingly short, or a known fluency-enhancing condition. Rules for the types of utterances to exclude from the analysis set are as follows:

a. Direct quotes (precise imitation) of another person
b. Words spoken or listed in a series ("One, two, three . . . A, B, C, D . . .")
c. Words that are sung or automatically recited
d. Isolated single-word utterances indicating "yes" or "no"
e. Unintelligible words or syllables

Disfluency Reference Data

Appendix 9.1 (see end of this chapter) offers a reference for disfluency type/frequency data per 100 words for nonstuttering speakers based on two sources. Participants in the Yairi and Clifton (1972) study were younger and older adults, males and females combined, who produced narrative speech samples of unspecified length in response to three picture cards. Participants in the White (2002) study were 30 men and women who produced narrative samples on the topics: a typical day in their life, how to drive a car, how to make a favorite meal, and how to change a car tire. Speech sample sizes ranged from 300 to 363 words. Note that, except for the category of interjection, the two studies provide reasonably similar data for the young adults. Disfluency data for reading (see Appendix 9.2) are based on the same set of participants in the White (2002) study, who read the 331-word Rainbow Passage (Fairbanks, 1960).

The reference data shown in the three appendices (9.1, 9.2, and 9.3) reveal that disfluency frequency in oral reading is typically much less than in narrative tasks. For this reason, if an adult who stutters is prone to stutter when she or he reads aloud, it may be particularly noticeable in contrast to what a normally fluent speaker would do. The White (2002) study also found that disfluency frequency for men was significantly higher than for women.

The only study found to provide disfluency data for nonstuttering adults in a metric per 100 syllables was Roberts et al. (2009). They reported reference data for 30 men from 20 to 51 years of age. The spontaneous speech tasks requested of participants were threefold: the job task, telling about hobbies, and explaining how a sport is played. No significant differences in overall disfluency frequency were found among the three topics or across three sample lengths, 300, 500, and 900 syllables. Based on a significant interaction between length and topic, it was concluded that the first 300 syllables for telling how to play a sport may elicit a higher relative disfluency frequency than samples based on the job and hobbies tasks. A table summarizing these data is shown in Appendix 9.3.

Appendixes 9.4 and 9.5 offer reference data for adults who stutter derived from two studies. First, Conture and Brayton (1975) reported disfluency data in oral reading of 17 participants (13 men and 4 women) based on a 500-word sample. Second, Silverman and Zimmer (1979) recorded spontaneous speech samples from 20 participants (10 men, 10 women) with a mean of 965 words for the women and 882 words for the men. Although females produced significantly more part word repetitions, word repetitions, and disrhythmic phonations statistically, the investigators concluded that women do not tend to have more severe stuttering than men.

There are surprisingly few disfluency type/frequency data reports for school-age children. Overall disfluency and within-word disfluency (similar to SLD) for 14 children (11 boys; 3 girls) who stutter, ages 5.5 to 11.5 years, based on 300-word conversation samples, were reported by Zebrowski (1994). Overall frequency of disfluency per 100 words ranged from 10 to 49 with a median of 16. Within-word (core) disfluency ranged from 4 to 36 with a median of 12 per 100 words.

Silverman (1974) published disfluency data according to frequency/type distribution for 56 school-age children who stutter and 56 normally fluent controls. Comparing oral reading and a story narrative, he concluded that the latter material provided better differentiation of the two groups. As reported by Silverman, the data presented in Appendix 9.6 are in the form of quartiles. The Appendix displays figures for only the first three quartiles (Q1 = lowest 25% of subjects; Q2 = the second 25% of subjects; Q3 = the third 25% of subjects). We suggest that the 50% (Q2) figures may be applied clinically for a diagnostic reference (comparing the child's data to the stuttering group) or for establishing a therapy target for a child who stutters (reaching the nonstuttering group).[4]

Overall, the important observation to make from the various sources is the large differences between those who stutter and those who do not stutter in the critical subset of disfluencies referred to as within-word, core, or SLD. These are the most characteristic of stuttered speech and also tend to be perceived by listeners as stuttering. Note that the total mean for this subset of disfluencies for the normally fluent speakers in oral reading is less than 1. It is about 10 for those who stutter. Typically, at least three SLDs or core disfluencies is seen as the minimum required to classify speech as stuttering.

Stuttering Severity

In its most frequent usage, the term *stuttering severity* refers to the level of disruption in the delivery of continuous speech. There is a high correlation between the objective quantity of stuttered speech and listeners' ratings of stuttering severity (Young, 1961). The number of times speech is disrupted, the specific characteristics of the disfluent speech, and the duration/length of the disruptions usually affect judgments of how much breakdown has occurred.

Overt stuttering severity, however, is independent of the impact of the total stuttering disorder. The independence mentioned earlier is seen in the case of a speaker who stutters rather severely yet has a mild disorder. That is, some speakers do plenty of stuttering but have minimal emotional reactions, and they have no disabilities or difficulties in social or vocational realms. Other speakers stutter mildly but experience

---

[4] It should be noted that Silverman's data were based only on male school-age children, second through sixth grade. As discussed in Chapter 13, preschool data yielded no significant differences between genders (Ambrose & Yairi, 1999). Some adolescent data revealed no significant differences between genders (De Oliveira Martins & Furquim de Andrade, 2008; Furquim de Andrade & De Oliveira Martins, 2007). We therefore suggest that the Silverman data are apt to be relatively applicable with either gender for children in elementary school.

a deep or intense disorder. The occasional overt instances of stuttering cause enough emotional distress to result in serious social or vocational debilitation. Although the impact of the disorder is ultimately important, this discussion is meant to highlight the point that the term *stuttering severity* is reserved for a description of the overt speech aspects rather than the disorder as a whole.

Clinicians may estimate the severity of stuttering in several ways. The simplest, devoid of any actual measurement or counting, is based on observing the client speak or read and then assigning a global rating on a subjective perceptual scale of stuttering severity. Clinicians seem to favor a 3-point scale with the most popular ratings being *mild*, *moderate*, and *severe*. Yairi and Ambrose (2005) used an 8-point perceptual scale, ranging from normal fluency (rated 0) to most severe stuttering (rated 7). They reported that some experience should yield high agreement with other clinicians. Clinicians, however, have been provided with several more analytical methods that take into account several factors in the assignment of a severity rating. For diagnostic purposes, Wingate (1976) recommended a 5-point scale (very mild, mild, moderate, severe, and very severe) that considers the frequency of stuttered events, the effort involved, and the presence of concomitant behaviors. This short instrument, the Severity Rating Guide, is presented in Table 9.3 for illustration purposes.

Two of the more well-known stuttering severity scales are the *Iowa Scale of Severity of Stuttering* (Sherman, 1952), and the more recent *Stuttering Severity Instrument*, also known as the SSI-4, by Riley (1994, 2009). Both are based on three components: frequency of stuttering events, their duration, and the intensity of

Table 9.3: Severity Rating Guide

	Descriptive Assessment		
Overall Rating	**Frequency (per words spoken)**	**Effort**	**Accessory Features**
Very mild	1/100 (1%)	No perceptible tension	None
Mild	1/50 (2%)	Perceptible tension but "block" easily overcome	Minimal (staring; eye blinks or eye movement or slight movement of the facial musculature)
Moderate	1/15 (7%)	Clear indication of tension or effort; lasts about 2 s	Noticeable movement of facial musculature
Severe	1/7 (15%)	Definite tension or effort; lasts about 2–4 s; frequent repeat attempts	Obvious muscular activity, facial or other
Very severe	1/4 (25%)	Considerable effort; lasts 5 s or more; consistent repeat attempts	Vigorous muscular activity, facial or other

Source: Adapted with permission from John H. Wiley & Sons, Hoboken, NJ: "Severity Rating Guide" in M.E. Wingate, 1976. *Stuttering: Theory and treatment*. (p. 319).

concomitant characteristics. The SSI-4, one of the most popular instruments, permits separate and independent ratings of each of the three components to arrive at an overall score. The examiner must obtain at least two speech samples, from spontaneous speech and oral reading contexts. Samples beyond the clinic setting are also encouraged. These samples are then analyzed in terms of the percentage of syllables stuttered, the average duration of the three longest stuttering moments, and the perceived level of distraction presented by any concomitant physical behaviors associated with stuttering. The total score summed across the three areas is then converted to a severity rating at one of the five levels: very mild, mild, moderate, severe, very severe. The SSI-4 also includes naturalness rating (Martin, Haroldson, & Triden, 1984) as well as set of self-reported rating scales for clinical purposes.

The *Iowa Scale of Severity of Stuttering* (Sherman, 1952) expands the ratings of severity to seven levels: very mild, mild, mild-moderate, moderate, moderate-severe, severe, and very severe. The larger range of ratings suggests increased discernment. Application of this scale can be challenging, however, because the descriptions may not fit clients' features too well. The scale presupposes that dimensions of frequency and duration of stuttering moments always increase together. If this is not the case, the clinician is forced to base the rating on only one of the two dimensions. No guidance is offered regarding the prioritization of the various dimensions.

Physical Concomitants

Various physical movements and postures can occur in the head and neck areas, and at times also in other parts of the body, in association with stuttering events. The terms *concomitant*, *secondary*, and *accessory characteristics* have been commonly used as referents to this dimension of stuttering. As we discussed in Chapter 4, they contribute to the impression of tense, struggled speech and to the overall perception of stuttering severity and abnormality. The number of variations in secondary characteristics is almost limitless among and within individuals who stutter. The list of the most common observable characteristics, taken from Chapter 4, is presented again:

Secondary Stuttering Characteristics

Head jerks	Head turns (side; up; down)
Forehead tension	Nostrils flaring/constricted
Eyes closed; squinting	Eyes widely open
Facial contortions	Lips pressured
Lip tremor	Jaw tremor
Jaw closed tightly	Teeth grinding
Jaw wide open	Rotational or sideways jaw movement
Tongue protrusion	Throat tightened
Body swaying	Hand and/or arm movements
Irregular exhalation (e.g., running out of air) during speech	
Irregular inhalations (e.g., gasping) in the midst of speaking	

During the interview, occurrence of these may be specified in the clinician's notes. Or they may be more carefully reviewed later from the recorded videotape. Prins and Lohr (1972), who studied physical concomitants in detail, reported that the number of areas within the head and neck region involved in stutter events had a significant weight on the severity factor. The clinician should consider secondary characteristics when assigning the overall severity rating of the observed stuttered speech. As already mentioned, the Stuttering Severity Instrument-4 (Riley, 2009) includes this factor in the final score. The information is also relevant for those clinicians who prefer specifically to target secondary characteristics in therapy. Certainly, it is also a good variable to include for assessing progress in subsequent evaluations.

Speaking Rates

A slower than normal speaking rate was pointed out in Chapter 4 as one characteristic of advanced stuttering, resulting directly from the extra time consumed by the stuttered portion of speech. Not surprisingly, speech rate is inversely related to the frequency and duration of disfluencies (Tomblin, Morris, & Spriestersbach, 2000) and potentially serves as an indicator of therapeutic progress (Tomblin et al., 2000; Walker, Archibald, & Cherniak, 1992). Slower rate is a common target in fluency intervention, as we discuss in Chapter 11, and influences perceptual judgments of speech naturalness (Onslow & Ingham, 1987; St. Louis, Myers, Faragasso, Townsend, & Gallagher, 2004). It is reasonable, therefore, to assess speaking rate as part of the initial evaluation of stuttering. Furthermore, it is a key element in the diagnosis of cluttering (see Chapter 15).

When measuring rate, clinicians should keep in mind that variations are expected with speech context. Adult speech rates have been observed to be significantly faster in conversation than in narrative contexts (Johnson, 1961a). Speech rates in the following contexts were found to differ significantly, in decreasing order: oral reading, conversation, and picture description (Duchin & Mysak, 1987, p. 256). Compared to general discussion topics, contexts involving storytelling and content sequencing may require greater language formulation processes, and therefore take more time. As to specific measuring procedures, there are two measures. The first *overall speech rate*, refers to how many words (or syllables) were spoken in the time needed to deliver an entire message or read a complete passage. It includes any pauses, disfluencies, or other variable dimensions of speech production. Syllables per minute is the preferred metric because the words per minute metric does not account for speaker differences in the numbers of multisyllabic words produced (Guitar, 1998; Pindzola, Jenkins, & Lokken, 1989). The second measurement, *articulatory rate*, refers to the speed of perceptually fluent utterances free of all disfluencies, hesitations, breaks, and detectible pauses longer than 250 ms (Yaruss, 1997a, p. 270). The typical metric for articulatory rate is either syllables per second or phones per second (Hall, Amir, & Yairi, 1999; Pindzola et al., 1989). Articulatory rates do not directly reflect oral movements for speech, but they do reflect those movements better than overall speech rates.

Rate Measurement Procedures

The procedures for measuring speaking rates begin with recording a speech sample, transcribing the words, and counting words/syllables as described earlier in this chapter. For most clinical purposes, the time taken for the speech sample, or segments of interest, may be measured in minutes and seconds using a stopwatch. If measures will be compared with published data, the clinician must ensure that methods and standards of measurement match what was applied. For *overall speech rate*, the time from beginning to end of the sample is clocked. The clock should not keep running when the conversational partner talks or during periods of 2 s or more of silence while thinking about what to say or while yawning, coughing, sneezing, or similar. To ensure accuracy, it is worthwhile re-clocking the sample twice, or even three times, find the mean, then calculate the rate by dividing the number of words or syllables spoken by the amount of time. The examiner must remember to calculate seconds using a 60-base, not decimal-base system. As stated in Chapter 4, Fairbanks (1960) reported that a satisfactory range of oral reading rate by more than 200 college students for a 300-word passage was 150 to 180 words per minute (wpm). A later study by Walker (1988) reported the mean oral reading rate for 120 young adults was 188.4 wpm (SD = 19.7), and it was 172.6 wpm (SD = 33.4) for conversational speech.

For *articulatory rate* measures, because the human ear is capable of detecting short silent intervals (e.g., 65 ms), even the slightest perceived break should disqualify an utterance from analysis (Prins & Hubbard, 1990, p. 495). Also disqualified should be utterances bounded by any disfluency either just before it begins or after it ends. When articulatory rates are measured, the clinician should select from the speech sample three perceptually fluent, uninterrupted utterances. An example of the calculation is presented in Table 9.4.

The clinician should bear in mind that articulatory rate measures are especially sensitive to factors such as utterance length, word lengths, and location within utterance. Longer stretches of continuous speech (e.g., 15 syllables) are apt to yield faster rates than shorter utterances (e.g., 5 syllables). Beginnings of utterances tend to be spoken more quickly than endings of utterances (Lehiste, 1972). Articulatory rates from spontaneous monologue contexts for nonstuttering adults for utterances of 7 to 8 words (8 syllables) typically range from 4 to 8 syl/s (unpublished research by CS; also consistent with converted data from Tsao & Weismer, 1997). There is some evidence to suggest articulatory rates in oral reading may tend to be on the slower end (approximately 4.35 syl/s) of this range (Logan, Roberts, Pretto, & Morey, 2002). In contrast, other reports of oral reading speech rates tend to be faster than spontaneous speech rates, probably because pauses are shorter and less frequent in oral reading.

If a client's speech rate is perceived to be faster or slower than expected, the clinician must consider what is leading to that impression. Naturally, when a speaker is disfluent, speech takes additional time and seems slower. Without disfluency, however, the perception of speech as fast or slow results largely from the placement and timing of pauses (Goldman-Eisler, 1961). The clinician would do well to also examine

---

Table 9.4: **An Example of Measuring Articulatory Rate**

1. Count the number of spoken syllables in each utterance:

Utterance A: "Can you find the answer for me"	8 syllables
Utterance B: "Was on the old table over there"	9 syllables
Utterance C: "Remembered to go the grocery store"	9 syllables

   (expected word "to" before "the" was not uttered; grocery said as: "gros-ry")

2. Measure the duration of each entire utterance 3 times and find the average duration for *each* of the utterances. For example:

Utterance A	Utterance B	Utterance C
1.60	1.72	1.67
1.58	1.75	1.65
1.57	1.72	1.68
Averages: 4.75 / 3 = 1.58	5.19 / 3 = 1.73	5.00 / 3 = 1.67

3. Find the articulatory rate for each utterance by dividing the number of syllables by the time. Next average the values from each utterance to arrive at the overall rate measure. For example:

	Artic. Rate
Utterance A: 8 syllables / 1.58 s =	5.06 syl/s
Utterance B: 9 syllables / 1.73 s =	5.20 syl/s
Utterance C: 9 syllables / 1.67 s =	5.38 syl/s
Overall Rate 15.64 / 3 =	**5.21**

---

which types of utterances are apparently faster or slower. Overlearned and previously prepared automatic sequences of spontaneous speech can be delivered at much faster rates than unrehearsed statements, especially those composed of new thoughts, unfamiliar words, or novel phrases (Goldman-Eisler, 1961; Levelt, 1989).

Voice and Other Communication Skills

Speech samples afford an opportunity for the clinician to screen other domains of communication besides fluency: articulation, language (syntax, semantics, pragmatics), and voice. The domain of voice requires particular attention in the evaluation of stuttering but is too often neglected or minimized because of the great concentration on the client's disfluency. The examination of voice (and other domains) can be made during the interview and later listening to the recorded speech. The clinician should remember to make note of such domains both in fluent and disfluent speech. Is the voice quality normal and relaxed, or is it tight or harsh? Are there notable changes during stuttering (e.g., vocal fry, sharp upward pitch breaks)? This is also the time to observe intonational variations: inflections and prosodic contours. A reduced range of these variations, in addition to the stuttering, may significantly affect the speaker's communicative effectiveness and the overall listener's impression of the disorder. This type of information is useful in planning goals for therapy.

Another aspect of evaluation not to be overlooked is the clinician's detection and appraisal of the client's communication strengths. Perhaps the client does well with nonverbal behaviors such as eye contact, facial expression, body postures and gesturing, or similar. Voice and intonational patterns may be particularly pleasant, stuttering aside. The client may do well with appropriate pragmatic uses of language compared to most speakers, have a strong vocabulary, pronunciation mastery, or display above-average command of grammatical constructions. The clinician should make a point to look for the client's strengths, being sure to discuss them in postassessment counseling. An awareness of these areas is important to enhance the client's self-understanding of his or her overall effectiveness as a communicator. Self-perceptions can often be distorted by a speaker's emotional frustration with stuttering.

Speech naturalness and speech quality have been common concerns about the outcome of stuttering treatment programs (Martin, Haroldson, & Triden, 1984; Onslow & Ingham, 1987). Speech naturalness is usually measured on either a 9-point or 7-point scale, where 1 represents highly natural-sounding speech, and 9 (or 7), highly unnatural-sounding speech. These ratings may be made by listeners such as the clinician or peers, or by the speaker in the form of self-ratings of naturalness. R. Ingham, J. Ingham, Onslow, and Finn (1989) demonstrated that adult clients can both rate and modify their speech based on the application of such scales. A later study revealed that speech quality could also be assessed through self-ratings of speech effort on a 9-point scale, where 9 is most effortful and 1 is least effortful (Ingham, Warner, Byrd, & Cotton, 2006).

Observations and Examinations: Other Domains

Having obtained speech samples for the multiple analyses just described, the focus of the initial evaluation shifts to other domains of the complex stuttering, those involving affective reactions. As discussed in Chapter 4, affective reactions become increasingly important with more years of experience with stuttering. Fear and discomfort may develop for specific types of social settings or in relation to speaking and stuttering, more generally. Following we present two classes of protocols, those related to (1) speaking situations and (2) more general attitudes and reactions to stuttering.

Situational Rating Protocols

The variability of stuttering across individuals and contexts is the main reason why clinicians seek information regarding the client's difficulties in different speaking contexts. This information is first gained during the case history interview but can be greatly enhanced through the administration of one or more available protocols. These include the *Stutterer's Self-Ratings of Reactions to Speech Situations* (SSR; Darley & Spriestersbach, 1978), the *Southern Illinois University Speech Situation Checklist* (Hanson, Gronhovd, & Rice, 1981), and the *Reactions to Selected Speaking Situations* (Prins, 1993, p. 138). These protocols are similar in that they use lists of situations, such as talking on the phone, introducing oneself, and so on, to which the client is to respond. What differs among them are the ways in which the client is to evaluate each situation.

In the *Stutterers' Self-Ratings of Reactions to Speech Situations*, 40 situations are each rated by the client on a 5-point scale corresponding to various descriptive statements for the following dimensions: (1) frequency—how frequently the situation is met, (2) stuttering—how much stuttering occurs in it, (3) avoidance—how much the client tries to avoid the situation, and (4) reaction—how much the client likes/dislikes speaking in the situation. An advantage to this scale is that a good amount of important information is obtained from the client. Also available are reference data (Darley & Spriestersbach, 1978, p. 314) for the scores in each of the four areas. A disadvantage is that some terms and expressions used in the situation list have become antiquated. For example, the descriptions refer to "parlor games," "a bull session," and "taking leave of a hostess."

The original version of the *Southern Illinois University Speech Situation Checklist* assessed 51 situation items. Its much shorter version is composed of only 21 items. In either version, situations are rated on a 5-point scale in only one dimension: how much it disturbs the client to speak in it. Clearly, the shortened version with fewer situations and only one area to rate offers greater efficiency. Another advantage is the research support for the item selection process for the shortened version. There are, however, no reference data against which scores can be compared, and a few items are worded in antiquated language. For example, there is a reference to "talking when high." In the past, it meant being very excited but because these words later became associated with intoxication from drugs, clients may find the item offensive or confusing.

The original version of the *Reactions to Selected Speaking Situations* includes 25 situational items, each of which is evaluated on a 5-point scale for three dimensions: (1) frequency (how frequently the situation is met), (2) level of difficulty (how much trouble speaking in it), and (3) level of confidence (how confident the client is in the situation). A modified instrument with 24 items is presented Table 9.5. Like the previous protocol, the small number of items makes for a more efficient use of time. In addition, none of the situation descriptions is worded in a way that is antiquated or ambiguous. A possible disadvantage is that clients might find it harder to evaluate levels of confidence than levels of disturbance, avoidance, or like/dislike of a situation. There also are no reference data for the scores obtained, but this should not necessarily detract from its clinical value. These protocols simply add more organized, more detailed information to that obtained in the interview. They also best serve for comparing a client's baseline ratings (pretreatment) with later progress (posttreatment) and not primarily as a differential diagnostic tool to distinguish the stuttering disorder.

Another meaningful way to engage in evaluating the client's concern about various speaking situations is the devising of an individualized situation hierarchy. Its advantage is that the client only has to deal with the situations that are meaningful to him or her, with immediate implications to own treatment. The client is first asked to list and describe as many situations as are meaningfully relevant to his or her life. The list should not be lengthy, and the clinician can offer suggestions of types of situations or permit the client to look at a list from a protocol for suggestions. After the list is constructed, the client ranks the situations in order from least to most difficult.

Table 9.5: **Reactions to Selected Speaking Situations**

Situation	Frequency[†]	Level of Difficulty[†]	Level of Self-Confidence[†]
1. Talking on the phone to family or friends.			
2. Talking on the phone to a stranger.			
3. Using the phone to purchase a ticket.			
4. Talking to a stranger in a social situation.			
5. Introducing myself.			
6. Placing an order in a restaurant.			
7. Talking to a close friend.			
8. Talking with parents.			
9. Talking with a sales clerk.			
10. Meeting someone for the first time.			
11. Asking for information.			
12. Being interviewed for a job.			
13. Talking with teachers.			
14. Making introductions.			
15. Speaking before a group.			
16. Saying a question or comment in class.			
17. Giving my name in a classroom situation.			
18. Giving a prepared speech.			
19. Talking to someone of the opposite sex.			
20. Participating at a meeting.			
21. Reading aloud to others.			
22. Conversation at meals with family.			
23. Conversation at meals with friends.			
24. Conversation at meals with strangers.			

[†] Scale Values:

Frequency	Level of Difficulty	Level of Self-Confidence
I encounter this situation:	This situation is:	In this situation I feel:
Q. Quite a lot each day	Q. Quite easy	Q. Quite self-confident
R. Regularly just a bit each day	R. Relatively easy	R. Relatively self-confident
S. Several times per week	S. Somewhat difficult	S. Somewhat self-confident
T. Twice or less per week	T. Tough	T. Thinly self-confident
U. Uncommonly	U. Utterly impossible	U. Unconfident

Modified version of "Reactions to Selected Speaking Situations" used with permission from Thieme Medical, New York, NY, and D. Prins, 1993 Management of stuttering: Treatment of adolescents and adults. (p. 138) In R. Curlee (Ed.) *Stuttering and related disorders of fluency*: Thieme Medical Publications.

Such a list is valuable when subsequent therapy is focused on desensitization. It is advisable to check in with the client later on, and on multiple occasions as necessary, to find out whether the sense of difficulty and ranking of the situations has changed.

The previous protocols evaluating the difficulty of speaking situations might also be viewed as assessments of client attitudes about speaking situations. In that light, two additional protocols also can be used. These are the *Self-Efficacy Scale for Adult Stutterers* (*SESAS*; Manning, 2001; Ornstein & Manning, 1985) and the *SEA Scale: Self-Efficacy Scaling for Adolescents Who Stutter* (Manning, 1994, 2001). The *SESAS* has the client rate the same 50 speaking situations on two dimensions: (1) approach attitude and (2) fluency performance. For either dimension, clients apply a 10-point scale from 10 to 100, where 10 is "quite uncertain" and 100 is "very certain." To assess approach attitudes, clients answer whether they would (1) enter the situation, and (2) how much confidence they have with their response. To assess fluency perform-ance, clients answer whether they would (1) be able to achieve fluency in that situa-tion, and (2) how much confidence they have with this response. Advantages of this protocol are that the descriptions use current terminology and the contexts are familiar, such as McDonald's, the shopping mall, or ordering a pizza. Also, rating con-fidence in a response could be easier than evaluating self-confidence, and reference data for stuttering and nonstuttering populations are available.

The *SEA Scale* requires adolescents to rate 100 situations on a scale from 1 to 10 to indicate confidence in the ability to enter and speak in each situation. All situational descriptions are worded with current and unambiguous statements. Responses can be evaluated with respect to 13 subscales related to telephone; arguments with familiar people; arguments with strangers; conversing with a family member; conversing with an authority figure; conversing with a familiar group; conversing with an unfamiliar group; formal presentations; making requests of a stranger; making requests of an authority fig-ure; time-pressure contexts; and memorized or unchangeable texts. Although making estimations of self-confidence can be challenging, the authors have provided clear descriptive statements to apply when using the scale. A disadvantage could be the time required for responding as well as for scoring the numerous responses.

Listed here are several possible choices of the method for assessing reactions to speaking situations. As we explained previously, the first two in this list address many situations but may use wording that confuses some clients. The next two offer rele-vant situations but still involve making a sizable number of ratings. An individualized hierarchy is quite functional but may pose the risk of overlooking some common sit-uations. When one of these tools is chosen, many other factors (e.g., time, cost, client age, etc.) must also be considered.

Tools for Assessing Speaking Situations
- *Stutterer's Self-Ratings of Reactions to Speech Situations* (*SSR*; Darley & Spriestersbach, 1978)
- *Southern Illinois University Speech Situation Checklist* (Hanson, Gronhovd, & Rice, 1981)
- *Reactions to Selected Speaking Situations* (Prins, 1993, p. 138)

- *Self-Efficacy Scale for Adult Stutterers (SESAS)* and *SEA Scale: Self-Efficacy Scaling for Adolescents Who Stutter* (Manning, 2001)
- Individualized situation hierarchy

It cannot be emphasized enough that whether the assessment is of reactions to speaking situations or of attitudes about stuttering, the clinician must have established a relationship of trust with the client prior to their administration. The clinician should judge whether a client is ready to disclose this kind of information, or if it would be better to wait until the client is more comfortable trusting the clinician with it. CS has seen multiple instances where clients have filled in responses according to what they believed they *should* answer, rather than what they actually experienced. In another occasion, a client marked all 25 situations with midscale ratings of 3 on the 5-point scale rather than reveal specific troubles. Rather than admitting the limitation, clients may also provide a rating for a situation despite insufficient basis for self-evaluation after years of avoidance of speaking in it. For this reason, the SESAS would be a preferable instrument to elicit informative responses. In some cases, it may be wise for a clinician to postpone administration to a later time when sufficient rapport has been established.

Attitude Rating Scales

Attitudes are one of the most important variables related to disfluent speech, yet they are among the most challenging to assess. Part of the challenge comes from the fact that there are so many potential attitudes that may be relevant, and individuals vary considerably in the extent to which certain attitudes are of concern. Clinicians should consider attitudes about stuttering, speaking, oneself, other people, and more. Naturally, the clinician's understanding of the client's needs begins with the dialogue that takes place during the case history interview. Attitudes need to be explored in a manner that is both respectful and sensitive to the feelings that may lie close beneath the surface. It can be difficult for a client to review the impact of stuttering and their attitudes about it.

Several formal instruments have been published for the purpose of assessing attitudes related to stuttering. These include *The Modified Erickson Scale* (Andrews & Cutler, 1974), which in its original form was referred to as *The S Scale* (Erickson, 1969), the *Communication Attitude Test* (Brutten, 1985; Brutten & Dunham, 1989), and the *Overall Assessment of the Speaker's Experience of Stuttering (OASES*; Yaruss & Quesal, 2006).

The *S Scale* consisted of 39 items, all in the form of statements to which clients must answer true/false about whether they agree with it. For example, "I find it easy to talk with almost anyone." Reference data are available to interpret the extent to which the score on the communication inventory is more similar to those who stutter or who do not. The *Modified Erickson Scale (S-24)* has only 24 items, and it also has reference data for comparing responses to those who stutter or who do not. Scoring of either scale is not straightforward. Instead of simply counting numbers of true or false answers, the numbers of expected answers are totaled. The scoring therefore requires comparison of each item's response with the expected answer, established during the construction of the instrument, as to whether it agreed (1 point) or did not agree (0 points). The 24-item version is a relatively efficient tool, with the exception of one item with such antiquated wording that people might not know what it means (i.e., "I am a good mixer.") Also, these Erickson scales have been criticized for yielding scores that are not independent of stuttering behavior (Ulliana & Ingham, 1984). That is, ideally a communication attitude inventory would assess thoughts and feelings operating independently of stuttering, but research suggests the answers are apt to be strongly influenced by stuttering.

The *Communication Attitude Test (CAT)* should be administered with adolescents, not adults. Appropriate for school-age children, 8 of the 35 statements make reference to "other children," "other kids," or being "in class" or with "classmates." Clients must answer true/false about their agreement with each of 35 statements. A revised version, the *CAT-R* with 32 items (De Nil & Brutten, 1991; Vanryckeghem & Brutten, 1992), yields reliable results with reference data for both stuttering and nonstuttering children, ages 7 to 14.

The *Overall Assessment of the Speaker's Experience of Stuttering* (*OASES*) includes both aspects of attitudes assessment and situation ratings. It is designed for adults who stutter, ages 18 and older, to assess the comprehensive impact of stuttering on the person's life. Clients respond to 100 items in four sections (General Information, Reactions to Stuttering, Communication in Daily Situations, and Quality of Life) using a 5-point scale that differs in meaning across sections. In the General Information section, 20 items address a broad overview of perceptions of speaking ability, knowledge about stuttering, and feelings about speaking and stuttering. In the Reactions section, 30 items address specific stuttering-related emotions, experiences, and attitudes. In the Daily Situations section, 25 speaking situations are rated for level of difficulty. The Quality of Life section contains 25 items about how much stuttering negatively impacts or interferes with the client's life, personally, socially, and vocationally. The scores for each section on the *OASES* are converted to Impact Ratings interpreted on a 5-level scale, ranging from Mild to Severe. There is also a Total Impact Score that is interpreted similarly. Score interpretation is based on published research and reference data. The questions and situation descriptions in the *OASES* are clearly worded, and its content has current relevance. Because the instrument is meant to be comprehensive, it is also lengthier than the rest. One limitation may be that, unlike the SESAS, clients do not indicate how certain they are of their responses.

To assess the quality of the instruments, Franic and Bothe (2008) reviewed 17 attitude and situation assessment instruments for psychometric properties. Ten of the 17 were evaluated in detail with respect to 15 measurement criteria. These criteria included conceptual model, validity, reliability, responsiveness, interpretability (reference data), burden (client respondent and examiner administrative), depth, and versatility. Of the instruments discussed, only the *CAT/CAT-R* and *Modified Erickson Scale (S-24)* met at least half of the standard criteria for application as a diagnostic tool. These were criticized for their low test-retest reliability, lack of being based on clear constructs, and insufficient research on their responsiveness to clinical change. The *SSR* and OASES met fewer criteria. The authors expressed concern that the OASES may overidentify problems. The *SSR* has not received adequate testing for validity and reliability. These were the only instruments reviewed among those that we have discussed in this chapter.

Like the assessment of speaking situations, rapport must be established first to ensure the client is ready to trust the clinician with the information prompted by attitude scales. Some scales are best suited to serve as pre- and posttherapy surveys with clients who have had previous experience with therapy. Some surveys, like the *OASES*, are best applied in the context of an interpersonal interview and not as a self-administered questionnaire given to the client to fill out. Because such scales prompt the sharing of highly personal emotional information, they may not be best to administer during the very first encounter with a client or in the context of a diagnostic clinic where the examiner will not be the one who is later administering the therapy. The following is a list of the attitude scale options:

- *Modified Erickson Scale* (*S-24*; Andrews & Cutler, 1974)
- *Communication Attitude Test* (*CAT-R*; Brutten, 1985; Brutten & Dunham, 1989)
- *Overall Assessment of the Speaker's Experience of Stuttering* (*OASES*; Yaruss & Quesal, 2006)
- *Self-Efficacy Scale for Adult Stutterers* (*SESAS*) and *SEA Scale: Self-Efficacy Scaling for Adolescents Who Stutter* (Manning, 2001)
- Individualized interview regarding attitudes and emotional reactions

Other Speaking Conditions

There are many other possible speaking conditions and factors related to the client's stuttering that the clinician may wish to observe and evaluate. Because often people who stutter are relatively more fluent on shorter, less complex utterances, it may be useful to observe speech on a set of sentences that are systematically increased in length and linguistic complexity. Similarly, the clinician may want to observe the client's speech in tasks such as picture naming, automatic series, imitation and unison, to appreciate which demands and conditions aid or stress fluency. If a client's stuttering tends to be mild, the client may agree that the clinician should observe speech under added stress factors such as speaking on the telephone, time pressure, interruptions, with groups, and so on. Therapeutic probes may be employed to observe how well the client responds to various fluency-enhancing techniques or to identification and modification instructions.

As with any speech-language assessment, the examiner should not neglect to note other possible disabilities or factors that may influence the client's speech and communication skills. These may be in areas of articulation, phonology, vocabulary, syntax, semantics, pragmatics, attention, cognition, word-finding, fine/gross motor, oral-peripheral/oral-motor, voice/resonance, intonation/prosody, respiration, and hearing/auditory processing.

Interpretations and Treatment Recommendations

Diagnosis

As explained at the beginning of the chapter, the diagnosis of stuttering in adolescents or adults is not apt to present much of a challenge. In the great majority of cases, the correct diagnosis has been made by the client. The clinician's main goal is to describe, quantify, and assess the various aspects of the stuttering disorder. In some cases, differential diagnosis from other fluency disorders (see Chapter 15), or faked stuttering, is called for. Other problems of communication or different suspected health issues may be revealed or just suspected. All these should be reflected in the final assessment. On occasion, when individuals with very mild stuttering seek intervention, the inexperienced clinician may be inclined to question whether the speaker's perception of the disorder is valid or out of proportion with the actual difficulty. The reality of the stuttering disorder in such cases should be apparent by means of the following analogy. Imagine that your knees suddenly and unexpectedly buckled under you about twice each week. Wouldn't it be enough to make you seek out a doctor? Similarly, even occasional stuttering episodes can be sufficient to generate a sense of great vulnerability for a speaker. In fact, it is precisely because these moments occur infrequently and surface when least expected that they pose such an insidious threat. The client with mild stuttering can still benefit from intervention strategies and counseling.

A related issue is how much of the client's stuttering is hidden or suppressed compared to what would be observed without the client's coping mechanisms. If advanced stuttering reflects a genetic factor for the individual, then the evaluation may need to focus more crucially on finding out the nature of a client's coping mechanisms. How well is the client able to describe and discuss characteristics of his or her coping mechanisms? Which coping mechanisms might best be left alone at this time, and which ones is the client most needing or wanting to change?

Treatment Recommendations

When all the assessment results are analyzed, clinicians should first determine if therapy is warranted and, if positive, how will they be useful toward selecting, or recommending, appropriate treatment. Naturally, one of the most important considerations will be what the client envisions as his or her goals in treatment. Are those goals realistic? How will the client's vision of the clinical intervention process need to be brought into alignment with how the clinician understands that process? The stuttering assessment should inform the clinician about how the client views the stuttering so that these questions can be addressed.

How do the speech characteristics guide the planning of treatment? In addition to providing a pretherapy baseline to evaluate progress, the clinician should have observed the speech characteristics in terms of the patterns of movement of various anatomical structures (i.e., lips, tongue, jaw, neck/larynx, and chest). How does their positioning, timing, and tenseness differ from what is associated with typically fluent speech?

Does stuttering tend to occur at the most common location of utterance initiation? Then a slower, easier approach to starting to talk may be an appropriate strategy to develop. Does the speaker have a high level of tension in the articulators? Then a more gentle, relaxed approach to their movement and contacts may be needed. Does the speaker hold his or her breath when starting to talk? Instruction for appropriate breath support may help. Are reactions and attitudes toward speech and stuttering preventing progress with speech change? Then these fears and avoidances may need to be addressed through counseling and desensitization activities. Do nonverbal behaviors or suprasegmental speech characteristics (e.g., irregular rate patterns, awkward phrasing, lack of eye contact, etc.) interfere with communication? Then these may need attention in therapy. How big is the factor of secondary characteristics? Although these tend to lessen or disappear of their own accord as the core stuttering and avoidance behaviors are decreased, occasionally secondary characteristics may need to be dealt with directly through awareness and self-monitoring. Additionally, each individual will have specific situations to address depending on their life roles (e.g., student, family relations, etc.), vocation, and recreational/social interests and needs. Finally, information obtained regarding past therapy experiences should be taken into consideration in deciding the future course of therapy.

The Diagnostic Report

The example of a speech evaluation report in Table 9.6 reveals the types of information obtained from a stuttering assessment. It also offers a model of possible wording and content organization for professionals who are new to reporting in this area.

Table 9.6: Sample Diagnostic Report

The Greater Midwest
Speech & Hearing Center

1818 Mid-continent Blvd.
Chatter City, USA 77778

SPEECH EVALUATION REPORT

Name: Basil Karger
Birthdate: 01/01/10
Age: 23
Gender: Male
Address: 510 Snow Rd.,
Chatter City, USA, 77778

Date of Evaluation: 01/01/10
Informant for History: Self
Clinic File No.: 1111112
Diagnosic Code No.: 333
Diagnosis: Stuttering

COMPLAINT AND REFERRAL

Basil, a 23-year-old male, was seen at his request at The Greater Midwest Speech and Hearing Center for evaluation of his stuttering. Basil, a college graduate who works in the receiving department of a major furniture store, feels the stuttering is distracting to other workers in the facilities, delivery drivers, and personal friends, and interferes in his career development.

HISTORY

Basil was raised on a farm near Chatter City. He is the youngest of four siblings, with only one of them being a full-blooded sib. He is the only one of the four who has ever stuttered. Basil did state, however, that his father had a stuttering problem that he overcame on his own after college. No other relatives were known to stutter.

Basil could not recall exactly when he began stuttering, but said he was aware of it at approximately 8 years of age. There was no recollection or knowledge of any medical or traumatic experience that precipitated the onset of stuttering. He also related that his family has always accepted his speech problem and that rarely have there been comments made on it.

Table 9.6: Continued

During high school years, tension was intensified due to meeting new teachers and peers, as well as increased academic responsibilities, resulting in Basil's stuttering becoming more severe. In college, familiar speaking situations and speaking with friends were thought by him to be relatively easy, whereas speaking to professors and in front of classes posed more difficulties.

Basil received previous speech therapy at another clinic for approximately 2.5 years during his high school senior year and his undergraduate years at a community college. He recalled "cancellations" and "pull-outs" as the major therapeutic techniques and felt that they were effective. Therapy was terminated by mutual decision of the clinician and client after they felt sufficient progress had been made. Recently, however, stuttering had increased.

EXAMINATIONS AND OBSERVATIONS

Disfluent Speech: An analysis of a 566-word sample of Basil's conversational speech revealed a total of 147 disfluencies, an average of 25.97 per 100 words. The breakdown of this figure according to specific disfluency types and categories is shown in the chart:

	Conversation (566 wds.)	Reading (463 wds).
Part-word repetitions	7.95 (45)	1.94 (9)
Whole-word repetitions	3.36 (19)	0.65 (3)
Disrhythmic Phonation	5.83 (33)	0.65 (3)
SLD Subtotal	**17.14 (97)**	**3.24 (15)**
Phrase repetitions	2.12 (12)	1.51 (7)
Interjections	6.01 (34)	4.31 (20)
Revisions	0.71 (4)	0.04 (2)
Other Disfluency Subtotal	**8.83 (50)**	**6.26 (29)**
Disfluency Total	**25.97 (147)**	**9.50 (44)**

As can be seen, the predominant types of disfluencies in Basil's speech were part-word repetitions and disrhythmic phonation (sound prolongations and blockages). The clinician estimated the average repetition contained two additional units (e.g., bu-bu-but), although sometimes three and four extra units were produced. Sound prolongations often lasted 2 s or more. Although Basil indicated no specific phonemes on which he had more disfluencies, it was noted that they occurred quite consistently on words or syllables beginning with the vowel /a/. Basil exhibited relatively fluent speech in reading both The Rainbow Passage and My Grandfather, a 463-word combined sample. The total SLD in this task was 3.24 per 100 words. Postponement behaviors observed were primarily in terms of interjections that tended to precede instances of severe stuttering. His disfluency in reading was less severe than in conversation.

Secondary Characteristics: Physically tense movements that typically accompany stutter events were observable as Basil spoke. Eye blinking, poor eye contact, and neck and facial muscle tension occurred quite consistently during moments of disfluency. He was often observed wringing his hands and fingers while he held the rest of his body rather still.

Severity: Judging the impact of both the disfluency and the secondary characteristics on a 7-point scale for an overall rating severity of stuttering, with 1 being very mild stuttering and 7 being very severe stuttering, Basil's speech was rated by the clinician at 5, although moments of more severe stuttering did occur.

Speaking Rate: Basil's conversational speech was timed. His average overall speaking rate, 132.5 words per minute, was below normal range.

(continued)

Table 9.6: Continued

Voice: During testing, Basil's voice quality was characterized by glottal fry and voice breaks. His optimal pitch was assessed by estimating the pitch level approximately a fourth from the bottom of his total pitch range. In conversational speech, Basil spoke at a lower pitch than the estimated optimal. Indeed, when asked to read in a monotone, the pitch he used was the same estimated as the optimal.

Speech Mechanism: The speech mechanism appeared both structurally and functionally adequate for speech.

Language: Although no formal language assessment was done, Basil used both vocabulary and syntax appropriate for his age and education level.

Hearing Screening: An audiometric screening was administered at both 25 dB HTL and 15 db HTL (re: ANSI 1969) with a portable Beltone audiometer. The following frequencies were tested bilaterally: 250, 500, 1000, 2000, 4000, 8000 Hz. Responses to all stimuli were consistent.

Client's View: Asked to describe the experience of a stuttering block, Basil said he felt "tension and inability to speak." He felt like "a hundred things were going on in his mind at once." After the moment had ended, he experienced a great relief, "like a weight off his chest." Basil stated that he felt the cause of his stuttering was nervousness. Asked what he does to change his stuttering, he said, "Trying to relax, slow down, and sometimes take aspirin hoping it would calm me down." Basil felt that some situations increase the severity of his stuttering. It is more difficult for him speaking to a group than to individuals, also speaking to strangers (e.g., various people with whom he has to communicate on the job) than to familiar people. He added, however, that he feels most people generally ignore his stuttering, although some former colleagues in college expressed difficulty in listening to, and understanding him, at times. He is often afraid to talk when expected to. On a 9-point scale of speech naturalness, Basil self-rated his speech as 7, which is rather unnatural. Among anxiety-producing situations he also listed speaking with people having authority, such as former professors and current superiors at his work environment; having to talk after arriving late to a meeting; and some phone conversations. It was also mentioned that Basil's stuttering seems to increase when he does not sleep enough.

Attitudes: Basil was administered the Modified Erickson Scale (S-Scale) and received a score of 37 points out of a possible 39, which would seem to reflect a very low attitude toward speaking when compared with normal speakers.

Social Effects: Asked about how stuttering influences his life, Basil replied that he feels avoidance reactions to various situations. In discussing plans for the future, he stated that he would prefer jobs that required less frequent speaking then his current one. He felt it would be unrealistic to do otherwise because the stuttering would always be there. As far as dealing with current social situations, Basil did not feel that his stuttering keeps him much from being more socially active than he currently is. Still, he is rather comfortable with a number of his friends, and stutters less when he is talking with people he knows. Although he dates women, he admits to some obstacles in this domain.

CLINICAL IMPRESSION

Throughout the diagnostic session, Basil exhibited moderate to severe stuttering in terms of the frequency, types, and length of disfluencies that were accompanied by several secondary characteristics and the usage of an inappropriately low voice pitch and significant components of glottal fry. His stuttering during oral reading was less severe in frequency and intensity than in conversation. The affective reactions to the stuttering are strong. Basil's stuttering clearly interferes with his personal life and professional career and aspirations. Although the speech therapy he received 2.5 years ago provided improvement, it is apparent that Basil needs additional therapy that will target the overt stuttering, voice, and affective reaction. Basil has expressed a desire to begin speech therapy, and stated his main goal to accomplish is to be able to go before a group of people without stuttering much and be able to handle it better.

Table 9.6: Continued

RECOMMENDATIONS

It is recommended that Basil Karger be enrolled in therapy for remediation of stuttering, voice, and affective reactions.

Student Clinicians _____

_____

Supervising Clinician _____

Summary

Stuttering assessment typically involves the major components of case history and client interview, speech sampling and analysis, supplemental speech tasks, emotions related to speaking and stuttering, and other factors impacting the client's personal, social, and professional life. To individualize assessment appropriately, the clinician considers the selection of speech sample contexts, speech characteristics and nonverbal concomitants to be analyzed, frequency measures, severity scales, speaking rate measures, and protocols for the examination of attitudes and/or reactions. The clinician has considerable choices of procedures and measures of the various aspects of the overt stuttering as well as an array of instruments to evaluate the emotional component. A thorough assessment involves informal screenings, such as of the parameter of voice, and an appraisal of the client's overall profile of communication abilities, especially his or her strengths. An in-depth assessment provides an essential foundation for the selection of treatment goals and objectives.

STUDY QUESTIONS AND DISCUSSION TOPICS

1. Which assessment procedures help the clinician discover the extent of the client's stuttering variability?

2. Pretend you are administering the stuttering evaluation, and explain to your client the reason for including each of the components in your assessment: speech samples, attitude protocols, and so on.

3. In what ways is the client required to engage in self-assessment during the clinical evaluation? How can the clinician help to ensure that the client uses that self-assessment constructively?

4. Compare and contrast the two measures: percentage of syllables stuttered and frequency of disfluency per 100 syllables.

5. Clinicians sometimes adopt an alternative reporting format showing the relative proportions of the various disfluency types as in the following chart. Note the absence of any information about the size of the speech sample. Why is it important to report the disfluency frequency relative to the size of the speech sample, as demonstrated in the chapter? Explain how this alternative format may enhance some specifics but lacks the contextual information necessary for an appropriate interpretation of the data.

Disfluency Type	Percentage
Part-word repetitions (45/147)	30.6%
Whole-word repetitions (19/147)	12.9%
Disrhythmic phonation (33/147)	22.4%
SLD Subtotal (97/147)	**66.0%**
Phrase repetitions (12/147)	8.1%
Interjections (34/147)	23.1%
Revisions (4/147)	2.7%
Other Disfluency Subtotal (50/147)	**34.0%**
Disfluency Total (147/147)	**100.0%**

SUGGESTED READINGS

Hillis, J. (1993). On-going assessment in the management of stuttering: A clinical perspective. *American Journal of Speech-Language Pathology, 2*, 24–37.

Manning, W. (2001). Assessing adolescents and adults. In *Clinical decision making in fluency disorders* (2nd ed., pp. 113–184). San Diego, CA: Singular (Thomson).

Riley, G. (1994). Manual for the *Stuttering Severity Instrument for Children and Adults* (3rd ed.). Austin, TX: Pro-Ed.

Yaruss, S., & Quesal, R. (2006). Overall Assessment of the Speaker's Experience of Stuttering (OASES): Documenting multiple outcomes in stuttering treatment. *Journal of Fluency Disorders, 31*, 90–115.

Appendixes

Appendix 9.1

Frequency of Disfluency Types per 100 Words in Narrative Contexts for Younger and Older Adults Who Do Not Stutter

Disfluency Type	White, 2002 Ages 20–22 (N = 30)		Yairi and Clifton, 1972 Ages 17–18 years (N = 15)		Ages 69–87 (N = 15)	
Part-Word Repetition	0.06		0.18		0.39	
Whole-Word Repetition	0.56		0.41		0.81	
Disrhythmic Phonation	0.03		0.15		0.28	
Tense Pause	NA		0.04		0.02	
CORE Subtotals		0.65		0.78		1.50
Interjections	4.69		1.66		2.92	
Phrase Repetitions	0.21		0.30		0.30	
Revisions	1.13		1.10		1.47	
ACCESSORY Subtotals		6.03		3.06		4.69
OVERALL Totals		6.68		3.84		6.19

Reprinted with permission from Disfluent speech behavior of preschool children, high school seniors, and geriatric persons by E. Yairi and N. Clifton. *Journal of Speech and Hearing Research, 15*, 714–719. Copyright 1972 by American Speech-Language-Hearing Association. All rights reserved. Adapted from E. White, 2002. *Normal disfluency in young adults across three speech tasks.* Unpublished master's thesis, University of Wisconsin-Milwaukee, Milwaukee, WI.

Appendix 9.2

Frequency of Disfluency Types per 100 Words in an Oral Reading Context for 15 Male and 15 Female Adults Who Do Not Stutter, Age 20–22 Years

Disfluency Type	Males		Females	
Part-Word Repetition	0.40 (0.45)		0.16 (0.19)	
Whole-Word Repetition	0.34 (0.37)		0.22 (0.35)	
Disrhythmic Phonation	0.06 (0.12)		0.04 (0.11)	
Tense Pause	NA			
CORE Subtotals		0.80		0.42
Interjections	0.41 (0.60)		0.20 (0.27)	
Phrase Repetitions	0.56 (.0.57)		0.52 (0.45)	
Revisions	0.56 (.0.58)		0.68 (0.47)	
ACCESSORY Subtotals		1.43		1.40
OVERALL Totals		2.23		1.82

Standard deviations are in parentheses.

Adapted from E. White, 2002. *Normal disfluency in young adults across three speech tasks.* Unpublished master's thesis, University of Wisconsin-Milwaukee, Milwaukee, WI.

Appendix 9.3

Mean Frequency of Disfluency Types per 100 Syllables for 500-Syllable Samples of the Job Task (Spontaneous Monologue) by 30 Adult Men

Disfluency Type	Mean	
Part-Word Repetition	0.23	
Whole-Word Repetition	0.58	
Prolongation	0.24	
Tense Pause	NA	
CORE Subtotals		1.06
Interjections	3.96	
Phrase Repetitions (and Multisyllable Word Reps)	0.26	
Revisions	1.08	
ACCESSORY Subtotals		5.30
OVERALL Totals		6.36*

* This value represents the total of these data. It differs, however, from the 6.52 they report.

Source: Adapted with permission from Elsevier (New York) from P. Roberts, A. Meltzer, and J. Wilding, 2009. Disfluencies in non-stuttering adults across sample lengths and topics. *Journal of Communication Disorders, 42*, 414–427.

Appendix 9.4

Frequency of Disfluency Types per 100 Words in an Oral Reading Context for 13 Male and 4 Female Adults Who Stutter

Disfluency Type	Mean	
Part-Word Repetition	5.34	
Whole-Word Repetition	0.41	
Disrhythmic Phonation (prolongation + broken word)	5.06	
Tense Pause	NA	
CORE Subtotals		10.81
Interjections	0.60	
Phrase Repetitions	0.30	
Revisions	0.72	
ACCESSORY Subtotals		1.62
OVERALL Totals		12.43

Source: Adapted with permission from The influence of noise on stutterers' different disfluency types by E. Conture and E. Brayton. *Journal of Speech and Hearing Research, 18*, 381–384. Copyright 1975 by American Speech-Language-Hearing Association. All rights reserved.

Appendix 9.5

Frequency of Disfluency Types per 100 Words in Spontaneous Speech for 10 Male and 10 Female Adults Who Stutter, Ages 19–48 Years

Disfluency Type	Males		Females	
Part-Word Repetition	3.08 (2.74)		4.50 (7.23)	
Whole-Word Repetition	1.89 (0.75)		2.85 (3.24)	
Disrhythmic Phonation	2.70 (2.07)		4.42 (6.03)	
Tense Pause	0.22 (0.25)		0.29 (0.87)	
CORE Subtotals		7.89		12.06
Interjections	4.29 (1.93)		5.47 (8.45)	
Phrase Repetitions	0.66 (0.35)		0.46 (0.37)	
Revisions	4.43 (2.38)		2.52 (1.77)	
ACCESSORY Subtotals		9.38		8.45
OVERALL Totals		17.27		20.51

Standard deviations are in parentheses.

Source: Reprinted with permission from Women who stutter: Personality and speech characteristics by E. Silverman and C. H. Zimmer. *Journal of Speech and Hearing Research, 22*, 553–564. Copyright 1979 by American Speech-Language-Hearing Association. All rights reserive.

Appendix 9.6

Frequency of Disfluency and Types per 100 Words in Story Narratives for 56 Male Children Who Stutter and 56 Male Children Who Do Not Stutter

Disfluency Type	Stuttering Males			Nonstuttering Males		
	Q1	Q2	Q3	Q1	Q2	Q3
Part-Word Repetition	1.2	3.0	6.8	0.3	0.8	1.2
Whole-Word Repetition	1.3	2.5	4.4	0.4	0.8	1.3
Disrhythmic Phonation	0.2	0.6	2.6	0.0	0.1	0.3
Tense Pause	0.0	0.0	0.4	0.0	0.0	0.0
Interjections	0.2	0.8	1.9	0.3	0.5	1.5
Phrase Repetitions	0.2	0.5	1.3	0.0	0.3	0.9
Revision-Incomplete Phrases	1.5	1.9	2.7	1.7	2.8	4.2
All Categories	6.9	11.3	21.4	3.6	5.8	9.5

Figures are for the first (Q1), second (Q2), and third (Q3) quartiles.

Source: Reprinted with permission from Disfluency behavior of elementary-school stutterers and nonstutterers by F. Silverman. *Language, Speech, and Hearing Services in Schools, 5*, 32–37. Copyright 1974 by American Speech-Language-Hearing Association. All rights reserved.

Chapter 10: Adult Therapy: Focus on Emotional Reactions

LEARNER OBJECTIVES

Readers of this chapter will be able to:

- Recognize distinguishing characteristics of adults who stutter and their prognostic outlook.
- Examine the potential role of psychotherapy as a form of stuttering intervention.
- Describe the objectives and rationales for a variety of techniques aimed at decreasing or increasing the emotional reactions of the person.
- Understand the benefits of group therapy.
- Evaluate past and present efforts to use drugs for the treatment of stuttering.
- Discuss the results of research related to the treatment approaches covered in this chapter.

Adults Who Stutter

You may wonder why the discussion of therapy for the three age groups covered in this part of the book reverses the chronological order, presenting therapy for adults first. The reason for this reversal is that the discussion of therapy for adults allows for a broader exposition of issues, principles, and methods, some of which are also relevant to treatment of preschool and school children. In this regard, it is interesting to point out that for many years the clinical literature on stuttering focused on adults rather than children. At the time, this trend mirrored activities in the stuttering research literature. Of course, before adult treatment is considered, a basic definitional question arises: Specifically, at what age are adult therapy methods appropriate? Or, when do children cross the threshold into adulthood? From a biological perspective, physical growth continues until as late as age 22. From a cultural perspective, where Western civilization is predominant, age 18 is a common milestone. From yet another perspective, puberty has been regarded as the transitional period to maturity. From the standpoint of the developmental course of stuttering, Bloodstein (1995) noted that its most advanced stage was typically reached during the range of years spanning high school. Similarly, Conture (2001) suggested that individuals in later years of high school and beyond could qualify as adults who stutter. We propose that adult therapy methods may be appropriate a year or so earlier, perhaps at age 15, provided there were no limitations in cognitive or emotional development.

Another important issue when working with adults is their history of past treatments. Because the number of school speech-language clinicians in the United States has substantially increased over the past several decades, it is safe to assume that the numbers of children they have served has increased as well. This logical inference was substantiated by a survey of adults who stutter that showed over 94% of respondents had received therapy in the past, with the majority reporting more than one treatment experience (Yaruss et al., 2002). Therapy experiences were especially common between the ages of 6 and 12 but often continued into adulthood, mainly prior to age 35.

The prognosis for adult treatment expressed in the literature appears to be rather guarded. Because adults tend to have long histories of stuttering therapy, often they are expected to be more skeptical about their chances for better results "this time around" or to possess well-entrenched stuttering patterns, attitudes, and beliefs about the disorder. One scholar of stuttering stated, "The habituation that adult people who stutter often exhibit implies that their stuttering and related concerns will be fairly resistant to change" (Conture, 2000, p. 284). Other factors besides attitudes and habituation, however, should be considered.

> The prognosis for adults must take into account the critical role of the epidemiological factors that contributed to their persistent form of stuttering. As discussed in Chapter 3, at least 75% of those who begin to stutter exhibit natural recovery in subsequent years. Adults who stutter therefore represent a small remnant of those who have ever stuttered. Their persistence most likely reflects a more robust disorder. In fact, genetics is an important factor underlying both natural recovery and chronic stuttering (Ambrose, Cox, & Yairi, 1997). Therefore, adult stuttering may be difficult to treat not mainly because of attitudes and resistance, but because of the tenacious nature of this subtype of the stuttering disorder. Clinicians must keep this information in mind before jumping to the conclusion that difficulties in progress are related to clients' attitudes.

There is also an optimistic side to the prognosis for adults who seek therapy. Adult maturity, compared to adolescence, is more apt to support a satisfying process of change. The tendency for greater emotional and social stability with increased age can lead to more "productive attempts at recovery" (Starkweather & Givens-Ackerman, 1997, p. 54). When an adult who stutters continues to seek help, despite a moderate or long history of therapy, it is a positive sign. It suggests hope, motivation to improve, and persistence in spite of past failures. Clients may be ready to change habits of avoidance and more boldly attempt new speaking experiences. The information about past treatments, their results, the client's feelings about speech therapy, and their clinicians all can be useful toward setting and attaining realistic goals in the present.

Treatments

In presenting the various treatments for adults who stutter, the current chapter is focused on psychologically oriented and drug therapies. Motorically oriented therapies, as well as instrument-based treatments, are presented in Chapter 12. This order also reflects our clinical orientation to stuttering treatment in adults. Unless otherwise indicated, we prefer to begin with some work pertaining to the client's stuttering-related emotional reactions and attitudes, preparing the grounds for what we believe to be more productive and stable results of speech-focused therapy.

Chapter 6 presented theories that portrayed stuttering as caused by deep-seated emotional problems, if not disturbances. Whether this is true or not, there is no doubt that in many afflicted individuals there are emotional components (various reactions) to their stuttering disorder (see Chapter 4). Clinicians know that in no small number of individuals who stutter, the emotional component is so obvious and so strong as to overshadow the stuttered speech. This is one reason why many laypersons think that "stuttering is psychogenic," and why some clinicians treat it as such, attempting to eliminate the psychogenic cause of the stuttering. Most scholars, however, believe that emotionality is not the cause but the result of stuttering, learned and reinforced through unpleasant experiences (see Chapter 6). Being a part of the problem, reduction of emotionality can, and should be, included on the therapeutic agenda. Clinicians, however, must be careful of making undue generalizations because of the wide range of emotional reactivity associated with stuttering. In our experience, some clients report little speech anxiety or emotionality. To them, stuttering is uncomfortable, an unpleasant irritation, but they do not hesitate to speak. Many others, however, are severely oppressed by the disorder.

Treatments to improve the psychoemotional responses of people who stutter do not neatly separate into subcategories of personal and social adjustment, because these two domains are closely related. Nonetheless, based on their major emphasis, the following therapy approaches are organized according to a focus on psychotherapy, relaxation, desensitization, social adjustment, and drug therapies. Following, we discuss a variety of psychological methods that have attempted to address personal adjustment and emotional reactions.

Psychotherapy and Relaxation

Over the past century, the meaning of the term *psychotherapy* has broadened to include procedures designed to (1) relieve emotional stress, anxieties, and their associated symptoms, (2) alleviate more serious emotional disorders such as depression, (3) develop positive self-concept and confidence, and (4) improve social adjustment. It involves an analysis of the client's thoughts, feelings, and behavior. The technique seldom requires the client to experiment actively with direct changes in behavior. More typically, psychotherapy aims at bringing about a new awareness concerning the nature or source of the problem, and this insight is expected to alter the client's experience and habitual responses. Thus the psychological awareness transforms the behavior as the client acts in accordance with new insights. In this light, many, if not most, stuttering therapies include certain elements of psychotherapy.

Purposeful, theory-based psychotherapy began toward the end of the 19th century with Sigmund Freud's (1899) techniques of psychoanalysis. Because these ideas were in ascendance in the early decades of the 20th century, one explanation of the stuttering disorder focused on personality conflict within the individual, referencing Freud. In Chapter 6, we explained that this theory viewed stuttering as an overt symptom of an unconscious, deep-seated neurosis.

> Logically, when stuttering was considered a psychoneurotic disorder, psychotherapy was the method to treat it. Although by current standards there is no, or only weak, evidence to support the neurosis hypothesis, anyone who works with clients who stutter would agree that the disorder can strongly affect the mind and emotions of a person who stutters. Having knowledge about psychotherapeutic methods is therefore important for practicing clinicians.

Psychotherapies are extremely diverse. Wikipedia (2007) lists approximately 140 different methods, reflecting various theoretical orientations and specific techniques. To illustrate the range, among those listed are psychoanalysis, humanistic psychology, cognitive behavioral therapy, existential therapy, person-centered therapy, holistic therapy, rational emotive behavior therapy, reality therapy, and primal therapy. Treatment is provided in different formats, such as individual, couples, family, group, and experiential therapy. As for the mode, most psychotherapies rely on spoken conversation, but some employ artwork, drama, playing a narrative story, dance, and others. Although sometimes the terms *psychotherapy* and *counseling* are used interchangeably, generally the first term applies to intervention for a serious mental health problem, whereas the second term implies assistance for coping with everyday problems or various difficulties.

Psychoanalysis

Classical Freudian psychoanalysis is aimed at the root problem, not the symptoms. Its ultimate objective is to elevate the unconscious to the conscious level. The clinician creates a relaxed situation, with the patient lying on a couch, where she or he is encouraged to let thoughts flow in a completely free manner, and in turn speak whatever comes to mind in total honesty. The open verbalization of thoughts as they float from one to the next is referred to as *free association*. Whatever the patient says is accepted without criticism. It is assumed that free association in the presence of a neutral therapist, supplemented with dream interpretation, will cause unconscious conflicts to surface so they can be confronted and resolved.

E. Yairi: "I subjected myself to classical psychoanalysis on a weekly basis for a two-year period while an undergraduate majoring in psychology. To pay for this expensive program, I took hard labor, literally dirty jobs, cleaning multifloor apartment buildings as they went up. I worked odd hours, e.g., 4–7 AM, so that I could make it to classes.
To me, therapy was an interesting process but a rather boring experience after a while. My free associations were dull or I was too inhibited to travel to exciting ones. In any event, although I felt better, psychoanalysis had no effect whatsoever on my stuttering. In short, therapy made me a happier stutterer."

Early on, in 1923, Brill reported that among his 600 patients who stuttered, 69 received psychoanalysis with considerable initial success. An 11-year follow-up, however, indicated that only 5 of the 69 patients (7%) were doing "really well." Conceding the large relapse factor, Brill concluded that some subtypes of stuttering will respond well to therapy, whereas the majority of "true stutterers" are very difficult to treat with the method. In the years that followed, others applied one of several psychotherapies in either individual or group settings (e.g., Barbara, 1962; Brody & Harrison, 1954; Glauber, 1958; Honig, 1947; Murphy & Fitzsimons, 1960; Sadoff & Siegel, 1965) but produced little quantitative data. In 1971, however, Travis reported on clinical experimentation with 30 adult individuals who stutter, all appearing to have conflicts over unmet early childhood needs. The psychotherapy, extending up to 3 years for some clients, yielded mixed results. Only six were considered cured, and five showed substantial improvement. If this subjective assessment is valid, just 35% of the entire group enjoyed a positive to very positive outcome.

In a more extensive study, Webster (1977) examined the clinical records of 648 people treated specifically for stuttering by a team of six psychotherapists at the Speech and Hearing Institute in New York City between 1969 and 1972. No objective counts of disfluencies were made. Outcome was indicated on the following scale: disorder corrected, moderately improved, slightly improved, and unimproved. The disappointing findings indicated that 0% of the clients fell in the "corrected" category and that moderate improvement in fluency was limited to only 8% of this large sample. In other words, 92% showed either no or only slight improvement. Webster commented that "while psychotherapy may have had some positive effects on the stutterer's psychological well-being, the same treatment seems to have done little to ameliorate the fluency problems of the vast majority of these individuals" (p. 254). Clinicians in the field with extensive experience treating teenagers and adults who stutter also reported that most of their clients who received psychotherapy for their stuttering evaluated it as noneffective as far as their disfluent speech is concerned (e.g., Dodge, personal communication, 2009). As psychopathological perspectives of stuttering began to flourish at the end of the 19th century, so did psychotherapies for the disorder. Those therapies were aimed at curing presumed deep-seated personality neuroses traced back to early childhood. Overall, their effectiveness in reducing stuttering has been limited, and research support for emotional disturbances underlying stuttering has been inconsistent and relatively weak. During the past 30 to 40 years, the application of psychotherapy as the sole or main therapeutic approach for stuttering lost much ground for two reasons: the failure of research to provide the necessary level of support for the claim that stuttering is a neurotic disorder, and the realization that psychotherapy has had very limited success. At present, the use of psychotherapies as the sole treatment for stuttering appears to be rare. Nevertheless, in assessing obstacles to therapeutic progress, clinicians should consider the client's overall emotional health and the need to obtain other expert evaluation.

Rational-Emotive Therapy

Rational-emotive therapy (RET), originated by Albert Ellis (1973), represented a significant departure from psychoanalysis because in this method, the patient does not merely note and express thoughts but actively takes charge of them. It is considered to be one of the earliest forms of cognitive-behavioral therapy (Phares, 1979). The viewpoint of cognitive-behavioral therapy is that when a person's way of thinking changes, their behavior changes. To understand behavior, examine the underlying thought processes. Detrimental thoughts lead to detrimental behaviors. Beneficial thoughts lead to beneficial behaviors. So one of the premises of RET is that psychoemotional distress arises from the irrational negative thoughts and beliefs people have about themselves, others, or life itself. These thoughts or beliefs can be particularly important if they take on the role of being *self-fulfilling prophecies*. A self-fulfilling prophecy is a prediction that influences its own outcome. Negative thoughts can set a person up for failures, whereas positive thoughts help to bring about favorable outcomes.

RET emphasizes a reorganization of the person's cognitive and emotional functions. That is, by reexamining beliefs and redefining problems, more suitable patterns of behavior will result. Hence central to this approach is a focus on positive self-talk. Self-talk is the inner dialogue that a person has with his or her self throughout waking hours. An example of negative self-talk might be "I sure am stupid. I hate myself." An example of positive self-talk might be "I like being human. I am a worthwhile person." The principles of RET likely were a precursor to the popular practice of rehearsing daily affirmations. One of the assumptions of RET is that by changing irrational (negative) self-talk into rational (positive self-talk), consequent emotions can be strengthened as a result. That is, one's thoughts have a direct influence on one's feelings and also on one's behaviors.

RET may be conducted with individuals or with groups. There are five steps in RET: (1) Identify the self-talk that occurred when there was an event that activated a self-statement (e.g., after making a mistake, the person tells himself, "That was stupid."). (2) Look deeper to examine the underlying assumptions and beliefs behind the self-talk (e.g., "I believe I must do things right all the time in order to think of myself as worthwhile."). (3) Acknowledge the associated feeling/s (e.g., "I feel depressed and discouraged."). (4) Challenge the irrational assumption and belief (e.g., "It's not reasonable to expect perfection from myself. No one always manages to do the right things."). (5) Replace the ineffective self-talk with effective self-talk (e.g., "I am a worthwhile person. I have permission to be human, and forgive myself when I make

Table 10.1: **Example of the Five Steps in Rational-Emotive Therapy Applied to Stuttering**		
Focus	**Step**	**Stuttering-Related Example**
Activating event	Identify the negative self-talk	"If I stutter now, it will be horrible."
Belief system	Examine underlying assumptions	"Stuttering makes me inadequate."
Consequent emotion	Acknowledge the feeling	"I feel ashamed and helpless. Poor me."
Dispute irrational thinking	Challenge the belief	"Is stuttering what matters most about who I am? No."
Effective self-talk	Replace with positive self-talk	"I am a worthwhile person, stuttering or not."

mistakes. It benefits nobody when I put myself down."). Table 10.1 provides an example of how the steps in rational-emotive therapy might be applied to stuttering.

The approach obviously involves an ongoing practice of self-monitoring and self-questioning one's thoughts and beliefs. The changes in emotions or stuttering itself are the indirect result of these cognitive processes. The client's active participation in the rational-emotive therapy is more in line with conventional speech therapy methods and should be given more consideration by speech clinicians treating stuttering. One study found this technique was more effective than systematic desensitization (Moleski & Tosi, 1976).

Relaxation

The previously described therapies emphasized the impact of psychoemotional adjustments on physical responses and behaviors. Relaxation therapies emphasize the reverse process. The reduction of physical tensions and responses can deliver a psychoemotional benefit. Thus the dynamics may work in either direction. The physical affects the emotional as well as the emotional affecting the physical.

As we discussed in Chapter 3 about the development of stuttering and in Chapter 4 about its advanced symptomatology, excessive muscle tension may appear in association with moments of stuttering from an early stage of the disorder. It becomes more pronounced as stuttering persists over the years. Physical tension in the speech mechanism and the entire head and neck are the most commonly observed locations. Frequently it spreads to other parts of the body, with tightness in the chest, abdomen, and even the extremities. One person who stutters related that even his toes tightened and curled before and during stuttering. We observed a person who used to crush objects held in his hand (e.g., a soda can) when stuttering severely.

Apprehension in anticipation of stuttering and the mixture of affective reactions during its occurrence also add a strong component of emotional tension—anxiety. Anxiety is associated with various neurological-physiological changes (e.g., muscle tone and sweat). The physical and emotional tensions are seemingly impossible to separate as one leads to the other. It is difficult to feel mentally relaxed while physically tense. It is well known that anxiety, phobias (unrealistic fears), or panic attacks are associated with physical tension. People with high anxiety have difficulty learning how to release the tension in their muscles, which, in turn, contributes to their experience of anxiety.

Reducing Muscular Tension

Whatever causes it, tension appears to be one of the final expressions of the abnormality of stuttering, presenting a direct obstacle to the necessary smooth movement for speech production. Excessive muscular tension can trigger or intensify the impression of "getting stuck." Here enters the concept of relaxation, which releases both the anxiety and skeletal muscle tension. The rationale for lessening emotional and physical tension is the assumption that this will (1) reduce the frequency and severity of stuttering, and (2) allow the client to attend to modifying speech in a constructive manner when the therapy reaches that stage.

> The advice "just relax" is one of the oldest informal instructions offered by laypersons to those who stutter. Although such advice usually puts someone on edge rather than being helpful, the aim of relaxing, if possible, may have value. The stiff and uncomfortable sensations of excessive tension seem incompatible with fluent speech movements. There is limited evidence, however, for the inverse assumption that a program of relaxation alone prevents stuttering. Peter Kupferman described his unfulfilled expectations of relaxation exercises in the video *No Words to Say* (Holzman, 1988), stating, "I was really relaxed, but I was still stuttering." Even when a speaker has reduced tension or anxiety to minimal levels, it is still possible to stutter. Thus stuttering therapy usually must involve more than relaxation or desensitization methods alone.

A relaxation component is found in many formal treatment programs. Reference to relaxation can be found in clinicians' writings from the first half of the 19th century. Van Riper (1973, p. 41) cited Hoffman, who, in 1840 stated that "The patient must use no muscular effort in the throat, tongue, or lips. Further, he must avoid working other parts of the body, such as the arms, feet, etc. . . . The greatest relaxation of the body must occur during speech." Some clinicians went as far as to propose that relaxation should be the basis for all stuttering therapy regardless of its format (Boome & Richardson, 1947). A comprehensive review of the relevant literature was published by Gilman and Yaruss (2000). Two formal avenues to achieve relaxation include authoritative suggestion and blending mental and physical techniques. A temporary state of relaxation can also be induced with various drugs (discussed later in this chapter).

Authoritative Suggestion and Hypnosis

Strong suggestion by an influential clinician that the client can be relaxed when entering a speaking situation may convince some to the point of success in achieving this goal. Persuasive literature, encouragement by fellow clients in a group setting, as well as other sources may also exert the power of suggestion (Silverman, 2004). When an authority figure, such as the clinician, influences client behavior through the power of suggestion, the technique is called *authoritative suggestion*. Bloodstein (1995) attributed the potential for almost any form of therapy to have temporary success in reducing stuttering to the power of suggestion. He cautioned that this factor complicates the evaluation of any new treatment that may be introduced. Sometimes clients can convince themselves of their ability to rein in a situation, a phenomenon known as *auto-suggestion*. Although a considerable amount of suggestion is applied routinely in clinical contexts, its use specifically to induce relaxation is not too common and its effect in stuttering therapy has not been very well evaluated.

Suggestions for keeping calm and relaxed may also be offered under hypnosis. Such posthypnotic commands instruct the client how to behave after waking up from the hypnotic state. The use of hypnosis in stuttering therapy, however, has been minimal. Several clinicians published descriptions of individual cases (e.g., Nao, 1964). In a rare clinical study with a commendable number of 40 participants, Moore (1946, 1959) reported mixed client responses and improvement that lasted only 2 to 3 days. Also Van Riper (1973) reported disappointing experiments with the technique. Although the use of hypnosis in stuttering therapy has been minimal for a long time, clinicians should keep in mind the poor results because some people who stutter are always seeking quick cures.

Blending Physical Relaxation and Mental Desensitization

Much more popular have been relaxation techniques, such as *progressive relaxation* (Jacobson, 1938), that require more direct, active physical and/or mental client participation. Employing the Jacobson technique, the initial sessions begin with the client sitting comfortably in a chair, eyes closed, hands in lap. In a soft relaxed voice, the clinician instructs the client to tighten the fists for a few seconds and then relax, observing the contrast between the tension and the feelings after muscles are released. Similarly, other muscle groups are targeted. Next, the client moves on intentionally to achieve a relaxed sensation (without first tensing) in one muscle group at a time, starting with the feet, progressing upward to the legs, abdomen, chest, shoulders, neck, face, and mouth, breathing slowly in a relaxed manner. The first round may take approximately 5 minutes, but the sequence is repeated several times, checking each muscle group until all reach complete relaxation. Throughout the sequence, the clinician, in a soothing voice, encourages the client to focus on each muscle group until the client reaches a state of being very relaxed, the muscles feel "heavy," and breathing is slow and easy. At the end of the session (20 to 25 minutes), the eyes are opened and there is a definite sense of calmness.

Following a few sessions, the client learns to quickly achieve relaxation in response to clinician's directions, then becomes capable of inducing self-relaxation by repeating the commands mentally. We have routinely demonstrated the procedure during classes, watching many students thoroughly enjoy the experience. Some clinicians have incorporated relaxation in their complex treatment programs with the idea that clients will thereby be better able to implement the various speech techniques regarded as the center of the therapy. Although the skills of relaxation can be learned, implementation in real-life situations can be difficult.

The practice of progressive relaxation has been used in conjunction with the therapeutic program known as *systematic desensitization*. Tyre, Maisto, and Companik (1973) described procedures for systematic desensitization used successfully with a young adult male client with moderate stuttering severity. The client was seen for two 55-minute sessions per week for 8 weeks. The first five sessions were spent with training in Jacobson's (1938) deep muscle relaxation techniques. The client was told to practice these techniques daily from that point on. The remaining sessions focused on a reciprocal inhibition program (Wolpe, 1958). This is a behavior therapy aimed at inhibiting one response by pairing it with the occurrence of another, incompatible response. For example, when anxiety-evoking stimuli are paired with relaxation, the power of those stimuli is weakened. It is discussed in more detail in the next section. The client was taught nonverbal signals of raising the right forefinger to answer "yes" to yes/no questions, and raising the left finger to indicate feeling anxiety, to accomplish communication while deeply relaxed. He was then advanced through imagery exercises for two situational fear-related hierarchies while concentrating on deep muscle relaxation. At the end of the 16 weeks and at the 6-month follow-up assessment, the client's stuttering severity improvement scores remained more than 2.5 standard deviations from the pretreatment level.

Summary of Psychotherapy and Relaxation

Various ideas that stuttering is caused by deep emotional problems traced back to early childhood spurred some interest in psychotherapy as the choice avenue for its treatment, especially as Freud's psychoanalysis approach gained in popularity. The negative findings of research concerned with personality characteristics and emotional adjustment of people who stutter, and clinical reports suggesting that traditional psychoanalysis has had only limited success in the treatment of stuttering, have considerably diminished enthusiasm for this therapeutic approach. Although the speaker's psychoemotional adjustment, more broadly, may be enhanced by a variety of psychotherapeutic approaches, the overt stuttering seems to be unchanged. Rational-emotive therapy that improves psychoemotional adjustment by replacing irrational beliefs that lead to negative self-talk with rational thinking and positive self-talk appears to be worth further study in stuttering therapy.

As we discussed in Chapter 4, the fearful expectation of stuttering causes considerable apprehension, distress, and anxiety. Such emotional tension is closely linked with physical tension. Physical tensions can be addressed directly through relaxation techniques or indirectly by auto-suggestion and hypnosis. The combined application of physical relaxation techniques and mental desensitization has been successful in reducing stuttering. Desensitization principles have played a major role in stuttering therapy over the years and are covered in greater detail in the following sections.

Desensitization

Considerable evidence supports an interaction between stuttering and anxiety or emotional stress. Recall that the review of the literature in Chapter 6 showed a tendency for people with a stuttering disorder to have greater state and trait anxieties.

Although the nature of the interaction between those anxieties and stuttering, and the specific implications for intervention have been controversial, many clinicians devote a substantial portion of therapy to the area of emotional reactions. The reason for this clinical focus is not that emotions are believed to be the root cause of the problem, but that they are an integral part of the disorder that interferes with reduction in the overt stuttering.

Although different emotions are experienced prior, during, and after moments of stuttering, it seems that clients and clinicians alike have been concerned primarily with general anxiety and specific fears about anticipated speech (e.g., Brutten & Shoemaker, 1967; Sheehan, 1958; Van Riper, 1973). Hence the focus of therapy has been on lessening psychological difficulties and reducing anxiety and fears to the neglect of increasing positive emotions and behaviors, such as assertiveness, self-confidence, and self-image. To this end, behavioral desensitization or anxiolytic drugs have been used. This section deals with the behavioral management of stuttering related anxiety, namely desensitization.

> Desensitization is the process of disassociating negative emotional responses, especially irrational fears (phobias) from the stimuli that evoke them. It allows the person to master anxiety in small doses (Rothbaum, Hodges, Smith, Lee, & Price, 2000). This is accomplished by being exposed to anxiety-provoking stimuli in a carefully arranged hierarchy, moving from weaker to stronger stimuli, and from a shorter to longer time of exposure. This can be enhanced using reciprocal inhibition techniques. As clients achieve the goal of remaining minimally affected by each of the weaker anxiety-provoking stimuli, they progress to greater challenges.

Two approaches are be discussed in this context: systematic desensitization and desensitization in vivo.

Systematic Desensitization

Systematic desensitization is a specific technique developed by the psychiatrist Joseph Wolpe (1958) and adapted for stuttering therapy by Brutten and Shoemaker (1967). It is based on the principle of counterconditioning (or reciprocal inhibition). As explained earlier, it seeks to weaken anxiety-provoking stimuli by pairing them with incompatible relaxation states. Therefore, the first step is to teach the skills of relaxation (the incompatible response), especially through the method of progressive relaxation described earlier.

Having mastered relaxation skills during the first few sessions, the second component of systematic desensitization is introduced by asking the client, while in a state of deep relaxation, to imagine a stimulus (a person, place, situation, and others) that habitually triggers fear and stuttering. The client quickly realizes that she or he experiences considerably milder anxiety facing the situation while relaxed and imagining it. With sufficient repetition, the situation loses its anxiety-provoking power also in reality.

In therapy, the client, with the guidance of the clinician, ranks a large set of stuttering-provoking situations from least to most distressing. The program then proceeds in a hierarchy of increasing difficulty both within and between levels of difficulty. In an anxiety-producing situation, like answering the telephone at home, several steps are involved, such as the ones listed here. At first, each of these steps is only imagined while the client focuses on remaining relaxed:

1. A telephone ringing from the basement of one's home.
2. A telephone ringing at the far side of the same floor of the house, but another person answers it.
3. A telephone ringing in a nearby room, but another person answers it.
4. A telephone ringing in the client's room, but the ringing stops as the client moves toward it.
5. A telephone ringing, and the client picks up the receiver but the caller says it was a wrong number.
6. A telephone ringing, and the client answers it and carries on a brief conversation.

The entire sequence proceeds in one session. When the client feels more comfortable, real telephone calls are planned in progressive steps. Once the client is capable of handling telephone calls, a situation at a higher level of difficulty of the hierarchy is targeted. The clinician must ascertain that no anxiety is experienced at each level before moving on to the next. The client remains at each step until a relaxed state is reliably achieved. An important advantage of systematic desensitization is that the client can practice reducing the anxiety in many situations in a short time without actually being there. Additionally, clients learn to self-administer the process and maintain the gains through regular practice. From this standpoint, the technique is very efficient. Several studies have reported its effectiveness in reducing stuttering (Fried, 1972; Lanyon, 1969; Tyre, Maisto, & Companic, 1973). The main drawback is the client's passive role with no speech included in the exercise. Therefore, we recommend that after the client feels comfortable with the imagined situations (e.g., telephone calls) that a sequenced hierarchy of real situations of talking is targeted.

It is not clear why systematic desensitization has had limited acceptance by clinicians treating stuttering. Perhaps this is because the technique has been perceived to belong in the realm of psychologists. In addition, research studies of systematic desensitization may be difficult to interpret because the relative contributions of its multiple dimensions (i.e., relaxation, situational hierarchy, cognitive confrontation, etc.) are not clear. Some research suggests that anxiety-focused approaches to treatment may successfully reduce the speaker's anxiety but not necessarily the stuttering (Blomgren, Roy, Callister, & Merrill, 2005; Gray & England, 1972).

Several means of confronting feared situations are possible. Before the computer era, the exposure occurred either through imagery (e.g., imagining a plane flight) or through real-life, or so-called *in vivo*, encounters with the feared situation (e.g., taking an actual plane flight). More recently, computer-simulated exposure (virtual reality) can be used in lieu of in vivo exposure. Research findings indicate that these methods are effective in resolving various anxieties (Rothbaum et al., 2000).

Desensitization in Vivo

This technique is used in behavioral therapy when the individual is exposed, in a hierarchical order, to feared, habitually avoided stimuli in real life. It is applied when avoided fears are not regarded as objectively appropriate. Clients learn to face fears directly, stay in the feared experience while remaining calm, proving to themselves that the "danger" is not as bad as they believe it to be. The aim is to lower the level of anxiety and other "negative" emotions although not completely eliminate them. No one can expect to reduce either emotional or physical tension completely or constantly, and sometimes a speaker must feel the intensity but resolve not to hold speech back. In essence, habitual responses to certain stimuli are replaced.

As mentioned earlier, desensitization has a double purpose. The first is to decrease the frequency of stuttering on the premise that the less fearful the client, the less stuttering is apt to occur. The second is to facilitate an ability to modify moments of stuttered speech because it is difficult to attend to constructive speech changes when a person is anxious. Van Riper (1973) suggested three major objectives when applying the technique in stuttering therapy: (1) open confrontation with the disorder, (2) desensitization to the client's own stuttering core behavior, and (3) desensitization to listeners' reactions. To these, one may add desensitization to time pressure, feared speaking situations, size of audience, people in authority, the opposite sex, and more. Next we elaborate on these objectives and provide a brief description of procedures, adapted after those of Van Riper, several other sources, and our own experience.

Being Open About Stuttering

Many adults who stutter do not like to look at, listen to, or talk about their stuttering. We have learned from our clients that most parents did not openly discuss stuttering with them except for suggesting to "slow down," "say it again," and so on. Nor did most stuttering children share with parents or siblings their difficulties and the pains brought about by their speech impediment. In one case, a mother of a kindergarten child who stuttered, watching behind an observation mirror, was shocked to learn how upset her child was with children making fun of his speech. She had no idea. The mutual silence usually continues into adulthood. Typically, adults who stutter do not talk about stuttering with friends, co-workers, or even spouses and children. Rarely do they look at themselves in the mirror when speaking. Although the overt stuttering, sometimes severe, is evident and making listeners uncomfortable, whole conversations may be carried on without someone saying a word about the person's stuttering. This reinforces the early-formed taboo. Therefore, early in therapy the client should be encouraged to confront the stuttering head on by breaking the silence. For this purpose we prefer Sheehan's (1970) idea of "bringing stuttering out in the open" so that the uncomfortable role of being a stutterer is better tolerated. We have developed this approach in three steps.

First, clients do ample talking with the clinician about their experiences with stuttering during childhood, school-age years, and as an adult, discussing many memories of specific situations, avoidance behaviors, people's reactions, and social impact. Clients may be asked to talk about how children made fun of them in school, or about adults who mocked them, general or specific fears of talking, ordering in restaurants, talking on the telephone, tricks they have used to minimize or hide stuttering, problems with job hunting, and more. We suggest to clients to talk about stuttering as if the listeners have no idea what it is, as if they came from another world. (In truth, this assumption is quite valid for most listeners.) In the second step, friends or relatives are invited to sit in a therapy session or two as the client shares with them what it means to grow up and live with stuttering. Interestingly, some adults who stutter are initially more uncomfortable sharing with people they know than with strangers. This, however, is the challenge.

In the third step, clients are encouraged to talk about stuttering with other people in various situations and opportunities out of the clinic (e.g., the workplace or in front of classes). The more clients talk about their stuttering, the more courage is gained as the habitual avoidance response weakens. Sheehan also viewed the procedure as a means to reduce guilt feelings that trigger stuttering. In a similar vein, Van Riper (1973) conceptualized the process of making a detailed analysis of the features of the client's stuttered speech (identification) as part of the desensitization process, especially in confronting the problem. In our opinion, however, identification procedures are better placed in the section concerned with stuttering-oriented therapy methods.

Role Play

Another useful procedure for confronting the problem of stuttering is *role play*. Participants could be members of group therapy sessions or just the clinician and client dyad during individual therapy sessions. In some cases, as it fits in the hierarchy of treatment aims, additional persons such as family members, peers, or others could be invited to individual or group therapy sessions to assist in role-play activities.

Role-play participants adopt and act out the roles of people having backgrounds, points of view, personalities, or motivations that are different from their own. Such exercises have been long incorporated in various educational programs, conflict resolution tasks, as well as in psychotherapeutic interventions, for example, *psychodrama* (Moreno, 1953) and *Fixed Roleplay* (Kelly, 1963). An important element in a successful role play is the creation of dynamic scenarios that fit the objectives of converting relevant feelings and information into a communication discourse. Participants gain insights about other people's beliefs, attitudes and values, and how and why others perceive and react to them as they do. Admittedly, employing role play in the context of facing the stuttering problem is a bit unusual because a person who stutters cannot be asked to play the role of a stutterer. Nevertheless, the client can see himself, and stuttering in general, through the eyes and perspectives of others when they play the role.

In practical terms, the clinician may assume the role of the person who stutters, simulating the client's stuttering patterns while the client plays various roles, such as a friend, employer, professor, telephone operator, waitress, police officer, and others. Depending on the client's and clinician's genders, another person of the opposite sex may be recruited to assume parts as needed. During his or her various role acting, the client has ample opportunities to confront the stuttering as portrayed by the clinician or others. As the client converses with the play partners, he or she is encouraged to verbalize impressions of and feelings about the stuttering observed. The clinician can also contribute by acting and expressing attitudes and beliefs that she or he knows are held by the client.

Desensitization to Stuttered Speech

No matter how many years and how frequently a person has stuttered, each experience of a stutter event may trigger multiple unpleasant feelings in the person who stutters, ranging from embarrassment to tension, entrapment, loss of control, and anxiety (see Chapter 4). Years of strained experiences form a strong association: stuttering → anxiety. Although people who stutter may learn to live with it, all too often the feelings associated with stuttered speech are fresh and acute. After more than 68 years of stuttering history, one of us (EY) can personally testify to this. Again, the desensitization process seeks to break the established association between stuttered speech events and emotional reaction. The client is to change his or her automatic reactions and learn that it is possible to be in the midst of a stutter while maintaining a substantially lower reactivity level. What the client needs to understand is that although the long-term objective is to diminish stuttering, this phase of therapy actually requires plenty of stuttering instances for practice to reach the intermediate goal. Many procedures are available, and several common ones are elaborated here.

Negative Practice

To provide quick appreciation of what is meant by experiencing stuttering with diminished emotionality, a technique known as *negative practice* may be used. Negative practice is when an incorrect or opposite behavior is performed in contrast with a target behavior. It rests on the idea advanced by Dunlap (1932) that purposely practicing an undesirable behavior can actually enhance a person's ability to change and eventually eliminate that behavior. The technique is also supported by Viktor Frankl's (1963) principle of *paradoxical intention*, as well as Wolpe's (1990) *reciprocal inhibition*.

In the field of speech pathology negative practice has been used in treating voice and articulation disorders, such as contrasting minimal word pairs (e.g., wug – rug) to highlight target speech sounds. In stuttering therapy, negative practice may also be described as *voluntary stuttering* or *pseudostuttering*. The technique can be applied in a multiple ways, described in the next section, and with a variety of rationales. Historically, it was recommended by Bryngelson (1931) at a time when the prevailing theory was that abnormal hemispheric dominance caused stuttering, and that the stutterer's emotional reactions exacerbated abnormal brain functioning. Regardless, the rationale for voluntary stuttering was reduction of emotional reactions. The client was to closely display his real stuttering patterns while remaining "objective."

Gregory (2003) recommended negative practice in a form that he referred to as "two degrees of tension" (p. 195). First, the client imitates the actual stuttering as closely as possible, monitoring the amount of tension, and then imitates the same stuttering but reducing the tension by 50%. Care should be taken not to ease up on the second

(continued)

imitation too much. According to Gregory, the process of gaining control and establishing change is best served if the speaker retains about half of the initial tension. In one sense, any use of voluntary stuttering is also a type of negative practice.

Voluntary Stuttering

For the same desensitization purposes described earlier, three rather different versions of voluntary stuttering are suggested. These versions are referred to as *easy stuttering*, *simulated real stuttering*, and *freezing*. Any one, two, or all three may be incorporated in treatment, depending on the phase and particular needs of the client.

The first form is a relaxed or *easy stuttering*, as it is often referred to, in the form of repetitions and prolongations devoid of tension. Our clients have reported that stuttering voluntarily in this manner lowers their anxiety, especially when the speaking rate is also a bit slower. After presenting the objective, rationale, and basic procedure, the clinician begins by demonstrating easy repetitions embedded in sentences of her own speech. For example, asking the client "Wha-wha-wha-what ta-ta-ta-time is it? Or "Te-te-te-tell me abou-bou-bou-bout your job," and "Do you have a ffffreshly baked whole-wheat bread?" Next is the client's turn to practice the technique in short sentences, copying the clinician's speech patterns and reporting impressions after each one. It is essential to reemphasize and monitor the easiness of the repetitions or prolongation, reminding the client of the rationale for the practice: to experience stuttered speech without the habitual negative emotionality. As therapy progresses, the client is to easily repeat and prolong in several locations per sentence. Repetitions may vary in length (e.g., three to six iterations per instance and prolongations from 1 to 3 s). After satisfactory results, easy stuttering is practiced in a variety of situations. Assignments begin in the clinic with the client phoning various places to ask brief questions while employing the technique. There is no need to be concerned if the easy stuttering is not perceived as "real." The practice will have its intended impact as well supporting the client's realization that it is possible to change.

The second version of voluntary stuttering for desensitization purposes has common roots to the one just described. We refer to it here as *simulated real stuttering*. The objective is to train the client to consciously remain calm while engaging in the typical pattern of stuttering complete with all the tensions and secondary body movements. The client engages in various speaking tasks and at each stutter event is to focus on remaining calm. Initially, the clinician facilitates the experience by softly saying "remain calm, remain calm" whenever the client stutters, gradually letting the client perform without any external prompt.

A novice observer may wonder why a clinician's instruction to "remain calm" during *simulated real stuttering* is different from the layperson's naive and ineffective admonition of commenting "relax" when stuttering occurs. There are vital differences. A layperson usually feels uncomfortable and intends the advice to alleviate the stuttering. The clinician, by contrast, feels comfortable and gives the instruction to permit and encourage stuttering. Each stutter event is a positive opportunity to practice a more calm response in the face of its occurrence. The client must, by all means, be prepared for the full extent of nonavoidance and open confrontation of stuttering involved with this technique. As always, frequent evaluation by the clinician and client of the performance and level of success is warranted.

The third useful technique to introduce here is referred to as *freezing*. The client is instructed to hold on to the stuttering posture, natural or voluntary, for as long as the clinician's hand is raised. During this time, he or she is to focus experiencing an unaffected calmness in the presence of the stuttering behavior. The client can continue talking as soon as the clinician's hand is lowered. Using a hierarchical progression, freezing may be started by holding the stutter for 2or 3 s, working up to 15 s or longer. As usual, after the desired skill of remaining calm during stuttering has been achieved in the therapy room, the next step is to practice in real-life situations. One client related to us that after he stopped to talk with someone, he kept stuttering on the one word until the other person just walked away. This illustrates why there is also a need for therapy to address how the client deals with the reactions of others to their speech and stuttering.

Desensitization to Listeners

One of the remarkable facts about stuttering is that it occurs almost always when the person who stutters talks to other people, not when talking to self or to companion animals. More speech difficulties are experienced in speaking to perceived unfriendly listeners or groups. Hence desensitization should also directly address this factor in terms of listeners' reactions and audience size. The goal is for the client to achieve the competing response of a comfortable feeling in the presence of various listeners (i.e., the previously anxiety-provoking stimuli), a goal achieved by employing principles similar to those described in the previous sections.

Desensitization to listeners is characterized by its important contribution to the generalization of the therapeutic success. It proceeds by bringing visitors into the safe environment of the therapy room. They may be instructed intentionally to engage in unreceptive responses to stuttering (e.g., smiling, looking down, appearing impatient, helping him or her say a word). The client is to watch the listener/s carefully for their reactions, remaining calm and unaffected by them. A hierarchy made up of various types of voluntary stuttering can be used to ease the client into observing listeners' reactions. The sequence may begin with accessory disfluency types (e.g., many 'um's), progress to repetitions or brief prolongations, and eventually move to longer and more severe stuttering, all while studying listener responses.

Outside activities can be designed to help the client be successful in remaining calm while watching different types of listeners in situations with gradually increased levels of perceived difficulty. The listener hierarchy may first involve an older person walking in the street, a young man in hurry, a police officer, and so on. Likewise, a hierarchy of audience size from two to three people to a class size can be arranged. Of course, the clinician should work with the client to design unique hierarchies tailored specifically to the set of potential listeners relevant to the client's life and needs.

> One client described a rather classic therapy assignment that reduced his anxiety about listener responses to stuttering. He stood in a public corridor (i.e., at the student union of a university) with a clipboard in hand and asked people passing by to participate in an opinion poll. The polled opinion, in this case, was what people thought about stuttering and about talking with people who stutter. His feelings were transformed by the realization that the vast majority of the people he met were not carrying around negative thoughts about stuttering or people who stutter.

One example of such an intensive exposure (also referred to as *flooding* or *implosion*) might be experienced by students and clinicians engaged in making telephone calls to people's homes in conjunction with a fundraiser for their university or various charity organizations. After 12 calls during 60 minutes, an individual's feelings can be transformed from hesitancy and embarrassment to comfort and confidence, demonstrating the strong effect of such experiences. It is good to keep in mind, however, that, adults with long histories of stuttering may harbor a certain amount of speech anxiety regardless of the intensity of the desensitization process or how fluent they become. The feeling that "it" may come back often remains just below the surface.

Summary of Desensitization

Desensitization reduces the person who stutter's negative emotion associated with stuttering. It is based on the principle that the power of a stimulus (e.g., the sight of a telephone) to evoke anxiety (and its stuttering consequence) is weakened when the person experiences the stimulus while in a relaxed state. A hierarchy of anxiety-provoking situations, often including imagined experiences, are used in a *systematic desensitization* approach. Real-life experiences are used for *desensitization in vivo*, where the client learns to gradually reduce anxiety. Psychoemotional adjustment often improves when the speaker learns to confront the stuttering disorder rather than suppressing or concealing it. Techniques for confrontation of stuttering include being open about stuttering, use of role play, negative practice of stuttering, and other uses of voluntary stuttering. Various methods of achieving physical and mental relaxation can help in the desensitization process.

Assertiveness Training and Group Therapy

Assertiveness Training

Whereas the previous discussion focused on the personal experience of emotions, particularly anxiety, and modifications of the speaker's reactions to stuttering and oneself as someone who stutters, how these adjustments translate into social experiences may need some direct attention. Improvements in social adjustment are evident when the speaker conveys self-confidence and assertiveness in social situations. These enhance the speaker's overall effectiveness as a communicator and as a self-advocate.

Most normally speaking people find themselves occasionally in situations where they feel uncomfortable, mistreated, and upset by what others, unjustifiably, say or do to them or to others. They feel wronged, that their dignity or rights were violated, but they are inhibited from making adequate responses. Consider the person who is watching a movie at the theater where a few spectators are making noise nearby that spoils the enjoyment. The person may want to say something to the inconsiderate neighbors but instead holds in the frustration and suffers for 2 hours. In another situation, customers may be served a "well-done" hamburger, although they ordered it "medium." Some people would be reluctant to be so particular as to send it back. These are examples of lack of assertiveness. People who stutter have more inhibitions with behaving assertively because added to the concern with speaking up is the embarrassment of broken speech. Furthermore, they are also likely to encounter behaviors directly related to the stuttering, such as being mocked, that call for appropriate response. Difficulties with assertiveness also interfere with therapy, especially with outside assignments. Some clients are reluctant to make telephone calls or stop people in the street to practice certain speaking assignments, such as stuttering on purpose, not necessarily because of stuttering-related anxiety but because they did not feel right "bothering" others.

> A *fight or flight* response to an adverse situation is natural. A person actually has not just two, but three choices: aggression (fight or blame the listener), passiveness (flight or avoidance of the listener), or the most constructive response—assertiveness (reclaim the right to speak up to the other party on equal ground). Assertiveness is the skill of taking positive action toward resolving one's needs without insulting or violating the rights of others.

Manual Smith (1975) refers to some assertiveness techniques such as fogging and negative assertion that are helpful at disarming criticism directed against us: People who stutter are apt to benefit by learning these techniques. The first one, *fogging*, is agreeing with the criticism. When an object is thrown into a fog, it is quickly lost from sight. Similarly, fogging is used to make criticisms fade away. An example of fogging by a client who stutters might be to respond to the listener who chides, "Don't you know your own name?" with replies such as "It sure seems like it, doesn't it?" or "I don't know my name or my serial number." Whereas fogging can deflate invalid criticisms, *negative assertion* is used to deflate valid criticisms. It consists of agreeing with or confessing to the shortcoming. For example, the client who stutters could respond to a listener's startled facial expression with the comment "Maybe you've noticed that I stutter."

Another aspect of assertiveness is the exercise of one's right to express feelings and wants. Unfortunately, stuttering often induces a desire to retreat from communication.

People who stutter may need to recognize and reclaim their right to state their feelings and wishes. For example, he or she may at some time want to express: "I like it when people don't try to finish my words," or "I do best when people just listen patiently." Such needs for assertive expressions can be met through training programs in which familiar situations, like the two mentioned earlier, can be initially used in role-play fashion. The situation is planned in the broad sense to preserve some spontaneity. The client orders a medium-rare hamburger while the clinician acts as the server. The client takes a bite and realizes it was cooked too much. He motions the server, who initially ignores him. She finally responds and he complains. She first argues that the hamburger is just right, the client gets angry, and she complies, ordering another hamburger. At the end, clinician and client analyze the verbal responses, body posture, manner, and so on. Improvements are planned and the situation is replayed. Several rounds may be necessary to obtain satisfactory behavior: assertive yet not aggressive nor submissive. Finally, situations more pertinent to the client are selected.

Sources concerning assertiveness training are numerous and can be found in the scientific literature as well as lay publications. See, for example, Tom Stevens's Web page (Stevens, 2005). Applications concerned specifically with stuttering were reported by Blood (1995). Gendelman (1977) described an assertiveness/confrontation treatment used with at least 200 adolescents who stutter, examined specifically in 40 of them. The approach was based on the theory that stuttering is a conditioned anxiety response (Brutten & Shoemaker, 1967) and a premise that verbal interactions are the stimuli to which speakers must be deconditioned. No time was spent desensitizing clients to stuttering itself, nor to words or sounds that evoke fear. Instead, clients were desensitized to interview situations in which they confronted their listeners with assertive statements related to their underlying fears. The clinician helped the client plan how to express fears in ways most apt to be received favorably by a listener. For example, "It's hard for me to talk with you because I think you don't like me" (p. 87). The subsequent discussion typically brought about explanations and reassurances that made for a more comfortable relationship. Each positive experience created confidence for the next one. Gendelman reported that more than half (23) of the 40 adolescents were normally fluent at the end of treatment, and another fourth (13) had improved. Several months or years later, 22 were either normally fluent or improved. The report is significantly weakened, however, by lack of details and the absence of data pertaining to stuttering frequency and reliability.

Group Therapy

Psychological group therapy sometimes comes in conjunction with individual therapy; at times it is the only available service because of the time and costs factors. Group therapy presents several advantages. First, a group of people with similar problems provides comfort and support to its members. Second, it provides opportunities and a safe environment for members to express their feedings openly and honestly and share their experiences with others. Members simultaneously give and receive feedback. The open self-expression, feedback, and interaction among members allows the person to view his or her personal and social issues in new perspectives.

Members can discover new interpretations of their problems and find alternative solutions. Third, it can serve to actually practice new responses in interpersonal and social situations. For people who stutter, group therapy can facilitate transfer of learning, in that it presents opportunities to practice speech patterns and other behaviors acquired in individual therapy. They can also share their recent successes and failures in working to overcome their stuttering. For the clinician, the group presents opportunities to observe the clients' performance and progress in a social situation. At times, group members may subdivide into smaller subgroups or pairs to accomplish beyond-clinic speaking assignments together, tasks that greatly benefit from mutual on-the-spot support. Manning (2001) put it aptly, stating that "The group setting provides opportunities for enhancing as well as maintaining change in both the surface and intrinsic aspect of the syndrome" (p. 297). Clinicians, however, should be careful not to turn group therapy into purely a support group. Nor should it be turned into just a speech practice event. Although group experiences should be supportive, the aim of group therapy is to enhance learning and the process of change.

Therapy groups vary in size but we recommend 5 to 10 members as the ideal. Smaller groups of less than 5 limit the sense of having "a group" and pose heavier demands for participation on those who attend. There also tends to be less variety of backgrounds and input. Larger groups of more than 10 will limit the potential participation of members. It is important to avoid a situation where one member dominates the discussion by taking too much talking time. The clinician must announce that a reasonable time distribution of group members' participation is desired. Leadership of the group therapy may be handled with different styles. For example, the clinician may select the theme for the session and be active in directing the interaction (e.g., prompting a quiet member to contribute), or the clinician may take a more passive role, letting members steer the session with minimal intervention.

It has been suggested that group experiences for people who stutter serve the dual purposes of therapy and counseling (Luterman, 1991). Some structure and rules, however, are necessary. St. Louis (2007) proposed four characteristics for a typical group therapy session. It should (1) feature a theme and a "lesson," (2) include something fun, (3) involve some real experiences for the participants, not just ideas, and (4) must "stand alone" as a onetime experience for the participant who shows up only to that one session, even though themes may be ongoing or sequential. Ham (1990) advised clinicians that "Each member of the group must be planned for, observed, and reacted to as an individual" (p. 253).

Group therapy for stuttering has been employed and described by a number of clinicians. A rare session-by-session account of group therapy with 14 college students who stuttered that provides a useful sample of a structured program, as well as of topics covered, has been presented by Cypreansen (1948). The author reported several indications of positive outcomes. St. Louis (2007) also provides several detailed illustrations of session content and dynamics. Group therapy has been employed in our own respective clinics. Among favorite discussion topics (in question format) we suggest are these: (1) How do you feel and what goes through your mind during a moment of stuttering? (2) What does being a person who stutters mean to you?

(3) What have been people's reactions to your stuttering: strangers, friends, family members? (4) What motivated you to seek help at this time? (5) Has therapy been helpful? If yes, how? (6) Where would you like to go in therapy? (7) What leads to relapse and what can be done about it? and (8) What are three of your strengths or most positive personal assets? Manning (2001) suggested that group activities may involve relaxation exercises, role playing, and public-speaking activities.

Guitar (2006) describes his own experience as a client in a group of seven where Van Riper served as the clinician. Typically, 5 years after termination of therapy, Van Riper measured the treatment outcome using several criteria, such as being rated below 0.5 on the Iowa Severity Scale, showing no avoidance behavior, near zero word or situation fears, and others. Guitar estimated that his group members would have done well if they had the opportunity to be rated. In Australia, group therapy was reported as the vehicle to teach replacement of stuttering with slow stretched speech, gradually shaping it into near normally sounding speech (Guitar, 1976; Howie & Andrews, 1984). This, however, was not the psychological group therapy as described earlier. Instead, the group setting was used primarily as an efficient method to present and practice the new speaking patterns. It is not known, however, whether the significant reduction in stuttering they reported had anything to do with the group setting.

Summary of Assertiveness Training and Group Therapy

The speaker who stutters may benefit from an approach that deals more directly with the social interactions impacted by the disorder of stuttering. Two therapeutic applications that address social adjustment are assertiveness training and group therapy. In assertiveness training, the person learns to manage challenging social situations by expressing needs directly and requesting respectful behavior by others. Group therapy affords a variety of benefits including social support and practice of speech strategies in a social situation. Both group size and session format should be considered during therapy planning.

Antianxiety Drugs

It is difficult to determine the most appropriate site in our book for this topic aside from having a special chapter, an unwarranted option in view of the limited scope of the current presentation. Drugs have multiple impacts, including physiological, motoric, emotional, and unknown. Some drugs used in stuttering treatment were intended to relieve physiological symptoms (i.e., tension and disfluent events), but most have been aimed mainly to control emotionality associated with stuttering, often for antianxiety purposes. Therefore, we have placed their discussion within this chapter pertaining to the emotionality involved in stuttering. We admit, however, to being somewhat arbitrary in choosing this location.

Why Drugs?

Most stuttering therapy approaches described earlier, as well as those we discuss in the following chapters, involve regular face-to-face contact between client and clinician over a period of time. In fact, the ASHA Code of Ethics states that when treatment is carried out through correspondence, clients must be diagnosed by a speech-language pathologist (SLP). Considering the large number of people who stutter in the world, the lack of clinical services for so many of them, and the poor economic status of most of the world population, one hopeful promise is seen in effective drugs, if they can be developed and be available at affordable price. During the past 25 years, consumption of prescription and over-the-counter drugs for every conceivable problem has mush-roomed, becoming part of the daily life and culture of the Western world. In light of this, the search of people who stutter for a relief, if not complete cure, by means of drugs, is understandable.

Potentially, drugs could reach large numbers of people who stutter worldwide and could easily be self-administered. Furthermore, availability of safe drugs would change considerably the treatment of stuttering even in conventional clinical settings. Of course, drug distribution and use is not a simple matter. It is expected that for many years to come, drugs for stuttering will require a physician's prescription as well as some monitoring. Unfortunately, many areas in the world are served by but a few physicians or qualified nurses who are very busy combating life-threatening diseases. Also, some patients may exhibit negative reactions to the drug. Others may be incon-sistent with its timely consumption. There is also the risk of misuse. Nevertheless, modern technology and services have been transforming medical care, for example, with the use of computers for medical consultations, mail-order drugs, and so on. Thus some of the major issues just mentioned will be gradually resolved. Finally, it is not unrealistic to contemplate that scientific progress will yield vastly improved safer drugs that may, in the future, be perhaps sold over the counter.

For the time being, although experimentation with treating stuttering with drugs during the past 100 years has not produced a satisfactory product, recent research progress in several related scientific domains (e.g., physiology, genetics, and pharmacology) make it reasonable to suggest that some pharmaceutical promises could materialize in the near to intermediate future. Therefore, clinicians should become familiar with information as it comes out and be prepared to discuss pros and cons with inquiring clients. Furthermore, because at least for some time to come, drugs will not provide complete cure, they would probably be most effective when integrated with conventional speech therapy.

Drugs for What?

Some drugs are designed specifically for quick relief of symptoms, for example, aceta-minophen for relieving headaches. They do not address the cause of the problem. Other drugs, such as insulin, provide a substance the body is no longer able to produce itself, whereas others, for example, Fosamax, actually help rebuild bone density, pre-venting osteoporosis. In other words, drugs may directly address a disorder or simply relieve symptoms. A basic question arises concerning the specific purposes of drugs for stuttering: What system of the individual who stutters should a drug be directed to?

What are its specific intended effects on the organism? The answer can be expected to reflect either one's theoretical outlook on the etiology of stuttering or one's urgency to deal with the symptoms. If stuttering were to be identified as a motor disorder associated with brief muscle spasms, would muscle relaxant drugs be a reasonable avenue to pursue? If stuttering were associated with underlying anxiety, then one of several antianxiety drugs might provide relief. If stuttering involves dopamine levels in the brain's speech control areas, drugs affecting these levels would seem to be a reasonable choice. Or, if we believe in multiple etiologies of stuttering, then perhaps more than one drug should be prescribed (e.g., one which controls emotional reactions and one which regulates motor functions). Also, regardless of other considerations, should we pursue drugs that have the properties of altering speech characteristics, for example, to induce slow speech that is known to facilitate fluency?

A question to consider in developing drugs for stuttering is the general strategy for the drug usage. Is the purpose to achieve a constant, long-term effect in the reduction or elimination of stuttering or to trigger the effect intermittently as needed? Would the drug be taken for a short period to produce permanent changes after the drug is withdrawn or will it continue to be consumed if it is effective? This is a rather fundamental question that should also involve a patient's choice but has not been adequately discussed in the literature. Of course, this issue has implications for the frequency of drug usage. Treatments of many health problems involve multiple daily doses for either short- or long-term use. Some long-term treatments involve once a day or once a week drug consumption, whereas other treatments involve taking the drug once a month. A related consideration is the time required for a drug to take effect. Some drugs may take 2 to 3 weeks for a gradual buildup, others may take an hour or so, whereas some become effective in 1 or 2 min. This has important practical implications for the consumer.

> A short-acting calming medication, for example, taken prior to an oral presentation, may have its effect wear off before the speaker even begins. Many years ago, one of us (EY) took such a drug before a presenting at an ASHA convention. With the particular dosage taken, its full-strength effect lasted about 30 to 40 minutes. Being the fourth presenter in the scientific session, much of the drug's calming effect had evaporated by the time it was his turn to speak, creating a last-minute experience of great distress.

Examples of Research Experimentation with Drugs for Stuttering

Experiments with medical drugs for the treatment of stuttering were reported in Europe as early as the late 1800s. In Germany, Gutzmann (as described by Hogewind, 1940) prescribed one of several drugs, including a bromium preparation, ergotine preparation (with some hallucinogenic properties), and others, depending on his classification of the client's physical constitution. During the first half of the 20th century, reports of drug use appeared sporadically in the literature, often in a less than reassuring scientific context. For example, in 1940, Hogewind, a Dutch physician, published an article in the *Journal of Speech Disorders*, reporting the administration of Bellergal (a combination of several sedatives) to adults who stutter. Starting with a large daily dosage of 3 to 4 tablets for the first fortnight, it was gradually reduced and sometimes stopped for a while. Hogewind commented that "On the whole, the results were satisfactory, sometimes even very good. The patients became calmer, and during the intervals, several asked on their own accord to be allowed to begin with the tablets again, so that they could speak better" (p. 207). He felt, however, that speech therapy should also be given and that the drug was especially useful during the early phase of the speech therapy as well as in reducing duration and severity of relapses. The Hogewind report is a revealing example of the unsatisfactory quality of the older literature in that it does not provide information about the number of participants, duration of treatment, or the specific dosage contained in the tablets. Similarly, no mention is made of measures of stuttering, or other relevant parameters, before and after treatment. Moreover, there were no follow-ups and no control groups.

Activity in drug treatment for stuttering continued during the 1950s. The belief that stuttering is caused by anxiety prompted a good number of experiments with anxiolytic drugs, that is, drugs prescribed for the treatment of symptoms of anxiety. Following this reasoning Winkelman (1954) used chlorpromazine. Clinicians used meprobamate, which works directly on muscles to induce relaxation, as well as having a sedative effect. Di Carlo, Katz, and Batkin (1959), for example, administered the drug to adults who stutter over a 4-week period. They write,

> Ten stutterers who were given 600 mg. of meprobamate per day for the first week, 1,200 mg. per day for the second week, 1,600 mg. per day for the third week, and 2,000 mg. per day for the fourth week, showed a reduction in the mean number of stuttered moments. This reduction, while not achieving statistical significance, did show a definite trend and was significant at the .10 level of confidence for the group that received the meprobamate. Nonparametric statistics revealed a statistically significant amount of progressive success with each trial for this group. Their own subjective evaluation confirmed the findings. On the basis of these results, further study is indicated. (pp. 560–561)

The preceding extract reflects the typical findings in this area. A number of other antianxiety drugs, such as *alprazolam*, were reported to yield some positive results in a minority of the participants. Those who responded positively, however, showed only a very modest reduction in stuttering (see review by Brady, 1991).

A different approach began in the 1960s, after haloperidol was introduced in 1958. Haloperidol is a highly potent antidopamine drug, used primarily in the treatment of psychotic conditions, delirium, and schizophrenia. Dopamine is a hormone and neurotransmitter (a substance that mediates impulses between nerve endings and muscles) that activates five types of dopamine receptors referred to as D1, D2, D3, D4, and D5. It has important roles in brain functioning, including regulation of behavior, cognition, control of movement, mood, attention, and learning. Dopamine dysfunction in the brain, such as depletion from normal level, has been viewed as associated with Parkinson disease, attention deficits, hyperactivity disorders, autism, and schizophrenia (Arias-Carrión & Pöppel, 2007). An important driving force behind the interest in haloperidol for treatment of stuttering has been the hypothesis that excessive levels of dopamine result in abnormally low metabolism of the cortical speech areas as well as in the *striatum*, a deeper brain structure. Indeed, the presence of considerably larger than normal quantities (50% to 200%) of dopamine in the brains of people who stutter was reported in 1997 by Wu et al.

Because excess dopamine has been suspected as a causal agent in stuttering, drugs that lower dopamine, such as haloperidol, a dopamine D2 receptor blocker, have been studied experimentally. Research studies of these older generation dopamine antagonists (they were previously used mostly as antipsychotic medications for hospitalized patients) were reported to improve stuttering symptoms, mainly severity, but typically only in a minority of the participants who stuttered. Andrews and Dozsa (1977), for example, reported improvement in fewer than 20% of the participants. Additionally, the drugs caused poorly tolerated adverse effects, including involuntary movement, drowsiness, and blurred vision, which limited their usage by outpatients, such as people who stutter. Hence a good number of subjects who stuttered ceased participation in the middle of the experiments (e.g., Andrews & Dozsa; 1977; Quinn & Preachy, 1973; Rantala & Petri-Larmi, 1976). A few years later, Prins, Mendelkorn, and Cerf (1980), in a double-blind study, found that whatever statistically significant effects the drug had on reducing the frequency of disfluency, they were too small to be clinically meaningful. Also, reduction in speech interruption occurred primarily on disfluency types more typical to normal speakers, not on the core behaviors of stuttering. All in all, at the time, it appeared that the limited influence on the amelioration of stuttering combined with an unwarranted level of side effects made haloperidol an undesirable choice for the treatment of stuttering in adults.

A noticeable development occurred in the late 1990s, when second-generation atypical antidopamine drugs, risperidone and olanzapine, were created, which blocked serotonin 5HT2 receptors as well as dopamine D2 receptors and were associated with fewer Parkinson-like side effects of stiffness and tremor. Experiments with these drugs in treating stuttering indicated some improved fluency (e.g., Maguire, Riley, Franklin, & Gottschalk, 2000; Maguire, Riley, Franklin, Maguire, Nguyen, & Brojeni, 2004). Stager et al. (2005) concluded from their data that olanzapine is a promising medication for the treatment of stuttering and further research is warranted. It must be noted, however, that olanzapine, risperidone, and similar medications are often associated with substantial weight gain.

Another group of pharmaceuticals, including paroxetine, and those targeting obsessive-compulsive symptoms as well as generalized anxiety, such as citalopram and clomipramine, collectively referred to as *selective serotonin reuptake inhibitor*, or SSRIs, have been experimented with in the treatment of stuttering. These medications are based on *serotonin*, another neurotransmitter that activates neural receptors known as 5-HT. These are different from the neurotransmitter blocked by haloperidol. Another term that better fits this group of drugs is *potent serotonin reuptake inhibitors* because a low dose of all of them has a strong effect in blocking serotonin reuptake. Serotonin is believed to play an important role in inhibiting anger, aggression, moods, and sexuality. Therefore, low-level serotonin may underlie aggressive and angry behaviors, clinical-level depression, obsessive-compulsive disorders, and anxiety disorders. The primary logic for using them in treating stuttering is the possibility that stuttering may share some underlying factors with obsessive-compulsive disorders, given that both involve intrusive repetitive behavior or thoughts. The few experiments conducted with this group of drugs yielded an unclear picture (Burns, Brady, & Kuruvilla 1978; Stager et al., 2005). The data are too few to reach a conclusion but seem to lack promise.

Finally, for the purpose of this brief review, an interesting concept was offered by Brady and Ali (2000) suggesting that two medications might be necessary, especially in severe cases, to deal with the multiple sources of stuttering. They experimented with a combination of alprazolam to reduce anxiety and citalopram, a serotonin reuptake inhibiting drug, to deal with the core symptoms of stuttering. Marked improvement was reported for three adults who stutter. The authors reported that as clients' anxiety subsided, it was possible to gradually eliminate the alprazolam. To sustain improvement in the level of stuttering, however, it was necessary to continue consumption of the citalopram. Regardless of the wisdom of combining these two drugs, the literature indicates that many patients reported trouble with alprazolam and discontinued it.

Recent Developments

In recent years, there has been substantial effort to experiment with pagoclone, a relatively new anxiolytic drug related to the sleeping medication zopiclone. But pagoclone, in contrast to zopiclone, produces its antianxiety effects with little or no sedative or amnestic actions when taken with low doses. The precise action of the drug is not known but it enhances the activity of the $GABA_A$ receptors, a neurotransmitter receptor in the brain that may be disrupted in people who stutter and is also targeted by meprobamate and alprazolam. The Indevus pharmaceutical company, which holds the patent for the drug, has conducted controlled clinical trials with the cooperation of several U.S. clinical and academic institutions. In 2006, Indevus released results of the largest pharmacologic trial of stuttering ever completed: a 8-week, placebo-controlled, double-blind, randomized design with 132 adults who stutter. Pagoclone improved stuttering symptoms in more than 50% of the individuals treated, which was statistically greater than the improvement in those receiving a placebo. Pagoclone not only improved the fluency of speech but also reduced the social anxiety that often accompanies stuttering. It was reported that pagoclone was well tolerated with only minor side effects of headache and fatigue reported in a minority of those treated. At this point, however, the findings have not been published in a scientific journal.

Summary of Antianxiety Drugs

We have proposed that the development of drugs for the treatment for stuttering holds great hope for the majority of people who stutter who are unable to receive speech therapy, and that conventional therapy will be enhanced by complementary drugs. Although a substantial number of reports on the use of drugs in the treatment of stuttering have been published, many presented observations on a small number of people who stutter, including single cases, during a short period of several weeks. Also, most group studies were not properly controlled according to acceptable high standards for drug research. In a recent analysis of the scientific quality of past work in this area, Saxon and Ludlow (2007) stated that of 75 reports they covered, the vast majority were uncontrolled studies. None were rated at the highest of four possible levels of research quality.

Our brief review shows that although most of the experiments indicated some positive effects, these usually occurred for a minority of the participants. Even when reports could be considered valid, the level of improvement varied from little to moderate and, quite critically, was associated with side effects that are too difficult to cope with by outpatient users, such as people who stutter, engaged in normal life activities. The specific drug effects on overt characteristics of stuttering are also not sufficiently clear. Thus far, speech symptoms have not uniformly improved with drug treatments. Van Borsel, Beck, and Delanghe (2003) concluded that, under medication, the most consistently affected stuttering symptom was reduction in repetition. Other data reviewed, however, indicated that much of the diminished behaviors could be classified as normal disfluency (e.g., interjections, phrase and word repetitions) and to a lesser degree the core stuttering-like disfluencies. Also not too clear is whether the frequency of stuttering or the severity of blocks is most affected. Our guarded view of the current state of the art is reinforced by another critical review of 35 publications pertaining to the use of drugs in the treatment of stuttering. The authors, Bothe, Davidow, Bramlett, Franic, and Ingham (2006), concluded, "None of the pharmacological agents tested for stuttering have been shown in methodologically sound reports to improve stuttering frequency to below 5%, to reduce stuttering by at least half, or to improve relevant social, emotional, or cognitive variables. These findings raise questions about the logic supporting the continued use of current pharmacological agents for stuttering" (p. 342).

> Although limited in success thus far, the effort to develop drugs for the treatment of stuttering should continue. As additional knowledge about the genetics and brain biochemistry properties of the stuttering population is expanded, perhaps it will even allow stuttering-specific drug formulations. Not less important would be efforts to test drugs using more rigorous scientific regimens, such as in the recent study of pagoclone. The current state of the art of drugs for treating stuttering may soon be changing if recent promising findings with pagoclone are substantiated and reported in prestigious scientific journals.

Finally, the literature on the applications of drugs for the treatment of stuttering is quite large. Interested readers will find a wealth of organized information in several sources, especially Bothe et al. (2006), Brady (1991), Maguire, Yu, Franklin, and Riley (2004), and Saxon and Ludlow (2007).

Summary

Although research evidence suggests that emotional and psychological conditions may serve only a rare or minor role in the cause of stuttering, it is clear that stuttering moments and their consequences cause many strong and negative emotional responses. These negative emotions can be debilitating to the speaker's courage to attempt speech change. Only a subset of people who stutter may need psychotherapy, probably for reasons other than stuttering. Most, however, will benefit from attention to their psychological and social adjustment. A variety of procedures have been developed to improve the management of emotional responses by people who stutter. The specific types of techniques include relaxation, desensitization, voluntary stuttering, and assertiveness training. For some individuals, antianxiety medications may be helpful. Future research also may uncover drug treatments for reducing stuttering. Attention to the psychological adjustment of the person who stutters may be no less important to a holistic stuttering treatment than the speech modification and fluency-shaping techniques described in the next chapter.

STUDY QUESTIONS AND DISCUSSION TOPICS

1. For discussion or essay: Unlike articulation treatment, the intervention approaches for stuttering target a wide range of dimensions, including emotional, physical, and cognitive aspects. Why do you think that is the case?

2. Explain the rationale for desensitization techniques in stuttering therapy. Why might some clients be resistant to such techniques?

3. List as many applications of voluntary stuttering as you can find. Do these all serve as means of desensitization?

4. Describe a time when you did not exercise assertive behavior. Role-play the situation with a fellow student, and act out how you would have liked to have responded with assertiveness.

5. What are the potential benefits and challenges associated with the use of drug treatments for stuttering?

SUGGESTED READINGS

Bothe, A., Davidow, J., Bramlett, R., Franic, D., & Ingham, R. (2006). Stuttering treatment research 1970–2005. II: Systematic review incorporating trial quality assessment of pharmacological approaches. *American Journal of Speech-Language Pathology, 15*, 342–352.

Davis, M., Robbins-Eshelman, E., & McKay, M. (1988). *The relaxation and stress reduction workbook*. Oakland, CA: New Harbinger Publications.

Ellis, A., & Harper, R. (1975). *A new guide to rational living*. North Hollywood, CA: Wilshire.

Stevens, T. (2005). Assertion training. Retrieved May 1, 2008, from www.csulb.edu/~tstevens/assertion_training .htm

Van Riper, C. (1973). Desensitization: The reduction of negative emotion. In *The treatment of stuttering* (pp. 266–300). Englewood Cliffs, NJ: Prentice-Hall.

Chapter 11: Therapy for Adults: Focus on Stuttering and Fluency

LEARNER OBJECTIVES

Readers of this chapter will understand:

- Objectives, rationales, and techniques for managing events of stuttered speech.
- Objectives, rationales, and techniques for managing fluency.
- Interventions that rely on instruments.
- Approaches that integrate stuttering and fluency management.

Introduction

As the chapter's title implies, therapies in this grouping deal more directly with the apparent main impediment and disability involved in the disorder of stuttering. Although for some people who stutter the emotional aspect of the problem assumes dominance, it is prudent to keep in mind that, as we know and define it, there would be no stuttering disorder without stuttered speech. Even covert stutterers sometimes experience stuttered speech. Understandably, many people who stutter view speech-oriented therapies as more relevant for them than desensitization. In our experience, the desire to speak without stuttering is expressed more frequently by people who stutter as their stated drive for seeking help than any other motivation. Among the several major therapy approaches that tackle speech directly is that of *stuttering management*, which enjoyed wide acceptance by speech-language clinicians from the 1940s into the 1970s and is still employed by many. Clearly, this is a symptom-oriented approach to the resolution of the stuttering disorder. Its focal point is stutter events, and therefore the client and clinician need stuttering to occur in order to pursue the therapy objectives.[1] Note, however, that in many clinicians' programs, stuttering management is a stage that follows desensitization.

---

[1] Some clinicians, for example Van Riper (1973), have included desensitization as a preliminary phase in a stuttering management program. According to our conceptualization, however, it has been placed within the adjustment-oriented therapies.

Although symptom oriented, another important aspect underlying the stuttering management approach is the ability of the clinician to help the person who stutters develop a sense of power: that she or he can overcome well-entrenched, stereotyped panic and struggle responses to old cues that yield fluency breakdown, replacing them with planned, controlled speech movements. Prins (1993) asserted that "Concerning treatment, self-efficacy theory[2] states that various approaches succeed because individuals become convinced they can successfully execute (i.e., control) the behavior required for a desired outcome. The emphasis, here, is not upon level of skills but on the conviction about their adequacy" (p. 116). Indeed, the motor skills required are not too complicated and can easily be learned. But what is important is to alter the speaker's belief in what she or he can do.

> The objective of the extensive practice, then, is not so much as to refine motor skills but to alter the client's entrenched belief that stuttering "just happens" to him and is beyond the person's control (see Williams, 1957). The aim is to develop a cognition that, indeed, the person is the master of his or her speech and, as such, is able to change it at will.

Although we began the chapter stating the focus is symptom oriented, our discussion and the preceding citation point out that even these approaches still involve significant psychological elements. Van Riper's (1973) traditional program for stuttering management comprises multiple phases. In contrast, the stuttering management program presented here includes just two parts or phases, *identification* and *modification*. Both, however, are rooted in his ideas.

Identification

The overall goal of *identification* techniques is to raise clients' level of cognition about their speech errors so they can be more efficient correcting them. With stuttering, the objective, of course, is to identify all the features of the stuttered speech, becoming closely familiar with all their small details. In the treatment of stuttering, identification has been known, at times, to have significant merit by itself. We have known several adults who showed a large reduction in the overt stuttering just going through it, without practicing any speech modification techniques. Van Riper, too, reported similar experiences. But we have also seen the opposite reaction, especially with mild cases, where the stuttering increased, or at least seemed to intensify for a while, as the client's awareness and attention to stuttering grew. Perhaps it may be wise to advise clients of the possibility that stuttering may appear to intensify, so they do not become alarmed if it does. Identification, though, is particularly important as groundwork for the subsequent direct management of overt stuttering through modification. There are two parts to the therapeutic program involved in identification: *awareness* and *analysis*.

---

[2] Bandura's (1986) work is an important reference in this respect.

Rationale

What is the rationale for identification? How does the clinician explain it to the client? Several important reasons for the approach are listed and elaborated here:

1. Familiarity with a problem is required for devising an effective means of resolving it (Van Riper, 1973). Although people who stutter are aware of the occurrence of many stuttering moments as they speak, they still miss quite a few events, especially mild ones. Some are surprised to hear so much stuttering in their tape-recorded speech. Additionally, awareness may be general in the sense that the speaker merely knows he just stuttered rather than the specifics of how that event occurred. People find it difficult to correct something that is unknown to them. Identification reveals the behaviors that should be targeted for modification, and thereby also illuminates specific objectives for therapy.

2. Identification requires the client to take an active role in therapy early on (Van Riper, 1973). People who stutter are often under the impression that something will be done, or given to them, in therapy that will make their stuttering go away, similar to experiences they might have had with medical treatment of physical ailments. It is essential, therefore, to instill the idea that behavioral therapy depends almost solely on the client doing the changing. The identification tasks that involve considerable verbal input from the client describing and analyzing his or her stuttering contribute significantly to creating the desired mindset.

3. The descriptive language used in identification enhances the ability to take responsibility for one's own stuttering. This is based on Williams's (1957) keen observation that people who stutter often relate to stuttering with animistic views. Such views are apparent when a person refers to "my stuttering" as if it is a living entity located somewhere in the body, acting independently, appearing on its own. Or, the person acts as if there is an outside force that makes him or her stutter. People who stutter often say "words get stuck in my throat" as if words are small objects, not sounds resulting from muscle movement. They need to realize that stuttering occurs only when they act to tense their speech muscles, hold their breath, and so on. This can be achieved by analyzing stuttering using language that describes what they do during each instance of stuttering (e.g., "I tensed my jaw").

4. Identification, as mentioned earlier, also contributes to desensitization. The more stuttering is discussed openly and objectively, the more the client's associated emotional reactions lessen. This concept is easily understood because most people, children as well as adults, have experienced that the mere talking to a sympathetic listener about what upsets them makes them feel much better.

Awareness

The objective of awareness is to increase the client's accuracy in recognizing the occurrence of stutter events. Van Riper (1973) referred to this process as "detection."

After discussing the objectives and rationale, the therapy takes on a hierarchical course, progressing from easier to more difficult tasks. An example of a reasonable sequence may include the following steps: (1) the clinician stutters on purpose while the client points out each of these instances of pseudostuttering, (2) the client speaks and the clinician points out instances of stuttering by saying "there" or using clickers, flashes of light, or other signals, (3) the client identifies his or her own stutter events from audio- or videotaped speech while a tally of identification is kept by both client and clinician for comparing the client's accuracy relative to that of the clinician's count, (4) the client identifies his or her own stuttering in running conversational speech while the clinician keeps a silent count for comparison at the end of the task, and (5) the client makes mental notes of stuttering in various speaking situations without the clinician's presence, for example, talking on the telephone while looking at the mirror and speaking face to face to people. It is self-evident that audiovisual feedback can be very useful. Simple counters also facilitate the task. Typically, 95% accuracy is accepted as the criterion for success at each level in the hierarchy, prior to progressing to the next level. Minor, brief stutter events should also be detected and counted. Although these often go unnoticed by the client, they could be important because tension builds up from mild blocks becoming more severe ones.

Analysis

Having successfully met the first goal of awareness training, the client moves on to the second part of identification, that of *analysis*, with the objective of becoming familiar with the details of the stutter events. Typically, the client is instructed to talk, pause after each stutter event, and describe what she or he was doing while stuttering—what were the various incorrect and unnecessary component behaviors. In line with the rationale just outlined, emphasis is placed on using descriptive language ("language of responsibility"). For example, instead of saying "my throat and lips got tight and my breath was cut off," a common language used by people who stutter, the client is guided to reflect his or her active contribution by describing the event as "I tightened my throat. I tensed my lip, and I held my breath." The clinician no longer lets the client talk about stuttering as though it is something that happens to him or her.

Whether stuttering is perceived as something that happens or as something one does may be related to a person's sense of whether clients have any control over their life more generally. A person's *locus of control* is what one believes about what has an influence over life experiences. An external locus of control is the belief that outside forces have great influence on life events, whereas an internal locus of control is the belief that one's self has a great influence on life events. A few scale measures of locus of control have been developed (J. Riley, G. Riley, & Maguire, 2004). Some research has shown relapse is more likely among those who exhibit an external locus of control (Andrews, G., & Craig, A., 1988; Craig, Franklin, & Andrews, 1984). In clinical practice, some programs compare pre- and posttreatment measures of locus of control to evaluate progress toward an increased internal locus (Guitar, 2006).

Ask a person who stutters to describe what took place during a stuttering moment, and the individual is apt to say something like "My tongue tightened up." By contrast, *language of responsibility* reframes stuttering as an active rather than passive experience. The speaker instead states, "I tightened my tongue." This change in language has a great influence on the client's point of view. It minimizes the thinking and feeling that something beyond control makes stuttering happen, and it instills a sense of responsibility for the behavior and thus, that one can change it (Williams, 1957).

The analysis of stutter events proceeds systematically, including movements directly involved in the disfluencies and those involved in the associated secondary characteristics. First, the client describes and keeps a list of as many behaviors involved in the stuttering as she or he is capable of perceiving without external help (e.g., "I pressed my lips together on the *p* sound in the word *picture*, then closed the right eye and tilted my head forward"). Because secondary characteristics often are easier to identify, more of these may be analyzed first. Next, the clinician may introduce again the *freezing technique* by having the client hold on to the stuttering events for several seconds, focusing maximum attention on his behaviors, then proceeding with the verbal descriptions. Next, the client continues the process by performing the analysis task in front of a mirror to facilitate identification of more subtle, or not so subtle, behaviors missed before. The clinician may provide additional refinement by pointing out still additional behaviors missed by the client. Audiovisual forms of feedback (e.g., mirror, recordings, etc.) are particularly helpful for pinpointing the details. Thus all the tense, unnecessary movements that constitute the stutter event are identified. Finally, the client may wish to recreate the stutter event just analyzed, observing again the movements involved, and drawing conclusions as to what should be done to redirect the actions to result in the goal of unimpeded speech, (e.g., start in easy on the vowel, keep the vocal folds open to permit airflow, bring the lips loosely together, etc.). This, in fact, is getting close to the stage of stuttering modification.

Typically, not all steps in either the awareness or the analysis parts are covered in a single session. Time and repeated practice (hundreds of analyses) are needed not only for accurate awareness and analysis but to impact the client's attitude, understanding, and insight into the problem. It is possible for a person who stutters to demonstrate accurate stuttering analyses early on. Still, it is extensive practice that brings about change in old beliefs and attitudes: taking the mystery out of stuttering and developing a strong realization that she or he is indeed doing the actions that constitute stuttering.

Summary of Identification

The exploration, detection, identification, awareness, and analysis of stuttering from an objective, nonemotional perspective has the potential to be the foundation for speech change. Through this process the client and the clinician discover what specific stuttering behaviors interfere with speech that should be modified, as well as alter the client's point of view of the nature of his or her problem. When attention is given especially to proprioceptive dimensions of speech during exploration, the speaker can start to gain a sense of his or her own controls. Next, those controls are developed through either the modification of stutter events or the production of a whole new manner of fluent speech (i.e., fluency shaping).

Modification

The overall objective of *modification* is to develop the client's skills for changing the habitual stuttering into easier, more relaxed, less abnormal patterns. The changed pattern will be characterized by more continuous, less interrupted speech movements. The basic tenet is that if a person has to stutter, the stuttering should at least be more acceptable to self and listeners. Such changes are cognitively based and achieved by self-monitoring and redirecting speech movements just after, in the midst of, or in anticipation of stutter events. In short, the aim is more "fluent stuttering."

Prior desensitization training equips the client to respond more calmly and constructively to the stuttering block and change behaviors instead of reacting with a panic that makes the stuttering more severe. Following weeks of extensive analysis as described in the preceding section, the speaker can quickly identify superfluous positioning, and transform the stuttering-related movements into appropriate speech-related movements. The theme of *taking responsibility* for stuttering behavior continues to be upheld.

> The learning challenge at this point is how to change speech and, not less importantly, how to be confident of an ability to take charge of speech. These priorities should be transmitted to the client. The clinician should emphasize another theme, that of "exploring alternatives" to the client's old rigid struggle responses in anticipation of, or during, moments of stuttering. Having the will to explore alternatives is an extremely important therapeutic achievement. It is a significant milestone when the client's strong tendency to panic at each moment of stuttering is replaced by a focus on intentional, positive action. It is, as one client summarized "a feeling of power."

The modification phase of stuttering management typically includes three procedural steps, all referenced in time with respect to the stutter event.

Post-Block Modification

The essence of the first procedure, referred to as *post-block modification* or *cancellation*, is changing the stuttering after it has occurred. In this procedure, the client should complete the stuttered word and then pause. The clinician ensures that the stuttered speech continues and the client pauses only *after* the stuttered word is completed. Pausing too soon exploits an opportunity to avoid either the stuttering or the word being said. Avoidance of stuttering, however, is not the goal of the technique. Analysis of the stuttering and selecting new behaviors are the aim. Based on behavioral theory, the pause is key because the time-out period interrupts the pattern of undesired reinforcement that results each time stuttering is followed by further progress with communication. Procedurally, the pause affords time to quickly (1) identify and analyze counterproductive behaviors, (2) reduce tension, and (3) plan necessary changes. Inasmuch as the client has had ample practice analyzing stuttering during the previous identification phase of the therapy, now he or she can do this very quickly. Having paused, the client next reproduces the stuttered word but with the appropriate changes, such as light contact at the lips for the sound /p/ in "picture," easy voice onset on vowels such as 'o' in "ocean," and/or a slower progression of movement. Initially, the pause may last as long as needed, at least several seconds, to achieve the multiple tasks. The reproduction may be exaggerated to enhance initial learning, by elongating or stretching out the word. Attention is focused on the oral sensation of speech movements and how these may guide adjustments. Sometimes the speaker may pantomime the word before speaking aloud. That is, silently mouthing how the word will be formed is used prior to speaking it again out loud. Sometimes the stuttered segment can be changed on reproduction using the *bouncing* technique. Bouncing is when a stuttered word or syllable is repeated several times with an easy, very relaxed production on each reiteration, such as in "pi-pi-picture." Because a major goal is to break the client's stereotypic response, emphasizing variations in the new behaviors is important. Clinicians do well to see that the client can restate the rationale for the cancellation technique in order to ensure its success. The client may be adequately motivated if the procedure is not found to be more embarrassing than stuttering itself, and if the gratification found by confronting and dealing with stuttering exceeds what is felt by avoiding it.

Clinicians should monitor cancellations carefully because clients could tend to hurry through the procedure, pausing very briefly, with little analysis, slight reduction in tension, and minimal alteration in the movement. All too often the process, especially the pause, seems inconvenient, even embarrassing to a client. It also interferes, although only temporarily, with interpersonal communication. Clients often prefer to bear with their old familiar stuttering than to engage in the pause and awkward new behaviors that deliberately call attention to the act of speaking. This is a time when clinician support is important, as well as the time to review again the rationales for the procedure. Overall it is a means for developing essential management skills as well a realization of being the master of one's own speech. Clients do not just wait for the word to "come out"; they do something about it.

In-Block Modification

Building on skills acquired with the post-block technique, the second step, *in-block modification*, also referred to as *pullouts*, is introduced. Assuming the client can now quickly identify and analyze the abnormal movement and tension on the stuttered word, the pause after it is eliminated so that changes are made earlier, as soon as the stuttering occurs. At this point, or mid-word, the client identifies and reduces the tension, and "pulls out" of the block with relaxed, elongated, or easy repeated movements like those described before. For example, an instance of tense repetitions a-a-a-a-ai is altered "on line" into an easily prolonged "a→I."

The elimination of the conspicuous pause after the stuttered word greatly improves overall communication and naturally is preferred over the cumbersome post-block procedure. Of course, when an in-block attempt fails, the client should immediately switch to a post-block modification as described earlier. Again, intensive practice provides an invaluable boost to the person's feeling of power over his or her speech.

Pre-Block Modification

The third step is the *pre-block* procedure that shifts modification to an even earlier time, prior to the occurrence of the stutter event. As discussed in Chapter 4, people who stutter frequently anticipate upcoming stutter events. Typically, some alterations in speech, such as respiratory changes, change of speaking rate, and tension, build up simultaneously with the anticipation. Van Riper (1971) referred to pre-block preparations as *preparatory sets.*

After spending many hours in therapy analyzing a large number of stutter events, the client can be expected to know much more about what malformed movements will eventually evolve into full-blown stutter events. Having this knowledge and the skill to generate easier speech, the client is now ready to alter those movements, for example, easing off tension in the jaw and lips, starting in with ease, and elongating the word, just in time to prevent the appearance of a block. The overall impression might be that of a somewhat more gradual entry into the act of speaking. If the moment passes by too quickly, then either a pull-out (in-block) or a cancellation (post-block) procedure is applied.

> The detailed procedural aspects should not create the impression that therapy is, by and large, just a technical matter. Above all is the importance of being there for the client. The clinician must be a keen observer of the client's feelings and reactions to shift readily from the role of a coach to a counselor. The counselor role requires understanding difficulties as they arise, easing frustrations, and offering encouragement when self-doubt and disappointment about progress are experienced. Also, the clinician-counselor redirects unrealistic expectations for therapy (such as insisting on perfect fluency, or unwillingness to accept gradual progress) and is supportive with other personal issues that may surface.

Summary of Modification

Following intensive identification and analyses of stuttered speech events, therapy proceeds with three modification steps of post-block (cancellation), in-block (pull-out), and pre-block (preparatory set) procedures, each requires changing the stuttering event at a different time in relation to its occurrence: after, during, and prior to. The purpose is to reduce the severity of stuttering rather than to speak fluently. These modification activities aid speakers because they present alternatives to old painful habits and provide them with the sense of an internal locus of control, more specifically, the power to control their speech. It also reminds clients that speech is movements, and that oral sensations can guide those movements. These two principles are also central to the fluency-focused therapies described next. Additionally, it conveys the view that easy stuttering is a better choice than forcing the word out regardless of imperfect speech delivery.

Fluency-Focused Therapies

Unlike the stuttering management approach that relies on the presence of stutter events to practice modification, a fluency management approach strives to afford people who stutter with completely fluent speech from the start. Rather than changing only the stuttering event, the whole manner of speaking is altered. Although the slow speaking rate, gradual voice onset, articulatory imprecision, and degraded suprasegmentals (e.g., flat intonation) of smoothed speech are unusual at first, more natural-sounding characteristics are eventually reinstated as long as fluency is maintained. Little or no attention is given to preparing clients for how to handle stuttering should it occur, and usually little emphasis is placed on managing emotional reactions. The assumption is that when the person speaks fluently, negative emotionality, such as anxiety, will dissipate on its own.

> The treatment of stuttering via a focus on a fluency-enhancing (or "managing") approach represents both old and modern thinking. The main objective is to employ techniques, such as stretched speech, capable of quickly instating fluency in the person who stutters, even if, at least initially, the new speech is often characterized by distorted patterns. These patterns are incompatible with stuttering, however. Once fluency is achieved and stabilized, speech is progressively shaped until it approximates normalcy, with the clinician ensuring that fluency is maintained throughout the various stages. At some point in the shaping process, generalization to the clients' everyday environment is initiated.

Among the obstacles encountered in pursuing this approach is the fact that although some forms of deliberate fluency may not sound too abnormal to listeners, it still may be so to the client because it does not sound like his or her own voice. Because typically all speakers sense comfort with the familiar sound of their own voice/speech, success with this form of speech can be challenging. A client must be ready to embrace a new sense of self and keep practicing the new speech pattern despite very strange, awkward feelings.

There has been a long history of attempts to have people who stutter produce fluent speech, often using unusual means. The classic technique of rhythmic speech, paced by metronomic instruments, was practiced in Europe during the early part of the 19th century (see review by Wingate, 1976) or even earlier. In the modern era, several fluency management techniques have incorporated instruments to facilitate, instate, and shape fluency. Other approaches, however, assign considerable responsibility to the clients' active participation and intensive practice. The latter is reviewed here. Therapies that are mostly instrument-dependent are discussed in a separate section.

Fluency-Shaping Basics

Fluency-shaping therapy emerged from three major roots. First was the observation of speech change during externally imposed fluency-inducing conditions (e.g., noise, speaking in chorus), suggesting that a common underlying production technique might be the key. A related assumption was that the abnormal motor articulatory, phonatory, and respiratory functions associated with stuttering could be overcome through careful retraining of basic speech gestures. Second, this approach was developed at the time when applications of operant conditioning principles to the area of stuttering became popular. These applications emphasized speech modification through reinforcement of behaviors that gradually approximated the target. It was a behavioral shaping approach to speech change. Finally, a third influential factor was the favorable experience of people who stutter with other speaking strategies that provided relief from stuttering, such as slow speech.

Typically, fluency-shaping programs begin by having the person who stutters speak in a novel but totally fluent manner. For example, if the speaker uses a very slow rate, elongating ("stretching") the vowels or the interval between speech segments (e.g., syllables), it induces complete fluency. Because the remarkable change begins with rather abnormal speech, clients may express pessimism or even resentment at being trained to talk in a way that would call as much attention to speech as stuttering itself. Therefore, early counseling is essential to point out that the exaggerated slow speech is temporary. It is only a means to learning correct speech gestures and other fluency skills, and speech will eventually approximate the normal manner. Other factors that enhance fluent speech, such as breathing and articulation patterns, as well as vocalization, may be introduced, incorporated, and practiced simultaneously with the slow rate. Subsequently, with gradual steps of reinstating normal prosodic parameters, intonation, stress, and rhythm, the slow novel fluent speech pattern is shaped toward increased naturalness.

Ideally, the behavioral skills learned from a fluency-shaping approach should continue to support the smooth flow of speech after treatment. Typical to stuttering therapy for adults, however, this is not always the case. Examples of these skills include slower transitions between syllables, easier vocal initiations, gentle contacts of the articulators, additional airflow to carry the sounds, chunking spoken utterances into shorter phrases, and connecting across words within the phrases. The role of the clinician, therefore, is similar to the music teacher who must help the player (i.e., client) learn to play a new instrument and practice until the skills are ready for public performance (i.e., situations of communicative pressure). Several fluency-enhancing techniques and programs are presented next.

Rhythmic Speech

Normal speech is characterized by varying rhythm within and between utterances. As discussed in Chapter 4, when the client substitutes a uniform rhythm by keeping equal intervals between the stressed impulses of spoken syllables or words, the resultant fluency promises to be useful for treatment. Under uniform rhythms, fluency can be maintained across a wide range of speaking rates, whether the intervals between speech units are fast or slow. Slow rhythmic speech has a very different quality from the slow-stretched speech typically induced in fluency-shaping programs described later in the chapter. This is because prosodic variations are possible and even encouraged during slow-stretched speech, but not during rhythmic speech. Even when rhythmic speech is produced at normal speeds, it still sounds robotic.

In an extensive analysis of rhythm and stuttering, Wingate (1976) traced the realization that speaking in rhythm yields fluency to ancient times. After the invention of metronomic devices in the early 1800s, rhythmic speech, with or without metronome pacing, has been employed by clinicians in various countries. Since then, however, the method has been characterized by erratic trends in popularity, but it has never attained widespread implementation by clinicians. A rise in interest, for example, occurred in Europe near the middle of the last century. Dantzig (1940), in the Netherlands, advocated a *Syllable Tapping* program whereby each syllable was synchronized with a quiet tapping of the client's preferred hand fingers, progressing from the little finger toward the thumb. The therapy included three stages: (1) practice with deliberate finger tapping per each syllable, (2) minimize the tapping and obscure the view of the fingers, and (3) just imagine finger tapping.

> One of us (EY) received rhythmic speech therapy in the 1950s, during his school years in Israel. This was done with and without the aid of metronome pacing. At an advanced stage in therapy, he was asked to swing his thumb from side to side while hiding his hand in the pants pocket. Curiously, a second clinician insisted that swinging the thumb was not a good idea. Instead, he recommended folding the fingers, one at a time, still keeping the hand inside the pocket. In those days, EY was not particularly keen on collecting comparison data.

One rhythmic speech therapy program, implemented without the use of the metronome, was referred to as *Syllable-Timed Speech*. It was carried on in the United Kingdom by Andrews, Harris, Garside, and Kay (1964), who reported its use with 35 stuttering clients ranging in age from 11 to 45 years, divided into four age subgroups. The 10-day intensive program consisted of four stages:

1. *Baseline.* Case history and speech samples were recorded. Baseline measures of stuttering were taken.
2. *Teaching Syllable-Timed (S.T.) speech.* Speech was produced syllable-by-syllable, stressing each syllable evenly, in time to a regular, even rhythm. Practice began with simple sentences composed of one-syllable words. Clients progressed to reading prose and then to conversational speech. If stuttering occurred, the phrase was immediately repeated, paying more attention to timing. By the first 2 hours, most adults and adolescents were speaking fluently but at a slow rate of 80 syllables per minute. To become proficient, considerable practice was necessary, about 50 hours in individual and group therapy over 4 to 5 days.
3. *Generalization.* Over 10 days, every client retained S.T. speech in relaxed group practice sessions that focused on attitudes and concerns regarding

stuttering. The group decided when they were ready for practice of S.T. speech outside the clinic, especially in previously difficult situations. Toward the end, clients spent more time accomplishing speaking tasks alone. An important assignment required the client to explain the changes in his or her speech to family, friends, and people in places of employment. This was done in order to facilitate the person's commitment to speaking fluently upon returning to family or job. By the last day, speech approximated normalcy.

4. *Follow-Up.* For maintenance, a follow-up session for each group was held approximately once a week for 10 weeks. If stuttering occurred, clients were asked to continue talking in S.T. speech for the rest of the day and also practice at home. Next, tape-recorded formal interviews were held every 3 months across 1 year with an unfamiliar staff member. Speech samples were recorded so that speaking rate and stuttering frequency could be compared with respective base rates. Feedback was also obtained from clients' families by means of questionnaires and stuttering severity ratings.

Andrews et al. (1964) presented data showing that all four age subgroups exhibited substantial reduction (20%) in the frequency of stuttering as well as in its rated severity compared to pretreatment measures. The gains remained stable over 1 year after the termination of therapy. Improvement was higher among those who were free of neurotic traits and in groups that also were provided the opportunity to discuss their anxieties and attitudes about speech. Clients with the most severe stuttering showed the least improvement.

Stretched Speech

Whereas rhythmic or syllable-timed speech did not catch on with speech pathology circles, especially in the United States, several programs that emphasized slow, stretched speech were developed from the early 1960s and gained significant acceptance. A few are reviewed here.

Conversational Rate Control Therapy

In 1965, Goldiamond reported that when people who stutter read under delayed auditory feedback (DAF), many automatically slowed down and became fluent. Several years later, Curlee and Perkins (1969) were among the first to develop a prototype fluency management therapy program. Motivated by operant conditioning principles, motor speech coordination was facilitated primarily by focusing on speech rate control, often using a DAF device to help the client slow down.

> The delayed auditory feedback (DAF) instrument delivers the sound back to the speaker at a brief delay after speech is uttered. The longer the time delay, the more speech will be produced prior to the speaker's hearing it. This delay induces the speaker to slow down so as not to be ahead of himself. The capability to incrementally increase or decrease the delay is an important element in the Curlee-Perkins conditioning program.

During therapy, the client is prompted to engage in self-formulated conversation while the clinician limits her or his participation as much as possible. Fluency is first established with a 250-ms delay, resulting in an extremely slow speaking rate of about 30 words per minute, about six times slower than normal. When the client maintains total fluency for two 15-min talking periods, rate is increased by adjusting the DAF, gradually shifting to faster rates, usually in 50-ms increments, as long as the client is able to meet fluency criteria. Also incrementally, both the volume of the DAF and the use of the instrument are diminished until normal speech is achieved without DAF. From the beginning, the client is entrusted with responsibilities for all the program's steps, including criteria for progress and correcting failures. Operant principles are important in the generalization stage.

The initial program in which slow speech was the sole procedure resulted in considerable improvement in the clinical setting as well as in everyday situations. Relapse, however, occurred in more than 50% of the clients (Curlee & Perkins, 1969). Later versions of the therapy regimen (Perkins, 1973a, 1973b) were expanded to include other elements that appeared necessary to shape normal speech, including rate, breath stream management, prosody, and self-confidence. These changes reflected Perkins's position that stuttering is a disorder of timing, characterized by lack of coordination of the various components of the speech system, namely, respiration, phonation, and articulation. Hence therapy should advance compensatory skills that enable stutterers to talk fluently.

In the revised version of the program, fluency-enhancing skills were introduced and added during practice at the exaggerated slow pace. An important one was continuous airflow throughout the utterance, a behavior typical of normal speakers. While speaking slowly, the client is taught to maintain uninterrupted expiratory airflow on short utterances of three to eight syllables, assuring sufficient air support. Because the slow fluent speech pattern tends to be monotonous, it is further supplemented by practice of normal prosody and emphasis on clear voice quality. Although speech drill is the main aspect of the program, Perkins and Curlee also mention the importance of what they call "psychotherapeutic discussion" that encourage the client throughout the program to use positive language and discuss success. Although these early programs used DAF, it is important to point out that the instrument is not at all essential to pursue them.

> Of course, every procedural step in this and any other approach involves a significant amount of practice in the clinical setting followed by much work to generalize the objective to various environments. To this end, the clinician charts out the therapy goals, teaches the techniques, presents rationale, supervises the drills, provides feedback, and more. Clients need the clinician's support and encouragement to move behaviors beyond the therapy room to the street, the workplace, with friends, family, and strangers.

Precision Fluency Shaping

Devised by Webster (1980a, 1980b), precision fluency shaping has probably received more exposure and publicity than any other of its kind. Theoretically, it is based on the assumption that motor abnormalities in articulatory, phonatory, and respiratory functions underlie stuttering, but that these can be overcome through careful retraining of the basic speech gestures. It has been presented as an intensive 12-day residential program.

The Webster program initially instates fluency by having the client speak while stretching the vowels at an extremely slow rate of one syllable per 2 s. Thus a two-syllable word would be prolonged over 4 s, an even slower rate than what was used in the programs described earlier. Instead of managing rate with DAF, the client is trained to mentally estimate and monitor the different speaking rates. Estimates are aided initially by tracking the seconds on a wristwatch. DAF is reserved for when/if stuttering occurs, and it rarely does. The objective of the therapy is not just to achieve fluent speech but to have the client attain additional speech gestures that generate fluency. Thus, following extensive practice at an initially slow speaking rate, several articulatory and phonatory behaviors are introduced to enhance fluency that are even more critical, in his opinion, than the slow rate. These are referred to as *fluency targets*. Perhaps the most notable after slow speech are *gentle voice onset* and *light articulatory contact*.

Continuing with the program, and still using the initial rate of slow-stretched speech:

1. Each vowel is practiced with a gentle voice onset. A computer-controlled biofeedback loop consisting of a microphone connected to an earpiece provides the speaker with an immediate awareness (audible beeping) concerning the acceptability of the slope of the gradual voice onset. The instrument serves only as an aid and is not essential to skill learning.
2. Slow syllables beginning with voiced continuants (e.g., w, l, v, and z) are practiced in combination with gentle voice onsets on the subsequent vowel.
3. Slow syllables beginning with voiceless fricatives (e.g., s, f) are practiced with lower intraoral air pressures in combination with gentle voice onsets.
4. Slow syllables beginning with plosive consonants are practiced with light articulatory contacts in combination with gentle voice onsets.

Once each of these skills is mastered, it is implemented in practice on single-syllable words uttered very slowly. Next, all the skills (fluency targets) are incorporated into longer words and then into phrases, all spoken very slowly. As might be expected, the next phase in therapy is to gradually increase the speaking rate while maintaining all the fluency targets. Using a stepwise progression, the rate is raised from its initial slow-motion pace of one syllable per 2 s up to one syllable per second, then up to one word per second (60 words per minute), until finally a slow normal rate of 120 words per minute is reached. Although this pace is more than 10 times faster than the initial rate, it is still slower than the average normal speaking rate of 150 to 180 words per minute. At this point, transfer and generalization begin, including telephone calls, visits to stores, and so on. During the last stage of the program, systematic work on respiration, primarily the use of diaphragmatic breathing, is incorporated. For this purpose, another biofeedback device, a diaphragmatic breathing belt, is used.

In Webster's clinic, participants are reported to spend many hours per day practicing speech. Practice time can be in the context of individual sessions with a clinician, group sessions, or even by themselves with computer feedback. Although the classic approach involves an intense practice schedule, the basic principles with many similar procedures and steps have been adopted by clinicians in a variety of settings with much lighter schedules, including the typical one or two weekly sessions.

As stated earlier in this chapter, as well as in other chapters of this book, the clinical programs we cite were selected to represent the relevant principles, structure, and techniques for their approaches. Variations on therapy programs, both published and unpublished, have been devised and practiced by clinicians in the field. Other good examples of fluency-enhancing therapies that involve stretched speech, gentle voice, and so on, can be found in Neilsen and Andrews (1992), and Schwartz (1999). As for clinical effectiveness data, in a comprehensive analysis of 42 treatment studies in 1980, Andrews, Guitar, and Howie reported that among several principal treatment approaches, listed starting with the strongest effectiveness, were prolonged speech, gentle onset, rhythm, and airflow. Other evidence for rate reduction therapies comes from the study by Andrews, Howie, Dozsa, and Guitar (1982), who examined responses by three adult men who stutter to various fluency-enhancing conditions. Slowing, syllable-timed speech, and prolonged speech under DAF were found among the strongest of 14 conditions, reducing stuttering by at least 90%. The mean reduction in stuttering frequency, in order from most to least effective conditions, was prolonged speech/DAF (98%), slowing at half one's usual rate (95%), and syllable-timed speech with a metronome at 90 bpm (91%).

Another study compared the efficiency of fluency-shaping training with 20 adult and adolescent clients who stuttered, half of whom received 16 hours of therapy within 4 days, and the other half received the same amount of therapy over 8 weeks. Both formats produced significant improvement in stuttering and other measures, and both were equivalent on all measures. Generalization of treatment effects was also observed for both groups (James, Ricciardelli, Hunter, & Rogers, 1989).

Behavioral Reinforcement

In Chapter 6, stuttering was discussed within the framework of operant learning theory with an underlying assumption that stuttering is a behavioral response that may be modified by its consequences. Some support to this theory was provided by various experiments showing that stuttering can be diminished through several learning modes, for example, punishment, such as a 5-s time-out period (Martin & Haroldson, 1982), withdrawal of reinforcement (Lanyon & Barocas (1975), and withdrawal of aversive stimuli (Flanagan, Goldiamond, & Azrin, 1958). Indeed, several therapeutic regimens have been developed contingent on stuttering events.

Relevant to this section on fluency-focused therapies, it is worth noting that reinforcement of fluent speech, rather than punishment of stuttering, has been the popular clinical implementation of operant conditioning principles. Generally, such approaches seek to gradually increase the length of fluently produced speech segments as well as the length of time during which fluency can be maintained.

In the 1970s, early adult treatment studies (Andrews & Ingham, 1972; Ingham, Andrews, & Winkler, 1972) examined whether existing syllable-timed speech programs could be enhanced by application of *token reinforcement* systems. A token reinforcement system is applied when a client is given some tangible object (i.e., something seen or felt) to reward desired performance. Tokens, the "stimuli" in behavioral terminology, can take any form (e.g., pegs, wooden blocks, etc.) but typically refer to small coinlike pieces resembling poker chips. Clients do not receive tokens when the performance is attempted but not achieved; thus the token reinforcement is contingent on the client's behavioral response. In a token economy, tokens can be exchanged, like money, for prizes or privileges. The target behavior typically reinforced is fluent speech, but other behaviors may be rewarded too, for example, entering specified speaking situations from a sequential hierarchy (Andrews & Ingham, 1973).

Research has shown that token reinforcement systems can be beneficial both by decreasing the time needed to reach the fluent speech target—greater efficiency—and by the amount of the reduction in stuttering attained—effectiveness (Andrews & Ingham, 1972; Ingham, Andrews, & Winkler, 1972). Some studies, however, have been less supportive, suggesting that token management may be unnecessary if a highly structured intervention system using other forms of reinforcement, such as praise or other verbal feedback, is employed (Howie & Woods, 1982).

A therapy that integrated the slow-stretched speech technique with operant principles and schedules, referred to as *DAF-Prolongation Program*, was offered by Ryan (1974, 2001b). It contains 12 steps beginning with establishing slow fluent speech at 40 words per minute with or without the aid of a DAF device. Typical of the gradual progress principle, the client begins with reading or saying fluent speech in single sentences.

The contingent reinforcement is "good" or a token. Although the verbal punishment "stop" may be applied if the client stutters, it is used rather infrequently because the stretched speech or the DAF are likely to keep the speech fluent. Ten consecutive fluent responses is the criterion required to advance to the next step. Next, the client is to maintain fluent speech for one whole minute, then for 5 min at the rate of 40 wpm while reading or talking. Eventually, the speech rate is increased in stepwise progression up to 150 words per minute over 5 min. Of course, contingencies remain a cardinal feature throughout the program.

Ryan (2001b) stated that he favors the stuttering behavior management program of gradual increase in length and complexity of utterance (GILCU) over prolonged DAF methods because it is easier to teach, nearly as effective, and has "better generalization, and no negative side effects of abnormal speech" (p. 114). The GILCU program includes two main stages, establishment and identification, combined with home practice. The establishment program consists of 18 steps. Throughout the progression of steps, both verbal and token reinforcements are administered. The clinician models and instructs the target speech pattern, and evaluates the client's response. Fluent productions are encouraged by "Good" and a token; "Stop; speak fluently" is stated if the client stutters. Ten consecutive fluent responses is the criterion required to advance to the next step. The entire sequence of 18 steps is completed while the client engages in one of three possible activities: reading, monologue, or conversation. The 18-step series is repeated for each of the three activity types, as appropriate, for example, a nonreader would not engage in the reading activity. In steps 1 through 6, clients progress from speaking fluently one word at a time to saying fluently six words at a time. In steps 7 through 10, the progression advances from speaking a single sentence to saying four consecutive sentences at a time. In the final steps, 11 through 18, the progression is from speaking for 30 s to 5 min. The client is expected to discover his or her own strategies for speaking fluently, which typically involves some form of slowing speech rate.

After the first 18 steps are accomplished, instating fluency with one of the three activities (reading, monologue, or conversation), programs of identification (of stuttering), and home practice are initiated. This backward order of identification appears to serve as the means to develop the client's self-monitoring and self-administration of the program targets. The adolescent or adult client is trained to recognize and count his or her own stuttered words. The first step of the three-part Identification training sequence begins with a 1-min speaking activity (i.e., reading, monologue, or conversation) during which the clinician identifies the client's stuttering by stopping the client with the word "There" and then describing and imitating the stuttering while the client observes. In the second step, the clinician continues the audible remark "There" when the client stutters, and the client overtly counts the moments during another 1-min speaking activity. In the third part, the clinician covertly counts stuttering moments while the client counts covertly. To advance between steps, the client's and clinician's counts must agree within one stuttered word. Home practice, during which stuttering is identified and counted, is also included. As previously explained, the establishment stage continues with the other two modes of activities.

Other programs have offered variations on the administration of behavioral reinforcement. For example, James (1981) demonstrated that self-administered response-contingent time-out periods could successfully reduce stuttering in a young adult man. Recall that *time-out* refers to having a speaker stop talking for a short time (several seconds) after she or he stutters. James found that fluency improvement was maintained at 6- and 12-month follow-up assessments after the treatment program. Approximately 15 years later, Hewat, Onslow, Packman, and O'Brian (2006) also published a program for training clients in self-administered time-out for stuttering. In this variant, clients learned to make estimations, not only about whether they stuttered, but also about stuttering severity and the passage of time.

Summary of Fluency-Focused Therapies

Fluency-focused therapies are designed to teach a different speech pattern with strategies that are likely to elicit fluency. Most begin with a slowed or rhythmic fluent speech to which other features may be added, such as gentle voicing. The resultant fluent speech is practiced, reinforced, and gradually shaped to approximate more normal rate as well as incorporate more typical prosody. Clients who stutter progress from more basic to more demanding speaking tasks as they acquire the techniques. Several approaches were described, including rhythmic or syllable-timed speech, conversational rate control, stretched speech, precision fluency shaping, and behavioral reinforcement. Many variations on these approaches exist. Another potential means of generating fluent speech is with the aid of fluency-inducing instruments, such as those discussed next.

Fluency-Inducing Instruments

The discipline of speech pathology has seen a growing number of mechanical instruments employed for both diagnostic and treatment purposes. This trend has also left its marks on clinical management of stuttering as already alluded to in the previous section (e.g., the use of DAF as an aid in fluency-shaping programs). Our experience has shown that most people who stutter indeed wish to discover or obtain a powerful external means to reduce/control their stuttering. The quick, often immediate, and substantive results in achieving fluent speech, the saving in the required therapeutic contact, and the ability to use the instrument either on a permanent basis or when needed most are all attractive features. Although the trend has been growing, the extent of using instruments in stuttering therapy programs has varied from being supplementary to being the main, or even the sole, technique. Whereas in the early conversational speaking rate control of Curlee and Perkins (1969), DAF served as the exclusive means to induce and shape desired rates, it is only one component in the more complex behavioral program outlined by Perkins (1973b). Whereas the Voice Onset Monitor that helps control abruptness of phonation is only one component in a Precision Fluency Shaping program (Webster, 1979), the Edinburgh noise maker serves as the sole technique in the Dewar, Dewar, Austin, and Brash (1979) treatment program. In some cases the instrument is advertised as if it will be fully sufficient by itself, yet supplemental speech therapy and fluency practice is highly encouraged to enhance user satisfaction.

Instruments employed in stuttering therapy have varied in their background, principles, and purpose. As we discussed in Chapter 4, there are several natural conditions known to induce fluent speech in people who stutter, such as high-level noise, rhythmic speech, singing, and others. Although the reasons for their powerful, yet often temporary, effects remain obscure, investigators and clinicians have been motivated to design instruments, such as miniature noise generators and metronomes, to exploit their potential for practical use. There have been other instruments emerging from laboratory-developed stimuli rather than natural conditions. Examples include DAF, the Voice Onset Monitor (Webster, 1979), and the SpeechEasy (www.speecheasy.com), which provides both delayed and frequency-altered feedback. Instruments employed in stuttering therapy can be classified into four groups according to their principle of operation: (1) speech pacing, (2) auditory masking, (3) physiological feedback, and (4) auditory feedback. Representatives of these categories are briefly reviewed here.

Metronome Pacing of Speech

Although regulated rhythmic speech can be produced without a monitoring instrument, the metronome, often used in music training, is a device that has provided a significant boost to the therapeutic application of the technique due to its capability to regulate the length of the desired speech intervals in stuttering therapy. Wingate (1976, p. 154) traces academic records of this technique to the writings of Colombat de l'Isère in 1830, who believed that stuttering was caused by lack of harmony between nervous activity and musculature involved in speech. He discovered that rhythm was the most effective exercise for harmony and then developed a prototype of the metronome, called *muthonome*. Although clinicians have employed various metronomic instruments in therapy since the original invention, a fundamental drawback was the impracticality of carrying around the conventional spring-operated desk metronome into everyday situations.

A surge in the use of metronome-paced speech as a major technique in stuttering therapy occurred in the early 1960s when a miniature electric metronome that fit behind the ear (originally one unit behind each ear), like a hearing aid instrument, was first introduced by Meyer and Mair (1963). Based on initial experimentation they found that metronomic beats between 75 and 95 per minute provided the most effective rate. Using improved versions of the instrument, several therapeutic programs were developed, and studies of clinical applications of rhythm were published. In 1968, Brady described a single-unit device, the *Pacemaster*, in which the rate of the metronomic clicks and their loudness can be adjusted manually. Three years later, Brady (1971) described a systematic therapy program, *metronome conditioned speech retraining (MCSR)*, with accompanied results of most extensive metronome-paced treatment to date. The program's title reflects Brady's theoretical view that stuttering consists of two components: nonfluencies and anxiety/tension. The MCSR follows five phases and is presented here as a good example of the rhythmic speech method as well as a logically structured, systematic speech therapy program:

> Phase I: Obtain nearly 100% fluency using a desk metronome in the clinic. The client determines the most comfortable metronome rate for fluency when reading aloud easy materials. For example, a person with severe stuttering might prefer 40 beats per minute (bpm), whereas a person with moderate stuttering may prefer 80 bpm. The client is to practice speaking with the desk metronome at home for at least 45 min a day, first alone, then in the presence of others.
>
> Phase II: Shaping the speech to a more normal rate. Using the desk metronome, the speaking rate is gradually increased by changing the frequency of the metronome beats and by pacing longer speech units per beat, that is, moving from one syllable per beat to words, longer words, and even three to four words per beat. Natural pauses are added. Home practice continues, varying the listeners and their numbers. This phase takes 2 to 3 weeks, ending when

the client is able to speak fluently with the metronome at a normal rate of 100 to 160 words per minute and exhibiting no more than 20% of the original disfluency level when speaking without the metronome.

Phase III: The miniature metronome. Because of the excellent mobility of the instrument, the objective is relaxed, fluent speech in virtually all speaking situations. The switch-over to the behind-the-ear metronome, however, may result in a partial setback. In that case, the speaking rate is reduced until fluency is reached again. The client is to construct a hierarchy of speaking situations and practice them in that order. Again, if difficulties occur, the rate is lowered and then gradually increased. Brady sometimes used systematic desensitization techniques to help clients overcome difficulties transferring the metronome-aided fluency to specific situations.

Phase IV: Maintaining fluency without the metronome. The metronome is turned off in less stressful situations and gradually removed from higher stress situations. If stuttering is experienced, the client immediately returns to a strict speech pacing without the metronome. Should difficulties continue, however, the metronome is turned back on.

Phase V: Continuation of training based on responses at Phase IV.

Overall, in spite of several encouraging results of systematic clinical applications of speech pacing, with and without the metronome, the technique met resistance from clinicians in the United States educated within the newly founded profession of speech pathology in the late 1920s. Many regarded it as a "crutch"' rather than a "real" treatment (e.g., Boome & Richardson, 1932). In this respect, it is interesting to note that although Johnson and Rosen (1937) found regulated rhythmic speech to be the most effective of 12 methods they compared, the method aroused little interest in clinical speech pathology circles.

> In our opinion, speech pacing, like speaking in unison or DAF, should be considered a viable option for clinicians to use as a bridge to fluency. With selected adult clients EY has used the technique, when needed, in conjunction with other techniques, to support the development of fluent speech. A few clients who encountered difficulties with other methods responded so well to rhythmic speech that it became the primary means to improving fluency, even without a portable device. The technique is discussed again later in relation to the treatment of children.

Auditory Masking

The strong effects of white noise on the amelioration of stuttering have been researched extensively and have prompted theoretical implications (see Chapter 4). Although some people who stutter do not improve, as we have seen, or show only limited improvement speaking under noise (Andrews et al., 1982), as auditory-related instrumentation developed, attempts to use masking for clinical management of stuttering also increased. Similar to the metronome case, a critical requirement was that the instrument be small enough to be easily carried by the user out of the laboratory. A first attempt in this direction is seen in a portable noise generator, the Correctophone, constructed in 1939 in the then Soviet Union by Derazne (1966), who reported good results in treating stuttering. Using an instrument he developed, Van Riper (1973) concluded that whereas continuous masking noise met with clients' objections, turning on the noise only at the beginning of stuttering was more effective. He observed, however, that the fluency obtained exclusively with masking did not generalize, and concluded it was useful only as a supplementary technique to a comprehensive behavioral speech therapy.

A breakthrough occurred in 1963 with the development of a lightweight portable electronic noise generator by Parker and Christopherson (1963) that delivered noise through headphones. Following, other models were developed (e.g., Donovan, 1971; Klein, 1967), including types that delivered white noise and those that delivered pulsating signals, resulting in various clinical applications. For example, Perkins and Curlee (1969) had three clients use a masker for several days to facilitate transfer of fluency to outside situations. Trotter and Lesch (1967) reported the experiences of one person (Trotter) who used a masker for nearly 50% of the days during a 2.5-year period.

Perhaps the most systematic, long-term clinical program that relied exclusively on masking noise was reported by Dewar, Dewar, Austin, and Brash (1979) using a portable masking noise device, the Edinburgh Masker, and its heavier clinical bench model. The device provided an automatically triggered noise. The portable model consisted of a pocket-size noise generator that also housed the on/off switch and volume control. It produced a low-frequency noise but mean frequency varied, depending on the client's vocal fundamental frequency. The instrument was connected to a throat microphone as well as to a light "stethoscope"-type headset. Alternatively, it could be connected to individualized ear molds via short plastic tubes arising from behind the neck to minimize visualization. The noise was triggered as soon as the client began talking into the microphone; however, it was also possible to turn the noise on or off manually. The clinical bench model was considerably bigger, and it offered greater frequency and loudness ranges.

The Edinburgh masker is no longer in production, but because similar devices can be constructed, we provide here some details of the therapy program reported by Dewar et al. (1979). Their group initially included 195 clients (all but two were adults) of whom nearly 75% exhibited severe stuttering. The therapy proceeded as follows:

1. *Baseline.* A speech sample is recorded for future reference assessments and to evaluate stuttering severity.
2. *Client fitting and screening.* As the client talks, the bench unit is fitted to provide complete masking of his or her speech. A continuous sound is delivered binaurally. When fluency is achieved, the noise is lowered to a level that just covers normal conversational speech. The device is then switched to the automatic throat microphone. Because of the natural tendency to raise vocal volume when talking in noise (i.e., Lombard effect), the client practices reading until a normal intensity level is reached through instruction or with a sound meter. If a word or a phrase begins with a silent

block, the device is activated by the client saying "er" or "mm." Those clients who have problems adjusting to the masker are screened out and excluded beyond this point.

3. *Using the portable masker.* Clients are provided with the portable model and instructed to adjust the noise level until speech is fully covered by it. They learn that when the voice rises above the noise level, the effectiveness of the instrument is diminished. Most are able to maintain normal loudness and intonation.

4. *Generalization.* Clients are advised about the ways the masker can be used in everyday situations and are encouraged to experiment with it. The bulk of the therapy activities are concentrated on using the device in various situations. Clients are also encouraged to experiment periodically with turning off the noise while talking, thus testing the carryover effect. In this stage, close clinical monitoring continues.

In contrast to the rich body of laboratory studies on the ameliorating effects of noise on stuttering, nearly all our current knowledge about the application of masking in the clinical setting has come from reports that are not based on adequately controlled studies. The person who began using a noise instrument (the Correctophone) for stuttering therapy in 1939, years later reported good results (Derazne, 1966). According to Van Riper (1973), the instrument was used by many clinicians in Eastern Europe but with mixed outcomes. Dr. Trotter, a speech pathologist, described his personal use of masking devices during 50% of the days during a 2.5-year period, about 15 min per day. He reported very large reductions of stuttering in many situations with brief, temporary carryover to unaided speech (Trotter & Lesch, 1967).

The largest clinical study of masking noise was published by Dewar et al. (1979) reporting on 195 people who stutter; all but two were adult participants in the program described earlier. Of these, 174 responded well to the masker during the screening phase and proceeded with the program. Follow-up progress was possible in 67 participants who used the device from 6 to 28 months (median = 12 months). Of these, 42% reported the device to be of "great" benefit, 40% of "considerable." and 12% as "slight" benefit. Interestingly, 67% considered that as a result of using the device, their unaided speech had improved, too. One of the limitations of this study was the reliance on subjective reports rather than speech measures. A much smaller investigation with only three participants found that stuttering reduction varied considerably using noise at the 80-dB level over headphones. The two clients whose stuttering was moderate to severe showed the least benefit, 30% and 49% reductions, respectively, compared to the one with mild stuttering, a 77% reduction (Andrews, Howie, Dozsa, & Guitar, 1982). As is the case with most of these fluency-inducing instruments, individual responses are apt to differ. Nevertheless, the large number of participants who reported a positive outcome in the Dewar et al. (1979) study is impressive. Perhaps the unique combination of long-term and intensive daily use (3.3 hr on average) deserves additional research attention.

Altered Auditory Feedback

Over several decades clinical researchers have experimented with DAF devices to aid speech fluency (Goldiamond, 1965; Howell, Sackin, & Williams, 1999; Perkins, 1973b; Shames & Florence, 1980). Such instruments did not receive much popular attention until the 1990s when they were made small enough to be inconspicuously worn in or around the ear (Kalinowski, Guntupalli, Stuart, & Saltuklaroglu, 2004; Lincoln, Packman, & Onslow, 2006). A set of in-the-ear auditory feedback devices known as the *SpeechEasy* has been marketed widely and is reviewed here as an example of the general method. Developed by Drs. Joseph Kalinowski, Andrew Stuart, and Michael Rastatter, the patent for the SpeechEasy is owned by the East Carolina University in Greenville, North Carolina. The SpeechEasy fits into the speaker's ear canal and is indistinguishable visually from a hearing aid. It digitally processes and transforms the speech signal so that there is both a time delay (DAF = delayed auditory feedback) and a pitch shift (FAF = frequency altered feedback). Only the speaker's self-perceptions are altered; others do not hear the sound it delivers to the speaker. Because it is usually applied to only one ear, the speaker's general listening capacities for external sounds are not disrupted.

The SpeechEasy typically is worn monaurally in the speaker's preferred ear, although binaural fittings may also be applied. The time delay is often set to either 50 or 75 ms, with a maximum range up to 220 ms (Antipova, Purdy, Blakeley, & Williams, 2008; Lincoln, Packman, & Onslow, 2006). The frequency alteration may be shifted up or down at increments of a quarter, half, or one octave above or below the speaker's voice. Mostly, it is shifted either a full octave up or a half octave down.

Like hearing aids, the devices are custom-designed to fit each individual's ear(s). Clients are encouraged to wear them constantly, testing the effect in all kinds of speaking situations, returning to the clinic as needed for adjustments and follow-up assessments. At the time of this writing, the cost was several thousand dollars, not including expense of accompanying clinical services.

Frequently, use of the SpeechEasy instrument is supplemented with some speech therapy. Subsequent to the initial fluency assessment and customized fitting, clients may attend several therapy sessions that train them to listen to their altered feedback, adjust their sensorimotor responses, and move past their stuttering blocks. They usually receive literature with exercises and instructions for ongoing practice of fluency skills throughout use of the device. They may be taught to use starters such as "um" or "ah" or to slightly prolong their initial sounds so they can start to hear themselves with the altered feedback (Stuart, Kalinowski, Rastatter, Saltuklaroglu, & Dayalu, 2004). Information is lacking, however, about the extent such additional strategies are needed or administered.

The developers explain the effect of the SpeechEasy in terms of its similarity to choral (unison) speech. When a speaker hears both self (via bone conduction and air conduction with the uncovered ear) and altered speech (via the device), the condition may be considered comparable to talking along in unison (or shadowing) with another speaker. Unison or shadowed speech is commonly known to induce fluency in people who stutter (see Chapter 4). This account offers only a conceptual analogy, however. The theory underlying the effect has not been worked out. The analogy between the SpeechEasy altered auditory feedback effect and choral reading is questionable based on clinical observations. Whereas choral reading never fails, the effect of the device varies from person to person, sometimes within the same individual. Despite the many articles published in research journals related to this form of intervention, scientific bases for its application are still lacking.

Not all individuals respond with improved fluency to the SpeechEasy. Studies have not yet revealed the proportion of individuals who will respond at the "80% to 90%" reduction rates claimed by the developers in the media and at www.speecheasy.com in the year 2008. Research has yet to show how long the device can be expected to impact the speaker (weeks, months, or years) who hopes for a lifetime benefit. Many advertisements promise favorable outcomes. Because often the client must apply speech strategies along with the SpeechEasy, it appears likely that the speaker, not the device, still bears the weight of generating an enduring speech change. Although some may gain courage from exploring their own capacities with SpeechEasy or similar instruments, others are apt to be disappointed by its inability to eliminate the problem. In our opinion, if a speaker can learn to use proprioceptive (sensorimotor) feedback to smooth out speech movements directly, in the absence of a device, it is apt to be more satisfying.

One of us (CS) observed video marketing and local newspaper advertisements regarding the SpeechEasy that carried a strong emotional appeal and demonstration of dramatic speech change. Ads suggest relief from stuttering by merely applying it. CS has known four people who used the device. Two experienced minimal benefit almost from the beginning, despite seeking follow-up adjustments. Two others experienced an initial decrease in stuttering to about half their pre-device level. With time, however, they acclimated to the device and, despite repeated adjustments, did not sustain long-term benefits. One returned to the pre-device level of stuttering, and the other independent of the device went on to develop his own strategies for milder stuttering. The parents of one young man had been so impressed by the device, that they became distributors. Because it was their son who returned to pretreatment stuttering levels, they abandoned their role as distributors after 2 years.

Biofeedback

Biofeedback is the delivery of information about the status or function of one's biological system through an analogous sensory signal. The sensory analog may take the form of tactile, visual, auditory, or combined modes. For example, electromyographic (EMG) biofeedback involves the placement of sensory electrodes on the skin over muscle areas of interest. An electromagnetic gel aids the conductance. When the muscles are contracted, a series of lights are illuminated and a beeping sound increases in volume and speed to reflect the level of that activity (Baken, 1987).

The effectiveness of electromyographic (EMG) biofeedback for reducing stuttering frequency has been illustrated with a single-subject research design. The research demonstrated that (1) a speaker could be trained to reduce stuttering with the aid of feedback, (2) treatment could be accomplished in just 10 consecutive days, and (3) relatively lasting effects are possible (Guitar, 1975). The investigator examined the use of EMG feedback in stuttering treatment with three participants. Surface electrodes were applied to three sites: upper lip, jaw (under the chin), and neck (just above the thyroid cartilage). Participants were trained to speak with almost resting-level muscle activity. Next, an entire treatment regimen was applied with one participant, a 32-year-old man, who learned to reduce muscle activity just before words that might be stuttered. As treatment progressed, the EMG feedback was removed so the person had to depend on his own perceptions. Stuttering frequency diminished from a mean level of 17% syllables stuttered during baseline to 1% or less with the treatment regimen. This low level was maintained at reassessments both 5 weeks and 9 months posttreatment. At the time of this writing, we were not aware of further clinical applications of EMG for stuttering.

Summary of Fluency-Inducing Instruments

Several instruments have been developed to take advantage of the effect of fluency-inducing conditions. The portable devices are intended to alleviate stuttering anywhere so the speaker can focus on communication instead of the act of speaking. Nonetheless, a certain amount of attention to speaking is still required. Types of these devices include metronome pacers, auditory maskers, auditory feedback, and biofeedback instruments. Treatments using a mechanical apparatus such as an old-fashioned desk metronome, or electrical systems like DAF or miniature noise generators, usually require some face-to-face contacts between client and clinician, limited as they may be. Devices, even if used independently of clinician contact, present problems in that they can be costly, sensitive to environmental conditions or mishandling, and require ongoing maintenance (e.g., batteries, cleaning) and repair. Individual responses to these instruments vary widely, and not infrequently effects are not sustained over time. Admittedly, we have known a few clients who were pleased by the relief provided by one device or another. Much more long-term research is necessary for each of these instruments. At the time of this writing, research was under way to address clinical questions concerning the relative benefit of these instruments.

Integrated Approaches

The sharp contrasts between the stuttering management and fluency-shaping approaches have not prevented clinicians from realizing potential advantages in combining elements of both into unified eclectic therapeutic programs. Both authors of this text have been involved with such endeavors during their professional careers. We have seen satisfying results with both stuttering management and fluency management procedures. Furthermore, based on decades of experience, we hold to the position that a comprehensive approach that also includes early work on facing the stuttering, identification, and attending to the emotional aspects increase the likelihood of success in subsequent speech-oriented stages of therapy involving either stuttering modification or fluency management.

Successful long-term maintenance seems to be supported by attention, in therapy, to reducing the negative emotionality associated with stuttering and increasing the client's positive feelings of self-confidence, assertiveness, and so on. We have worked with clients who formerly underwent only fluency-enhancing therapies who immediately experienced great progress that, unfortunately, proved to be intermittent, if not short lived. Fluency collapsed in situations of relatively mild pressure because they were not skilled in how to calm themselves or take charge of speech-related movements when stuttering occurred. Their well-practiced fluency-enhancing techniques, such as gentle voice onset, could not be executed under stress.

With respect to integrated therapy, in the early 1970s one of us (EY) devised and implemented selectively such a program (unpublished) that balanced the cognitive-emotional and speech domains of stuttering. It consisted of the following components:

1. Identification and facing stuttering (bringing it out into the open)
2. Desensitization
3. Fluency-facilitating strategies
4. Stuttering modification

Specific procedures were already described in related sections of Chapter 10 and earlier in this chapter and are not repeated here. Admittedly, we have never quite made up our mind as to the question of order: Which should be introduced first, stuttering management or fluency enhancement procedures? It seems logical to begin with the positive approach of practicing fluent speech, shifting to stuttering managing techniques only when fluency fails. In practicality, however, the order has been changed depending on the client, or else techniques from both approaches have often been introduced simultaneously. Sometimes, instruments have also been used to facilitate work on fluency.

A different concept of integrated therapy was developed by the second author (CS) to merge fluency-shaping and stuttering management techniques. In this approach, fluency-facilitating behaviors (e.g., easy voice onsets, light contacts, etc.) are tailored specifically to the physical locations of tension produced by the client (e.g., easy voice onsets for glottal tension, etc.). These are employed either at the initiation of utterances (where stuttering is most apt to occur) or at the moments when stuttering occurs, as a form of pre-/in-/post-block management of saying the word. The methods are taught concurrently, not as fluency enhancement first and stuttering modification second. The fluency-facilitating behaviors are described as follows:

- Proper breath management—breathe in fully but not beyond; start exhalation just before initiating voice.
- Easy voice onsets—start voice gently with a gradual swell to appropriate loudness during the first vowel
- Slow rate—initiate the word gradually, stretch the vowel sounds, slide on to the next word
- Connect between words—continue voice throughout the words within a phrase, saying the phrase like it was one word; focus on moving forward to completion
- Light articulatory contacts—gently touch the lips, tongue, and other oral structures that come together for sounds; apply minimal pressure, release gradually to glide forward to the next sound

- Phrasing—group 3–6 syllables into a phrase; pause slightly between phrases; do not succumb to time pressure to start the next phrase right away; remember to connect between words within the phrase

Others have developed integrated therapies that are similar to those we have described. Schwartz's treatment approach teaches clients to apply speaking skills derived from a fluency-shaping orientation but borrows modification concepts of client responsibility and desensitization counseling to address and reduce emotional reactions. Especially beneficial to student clinicians, Schwartz (1999) offers plenty of examples of exact wording that may be used when teaching clients about topics such as the speech mechanism, slow and smooth speech initiation, connecting across word boundaries, counseling related to stuttering, and more.

Some other well-known examples of integrated therapies include Guitar (2006) and Manning (2001). It is interesting that simultaneously, but independently, the ISTAR Comprehensive Stuttering Program bears a striking similarity to EY's steps. It was first published by Boberg and Kully (1985) and recently updated by Kully, Langevin, and Lomheim (2007). This intensive 3-week program is typically conducted with groups but allows for individual delivery too. The acquisition phase progresses as follows:

1. Clients begin with learning to identify stuttering and reduce tension during stuttering.
2. Fluency skills, such as prolonged vowels, and light articulatory contacts are learned.
3. After all skills are acquired, they are refined and the speech rate is increased from 40 to 60 syllables per minute (spm) to 150 to 190 spm. Skills are practiced at each rate level.
4. Clients learn stuttering modification techniques, such as post-block, in-block, and pre-block.

An important feature of the program is the constant monitoring of progress through self-rating by clients, as well as their rating by peers and clinicians regarding performance and stuttering severity. There is also an effort throughout the program to develop cognitive-behavioral skills aimed at providing knowledge about stuttering, encouraging positive thoughts, understanding feelings, and self-acceptance.

With acquisition accomplished in the first few days of therapy, a very carefully structured maintenance regimen ensures fluent speech is implemented in many situations, with a variety of listeners, as well as in more formal presentations. The program ends with equally intensive preparation for the maintenance phase post-therapy with emphasis on daily warm-up and ongoing practice once the client leaves the clinic. Clinical outcome studies of 42 adolescent and adult participants indicated that after 1 year posttreatment, 10 clients relapsed. Of the remaining 32, 69% maintained a satisfactory level of stuttering frequency (under 3%) and 7% maintained a marginally satisfactory level (3% to 6%) of stuttering (Boberg & Kully, 1994). After 2 years, 80% of the clients reported that they were satisfied with their speech.

Summary

Speech-focused therapies are intended to teach a new way of managing either stuttering events or a style of speaking fluently. In either case, the client is challenged to abandon previous behaviors and adopt new ones, to stutter easier or apply strategies to speak fluently. The application of instruments, in contrast, appears to create conditions in which the speaker may talk fluently without specifically concentrating on the act of speech. Across individuals, the response to such devices varies widely, and a number have not found full or lasting relief. Speech clinicians must apply their independent professional judgment toward the selection of approaches among those described. It is expected that strategies and techniques will be adopted within the larger framework of a holistic process of change tailored to meet individual client needs. Although we cited data supporting some therapy programs, much of the current clinical research has not been particularly strong according to principles discussed in Chapter 9. Hence you should proceed with caution as you work with limited evidence, and be especially skeptical about media broadcasts with successful treatment claims. Research on treatment effects to date yields more support for forms of the fluency management compared to other approaches. The fact remains, however, that no intervention will work with all clients, and individual factors must be incorporated into therapeutic decisions.

STUDY QUESTIONS AND DISCUSSION TOPICS

1. What are the rationales for the identification and analysis of stutter events?
2. What are the rationales for the pause in the technique of post-block modification?
3. What are the major differences between stuttering management and fluency management approaches to stuttering intervention? Similarities?
4. What are the potential benefits and challenges associated with the use of fluency-inducing instruments for stuttering treatment?
5. What different techniques have been used to establish fluent speech in people who stutter?
6. Why is it not enough to simply establish fluent speech?
7. What different methods have been used to sustain fluent speech after it has been established?
8. What are the advantages and disadvantages of instruments in stuttering therapy?

SUGGESTED READINGS

Andrews, G., Guitar, B., & Howie, P. (1980). Meta-analysis of the effects of stuttering treatment. *Journal of Speech and Hearing Disorders, 45,* 287–307.

Guitar, B., & Peters, T. (Eds.). (2004). *Stuttering: An integration of contemporary therapies* (Book No. 16, 4th ed.). Memphis, TN: Stuttering Foundation of America.

Kully, D., Langevin, M., & Lomheim, H. (2007). Intensive treatment of stuttering in adolescent and adult. In E. Conture & R. Curlee (Eds.), *Stuttering and related disorders of fluency* (3rd ed.). New York: Thieme.

Ryan, B. (2001b). *Programmed stuttering therapy program for children and adults* (2nd ed.). Springfield, IL: Charles C. Thomas.

Schwartz, H. D. (1999). *A primer for stuttering therapy.* Boston: Allyn & Bacon.

Van Riper, C. (1973). *The treatment of stuttering.* Englewood Cliffs, NJ: Prentice Hall.

Chapter 12: Therapy for School-Age Children

LEARNER OBJECTIVES

Readers of this chapter will understand:

- Factors that distinguish school-age children who stutter from speakers at other ages who exhibit stuttering.
- Therapy techniques to manage the emotional and social aspects of stuttering in school-age children.
- Stuttering modification and fluency-enhancing techniques applied to school-age children.
- Methods for incorporating parents in the therapy program for school-age children.
- Current status of clinical research related to stuttering treatment for school-age children.

School-Age Children Who Stutter

Generally, the material discussed in this chapter pertains to children occupying the range between the first and sixth grades, typically ages 6 to 12. Although this is a useful frame of reference for organizational and didactic purposes, it is an arbitrary range in that some children at the lower end may be immature for their chronological age, whereas some at the upper end demonstrate advanced maturity for their age. Regardless of the extremes, it is impossible to address many issues discussed in this chapter as equally applied to first/second graders as to fifth/sixth graders. Just imagine a first-grade child and a sixth-grade child, and you will appreciate the differences. Hence you should understand that whatever is addressed here in regard to treatment of school-age children must be adjusted to the level of the individual. Besides the age-spread factor that is relatively large, there also is a relatively large spread in the length of the stuttering history within the group, depending on the age at onset and the current age. For example, a fifth grader who began stuttering at age 2 presents a 9-year history, whereas a second grader who began stuttering at age 4 has only a 4-year history. Their experience with stuttering and its consequences, therefore, are quite different.

Prior to discussing therapy, it would be sensible for clinicians to hone their knowledge of several characteristics of the stuttering disorder in school-age children and consider them when preparing to work with this group. These characteristics include aspects of stuttering persistence and awareness, emotionality and attitude, academic performance, overt speech characteristics and secondary body movements, social and peer responses, parental interactions, and therapy adaptations.

Because school-age children have stuttered for several years, they have bypassed much of the allotted chance for natural recovery, although some may still recover (Andrews & Harris, 1964; Yairi & Ambrose, 1999a). By now, these children exhibit chronic stuttering, more advanced both in its overt and covert manifestations, that is likely to persist for years.

> Those whose stuttering persists constitute a small minority among other children who began stuttering at about the same time as they did, most of whom have recovered. This minority apparently possesses extra genetic components, and perhaps also is influenced by additional environmental factors that result in chronic stuttering. All of these combine to make the disorder more resistant to amelioration, be it natural or in response to intervention. Hence the ultimate therapy prognoses are guarded and the therapeutic objectives are quite different from those set up for preschool-age children.

Awareness and Emotional Reactions

Being older, with a longer history and more developed cognition than preschoolers, the school-age child who stutters is highly aware of the stuttering (Bloodstein, 1960b) and in many cases has developed self-identification framed as "I am a stutterer." In turn, awareness of one's own stuttering is a major factor underlying the emergence of another important characteristic, a wide range of emotionality associated with the stuttered speech. It begins with feelings of frustration and embarrassment that are soon followed by much stronger reactions, such as shame and anxiety that lead to avoidance of speech. (See Chapter 4 for a more detailed discussion of the developing features of stuttering.) This emotionality also is nurtured by the heightened awareness of stuttering among the child's normally speaking peers, even at early grades as found in an experimental study (Ezrati-Vinacour, Platzky, & Yairi, 2001) and in response to a communication attitude questionnaire (De Nil & Brutten, 1991; Vanryckeghem & Brutten, 1997). Some classmates react overtly by mocking and bullying the stuttering child (Davis, Howell, & Cook, 2002). It is at this stage that the social impact of the disorder enters in and occupies a substantial portion of the picture. The fear and avoidance of speech, reinforced by peers and other people's reactions, can, and often does, spread to many situations, eventually leading to social withdrawal, the degree of which varies greatly.

One indication of others' attitudes is made evident in research findings showing that even speech-language clinicians working in the schools, the people who may be expected to be most understanding and accepting of children with communication disorders, hold negative stereotypes of school-age children who stutter (Yairi & Williams, 1970). All in all, a general alteration in the nature of the stuttering disorder is seen. Whereas at the very early stages, stuttering was primarily a disorder of speech difficulty, it now has become a disorder with significant emotional, social, and educational components that sometimes overshadow the speech aspect. As children advance to higher grades while they continue to stutter, more of them develop strong emotional reactions associated with stuttering (Rustin, Cook, & Spence, 1995). Furthermore, the child is likely to have only little, if any, understanding of the stuttering problem, adding to the complexity of emotions that appear in conjunction with the stuttered speech. Unrealistic explanations and erroneous beliefs take root. One child (EY) believed, perhaps correctly, that something wrong in his brain made him stutter and that if struck by lightning, his stutter would be cured. Thus he would walk in the empty streets during nights when particularly severe lightning storms brightened the sky. We worked with a second grader who, while circling his hand around his head, said in an emphatic tone that "something is wrong with my brain." Of course, children vary greatly in the speed and intensity of these new developments, which should be kept in mind as the clinician probes into the problem, planning therapy that deals with its significant variables.

Children may show complex emotional reactions to daily speaking demands at school that interfere with routine classroom tasks. Reading aloud or being called on to answer a question in class can be terrifying for a child who stutters. Fears are heightened regardless of whether the turns are up and down the rows so the child is able to anticipate what section of the material he or she is responsible for, or whether "popcorn" reading is required, where the teacher randomly picks children to read aloud. Some children who stutter intentionally drop their pencils as their turns come, thus creating a distraction that "causes" them to lose their place so the teacher will move on to the next child. Others will ask to be excused to the bathroom just as their turns come up.

It is reasonable to conclude that in addition to the overt stuttered speech, treatment may, or should, tackle the negative emotionality associated with (1) moments of stuttering and (2) self-image/self-confidence, as well as (3) social distracters, employing appropriate therapeutic procedures for the child's maturity level. Case Study 12.1 illustrates the emotional and social reactions of one child.

Case Study 12.1: *Emotional Reactions of a School-Age Child*

"As a school-age child, I (EY) had severe stuttering always hanging over my head. At times it was rather traumatic in its emotional and social impact. Progressing each year to the next grade, having new teachers and a few new children in the class with whom I had to deal (and stutter to), was repeatedly a tense period. I would be dreading the moment when 'they will find out' I stutter, especially those girls whom I happened to like. I avoided speaking in class as long as possible. Moving to another school was a real crisis for the same reasons, just twice magnified due to the larger number of new kids and teachers to meet and expose to my stuttering. When in the lower grades, I would at times cry in class when visitors, such as the principal or a supervisor, came

(continued)

Case Study 12.1: *Continued*

to the classroom and it was my turn to read aloud or answer a question. Throughout school, I used to carefully select my desk location, all in consideration of my stuttering and where I would be less likely to be targeted by the teacher to answer or read, or where I could minimize the impact of the stuttering on peers. A front seat was 'dangerous' because it exposed me directly to the teacher. Also, if I stuttered, the whole class behind me would smile or laugh. A back seat was also undesirable because if I stuttered, the stuttering would thunder over the entire class in front of me. I always ended up selecting a seat in the middle of a side row, by the wall or by the window. It took weeks of constant tension in a new classroom, being anxious that I might be called upon to recite in class, until I finally felt comfortable as the teachers 'learned,' more or less, how to deal with me, and the new kids 'learned' to accept my speech. Some teachers were really good and, in my judgment, contributed significantly to my eventual success."

Overt Stuttering

Another phenomenon or a characteristic of stuttering, mentioned briefly earlier (and in Chapter 4) can be seen as the disorder persists into the school-age years. For a good number of children, there is a significant alteration in the overt stuttering. Whereas repetitions were the most common disfluency type in an earlier period, now the proportion of sound prolongations and complete blocks increases, sometimes becoming dominant. Secondary characteristics, such as facial contortions and respiratory irregularities, increase in variety, frequency, and severity. These developments also contribute to the heightened awareness and emotionality. The implications to the treatment of school-age children are clear: Direct speech therapy should be a central approach. The children are capable of understanding and handling this kind of therapy, although they may be reluctant to apply the techniques outside the clinical space. This is quite different from past controversies regarding the propriety of direct therapy treatment for preschool-age children.

Academic Performance

One possible educational impact of stuttering is in the area of reading. A common practice for assessing the reading abilities of young children is by means of reading fluency measures, such as the Dynamic Indicators of Basic Early Literacy Skills, or DIBELS (Good & Kaminski, 2002). Reading fluency tasks include naming as many letters as possible, reading as many sight words as possible, or making as many rhyming words as possible in a minute. A child's results are compared to norms to determine whether he or she is developing important early literacy skills at a typical rate. For a child who stutters, performance on such tasks may be influenced by stuttering, leading to confusion regarding whether diminished performance is due to challenges with reading or with speaking.

Other possible areas of impact can be noted across a state's public school curriculum benchmarks. Iowa's core curriculum literacy benchmarks expect children in kindergarten to grade 2 to "demonstrate control of oral delivery skills, including using appropriate volume and vocal expression and attending to rate of delivery" (Iowa Department of Education, 2008). Virginia's English Standards of Learning (2003) require fifth-grade students to "maintain eye contact with listeners [English 5.2(a)]," and seventh-grade students to "communicate ideas and information orally in an organized and succinct manner [English 7.1(b)]." Stuttering may interfere with a child's ability to perform according to these benchmarks, potentially limiting his or her ability to make adequate educational progress. Furthermore, children who stutter who habitually say "I don't know," even when they do know an answer because "I don't know" is easier to say, may also risk lower academic grades that do not reflect their actual skills and knowledge. One high school student we know used the "I don't know" response so frequently in her chemistry class, her lack of oral participation points lowered her overall grade in the course to a D.

Keeping an eye on the child's academic achievements, therefore, is warranted because a few studies have reported that children who stutter were several months behind the average control group in either grade placement (Schindler, 1955) or standardized academic skill tests (Williams, Melrose, & Woods, 1969). Among other reasons, it is possible that these findings reflect avoidance of class participation by children who stutter, hence teachers' reluctance to call on them, and a resultant diminished academic effort on the child's part.

The School and Home Factors

As children who stutter progress into the school setting, they are transported from the relatively limited environment of home or day care center, with a small staff and a small group of kids of similar age, into a significantly expanded world of many children of different ages, larger number of adults, rules, more structured schedules, and so on. Although parents typically maintain centrality in the child's life, teachers and peers assume significant influence. Hence knowing the child's setting and circumstances in the class, including teachers' and peers' attitudes, can help the clinician terminate bad situations (e.g., peers imitating the child's speech). Furthermore, the clinician may be able to alter peers' attitudes in a positive way, recruiting their cooperation in protecting the child from others. As we discuss later, teacher cooperation may be employed as well in facilitating the work done in speech therapy. Therapy also should be oriented to train the child to properly handle adverse situations at school. Consideration must also be given to the setting in which treatment is delivered and its format. A child who attends speech therapy in the public school may receive shorter therapy time per week than in private settings. Not only may therapy time be shorter, public school treatment must often be conducted in groups, not in a one-on-one format. Hence the child may have fewer opportunities to practice new behaviors because treatment time is shared with other children who need opportunities to practice their own new skills.

Although the child's world has been expanded, as mentioned earlier, parents continue to play a central role in the child's life. Therefore, their participation in the overall therapy program always would be wise to consider. This can be in the form of counseling, as well as active participation in the carryover of the therapy to home (Mallard, 1991). Parents, for example, can remind the child to use the speech patterns practiced in therapy or can conduct brief practice sessions at home (which is actually required by some programs). We strongly believe that parental involvement in the therapy, even in small ways, can substantially increase its effectiveness.

The Age Factor

Lastly in this list of characteristics, the school-age child who stutters is, in most respects, like others of the same age. For example, because children have not yet developed adult levels of cognition, the clinician's explanations of stuttering, instructions, and rationales given for therapeutic procedures, and so on, should be brief, presented in simple, concrete language, and accompanied by lots of visible illustrations and demonstrations. Another example is in the level of responsibility assumed in conjunction with therapy. Whereas adult clients are expected to carry out their own various home assignments, such as making a set number of telephone calls each day, or voluntarily entering conversation with a set number of strangers, second graders should not be expected to perform these kinds of assignments.

Motivation also may be problematic. Whereas adults refer themselves to therapy, young children are referred and brought by parents. Although the child who stutters wants to speak better, other attractions (e.g., extracurricular sports activities) compete with going to the speech clinic. The decisions associated with activity selections often present major dilemmas for parents. Most parents want their child in therapy hoping to diminish the amount and impact of stuttering before the child gets any older. At the same time, they see the value of their child having a variety of interests and skills and the importance of other activities to their child's self-esteem. In an ideal world, the child does both, but in reality parents sometimes have to choose between the Tuesday-Thursday speech therapy session and the Tuesday-Thursday baseball league. There is not one right answer; the best decision will be different for each individual.

Prognosis and Objectives for Therapy

Why Is Stuttering in School-Age Children Difficult to Treat?

The literature on stuttering includes many opinions advocating clinical intervention soon after stuttering onset, typically during the preschool period (e.g., Ingham & Cordes, 1998). The main argument put forward by these scholars and clinicians is that difficulty achieving a cure, or even appreciable progress in stuttering therapy by the time a child enters school, stems from the failure to provide early intervention. They go on to argue that by the time children reach school age, they have bypassed the window of brain plasticity that would have enabled therapy to cause changes in brain processes responsible for speech. Thus stuttering becomes less amenable to treatment. Indeed, clinicians have concluded from experience that it is much more difficult to achieve successful treatment with this age group (also with adults) as compared with reported successes for preschool-age children (e.g., Conture, 2001; Ward, 2006).

If their assertion that school-age children do not respond to stuttering therapy as readily as preschool children is valid, as we believe it is, we hold to a different explanation. In our opinion, the prognosis for school-age children, like that for adults (see Chapter 9), must take into account the critical role of the epidemiological factors that contributed to the persistent form of stuttering. As explained in Chapter 3, school-age children are a small minority (25%, perhaps as small as 15%) of the original population who began stuttering about the same time. This minority failed to exhibit the natural recovery exhibited by 75% or more of their stuttering peers. Current research in statistical genetics as well as genotyping (Ambrose, Cox, & Yairi, 1997; Suresh et al., 2006) has shown that genetics is an important factor underlying both natural recovery and chronic stuttering. Hence the difficulties encountered in treating stuttering in school-age children may simply reflect a genetically based, tenacious, more robust, resistant form of stuttering: a different subtype of the disorder. Quite likely, it would have resisted therapy if provided in early years, an assumption supported by the findings that almost all preschool participants in the large Illinois project who persisted did receive therapy (Yairi & Ambrose, 2005). Therefore, the idea that treatment difficulty in school-age children is the fault of negligence to treat them earlier as young children, and that these difficulties should be assigned to lost brain plasticity previously available, not only fails to recognize the role of genetics, it could have some negative effects as well. First, it places undue pressure to begin treatment as early as possible after onset, when actually it might not be necessary in view of the high rate of natural recovery during that period. Second, if clinicians fail to appreciate that school-age children who stutter present a genetically different subtype of stuttering that is inherently more resistant, it may cause an unjustified sense of failure in clinicians and clients alike and promote misguided, unrealistically high therapeutic objectives. This also can contribute to clinicians' perceptions that they are "bad" at stuttering therapy, which can lead to negative attitudes toward children who stutter as a group.

Therapy Alternatives and Objectives

Both Van Riper (1973) and Williams (1971) opined that therapy for the school-age child who stutters frequently takes the form of adult therapy with some modifications. We believe that, in general, therapeutic objectives similar to those set out for adults also may be applied to school-age children who stutter. The main difference between therapy for the two groups is not so much in the objectives but in the procedures employed that are adapted to the child's level. As discussed in Chapter 8, there are three major alternatives to consider when setting up long-term therapeutic objectives for stuttering: increased fluency, reduced stuttering, and improved emotional and social adjustment. We believe that all three should be incorporated, or at least considered, in formulating the objectives for the individual client. For many years, we have practiced comprehensive therapy programs that incorporate these different major approaches.

Under the increased fluency alternative, two subcategories, *naturally fluent* speech and *deliberate fluent* speech, were listed. It has been shown experimentally that it is possible for preschool-age children who stutter to achieve naturally fluent speech that is indistinguishable from that of normally speaking peers (Finn, Ingham, Ambrose, & Yairi, 1997). This outcome also entails that the child feels, thinks, and behaves like normally speaking individuals. Unfortunately, close scientific examination of the normalcy of post-therapy speech in school-age children has not been documented. Although achieving naturally fluent speech patterns and all the psychological domains of normal speaking might be possible for school-age children,[1] particularly in lower grades, it is very difficult to erase the self-concept of a "stutterer" and the feeling that stuttering is still there, just waiting to resurface. We feel, therefore, that achieving *deliberately fluent* speech is a more reasonable initial objective. The tenacity of stuttering by this age means that for a fairly long time, fluency will be consciously "controlled" and self-monitored. The child will have to exercise a form of mental and behavioral activity to maintain fluency, which can be daunting at any age.

The idea behind the second alternative, lessening the abnormality of overt stuttering, is quite different. Here, the client does not strive to be fluent but strives to be able to manage speech movements during stuttering events, movements that yield milder, smooth stuttering that is more acceptable to listeners (Van Riper, 1973). Lastly, improved adjustment pertains to changing the broad spectrum of emotional and social behaviors related to speaking. This includes helping the child carefully confront a variety of difficult speaking situations, respond to and cope with potential teasing, and, above all, choose to continue to communicate even when stuttering. Such changes are important in strengthening the client's ability to either work on fluency or on modifying stuttering. Additionally, reducing emotionality also may result in less frequent stuttering as a by-product.

> Clinicians must strike a careful balance between encouraging the goal of easier, smooth speech along with fostering a positive emotional self-acceptance of experiences with stuttering. This balance is necessary because if a premium is placed on attaining fluency, the child may infer that his or her stuttering is unacceptable and be apt to develop behaviors that merely suppress stuttering. Suppression may be evident, for example, if after a few weeks of therapy, the SLD have significantly decreased, but the Other Disfluencies, such as interjected "ums," have increased. It is best therefore to conduct therapy in the safe environment where stuttering and its modification are acceptable by the clinician at the same time that strategies for fluent speech are explored and practiced.

Speaking partner behavioral adjustments commonly applied during intervention with preschool children are also appropriate with school-age children. Specifically, both the clinician and parents can serve as role models of a slower, relaxed approach to talking, of appropriate pausing and phrasing, of frequent easy initiations of speech,

---

[1] It has been reported that speech therapy can alter the brain waves of people who stutter (e.g., De Nil, Kroll, & Houle, 2001). The author (Yairi) believes future advances with medical treatments may yield an increasing number of complete cures.

and of showing restraint from interruptions and simultaneous talking.[2] A blend of these less direct strategies of environmental support can be combined with the direct instruction offered in treatment sessions. When a school-age child does not have firmly entrenched avoidance habits, objectives designed to prevent or reduce avoidance may be appropriate. Specifically, the child can be encouraged to go ahead with talking whether stuttering occurs or not, in safe environments created by the clinician and supportive speaking partners, to counteract the natural inclinations to hold back or struggle against the act of speech that serve to exacerbate stuttering. Treatment objectives for school-age children otherwise do not differ substantially from those set for adults. For example, objectives may be set for the child to learn about speech and stuttering, to reduce negative emotionality associated with stuttering, to develop assertiveness and self-confidence, to identify and modify stuttering, and/or to facilitate fluency-related skills. The main difference between therapy for adults and school-age children lies in the procedures employed to achieve these objectives and the cognitive and linguistic sophistication of the discussions held between the clinician and child. Of considerable importance, particularly for school-age children, is to promote and encourage appropriate forms of support in the child's home and school environments. Like adults, every child's needs will be different, and so therapy must be individualized.

School-based clinicians may be familiar with the phrase "adversely affects educational performance" (from IDEA, 1997), a key criterion indicating whether children who stutter are eligible to receive speech therapy. Unfortunately, the widely recognized phrase is often misunderstood. Some have interpreted it to mean that stuttering must adversely affect a child's grades in order for the student to be eligible for treatment. This, however, is not the case. The 2004 reauthorization of IDEA actually increased the accessibility of services for children who stutter by emphasizing not only academic performance or speech characteristics but also how stuttering affects other aspects of the child's life. In other words, school-based clinicians should broaden their focus to consider not only the academic issues but also the academic setting. Under IDEA 2004,[3] the academic setting is defined as encompassing regular education classrooms, other education-related settings, extracurricular, and nonacademic activities. This means that not only should the impact of the child's stuttering on performance in the classroom be considered, but also how it impacts success with communication at recess, on the school bus, at lunchtime, and in interactions with peers during school-sponsored clubs and activities. This broader view of the educational impact of stuttering allows for inclusion of a variety of goals in the child's treatment, such as improving communication attitudes, reducing negative reactions to stuttering, educating people in the child's environment, and minimizing the overall impact of the child's stuttering in many domains.

---

[2] The aim of involving parents as role models has a dual purpose. Parents are less apt to adopt unreasonable expectations of their child's ongoing deliberate fluency control when they have attempted ongoing speech changes of themselves and appreciate how difficult the endeavor actually is.

[3] For more information on IDEA 2004, visit http://idea.ed.gov/explore/home.

Too often, school-based speech-language clinicians have set up goals for a child who stutters aimed at the elimination of the stuttering. Because of the persistent nature of stuttering in this population, defining the stuttering disorder as only speech behaviors, and relying only on a decrease in those speech behaviors as therapeutic success, clinicians run into failure of their own making while also overlooking important areas where they can help the child in meaningful ways, such as developing more helpful attitudes about communication that lessen the social impact of the disorder. With the school-age population, what is the success rate for getting children who stutter to be normally fluent all the time? Likely, not very high. If we use a broad-based definition of the disorder, taking into account the child's overall communication experience, therapy can be much more successful. In other words, if stuttering is more than just stuttered speech, then treatment should be more than just speech-focused. Throughout the therapeutic process, parents and teachers need to understand that progress is not measured only in terms of fluency. Goals that are included on a student's Individualized Education Plan should reflect the view that progress can be shown in many ways, not just in decreased disfluency.

Goals designed to reduce the child's negative attitudes, as well as the behavioral and cognitive reactions that accompany stuttering, are essential to the creation of a broad-based approach toward stuttering management. For example, goals such as "stuttering easily, strengthen self-confidence, and feel good about self" seem to be more desired than just "no stuttering and using easy onsets." School-age children who stutter often are relieved to hear this, although parents may have more difficulty accepting the probability that their child will continue to stutter. This is another reason why parent counseling is such an important component to school-age stuttering therapy.

Another issue in stating goals is the criteria sought to achieve them. In speech-language pathology, many goals for clients, regardless of the disorder, are stated using a percentage-based metric (e.g., "client will do . . . 80% of the time"). Although this structure is legitimate for use in generating goals for a school-age child who stutters, clinicians also should consider other forms of measurement. One way is to develop a list of achievements the child can pursue along a hierarchy from easier to harder situations. For example, if the child's goal is for him or her to be able to educate others about stuttering, it does not make sense to state the child should be able to do this 80% of the time. Instead, the clinician could document that the child can demonstrate the skill in a variety of settings, such as with the teacher, peer, or parents. A criterion for this type of activity might be written as an all-or-none achievement, such as "the child will educate three individuals about stuttering." If the child does it, a check mark is made, indicating success; if the child has not done it, then no check. Using this method, both clinician and child can see the level of progress by counting up the number of checks on the goal chart, comparing it to the total number of situations listed in the hierarchy. Another example of an alternative measurement criterion may be used for documenting changes in a child's fear or anxiety about a particular speaking situation. The clinician can ask the child to rate the intensity of his or her fear/anxiety before and after entering the situation using a self-rating system on a 1 to 10 scale. The criterion could then be set to a change in self-rating of 2 or more points.

Home and School Environments

Although the school-age child's world is an ever-expanding experience beyond home and family, parents still constitute a major component of that world and should be included in the therapy scene if at all possible. The physical conditions, however, present challenges. Because most schoolchildren in need receive speech therapy on the school's premises during regular hours, parents are not the ones bringing them in, nor are they present after the session as is the case with many preschool children. Hence the clinician's opportunities for contact with the parents are greatly diminished. Furthermore, mothers of school-age children are more likely to work outside the home than mothers of preschool-age children, a fact that also limits their availability. Recognizing the difficulties, all efforts should be made to have at least one or two meetings with the child's parents early in the program, as well as at least some periodic contact throughout via brief written or e-mail (if available) notes sent to the home. Because the home environment is explored through parent counseling, attention should be given to three objectives: providing information about stuttering, venting parents' feelings, and reduction of interfering factors.

Counseling Parents

Information About Stuttering

We first probe parents concerning their knowledge about stuttering that they may have acquired from various sources, such as the Internet, newspaper articles, relatives, doctors, and others. Misinformation should be dispelled, followed by a brief presentation of the essential state-of-the-art information. One pair of parents suspected that their child stutters as punishment for *their* misbehavior, an inaccurate tax report. One father was convinced that his child stuttered to annoy him. Responding to the most frequently asked question, "What causes stuttering?" the clinician proceeds by presenting the main theoretical views about stuttering: psychological, learning, organic, and multiple causation, succinctly explaining each one. In this context, it is useful to point out that research has not provided reasonable support to the psychological and learning theories, although the two factors do play an important role in the further development and maintenance of the disorder. For example, emotional reactions often become an important part of the disorder *after* it has begun. These emotional components are the result of stuttering, not the cause of it as laypeople and some health professionals, e.g., pediatricians, tend to believe (Yairi & Carrico, 1992). Moreover, recent research findings have implicated intricate neurological and motor components. These data, combined with information about the genetic bases of stuttering, should serve to alleviate possible parents' guilt feelings, blaming their behavior as the cause of the stuttering.

Additional information about the variability of stuttering, what may trigger ups and down in its frequency, and the emotional and social implications of stuttering should be provided. Many parents are aware mostly of the overt stuttering. Because many, if not most, schoolchildren rarely share their concerns about stuttering with parents, and because parents often feel uncomfortable asking, they have a vague, or no, idea of the devastating emotional components of the disorder. They may not know, for example, that their child sits tense during class, dreading being called to answer a question or recite something, that he fears the ringing telephone at home, or that she suffers mockery by a few kids in school. Some parents were utterly shocked to discover situations like these when watching behind a two-way mirror as their child conversed with us. The fact that environment plays a substantial role in the shaping and maintenance of stuttering should be used to advise parents that they can create more favorable conditions at home that might improve the child's life. Later on, they may be asked to contribute in other ways to the therapy program. Simple suggestions for reducing undue stressful communication demands on the child, avoiding or minimizing other unnecessary pressures at home, stopping parents' and/or siblings' negative responses to stuttering, reviewing and alleviating other stressful family interaction patterns, and concrete suggestions for how to handle the child's moments of stuttering should be offered and discussed. It is also wise to teach and encourage parents to notice when their child is communicating well, such as telling a funny story, finishing a difficult word, being polite, or taking conversational turns. Focusing on desired communication behaviors is as important as focusing exclusively on stuttering, so that the child develops awareness of what he or she needs to do to be a good communicator whether stuttering or not. Because this may be a rare opportunity for having face-to-face communication with one or both parents, a brief and simple presentation of only several key suggestions is recommended.

Attending to Parents' Feelings

Having lived with the child's stuttering for several years, some parents may have toned down the initially strong emotional reactions they had at the time of onset. They may try not to call negative attention to it and have become accustomed to hearing their child's abnormal speech. It does not mean, however, that they are at peace with the handicap—nor does it mean that strong emotions will not resurface. It's not uncommon for parents to become highly anxious or upset when important life events present themselves, such as the child transitioning from elementary to middle school, because communication demands can be quite different. Other life events that may cause parents anxiety include religious rituals such as confirmation or a bar mitzvah, making a speech to earn Eagle Scout status, or trying out for a school play. Being worried about the social consequences of stuttering, parents may have become highly protective. Parents naturally want what is best for their child; they do not want him or her to experience the pain or shame of stuttering. Protectiveness may lead to limiting social interactions for those children who stutter, speaking for them in public places, and making decisions about social arrangements based on the stuttering. They (parents) may develop compensatory habits themselves, stepping in to bridge the gap for the child's difficulty initiating communication. Because public stuttering may bring pain and embarrassment to parents and family as well as the child, their nonverbal behaviors and management of situations may send a big message that stuttering is a stigma. But the problem is that the message to "avoid stuttering" will thereby suggest "avoid communicating." The child's avoidance of communication is worse than openly stuttering. Neither the family nor the child may realize they are taking this path.

Our clinical experience has shown that many parents remain concerned about the stuttering, disappointed in their hopes for recovery, frustrated by their inability to help and/or by unsuccessful treatment, concerned about the child's current suffering as well as his or her future (e.g., career), and sometimes continue to harbor guilt feelings about their possible contribution to the disorder. DiLollo and Manning (2007) opined that parents of children who continue to stutter can exhibit many grieving reactions, such as denial, anger, and depressions. Therefore, within the limited opportunities available for interacting with parents, spending a portion of the time to allow them to express their feelings certainly is beneficial. It also provides the clinician with insight into the child's more intricate and intimate home environment and the kind of cooperation that might be possible to gain from parents. A few simple questions are often sufficient to facilitate this avenue. Some of these may have been discussed as part of the initial evaluation if the parents participated. For example, (1) What happened when stuttering began? (2) What did you think caused it? (3) How did you react then? (4) How do you feel about it now? (5) What kind of a child is your son/daughter? Tell me about his/her personality, strengths, and weaknesses. (6) Does he/she spend time with friends? We have found these or similar questions enable most parents to talk at length. As DiLollo and Manning (2007) suggested, the next goal is to encourage the parents to redirect their emotional energy from grieving toward involvement in the treatment and supporting the child. Parental participation in a support group, if one is accessible, can facilitate understanding and support for the child (Manning, 2001). Parents are more apt to listen to the clinician and apply her practical suggestions if the clinician has developed sufficient rapport first, providing supportive listening and ample opportunity for venting of emotions.

Interfering Factors

Another objective to pursue with parents is the identification of factors that might interfere with, or facilitate progress. This can be achieved by directing a few questions that probe relations among the family members, such as: (1) How do your spouse and other children react to the stuttering? (2) How do the children get along? (3) Do you talk about the stuttering at home? (4) Do you and your spouse agree on how to handle the child's stuttering? And (5) Generally, how are things at home these days? As is the case with preschoolers, parents of school-aged children can enhance the child's progress by offering at home a number of practical support strategies. Research indicates that communication partners can support fluent speech with several behaviors: slowing the pace of their conversational speech, following rules of conversational turn-taking (i.e., not interrupting), and delaying their conversational responses (Bernstein Ratner, 2004). Perhaps more than anything else, just encouraging their child to go ahead and express what he or she wants to say, even if there is stuttering, is the most important type of support parents can offer. Providing an environment where the child feels free to talk openly about his or her speech and stuttering is another important way parents can support their child. Parents are often unsure that talking openly about stuttering with their child is a good idea. This is where a clinician can be especially helpful to the family. Schoolteachers as well as parents can be apprised of these strategies.

Teachers and Peers

If you talk with adults who stutter about their past experiences in elementary school as children who stutter, you may hear different stories about experiences with schoolteachers. Although some are remembered as sensitive, understanding, and supportive, others are remembered for responses to stuttering that brought pain to them as a child. Examples of the latter are anecdotes about teachers who made a child put marbles in his mouth or who stood by passively when peers mocked or laughed. Even when an infraction is minor and the teacher meant well, the pain of embarrassment or unfair treatment can be indelibly inked in a child's memories. These memorable responses by teachers can come from opposite sides of the coin, either circumstances for talking were unusually spotlighted or the child was unfairly deprived of an opportunity to speak. The findings of two studies illustrate some of the potential problems in the school environment. The first one asked school speech-language clinicians to assign adjectives to children who stutter, resulting in a list of rather negative personality descriptors and other unfavorable characteristics (Yairi & Williams, 1970). More than two decades later, a group of investigators used similar methods targeting schoolteachers with similar results: Teachers hold a predominantly unfavorable, stereotypic view of the characteristics of a child who stutters (Lass et al., 1992).

To help teachers and children avert these potential unpleasant experiences and painful memories, it is vitally important for the clinician to educate teachers and school personnel about stuttering. Teachers need to know about the need to check in with the child privately regarding the types of talking opportunities she or he will be comfortable with in school. They need to know that the child who stutters often wants and needs to talk even if he or she stutters but also to be sensitive to averting talking circumstances that can be too fear-filled and emotionally threatening. Having reached an understanding with the child, possible ways to facilitate class participation initially might be to ask the child questions that require short answers or to have the child demonstrate on the blackboard step-by-step solutions to math problems that can be done with minimal talking demands. Besides, it is quite likely that if the child talks while writing on the board, there will be no stuttering. They also may reach an understanding that the child will not be asked to read aloud to the whole class, if the child so wishes. Use of simple cues, such as the child raising a closed hand to indicate "I know the answer, but please don't call on me," versus an open hand to indicate "I know the answer and would like to be called on," can be negotiated by the teacher and child so that the child is encouraged to participate to the degree that feels safe. Teachers (or adults, parents, etc.) should not make a unilateral decision to exclude a child from a speaking task without checking in with the child. The speech clinician needs to communicate with the teacher and parents about the level of participation appropriate to the child's progress with therapy, and facilitate, with all involved, a hierarchy that moves the child toward greater classroom communication at a rate that keeps fear at a minimum.

Teachers need to understand the nature of the potential anxiousness that can build up prior to being called on, before having to say one's name, or when expected to take a turn talking in front of peers. This may be one of the difficult things to achieve because most people simply are unaware of the strong emotional component of stuttering. The teacher needs to appreciate his or her important role to instruct peers not to laugh at or tease or think less of the child who stutters. Teachers should be educated about the general objectives of the therapy program and the general procedure. When therapy is focused on certain behaviors (e.g., pullouts or gentle voice onset), a cooperative teacher is in a position to provide reinforcement, although not in front of the class. Teachers also may be advised that stuttering can be addressed in the class within units on diversity. Everyone has different characteristics, and how one talks is just one such difference, like height, weight, or skin color. A number of available curricular programs for preventing teasing and bullying apply to all students in a classroom, not just the student who stutters.

The speech clinician also needs to ensure that teachers and other school personnel are provided with basic facts about stuttering. They need to know that children can be very intelligent and still stutter and that periods of fluency do not mean the child has an ability to control or stop stuttering from occurring. It is important to dispel the misguidance of popular folklore that has been passed around, like the belief that stuttering was caused by the parents. School personnel need to have their questions answered, such as: "Can I look directly at the child when he talks, or is that apt to make him stutter more?" Teachers should also feel confident that if they have a question about how to handle a given situation with a specific child, that it's okay to talk with that child about his or her wishes. Here is our brief information sheet that clinicians may hand to teachers (and other school personal) who have a child who stutters in their class.

Children Who Stutter: Basic Information and Advice for Teachers

1. Most children begin stuttering between ages 2 and 4. The school-age child who stutters (CWS) has had several years of unpleasant experiences with the disorder.
2. Stuttering is not a "bad habit." Although the specific cause is not known, it is related to genetics but also is very sensitive to environmental forces, such as pressure and people's reactions to it.
3. The disorder afflicts the child in several ways, with the two most important being (a) the observable speech difficulties, and (b) the strong emotional reactions, often hidden, especially shame and intense fears of talking that lead to avoidance. If asked a question in the class, the CWS may reply, "I do not know" just because he or she is afraid of stuttering in front of the other children. The child's apprehension can rise substantially just anticipating

(continued)

that he or she will be asked to recite orally. An experience of severe stuttering in class may cause devastation for several days.

4. Aside from the overt stuttering and emotions associated with it, research has shown that CWS, as a group, are similar to children who do not stutter in nearly all other respects (e.g., personality and intelligence).

5. Children who stutter may experience serious difficulties when they move to a new school and face a new teacher and new peers who become acquainted with the fact that they stutter. They may feel extremely embarrassed, especially at the beginning of the year when their stuttering is first "exposed." The first 2 to 3 weeks are especially critical for teachers to be understanding and provide support and comfort to the child.

6. The testimonies of many CWS and their parents indicate that the teacher's understanding and cooperation can be critical to emotional experiences in school in ways that the speech-language clinician may be unable to impact. The most important areas where teachers can help are (a) peers' reactions toward the child who stutters, (b) class participation, and (3) cooperation and support (to varying degrees) with the speech therapy.

7. Not infrequently, the CWS is the subject of mockery, sometimes bullying. A single inconsiderate classmate can make life miserable for the child. The teacher should be alert to this possibility. You may observe such peers' behavior or you may learn about it through an open talk with the CWS. The offender should be confronted and counseled individually. Also, you may explain to the whole class about the damage that such behavior might inflict. Do so when the CWS is not in the classroom.

8. In regard to the child's verbal participation in class, it is best to have an open discussion with him or her privately and come to an agreement as to the desired type and frequency of oral recitation. For example, the child may prefer to respond to questions that call for brief answers but not like to read aloud. Alternatively, or additionally, solving math problems on the blackboard could be a desired mode of participation, for example. Teachers also may call on the child early before anxiety builds too much or when they know the child has the answer to the question.

9. There are several conditions in which the CWS typically experiences fluent speech. For example, singing, talking in chorus, talking in rhythm, making movement while talking, speaking in a different dialect, high or low pitch, whispering, and so on. These can be used to allow participation in plays and other class projects involving verbal performance.

10. Teachers can contribute substantially to the success of speech therapy in ways that require minimal time. As the child practices various ways of changing speaking behaviors in therapy, such as maintaining eye contact, slowing down, or reducing tension during a stuttered word, some feedback in class is important. You can employ two or three agreed-upon nonverbal

signals (e.g., one as a reminder to the child to use the technique, one for reinforcement of good performance, etc.). Again, this should be discussed with the child and the speech-language clinician.

Additional information for teachers may be found in several other sources:

Rind, P., & Rind, E. (1988). *The stutterer in the classroom: A guide to the teacher.* New Rochelle, NY: Stuttering Resource Foundation. Also see www.stutterisa.org/CDRomProject/teacher/teacher_main.html

Scott, L. (2008). *The child who stutters at school: Notes to the teacher.* Memphis, TN: Stuttering Foundation of America. Also see www.stutteringhelp.org/download/0042nttt.pdf

Stammering Association. Information for teachers at www.stammering.org/teachers_info.html

Therapy: Explaining Stuttering

As mentioned earlier, what is happening during stuttering is somewhat of a mystery to most people who stutter, certainly to children. An early goal to pursue in therapy is to provide the child with a reasonable understanding of the stuttering in the context of speech production in general (Williams, 1971). Some of the ways that this objective can be accomplished are described next.

The Speech System

Using a simple three-dimensional model or a good-sized diagram of the upper body, the clinician explains the sequence of events that result in speech: inhaling air, exhaling it through the two vocal folds ("voice box") that vibrate to produce voice, continuing upward into the throat and mouth. The air forces its way out through a series of moving parts in the mouth, such as the tongue, lips, and jaw, that results in many other speech sounds, depending on the shape and postures of these structures. The emphasis is on the continuous, smooth movement that characterizes normal speech. This can be demonstrated by the clinician as she talks, highlighting the ongoing movement of her lips, jaw, and tongue (Guitar, 2006; Williams, 1971). Simple and descriptive terms can be applied, such as the *speech helpers* suggested by Runyan and Runyan (1986).

What Can Go Wrong with the Speech System?

The clinician may count on the probability that many schoolchildren have had opportunities to observe babies as they start learning to talk by uttering many repetitions and stretching sounds and syllables (i.e., babbling), to eventually master short words and brief phrases. These disfluencies are normal. Many older children and adults continue to occasionally hesitate when talking or repeat and stretch sounds and syllables. This too is normal. We do not know why, but some children begin repeating and prolonging much more than the usual and also with much more tension. This is different. This kind of speech is made worse when the person becomes concerned about the repetitions and prolongations, gets even more uptight, and tries to force the words out by tensing up the speech muscles in many places (point to them in the diagram). The more one tenses, the more difficult it becomes to have the speech system move smoothly. *This is what stuttering is.* It is the tensing and forcing that causes much of the stuttering and the unpleasant feeling of getting stuck. In other words, an emphasis is placed on the idea that children are making talking harder for themselves. They need to go ahead and let themselves talk instead of investing so much energy fighting the stuttering. This also is an opportunity to point out other activities in which children are engaged that do not go well or even fail when the child gets panicked and uses excessive tension attempting to get out of it (e.g., activities like learning how to ride a bicycle or swim). Tensed, panicked, disorganized movement is what gets swimmers to feel they are drowning.

Experimentation

At this point, the child is encouraged to experiment with speaking behaviors that actually make talking difficult or impossible altogether. For example, inhale, then tighten the throat on purpose, then attempt to speak. Nothing comes out, neither air nor speech. Similarly, the child is asked to speak while purposely pressing the lips together, or talk while forcing the tongue against the hard palate. This is what Dean Williams (1971) wisely referred to as *hard speech*. Next, proceeding with additional experimentation, the opposite concept, *easy speech,* is soon brought into play by asking the child to first say a word the hard way and then say it again easily, without physical tension.

The difference between *hard speech* and *easy speech* also can be illustrated with nonspeech behaviors, say by asking the child to shake hands "really hard" and then do it again easily, gently, and slowly. Several comparisons of hard and easy speech are practiced. Children thus gain some insight into their own contribution to the stuttering and also may begin realizing that they can do something about it. Overall, such demonstration and experimentation are effective ways to have children comprehend more abstract explanations of the problem of stuttering that the clinician provides. The fact that they can change from hard to easy speech also should help in reducing the upheaval that the child often experiences during stuttering. At this point, limited practice is sufficient. At a later stage in the therapy, when the program is focused on identification and speech modification, much more extensive practice will be resumed.

> The process of strengthening the client's learning by contrasting two opposing behaviors is called *negative practice*. In fluency therapy, the experience of flexibly performing the *hard speech* versus the *easy speech* highlights the parameters of the easy speech that the child is endeavoring to learn. The procedure is similar to the negative practice employed in articulation therapy, where a child is required to contrastively produce a target phoneme in both the incorrect and correct ways to enhance learning of the new skill.

Therapy: Handling Emotional Reactions

School-age children who stutter present a wide range of emotions reacting to, and resulting from, stuttering. Clinicians, however, should exercise caution against undue generalization. Just because a child stutters, he or she does not necessarily possess strong reactions; some children show no hesitation responding to, or initiating, telephone calls, whereas others make themselves disappear as soon as the phone rings. Smith (1999) referred to this as the nonlinearity of the stuttering problem. Making assumptions about a child's emotional reactions based on the severity of the speech behavior should be avoided. We knew one child whose overt stuttering was approximately 4%, or very mild in severity. Her speech was very smooth and natural and only occasionally disrupted by brief repetitions. This child, however, was terrified to be called on in class and would engage in a number of avoidance strategies such as asking to go to the bathroom if she anticipated the teacher was going to ask her a question. Another child who presented with severe stuttering, including long blocks and visible facial tension, always volunteered to be the reporter for his small groups during class projects. Hence some prior probing of this domain is warranted. If problems are identified, a comprehensive stuttering treatment program should address them in a direct manner, in addition to whatever other approach(es), aimed at the speech aspect, are pursued. This is an example of a therapeutic objective that is similar to that encountered in adult therapy. The question, however, is how this objective can be best accomplished with children. As suggested earlier, taking a milder (less aggressive) approach is the key: simple presentation of the problem and the therapy objective, use of concrete instead of abstract language, avoidance of lengthy abstract explanations but use of ample meaningful examples, simplified procedures, and demands that are not too challenging. As with adults, we advocate a two-pronged approach when working on the emotional aspect. One approach is aimed at diminishing negative emotionality by means of desensitization. The second approach is aimed at increasing positive self-perception and assertiveness.

Adapted Desensitization Activities

Applying a milder approach, particularly with children in lower grades for whom desensitization is deemed necessary, procedures should not require the child to enter boldly into unpleasant or challenging situations as is sometimes employed with adults. For example, an 8-year-old should not be asked to go up to a stranger and hold on to a stutter for seconds while attempting to remain calm. Van Riper (1973) has commented that the *systematic desensitization* technique is not particularly useful with schoolchildren. For early steps, exposure to stuttering identification techniques is useful, such as having the child identify *hard speech* events made purposefully by the clinician, or in video or audio speech samples that she had recorded of her own speech. Van Riper (1973) also recommended that clinicians put stuttering in their own mouth for various purposes. These activities begin with exposure to mild-to-moderate rather than severe stuttering. If the child is ready to describe the feelings, reactions are elicited and discussed. Videos of other children and adults who stutter that are available for purchase as part of various clinical programs also are very useful for this purpose (e.g., *Stuttering: For Kids by Kids*, distributed by the Stuttering Foundation of America). Besides providing greater exposure to stuttering, selecting samples of gradually more severe stuttering, such videos help make the point that the child is not alone in stuttering. Children also may find comfort from age-appropriate literature containing characters who stutter. An example is the "Mary Maroney" book series by Suzy Kline in which the main character is a second-grade girl who stutters. Another is found in a story about a squirrel who stutters who learns about self-respect in *Stuttering Stan Takes a Stand* by Artie Knapp. A Web site with a list of children's literature that deals with stuttering can be found at: www.mnsu.edu/comdis/kuster/Bookstore/childrensbooks.html

Because a sense of isolation is one of the most difficult aspects of stuttering, finding videos of children, even older children who stutter, who talk about their experiences can be helpful. If a group therapy experience is possible, it too can help in this regard. (A range within one or two grades among group members seems to work best.) As the children converse, or as each, in turn, speaks about a given topic, they are to point out each time the speaker stutters but without any expectation that speech should be changed. Typically, this activity is rather entertaining to the children, creating a feeling that should reduce the pain of stuttering. "Playing" with stuttering behaviors, being willing voluntarily to produce some stuttered speech in the accepting clinical environment, with the clinician's participating in the activity, helps create an atmosphere of openness and also is desensitizing in that it makes the children feel more comfortable with stuttering (Healey, Scott Trautman, & Susca, 2004; Ramig & Bennett, 1997). This type of relaxed handling of stuttering is expected to be partially transformed into more calm reactions during genuine speaking situations when stutter events occur. As a contrasting activity, it has been suggested that children, especially in a group, may be asked to compete in a demonstration of the "most possible stuttering." Because of the artificiality involved, this tends to be an amusing and fun activity that, again, provides the child with experiences of stuttering without pain—the objective of desensitization (Emerick, 1970).

After several sessions, desensitization proceeds into more sensitive materials with the children being asked to share experiences they have had with adults or peers who have made fun of them. This more serious issue could be more difficult for some children and should be handled carefully. As often is the case, however, when a person talks about what hurts, the hard feelings subside. The aim of sharing their experiences is to express and release emotional tensions rather than bottling them up inside. Many other procedures have been suggested, such as telling jokes about stuttering. Another one presents the child with brief descriptions of several situations, accompanied with illustrating drawings, each involving a child who stutters and listeners. For each, the child is to select one of several listed emotional descriptors: shame, disappointment, fear, anger, pride, triumph, and confidence, in order to describe what the person in the situation feels (Guitar & Reville, 1997). This, as well as other sources, provides plenty of reasonable ideas concerning desensitization for children. Some are listed at the end of the chapter. Clinicians, however, should be capable to devise their own procedures to suit their clients, incorporating suggestions offered by the child or the group. In doing so, clinicians should keep in mind that the goal is to reduce painful feelings associated with stuttering.

In addition to becoming less reactive to the stuttering itself, children need opportunities to openly express their emotions, just like the parents do. Relevant activities may include drawing pictures of their stuttering, drawing pictures of people who scare them or make fun of them and then tear them up, writing essays about their stuttering, or becoming the experts who teach fellow classmates about stuttering (Emerick, 1970). More positive self-perceptions also can be encouraged by having children engage in activities such as making a list of things they like about themselves, things that they are good at, and in developing a talent that they can share with others. Also, having the child role-play responses that convey confidence and assertiveness can be beneficial. One of the best sources for activities to help children talk about their feelings is *The School-Age Child Who Stutters: Working Effectively with Attitudes and Emotions* by Chmela and Reardon (2001), published by the Stuttering Foundation of America. The Stuttering Foundation of America has other resources for addressing various topics, such as teasing, bullying, and self-perceptions.

Teasing and Assertiveness

Teasing is a rather frequent problem confronted by schoolchildren who stutter as our clients have reported to us. Among others, it indicates their lower acceptance by peers (Davis, Howell, & Cook, 2002). Teasing is making comments that embarrass and hurt. Often a teaser thinks everyone finds it fun to make light of a matter, and does not understand how feelings have been hurt. At times it is done purposely to hurt. Clinicians should be aware of the risk and probe the child in this regard because some children will not bring it up themselves. Here, the teacher's cooperation is of the utmost importance. Teachers should see to it that the teaser understands the seriousness of his or her negative behavior and stops it. The child who stutters also can be helped through assertiveness training. Many schools now have curricula that address teasing and bullying behavior.

Assertiveness and assertiveness training were discussed in Chapter 10 in relation to adults. It was suggested that most people occasionally find themselves in situations where they feel they have been wronged by others or that their dignity or rights were violated. Still, they are inhibited from making adequate responses. We offer the example of a person watching a movie at the theater while a few spectators disrupt the show with loud talk and laughs that spoil the enjoyment. The person badly wants to say something to the inconsiderate people but, instead, keeps silent, holding in frustration and suffers. Assertiveness is the skill of taking action toward resolving one's needs without insulting or violating the rights of others. The child who stutters, however, faces a double challenge: first, the typical anxiety of just speaking in a difficult situation and, second, speaking up assertively (e.g., protecting his or her rights).

Assertive responses can be developed typically through specific, short role-play programs in which familiar situations, such as peers mocking the child's stuttering, are rehearsed and the child's reaction are properly modified. As we explained in

Chapter 10, a situation is planned only in general outline to allow for some spontaneity. For example, the child who stutters is playing in the schoolyard during lunch break. Another child, played by the clinician or another child in the group, passes by saying "Hi, you stu-stu-stutter boy. You talk funny." Several optional responses are provided in advance (e.g., "So what?", "Better watch it, you may catch it," "Sticks and stones may break my bones, but words will never hurt me.") (see Van Riper, 1973, p. 435). The situation is replayed several times with feedback, reinforcement, and suggestions for improvements. The clinician emphasizes that the desired behavior is being assertive, not aggressive. The child is then asked to recall other situations, not necessarily involving reactions to stuttering, where more assertiveness would have been desired (e.g., standing in line at McDonald's when an adult is barging in front of him). These are practiced through role play until the desired behavior is achieved (Murphy, Yaruss, & Quesal, 2007b). We have employed this technique for many years and witnessed great enthusiasm and satisfaction expressed by children as they were practicing. The effectiveness of this method with children in achieving desired behavior has been shown experimentally. In one study with nonstuttering 8- to 11-year-olds, targeted behaviors included ratio of eye contact to speech duration, loudness of speech, and several new responses. Results indicated an increase in each target behavior, as well as in rating of overall assertiveness by judges not familiar with the study (Bornstein, Bellack, & Hersen, 1977). Several relevant sources are listed at the end of this section.

Bullying

Bullying perhaps can be viewed as a more intense and severe level of hurting people than teasing. It is intentionally harming another person emotionally through frequent verbal harassment, sometimes also through physical assault, or even forcing another person to do something against his or her will. This can be done by one person or a group ganging up on their victim. The bully may have a need to experience a sense of power and superiority over others. Usually, adults need to get involved to establish and enforce rules prohibiting the bullying. Although teasing of children who stutter is quite common, "hard bullying" is not too common. Nevertheless, teachers need to frame stuttering as one type of observable personal difference and instruct children to accept the stuttering without offending comments. Children who are bullied need comfort, support, and a clear message the problem belongs to the bully, not to them. Additional information regarding Assertiveness Training and addressing bullying/teasing may be found at the following web sites:

www.csulb.edu/~tstevens/assert%20req.html
www.stopbullyingnow.hrsa.gov/kids/

Therapy: Focus on Speech

Identification and Analysis

Earlier in the chapter, we referred to simple identification of stuttering procedures as one of several useful techniques applied in working on desensitization. For that purpose, activities were mostly in terms of observing others or self and pointing out stuttering events when they occur. For clinicians who feel comfortable with traditional approaches to stuttering therapy, continuing into more extensive, somewhat more detailed, identification activities may be a reasonable option as the program progresses closer toward a focus on speech modification. This time, however, stuttering events are not only identified as they occur, they are also analyzed for their special characteristics. Again, the objectives and rationale are similar to those for adults, but the procedures are adjusted to suit children's level and abilities. At this stage, the clinician explains to the child, in a simple manner, why it is a good idea to get to know his or her own stuttering by taking a closer look at it from different angles. Essentially, the question asked is, "What is going on when you stutter?" It is much more preferable, however, to word the question as, "What do *you* do when you stutter that makes speech more difficult?" The parallel procedure with adolescents and adults tends to explore stuttering in great detail. Analysis with school-age children, however, especially at lower grades, should be focused on a limited number, say three to five, of the child's main stuttering characteristics. Getting into too many details could be counterproductive.

Using mirrors and videos taken of him or her, the child is guided to examine the most frequently occurring disfluency types (e.g., repetition and prolongation) as well as the most obvious secondary characteristics and the focal points of tension associated with them. The child's readiness to observe audio and videos of self should be recognized in advance. For some children, seeing themselves stuttering on video may be too emotionally intense. Working in front of a mirror for some time may be a good intermediate step prior to introducing video observation and analysis. Some difficulties can be expected because, as Conture (2001) pointed out, many speech movements and postures involved are not observable. The clinician helps the child describe the behaviors, for example, "I stretched the '*Wh*' sound in the word '*where*' and at the same time I tensed my lips." Or, "I repeated '*I-I-I*' and at the same time twisted my head to the side." Of course, the use of the language of responsibility, for example, "I twisted my head to the side," is purposely injected to help the child realize that what he or she does can also be changed. (This concept was discussed in Chapter 11.) Additional help is necessary to provide the child with a better idea of the unseen behaviors, for example, when blocking on the sound /k/, pressing the back of the tongue against the palate. The clinician can demonstrate these movements and postures using one hand as the tongue and the other one as the palate. Models of the speech mechanism are useful for this purpose, as is the videotape *Stuttering and the School-age Child* (by the Stuttering Foundation of America). If extensive practice, that is, the many analyses of the main stuttering features that we pursue in therapy, leads the child to recognize additional characteristics, there is no reason not to permit him or her to expand the behavior repertoire being analyzed.

Another useful aspect of the analysis technique is in guiding the child to differentiate the severity level of stuttering events, for example "light," "middle," and "hard" stuttering. Greater awareness of the variability may drive home the point that, depending on the individual case, much of the problem is not as bad as the few severe stuttering events may lead the child to believe. With children, special terms can help add a more game-like feeling to the processes of therapy. Clinicians can involve children in making up their own terms. For example, an older child who likes golf might enjoy referring to a cancellation as a "mulligan." Examples of possible terms are shown in Table 12.1 based on analogies to video recordings, football games, show terms, and more.

Changing Speech

There is no clear demarcation line where work on identification ends and speech modification begins. Often, while working on identification, some practice on modification is incorporated. When a child identifies and analyzes a stuttering event, it sometimes is inviting to show him or her how to "correct" it, how to switch from "hard speech" to "easy speech." Nonetheless, when therapy has progressed to the point where speech modification calls for a more prominent focus, several options are available. First, as just described, the clinician may opt to proceed with the traditional Van Riper's (1973) approach aimed at having the client learn to modify the form of stuttering, making it more acceptable to listeners. The second option is to employ operant conditioning techniques to gradually increase the length of fluent speech segments (Ryan, 1979). Third, the clinician may pursue fluency-generating techniques, such as those developed by Webster (1980a, 1980b). All these were described in Chapter 11.

Stuttering Modification

We prefer to begin with at least a brief stuttering modification program following some of Van Riper's (1973) ideas because the skills acquired through the procedures provide clients with the feeling that they can do something that directly combats the stuttering, the source of the pain, frustration, and feeling of helplessness. (See Chapter 11 for a more detailed description of the stuttering modification techniques.) Adapted to the child's level, the modification procedures we select are easily demonstrable, well

Table 12.1: **Examples of Terms Used in Therapy with School-Age Children**

Behavior	Video Terms	Show Terms	Football Terms	For Young Children
Talking too quickly	"Fast forward"	"Run through"	"Rushing"	"Rabbit talk"
Repetition	"Rewinds"	"False starts"	"Fumbles"	"Bumpy talk"
Prolongation	"Long plays"	"Delays"	"Holdings"	"Sticky talk"
Stop talking	"Pause"	"Cut"	"Time-out"	"Red light"
Start talking	"Play" or "Resume"	"Roll 'em"	"In play"	"Green light"
Cancellation or pullout	"Erase" and "Record over"	"Restart" or "Take 2"	"Instant replay"	"Yellow light"
Talking slowly	"Slow play"	"Slow motion"	"Stretching"	"Turtle talk"

understood, and typically well received. It is worth pointing out that a child who is trained primarily with fluency-shaping techniques will benefit from some practice with stuttering modification because of the likelihood to be in situations when fluency is lost. It is then that the ability to also *manage* stuttering is extremely useful in helping the child get back on the fluency track. Without stuttering managing experience, the child may be incapable of regaining a hold on the fluency-generating techniques.

For the sake of simplification, with children in early school grades, the stuttering modification program may be limited to perhaps only the *in-block* procedure, also known as *pullout.* In our experience, young children do better with pullouts, preferring it to the post-block modification (*cancellation*). The pre-block procedure appears to be too abstract and difficult for them altogether. The clinician demonstrates a stuttering block while saying, for example, the word *picture*, with clear tensed lips on the /p/ sound. For demonstration purposes, the tension is reduced in the most obvious manner, as the word is uttered smoothly with some elongation or by easily repeating the syllable /pi/ 2 or 3 times. We tell the child, "Let's *pull out* of the stuttering," or "Let's switch from hard speech into easy speech." Visual illustrations, such as a drawing symbolizing the block with spikes that gradually decrease in size, turning into an arrow projected upward and forward in moderate angle, or making a fist for the block, slowly changing into an open hand to illustrate the release, might be useful with some children. The practice begins with releasing many purposeful stuttering blocks and then continues into changing an authentic stuttering event during reading or conversation. The child is encouraged to "feel the change" and recognize it is of his or her own doing. It is important here to note a small, although potentially significant, deviation from Van Riper's (1973) writings. Whereas he advocated "teaching the child to stutter easily" (p. 441) and "to show him how to stutter in a new way" (p. 442), Williams (1971) preferred altering the language used in presenting the task to the child, opining that the child must learn to "talk easily rather than hard." In particular, Williams favored teaching the child to modify a stuttering block into easy repetitions. In doing so, he did not advocate fluency-enhancing approaches. Using this language ("talk easily"), he explained, shifts the frame of references from that of a "stutterer" to that of a "speaker." As the child stutters, the clinician may join his stuttering and demonstrate the desired transition. With a young child, a demonstration is more effective than several explanations. With children at more advanced grades, say fourth to sixth, stuttering modification can be more elaborate, including the post-block procedure that requires the client to stop after stuttering, reduce tension, and say the word again in an easier fashion.

The practice of modification with the clinician should progress into a generalization program. Among the first people who should be included in this process are the child's parents. Their presence in some sessions can help significantly. Often, children are reluctant to use at-home techniques they have learned in therapy because parents and sibling might think it is odd and react in unpredictable ways. Parent presence in therapy sessions releases much of the pressure and also allows them to encourage the child.

Fluency Facilitating Speaking Skills

Following the traditional therapy approaches outlined here, including desensitization, identification, and modification, we proceed by shifting focus to the more recent fluency-generating approach as discussed in detail in Chapter 11. We have pursued such integration of approaches since the 1970s and have been impressed with the advantages provided by each. Other clinicians, however, may elect to employ only the fluency-generating approach.

The clinician explains the change in the direction of therapy, conveying the general idea that "now, when you have learned a lot about stuttering and have practiced techniques that let you release stuttering blocks without getting panicked, it is time to also learn what can be done to speak more fluently to begin with so that fewer instances of stuttering occur." The clinician states that four ways of talking will be practiced that help produce stutter-free speech: slow stretched speech, gentle voice onset, light articulatory contact, and continuous movement and airflow. (These are the *fluency targets*, as they are often referred to in the literature.) Each is explained and demonstrated. A general plan is outlined whereby each of the four speaking patterns will be practiced, then gradually merged into the ongoing speech.

1. Establish slow, stretched speech, about 1 word per second (with adults the initial rate is much slower, 1 word per 2 s). Start with one-syllable words and then move to two-syllable words. Clinician provides models until the child catches on.
2. Introduce gentle voice onset. Demonstrate by contrasting hard and gentle attempts at voicing. Have the child do the same. Simulate the desired vocal fold movement with the two hands lightly vibrating against each other. Then, practice easy voice initiation, starting with words that begin with vowels, sliding from near whisper to normal loudness. Next, practice words that begin with voiceless consonants.
3. Introduce light articulatory contact. Similarly to the earlier example, demonstrate hard and easy contacts, like in saying the /k/ and the /p/ sounds. Have the child do the same in order to feel the difference and become aware that the hard contact stops the airflow. Provide visual simulations, such as producing the /k/ sound by holding the fist of one hand (representing the tongue) against the second flat hand (representing the palate). The contact can be hard or the fist just slides easily along the hand surface while saying words like "kite," "take," and so on. Contrast hard and easy release of these and other classes of sounds.
4. Integrate gentle voice onset and light contact with slow speech, using one- and two-syllable words, keeping the same rate of one word per second. This complicated task requires more practice than the previous steps.
5. Increase the length of the utterances to three to four words but still keep the same initial slow rate.
6. Introduce continuous speech movement and continuous airflow throughout the phrase. As children practice talking slowly in short phrases, they are being

urged to attend to the constant ongoing motion of the speech mechanism: how the words blend into each other without stopping in between. This is the essence of normal speech. Most speakers do not stop in the middle of or between words. Again, models, videos, hand motions, and other illustrations should be used to highlight this important characteristic.

7. Proceed to practice longer sentences while also increasing the rate to two words per second. This rate is the low end where some parts of normal speech reach. All along, pay attention to the other basic targets of gentle voice, light contact. The continuous movement target is easier to practice in longer sentences.

8. Proceed to conversational speech, keeping the slow rate. Some useful exercises can be found in Guitar and Reville (1997, pp. 89–106).

9. Transfer to several selected situations, then to a range of life situations.

We again emphasize that considerable flexibility should be exercised in pursuing the program's steps. Some may need to be eliminated or altered; much depends on the child's age and ability to follow. For example, with an 8-year-old, the clinician may begin with a faster rate, although still perceptibly slower than normal, using short phrases rather than single words. We have had noticeable success with variations of this program, working with children ages 8 to 12. For the most part, however, this was done in a clinical setting, not in the schools, and we enjoyed excellent cooperation from parents who participated in the sessions when asked to, and also used slow speech while interacting with the child. Years later, one child who initially exhibited moderate-to-severe stuttering won a state speaking award.

Generalization

A significant number, perhaps most, of a school-age child's communication situations, take place in school. Thus the school setting presents a very real and appropriate setting for generalizing treatment goals into real-life settings. It is because school-based clinicians work directly in the school setting that they have a significant advantage over clinicians in other settings in terms of helping children who stutter. If possible, and when the child is ready, clinicians should attempt to get the child out of the therapy room and immediately begin to facilitate generalization of techniques: They walk with the child down the halls, for example. Then the approach is extended to other settings where the child spends time, asking the child to complete brief homework activities outside the school environment. More specific examples of strategies for generalization could include using materials from the classroom in all practice activities, bringing in a friend, sibling, or a teacher to the therapy session, teaching other people in the child's environment about stuttering, and so on, and holding parts of therapy sessions on the playground, in the gym, and/or the library. Learning to modify speech while engaged in activities that require divided attention, such as walking, participating in a conversation with multiple listeners, talking in environments with lots of background noise, or using different loudness levels like those in a classroom versus on the playground, are all hierarchies that should be explored and practiced.

Another interesting generalization activity, contract cards, is described by Chmela (2006). The child, clinician, and teacher (or other adult, such as a scout master) develop a contract for the child's participation. For the contract, the child agrees to demonstrate participation in a specific way such as using a speech tool to provide an answer in class during social studies. The contract is written on an index card, and following the social studies lesson, the child would take the card to the teacher and they would both sign it to indicate the child had fulfilled the contract. The card would then be returned to the clinician and discussed in the next therapy session. In a sense, methods like these bring the therapy into the real world.

Other Programs

The literature presents a number of other therapeutic programs for school-age children that reflect differences in approaches and scope. A few are summarized next, to demonstrate their range.

Conditioning Fluent Speech

In Chapter 6, stuttering was discussed within the framework of operant learning principles, such as positive reinforcement, punishment, extinction, and negative reinforcement, that were used to portray stuttering as a response modified by its consequences. Applications of these principles can be seen in several early therapy regimens (e.g., Haroldson, Martin, & Starr, 1968; Rickard & Mundy, 1965). Bar (1971) had parents trained in reinforcing fluent utterances in their child's speech using verbal contingencies. Two programs are presented here.

Gradual Increase in Length and Complexity of Utterance (GILCU)

The *GILCU* program (Ryan & Ryan 1995) was described in Chapter 11 in the context of therapy for adults who stutter. It also is suitable, if not more so, for school-age children. The main objective is to gradually increase the client's length of fluent speech by means of immediate positive or negative feedback about the speech behavior. The program includes three parts, oral reading, monologue, and conversation, each composed of a similar progression through 18 steps. In each case, the 18 steps are divided into four levels. Within a speaking context, the client gradually progresses from one-word fluent responses to 5 consecutive minutes of connected speech. The criterion for advancing between steps is 10 consecutive fluent responses. Table 12.2 lists the target responses corresponding to each set of steps. In practice, the client is instructed to speak fluently, and each fluent response is reinforced by the clinician's feedback of "Good" and/or delivery of a token. Stuttered responses are followed by feedback such as, "Stop; speak fluently." After the child has completed the first 18 steps to attain 5 min of fluent reading in the clinic, the parents are trained to apply the reinforcement system at home. The fluent reading responses are reviewed each session while the client proceeds through the same 18 steps in monologue and then ultimately in conversation.

The effectiveness of this approach was investigated in a study of 12 school-age children seen for 30-min sessions twice weekly for an average of about 8 weeks;

Table 12.2: Target Responses Corresponding to the Sets of Steps in the GILCU Program

Set of Steps	GILCU Target Responses
Steps 1–6	One word to six words
Steps 7–10	One sentence to four sentences
Steps 11–16	30 s to 3 min
Steps 17–18	3–5 min

9 showed a drop from 6.0 to 0.4 mean stuttered words per minute under the Establishment program administered in public school settings. Follow-up measures taken 14 months after the Maintenance program revealed a mean 0.6 stuttered words per minute for 6 of these children (Ryan & Ryan, 1995).

The Lidcombe Program

Developed by Australian speech-language clinicians, this program has been directed mostly to preschool-age children. Hence more detailed information is presented in Chapter 14. The Lidcombe program focuses on reinforcing fluent speech on the one hand and pointing out stuttered events on the other. Although the authors view responses to stuttering as "neutral," their corrective nature also can be characterized as "punishment" in operant conditioning terminology. That is, the stuttering response is followed by verbal stimuli designed to decrease that behavior. The program relies primarily on parents' administration of the procedures at home (Onslow, Packman, & Harrison, 2003). Although Onslow and colleagues opined that stuttering in children older than 6 years is less responsive to parental contingencies, the program also has been applied to school-age children and may be considered for those in the lower grades.

   The initial few sessions are conducted in the clinical setting as the clinician demonstrates to parents when and how to apply verbal contingencies: positive reinforcement to the child's fluent speech but requesting a reattempt or giving neutral feedback related to stuttered speech. Fluent utterances are rewarded with responses such as "That was smooth speech" and similar reinforcing praises. Stuttered utterances are met with corrective feedback such as, "That was bumpy speech." In addition to verbal contingencies, the child also may be instructed to correct the stuttering (e.g., "Say it again to smooth it out"). An overall 5:1 ratio of praises to corrections is maintained. When parents are thought to be proficient with the procedures, the therapy is transferred to the home, starting with a few brief structured practice sessions per day conducted by the trained parent. Shortly thereafter, contingencies are applied in various home situations. Parents monitor progress by daily rating of stuttering severity. Progress also is evaluated by the clinician during periodic visits to the clinic. A single study that evaluated the effectiveness of the Lidcombe program with school-age children demonstrated good results. All children exhibited reduced stuttering 12 months after termination of therapy (Lincoln, Onslow, Lewis, & Wilson, 1996).

Integrated Programs

Fluency Rules Program

Developed by C. Runyan and S. Runyan (1993, 2007), this program requires the child to adhere to three rule classes totaling seven rules that are basically instructional procedures. They appear simple to present to children and easily understood by them.

> *Universal Rules*: (1) Speak slowly (turtle speech), (2) Say a word only once, (3) Say it short.
> *Primary Rules*: (4) Use speech breathing, (5) Start voice box running smoothly.
> *Secondary Rules*: (6) Touch "speech helpers" together smoothly, (7) Use only "speech helpers" to talk.

As you can see, the therapy emphasizes fluency-enhancing techniques (rules 1, 4, 5, and 6) with additional important elements designed to control stuttering, mainly by limiting its occurrence or duration, that is, learning what not to do (rules 2, 3, and 7) rather than how to modify stuttering according to the traditional Van Riper techniques. For example, rule 7 directs the child to avoid making nonspeech behaviors, or secondary characteristics. The therapy is conducted twice or three times per week in the school environment in a nonstructured manner with the children sitting on the floor and engaged in conversational speech and games. Speech is kept slow although not abnormally slow. An example may be made of the children's TV host, Mister Rogers, who speaks more slowly than most people but remains within the normal range of natural rates. Symbolic therapy materials, such as turtles and snails to characterize slow speech, and a race horse to indicate that speech is too fast, are generously employed. Parents also are encouraged to speak at a normal slow rate. Significant attention is given to carryover and transfer to the classroom and home. This requires active cooperation of teachers who are to remind the child to adhere to the rules via agreed-on signals. The authors reported generally positive results for a total of 32 children, mostly in the lower school grades with treatment lasting 9 months on average.

A Comprehensive Stuttering Program for School-age Children (CSP-SC)

This program, which addresses both overt stuttering behaviors and the emotional domain of the disorder, was developed in Canada over a 20-year period, specifically for children ages 7 to 12 years (Kully & Boberg, 1991; Langevin, Kully, & Ross-Harold, 2007). It is designed to be delivered in a 4-week intensive format with groups of six to eight children. However, it has been delivered in other formats in the clinic as well as through interactive mass media e.g., telehealth therapy (Kully, 2002). In several aspects it bears significant similarities to our comprehensive program described earlier in the chapter. These are the *CSP-SC's* four main components:

1. Speech-related goals achieved through both fluency-enhancing and stuttering management techniques.
2. Attitudinal-emotional goals that include reduction in fears and avoidance on one hand and an increase in assertiveness, positive attitudes toward communication, and social skills on the other.

3. Self-management goals, such as developing problem-solving and self-monitoring skills, as well as the ability to plan and carry out practice activities.

4. Environmental goals that basically include parent counseling regarding the nature of stuttering and an understanding of and cooperation with the therapy program.

Work on each component proceeds along three stages: acquisition, transfer, and maintenance. Practice on fluency skills during the first two phases is delivered in small groups of two children. Emotional aspects are dealt with in several formats from larger groups to individual sessions. The authors reported therapy outcomes for four schoolchildren. For three of these, stuttering was reduced by 52% to 75% within 6 to 19 months follow-up. Later follow-ups with parents indicated good maintenance of the gains. The fourth child presented a relapse 2 months posttherapy.

Family Stuttering Programs

A unique and less well-known therapeutic approach that differs from the programs described earlier attempts to expand therapy significantly beyond the emphasis on the child who stutters to include a circle of people in his or her home and school environments (Mallard, 1991). We believe it contains some ideas that might be useful also to clinicians who prefer other programs. Influenced by the work of Rustin and her colleagues in England (e.g., Rustin & Cook, 1983), Mallard's approach reflects the belief that, inasmuch as communication is a social skill, therapy must take into account the social environment in which the child communicates. His program is "based on the assumption that intervention with individuals who influence the communication environment of the stuttering child is the critical component in the treatment of stuttering children" (Mallard, 1991, p. 22). According to this model, a successful therapy can only be achieved when the person who stutters and those in the person's communication environment work together. Hence the entire immediate family, including parents, siblings, grandparents (spouses in adult cases), and the home environment structure, as well as teachers and the classroom structure, and their respective modes of communication, are very relevant if carryover of improved speech is to take place. Therapy is focused on two main goals: speech control and the acquisition of social skills that enable the new speech patterns to be employed in the child's environments. Toward this end, parents must participate in the therapy, and they, as well as teachers, must be willing to cooperate to allow the process of carryover.

Therapy is delivered either in a 2-week intensive group program or a nonintensive format. Either program requires the parents. Hopefully, other important people in the child's environment will also contribute to the process. In fact, changes are expected both for the child and in the child's communication system as well. The program begins with an explanatory meeting in which the entire family is present. Next is a 3-week phase during which each parent must initiate twice a week a 5-min *Talk Time* with the child at home. Each parent submits a weekly evaluative report about these assignments. An important rationale for the *Talk Time* is that it establishes a routine for parent-child communication. It also creates the basis for home speech assignments.

Next, weekly therapy sessions are initiated with the family. Various discussion topics are offered by the clinician, beginning with problem-solving procedures, followed by exercises of resolving actual problems. The objective is to get the family to view stuttering as a problem that can be solved, not necessarily a disorder that must be treated. Many of the problems raised by the child and family appear to be in regard to coping with the stuttering. For example, a child who has to give an oral report in class may be more concerned about how to handle peers' teasing rather than talking without stuttering. Options are listed and considered, and a response to the specific problem is selected. Other topics/assignments include social skills training such as turn-taking, observation, and listening. These topics also can provide for home assignments as needed. In therapy, parents may be asked to mimic their child's stuttering in order to appreciate what he or she is experiencing all the time. They also could be asked to engage in this activity at home during Talk Times because it provides insight for why the child avoids talking. All sessions begin with an evaluation of the previous week assignments.

Work on speech begins after a few sessions. The first step is for the child and family to understand normal speech processes and what is happening during stuttering. Next, the participants, with the clinician's guidance, select a few techniques for changing speech, such as maintaining eye contact with conversational partners, stuttering voluntarily (for desensitization purposes), or stuttering in a relaxed manner. All therapy sessions are conducted with the family present (Mallard, 1998). The effects of these speech changes are discussed. The child and parents are to practice all speech modification techniques at home during Talk Time. The speech modification sequence generally begins with keeping eye contact during moments of stuttering and then moves to stuttering easily with control and maintaining eye contact. Emphasis is placed on stuttering without tension or avoidance (Dell, 1980). Training in social skills, such as turn-taking and problem solving, continues.

In a school setting, open discussion ensues to explain the child's stuttering to the teacher, the various nonobservable aspects of it, what is done in therapy, and how the teacher can help, for example, selecting a time for the child to use his or her speech control procedures and agreeing on reinforcement signals. According to Mallard, when following a family-based problem-solving model of treatment, the role of the speech-language pathologist changes from that of the primary service provider to that of a monitor of how the child, parents, and significant others in the child's communication environment are progressing. No formal research data have been published for this program.

Group Therapy

Principles and basic methods of group therapy were presented in Chapter 10 in regard to treatment of adults who stutter. Generally, group therapy also is applicable for schoolchildren who stutter, and several examples were presented earlier in the chapter. The school setting is conducive because the children are already under one roof, and clinicians often look for ways to economize their time. Groups typically are small because not too many children who stutter are found in a single school. Groups also are restricted in size because age/grade difference may cause problems.

We recommend group members come from a narrow range of no more than two grade levels. Many times speech-language clinicians group children who stutter with other children of the same age who are working on nonfluency speech goals because of constraints related to their time and availability. If handled well, a mixed group still can provide an effective forum for therapy, but care should be taken with this arrangement to ensure that it is a "safe" and comfortable environment in which to stutter. Leath (1984) advocated what he called a *shaping group* as part of stuttering treatment program in the school environment and listed several advantages of heterogeneous groups: The interaction among members is more natural, opportunities to practice new speech patterns in front of people who do not stutter are more like real-life situations, feedback to expressed feelings tends to be more objective from children who do not stutter, and all benefit from learning that children have other problems. The shaping group format requires all members to actively participate in the discussions, monitor the speech behaviors of the other children, as well as administer reward and penalties. The clinician assumes a less active role.

Clinical Research

In spite of the appreciable amount of clinically related literature pertaining to school-age children who stutter, it appears that research related to intervention with this age group has been limited. Considerably more research is available for treatment with younger children and adult populations. Very few reasonably controlled clinical efficacy studies were conducted exclusively with school-age children (6 to 12 years of age). This is partly due to the tendency in a good number of studies to use a wider age range of participants. For example, Ryan and Ryan (1995) included children between the ages of 7 and 17. It may also be a reflection of how school-age children who stutter access therapy; many of these children are served within the school setting, where conducting methodologically sound clinical research can be challenging. After a comprehensive review of 162 articles pertaining to stuttering treatment results for preschool-age children through adulthood, only 39 were found to satisfy four of five methodological criteria to be considered as meeting clinical trial quality (Bothe, Davidow, Bramlett, & Ingham, 2006). Perusing this list we found only five reported data for children between 6 and 14 years of age. Of these, three reports included only one to three participants.

Perhaps an exception is the exemplary investigation conducted in Australia by Craig and a large group of collaborators (1996). They compared effectiveness among three therapy methods: intensive smooth speech, intensive electromyography (EMG) feedback, and home-based smooth speech. Each group was composed of 25 to 27 children. These also were compared with a nontreatment control group of 20 stuttering children. Progress was assessed in terms of percentage of syllables stuttered and speaking rate (number of syllable spoken per minute). A 12-month follow-up was conducted. Comparisons were made in several speaking environments (e.g., clinic, home, and telephone). By the end of therapy, the frequency of stuttering in all treatment groups improved by 85% to 90%, decreasing to under 1% stuttered syllables. By the 1-year follow-up, there was a slight increase in stuttering to the 3% level on average. No change occurred in the control group. The authors concluded that the three approaches were very successful for 70% of the children, with the EMG and home treatment showing the best results. In a follow-up study, Hancock et al. (1998) compared the same children after a mean of 4 years posttreatment. Long-term effects of the therapy continued to be good in that the children in the three treatment groups maintained stuttering frequency similar to what they had demonstrated at the 1-year follow-up in the first study. Effectiveness was not significantly different among the three approaches. Later investigators, however, attempting to replicate the EMG portion of Craig et al.'s study, were not as successful (Block, Onslow, Roberts, & White, 2004). Given the initial finding that all three treatment approaches met with comparable success, it may be that the specific methods employed are less important than the broad aim of an approach to speech management with reduced tension. Similarly, it has been difficult to establish that any particular approach to treatment of phonological disorders is better than another as long as the sound targets have been selected appropriately (Kamhi, 2006).

Other studies have reported various degrees of success, although they fell short of tight methodology. For example, earlier in the chapter we referred to a study that tested the Lidcombe program administered to school-age children (Lincoln, Onslow, Lewis, & Wilson, 1996). Eleven children, ages 7 to 12, were treated using this method. The investigators reported that a median of 12 1-hr treatment sessions was required to reach 1.5% stuttered syllable in speech samples recorded within-clinic as well as in three everyday speaking situations out of the clinic. The reduced stuttering frequency at the end of the treatment was maintained by all the children at a 12-month follow-up. Parents were either "satisfied" or "very satisfied" with their children's speech posttreatment.

Another recent interest in treatment research involving school-age children took the form of a case study of a 9-year-old boy who, in addition to stuttering modification and fluency-enhancing therapies, was exposed to several techniques aimed at reducing emotional reactions. Following treatment, the child exhibited improved communication attitudes and reduced frequency and severity of stuttering (Murphy, Yaruss, & Quesal, 2007a). It is difficult, however, to determine whether changes in stuttering resulted from the attitude treatment or if attitude improvement could have resulted from the effect of reduced stuttering. Clearly, if clinicians are to practice data-based therapy, a considerably larger number of investigations looking at various approaches must be conducted employing rigorous scientific methodologies.

Summary

Clinicians who work with school-age children who stutter should be cognizant of the special characteristics of stuttering in this age group, the increased severity of the overt stuttering, the high level of awareness of stuttering, emergence of strong emotional reactions associated with the speaking difficulties, the growing impact of social forces on the disorder, and the persistent nature of the disorder that has set in. This last item has clinical implications to goal setting and expectation of progress.

For children within the age range of 6 to 12 years, therapy may vary significantly, depending on the age, level of emotional and cognitive maturity, and the potential for family and teachers' cooperation. There is certain degree of similarity among school-age children, adolescents, and adults who stutter in the broad therapeutic objectives and approaches. Management of the emotional component of the disorder, traditional stuttering modification, and fluency shaping all may be applied. A wide array of therapies was described. Individual as well as group therapy formats can be pursued successfully. Although objectives and general approaches are similar, therapy procedures must be adapted to the child's level. Many activities differ in that skills and strategies often are instructed in the context of imaginative terminology, games, and fun activities. To help prevent negative communication experiences at school, the clinician needs to be proactive to educate school personnel about stuttering and support the self-confidence and esteem of the child who stutters. Problem with teasing and bullying may need to be addressed. Parent involvement in the therapy process, if possible, remains extremely desirable.

There seems to be an overall clinical impression that improvement in stuttering in school-age children as the result of therapy is more difficult to achieve and sustain than it is in preschool-age children. We believe that this limitation reflects, in large part, a more resilient form of stuttering. Still, treatment efficacy research with school-age children has been very limited and the impression just mentioned should be viewed with caution. Although further studies are necessary to reach any conclusions, it is possible that specific methods are less important than whether the child learns to initiate and manage speech with reduced tension.

STUDY QUESTIONS AND DISCUSSION TOPICS

1. What are the particular stuttering characteristics of school-age children that should be considered in regard to therapy? In what ways do they differ from those of preschool-age children who stutter?

2. What are the particular emotional and social characteristics of school-age children who stutter that should be considered in regard to therapy? In what ways do they differ from those of preschool-age children and adults who stutter?

3. What are the potential roles of parents in the clinical management of school-age children who stutter?

4. Given the choice between employing the GILCU program or the Lidcombe program, which one would be your preference, and/or under which conditions? Explain why.

5. Given the choice between employing the fluency-enhancing program or a stuttering modification program, which one will be your preference and/or under which conditions? Explain why.

6. Compare your response to question 5 in relation to treating adults who stutter. Explain why it does or does not differ.

WEB SITES

Stutter Buddies: www.westutter.org/whoWeHelp/parents/Kids-Newsletter-Stutter-Buddies.htm

Friends—National Association of Young People Who Stutter: www.friendswhostutter.org

Stuttering Foundation of America, Just for Kids Web site: www.stutteringhelp.org/Default.aspx?tabid=25

Stuttering home page Just for Kids Web site: www.mnsu.edu/comdis/kuster/kids/kids.html

SUGGESTED READINGS

Chmela, K., & Reardon, N. (2001). *The school-age child who stutters: Working effectively with attitudes and emotions.* Memphis, TN: Stuttering Foundation of America.

Guitar, B., & Reville, J. (1997). *Easy talker.* Austin, TX: Pro-Ed.

Langevin, M., Kully, D., & Ross-Harold, B. (2007). A comprehensive stuttering program for school-age children with strategies for managing teasing and bullying. In E. Conture & R. Curlee (Eds.), *Stuttering and related disorders* (3rd ed., pp. 131–150). New York: Thieme.

Ramig, P., & Bennett, E. (1997). Clinical management of children: Direct management strategy. In R. F. Curlee & G. M. Siegel (Eds.), *Nature and treatment of stuttering: New directions* (2nd ed., pp. 292–312). Boston: Allyn & Bacon.

Runyan, C., & Runyan, S. (2007). A fluency rules therapy program for young children in the public schools. In E. Conture & R. Curlee (Eds.), *Stuttering and related disorders* (3rd ed., pp. 101–114). New York: Thieme.

Chapter 13: Assessment of Stuttering in Early Childhood

LEARNER OUTCOMES

Readers of this chapter will understand:

- Differences between the initial evaluation of a preschool child and that of older children and adults who stutter.
- The objectives and rationales for the initial evaluation of preschool children who stutter.
- The structure and content of the parent interview.
- Procedures and formal instruments for the measuring stuttered speech in young children.
- Criteria for differentiating early stuttering from normal disfluency.
- Criteria for making early assessment of chances of persistent and natural recovery courses of stuttering.
- How to offer parent counseling in conjunction with the evaluation.

Challenges, Objectives, and Settings for the Initial Evaluation

In Chapter 9 we stated that in health fields, a typical diagnostic evaluation involves an analysis of presenting symptoms, both objectively observed and reported by the patient. It is a process that eventually leads to the diagnostic finding: the identification of a disease or a disorder that was not apparent at the beginning of the process. Sometimes the diagnosis is substantiated by a single sign; in other cases there may be a pattern of signs. The primary motivation for isolating the condition or disorder from other alternatives is to facilitate decisions concerning suitable treatment. It was suggested that because the majority of adults who stutter correctly diagnose their own speech problem, the main purpose of initial evaluation for adults is to understand, describe, and measure the various dimensions of the disorder, rather than to identify it. Is this also true for preschool age children? Frequently, the answer is positive. By the time the speech-language pathologist is consulted, typically more than one caretaker has noticed the appearance of excessive and unusual disfluencies in the child's speech and correctly diagnosed it as "stuttering."

Occasionally disorders of phonology and/or language may be called "stuttering" by individuals unaware of the distinctions. At other times parents who expected greater fluency proficiency during the language learning process may express concern about "stuttering." In our experience, however, these are the minority of cases.

Stuttering Versus Normal Disfluency: A Diagnostic Challenge

Yairi and Ambrose (2005) stated that rarely did they have occasions to question parents' diagnoses of their child's speech as stuttering. Close agreement between the parents' and clinician's diagnosis of stuttering in preschool age children has been reported in several studies (e.g., Ambrose & Yairi, 1999; Yairi, 1983). Yet there can be exceptions to agreement as well as to clear evidence for a diagnosis. Sometimes referral occurs at such an early stage of the disorder that it is not fully formed at the time of the initial evaluation. Also, because speech skills are still developing, normal childhood speech characteristics, such as "placeholder" word and phrase repetitions, may blur the picture. Thus clinicians should exercise extra caution in determining whether a disorder of clinical significance exists, and which one. Occasionally there are exceptions to the close agreement between parents and clinicians in diagnosing stuttering. For example, based on objective evidence a clinician may be reluctant to diagnose borderline disfluency as stuttering, whereas overly anxious parents, perhaps with a familial history of stuttering, are more inclined to do so. Disagreement may also arise in the case where parents have had opportunities to observe more pronounced stuttering episodes that never occur even during two or three visits to the clinic. Finally, there are isolated instances where children are brought in because of parental concern about "stuttering," when actually they exhibit another communication disorder altogether. These few cases do present the classic challenges of the diagnosis process. Based on our experience and data, however, we disagree with several authors who overemphasize difficulty in differentiating early stuttering from normal disfluency (Conture, 2001; Gordon & Luper, 1992a, 1992b; Manning, 2001). They stand in sharp contrast to Curlee (1999, p. 3), who stated that "I can recall only a handful of parental misdiagnoses of stuttering in over 25 years of clinical practice."

How do we explain Curlee's and our observations? The answer: Whereas a normative study of speech disfluency in 1,000 preschoolers selected randomly from the general population might find a few children in the gray area between normal and stuttering to pose a diagnostic challenge, the clinical setting presents an altogether different picture. Preschool children seen for evaluation in the clinic, or sometimes by a school speech-language clinician, constitute a selective, not random subset. They have already been closely and intensively "*screened*" by their parents, who found them to exhibit speech characteristics that are beyond normal. Typically parents have observed these behaviors for weeks, if not months, prior to making a referral to the speech clinician. This is the main reason why borderline cases seen for evaluation are infrequent. Furthermore, according to a recent study, a substantial majority of preschoolers seen for initial stuttering evaluation exhibit moderate or severe stuttering that makes for unmistakable diagnoses (Yairi & Ambrose, 2005). Regardless, several disfluency measures, to be discussed later in the chapter, may be applied to make reasonably clear differentiation between normally fluency and stuttering.

Other Key Diagnostic Issues

The initial evaluation of preschoolers who stutter is different in several significant aspects from that of adults who stutter. Key aspects include the role of parents, the accuracy of stuttering history information, the lack of clarity regarding emotional factors, the possibility of concomitant disorders, and the challenge of eliciting representative speech samples to observe the stuttering.

The Parent Role

Whereas adults are typically self-referred for consultation and therapy and are the main source of information about themselves, parents are the ones who bring the child to the clinician out of their own worries, and the role of informant falls to them, typically the mother. Not only do they provide the background information, they also collect important data from the child. Being so close to the problem, parents become a second major focus of the evaluation. Their own background or family's experience with stuttering, their personality, the atmosphere they create at home, and their attitude and reaction to the child's stuttering are important for an understanding of the child's problem and factors that may aggravate it. Of course, potential positive parental resources also can be revealed and tapped for more effective handling of the problem. Finally, it is the parents who ultimately make the decision about the nature and timing of clinical intervention.

Accuracy of Information

Because of the short history of the disorder, information about onset and surrounding circumstances should be accessible from parents in greater detail and better validity than what typically is obtained for older clients. For some children such information may be only a few days or a few weeks old. Additionally, in the early years of life, most of a child's relatives are alive and available to provide extra information, greatly enhancing the accuracy of the history and familial incidence of stuttering that are important details for prognostic purposes.

The Emotional Domain

Whereas most adults are willing to share and verbalize their feelings about stuttering, assessing the emotional reactions of the young child is difficult. On the one hand, the child may not have such reactions. On the other hand, if emotional reactions do exist, preschoolers are often incapable of verbalizing them. True, some children clearly express their awareness and frustration. For many others, however, we simply do not know what goes on inside their minds. Age is a factor in the domain of emotional reactions. The percentage of children 4 to 5 years of age who appear to be aware of their stuttering is certainly greater than among 2-year-olds (Ambrose & Yairi, 1994). Other factors, such as severity of stuttering or environmental reactions to the child's speech, probably play a role. We may assume that the stronger the environmental reactions and the more severe the stuttering, the higher the likelihood for the child to respond emotionally. Unfortunately, the information available for this domain is very limited.

Concomitant Disorders

All children in the preschool age range undergo fast developmental growth in multiple domains. An appreciable number of them may exhibit either slowness or more serious problems in one or more of these domains. Therefore, the initial evaluation of a young child who stutters must also include comprehensive testing of hearing, language, phonology, motor, and cognitive skills that constitute an integral part of standard speech-language-hearing evaluations of children. This point is particularly important in light of information that a wide range of disorders, especially those of phonology and language, are present concomitantly with childhood stuttering more frequently than in children who do not stutter (e.g., Arndt & Healey, 2001; Blood, Ridenour, Qualls, & Scheffner Hammer, 2003).

Speech Elicitation and Stuttering

Not infrequently, eliciting an adequate speech sample from the young child is not a simple matter. Children may remain quiet during the first visit or two, speak little, and be uncooperative during the administration of various tests. Hence several visits are sometimes required to accomplish a comprehensive evaluation. Even if the child is cooperative, on a "good day" he or she may exhibit little stuttering, way below the typical level as described by parents. Thus at least two or three speech samples may be necessary, including one at home.

Objectives for the Initial Evaluation

Here is a list of specific objectives for the initial evaluation:

1. Obtain from parents a thorough history of the disorder: (a) exact time, circumstances, and type of onset (sudden, gradual, etc.), (b) description of the initial stuttering characteristics, including physical behaviors and emotional reactions, and (c) description of changes in the stuttering characteristics and severity from onset to date.
2. Describe/quantify the various aspects of the child's disfluency and other features of stuttering, including their fluctuation in response to various conditions.
3. Examine the child's language, phonology, motor skills, and hearing.
4. Identify other factors relevant to the stuttering (e.g., familial history of stuttering and current home environment conditions).
5. Assess the current stuttering in light of its history and the potential risk factors in order to reach a prognosis and suggested course of action.
6. Share findings and recommendations with parents.
7. Provide parents with information about stuttering and guidance for handling it at home, day care, and in other settings.

Setting and Preparations

In our experience, a comprehensive evaluation of a preschool child may require three sessions, depending on the child's cooperation and availability of a second clinician to assist with the testing. Keep in mind that it is necessary to record speech samples over at least two different days, and administer language, phonology, motor, and other tests in addition to the evaluation of stuttering. Also, initial parent interview may require a whole session, and, similarly, the parent conference at the completion of the evaluation. As with the evaluation with adults, both audio and video recording are desired. Special attention should be given to the child's typical daily schedule, especially in regard to naps, snacks, or other routines. Having the child scheduled for the evaluation at the time when he or she is most alert during the day can make an appreciable difference. Parents should be advised to bring with them notes about their child's developmental progress, birth and health history, the incidence and course of stuttering among the extended family, and, if possible, a recorded speech sample of the child. They may also bring along favorite quiet toys and/or books that the child would be inclined to want to talk about.

The evaluation is structured in three parts: the case history interview with parents, observing and testing the child, and a concluding conference with parents.

The Case History

The initial case interview with one or both parents is conducted without the child present so that the parent and clinician can focus on an open and comfortable sharing of information. The case history includes four components: (1) personal and family information, (2) time and circumstances of onset, (3) symptomatology at onset and at the present, and (4) general child development and health. Specific information items and interview questions are presented in our Case History Form. Comments on specific items are inserted at the end of each section.

Case History Form: Preschool Children

Part I: Client and Family Information

Client Information

Child's Name _____ _____　　File #_____
　　　　　　　　　Last　　　　　　First

Address _____

Home Phone (____)_____　　Parent's Work Phone (____)_____

email _____

Child's date of birth _____　　Age _____　　Gender _____

Race/Ethnicity _____

Informant _____　　　　Relation to child _____

Referral _____

Date of Evaluation _____　　　　Clinician: _____

(continued)

Family Information

Parents Married _____   Divorced _____   If yes, child lives with _____

Language(s) at home _____

Mother: Name _____   Age _____   Education Level _____

Occupation _____

Stuttering History: No _____   Yes _____   When/How long _____

Relatives on mother's side (her parents, siblings, nieces and nephews) who have had stuttering history. For each one who stuttered, indicate if/when recovered or if persists:

_____

_____

Father: Name _____   Age _____   Education Level _____

Occupation _____

Stuttering History: No _____   Yes _____   If yes, when/how long?

_____

Relatives on father's side (his parents, siblings, nieces and nephews) who have had stuttering history. For each one who stuttered, indicate if/when recovered or if persistent:

_____

_____

Siblings: List siblings by gender and age. Indicate if sibling has had a stuttering history.

_____

_____

Comments on Part I

Items referring to familial history of stuttering serve two purposes. First, they are critical in relation to the child's prognosis. As explained in earlier chapters, a child has about a 65% chance of matching the pattern of family history for stuttering. If there is a family history of recovered stuttering, there is about a 65% chance to follow the same pattern; if there is a family history of persistent stuttering, there is about 65% chance of following that same pattern. Hence both parents should be urged to check with the relatives of their respective families about stuttering history. Questions about familial history should be raised in subsequent opportunities because new information may surface. Telephone calls to these relatives may add significantly to the reliability of claims. A helpful means for tracking familial history of stuttering is to draw a pedigree (a family tree) that includes the relatives of both parents. A second purpose for pursuing this topic is that it may shed light on the feelings and attitudes toward stuttering at home.

> The importance of urging parents to ask questions of their relatives about stuttering must be underscored. It should not be assumed that stuttering would have been mentioned had it occurred. In our experience, relatives often do not offer the information until someone else raises the topic. For example, one young mother, who herself stuttered, was surprised when she learned that her own grandmother, with whom she was close, was someone in the family who had stuttered. She remarked how she might never have known this fact if she had not initiated a discussion of the topic.

Part II: Time and Circumstances of Onset

1. When was the stuttering first noticed? Probe for an accurate date through surrounding circumstances.

   Approximate date of onset _____   Child age at onset _____

   Child current age _____   Time since stuttering onset _____

   Notes regarding parent's estimation of date of onset: _____

   _____

   _____

2. Who first noticed the child's stuttering? _____

3. Was the onset sudden or gradual?

   ____ Sudden: 1 day   ____ Gradual: 2 weeks
   ____ Sudden: 2–3 days   ____ Gradual: 3–4 weeks
   ____ Sudden: 1 week   ____ Gradual: 6 weeks or more

4. Were there any illnesses, accidents, or physical traumas when he/she began stuttering or shortly (2–3 weeks) before that time?

   No ___ Yes ___ Which/When _____

5. Were there any identifiable emotionally upsetting events in the child's or the family's life just prior to or at the time of the stuttering onset?

   No ___ Yes ___ Which/When/ Explain? _____

   _____

(continued)

6. Did the time when the child began stuttering coincide with the arrival of a new baby, pregnancy of the mother, or other sibling rivalry?

No _____ Yes _____ Explain: _____

7. Was the child undergoing toilet training, giving up thumb-sucking, or changing other habits at the time?

No _____ Yes _____ Explain: _____

8. In general, was the child under some pressure/stress during the period when he/she began stuttering?

No _____ Yes _____ Explain: _____

9. Generally, based on the above, the clinician estimates the manner of stuttering onset as:

_____ Sudden, following emotionally stressful event
_____ Sudden, following physical illness
_____ Sudden, uneventful
_____ Gradual, following emotionally stressful events
_____ Gradual, following physical illness
_____ Gradual, uneventful

10. Was the onset of stuttering associated with noticeable changes or development in the child's general speech and language skills?

No _____ Yes _____ Explain _____

11. In your opinion, what was the most important cause of the stuttering? What other factors contributed?

_____

Comments on Part II

Question 1 ("When was the stuttering first noticed?") is the most important item because it provides the estimated time elapsed from onset to the date of the evaluation. This information is critical to determine the current status of the disorder, prognosis, and consideration of possible intervention. If the post-onset interval is short, say less than 6 months, and stuttering has slightly declined, an additional waiting period is a reasonable option in light of the possibility of natural recovery. The shorter the interval, additional waiting is more justified. However, as the post-onset interval increases, particularly when it is 9 months or longer, the smaller is the chance for natural recovery, and intervention may be given greater consideration. Also, there is a trend for children who had onset at an early age to have a greater chance for recovery as compared to those who reported late onset (Buck, Lees, &

Cook, 2002; Yairi & Ambrose, 2005). Parents should be guided to identify the time of onset with questions that systematically narrow the possible time range. To this end, they are encouraged to recall the onset in reference to other events, such as birthdays, holidays, trips, or illnesses. For example, if the child began stuttering in the winter, urge parents to recall whether the child had already stuttered during Christmas or was it closer to the end of winter (e.g., the month of March). Or, if the child began stuttering during summer, was it before or after the Fourth of July, before or after a birthday or other significant events.

Question 3 ("Was the onset sudden or gradual?") is pertinent in revealing the circumstances and the degree of parents' confidence in their diagnosis. It is not surprising that our data show that stuttering associated with sudden onsets tend to be perceived as more severe. Perhaps it is the severity that calls it more immediately to the parents' attention. Also, some significant differences have been found between children who experienced sudden and those who experienced gradual onset, such as a tendency for parents of the latter group to report recent spurts of language growth (Watkins, 2005). As we discuss later, rapidly emerging or precocious language skills is a potential risk factor for persistent stuttering.

Questions 4 through 8 are straightforward, helping the clinician assess physical health and emotional factors possibly contributing to the problem. The clinician asks questions that may lead parents to recall and consider stressors that either facilitated or complicated the onset. At the very least, the answers may shed light on the child's home environment and parents' evaluation of, and reaction to, the events that are discussed.

Question 11 is a broad wide-open question that invites parents to present their point of view and look at parameters that have not been discussed. Conditions, processes, and behaviors such as advanced language skills, nutrition, apparently unrelated medical issues, and other life factors, might surface. Although many of these explanations are typically rejected by most scientists, they should be evaluated for their merit in each case.

Overall, the very task of the parents analyzing the child's stuttering and its background might produce secondary therapeutic values, helping them take a good look and reassess their home environment and family style. Johnson et al. (1959) were convinced that the lengthy parent interviews they conducted for their study of stuttering onset were instrumental in the eventual improvement reported for many of the children.

Part III: Symptomatology at Onset and at Present

12. Describe and demonstrate the child's speech when he/she first began stuttering:

_____

_____

(continued)

13. Indicate which of the following speech disfluencies were observed near onset and now:

Disfluency	Onset	Now
Repeating sound/syllable (ba-ba-baby)	_____	_____
Repeating short words (and-and)	_____	_____
Repeating phrases or longer words (going to-going to)	_____	_____
Prolonging vowels (aaaall)	_____	_____
Prolonging consonants (sssso, mmmy)	_____	_____
Silent blocks (b-aby)	_____	_____
Incomplete words (ba-)	_____	_____
Revisions (it was it went)	_____	_____
Interjecting (ah, um)	_____	_____
Other _____	_____	_____

14. Classify the main disfluency type at the time of onset and now:

Onset: __ Repetitions __ Prolongations __ Blocks __ Interjections
Now: __ Repetitions __ Prolongations __ Blocks __ Interjections

15. Were there secondary characteristics associated with the stuttered speech?

Secondary Characteristics	Onset	Now
Facial grimaces	_____	_____
Eyes closing/blinking	_____	_____
Eyes wide open	_____	_____
Lip tension (e.g., on /p, b, m/)	_____	_____
Lip tremor	_____	_____
Tongue tension (e.g., on /t, d, s, z, l, n/)	_____	_____
Mouth wide open	_____	_____
Jaw tremor	_____	_____
Throat tension	_____	_____
Respiratory irregularities	_____	_____
Upward swings in vocal pitch	_____	_____
Head tilting	_____	_____
Arm/leg movement/tension	_____	_____
Other _____	_____	_____

Parent Scale of Stuttering Severity

16. Rate the severity of the **earliest** stuttering at onset (may select midpoints):

0	1	2	3	4	5	6	7
Normal		Mild		Moderate		Very Severe	

17. Rate the **current** severity of the stuttering (may select midpoints):

0	1	2	3	4	5	6	7
Normal		Mild		Moderate		Very Severe	

18. Where in the speech stream did the stuttering occurred at onset? Now?

   At onset: __ First word primarily   __ Words throughout the sentences

   Now: __ First word primarily   __ Words throughout the sentences

19. Were there indications of the child being aware or reacting negatively to the stuttering soon after onset? Currently?

   At onset: __ Not aware   __ Somewhat aware   __ Clearly aware and bothered

   Describe: _____

   Now: __ Not aware   __ Somewhat aware   __ Clearly aware and bothered

   Describe: _____

Comments on Part III

Questions 12 through 19 are designed to provide detailed information about the stuttering characteristics both at onset and at the present. Requesting an imitation of the child's stuttering is a good way to obtain a more valid description. The direct comparison of past and present characteristics is an excellent way to evaluate the child's progress in relation to the length of the stuttering history. Neither the description of the initial stuttering nor the present stuttering, each in and of itself, is as meaningful as the comparison of the type, amount, and direction of the differences that have taken place over time. The disorder's progression over time is a key component in the assessment and prognosis. For example, a current severity rating of 5 (on our 8-point 0 to 7 scale) should be alarming if the case history reveals that when stuttering began it was rated by the parent as 2. The same rating of 5, however, would be viewed as a positive sign, if the stuttering severity at onset was rated by the parent as 7 because of the apparent progress. Having this information may have a significant impact on the prognosis for the child and the counseling given to parents concerning decisions for intervention.

Although parents are initially encouraged to describe in their own words the general course of stuttering and changes they have observed in overt stuttering characteristics as well as the child's reactions, checklists of speech and secondary characteristics are used because many parents often are unable either to recall or express all the details. It is important to differentiate carefully between parent descriptions of stuttering at onset and at the present. When rating the severity of stuttering on the 8-point scale, parents should be instructed to evaluate their overall impression. The clinician makes sure to define 0 as normal speech, 1 as borderline stuttering, 2 as definite but mild stuttering, 3 as mild+, 4 to 5 as a range of moderate, 6 as severe, and 7 as very severe. Parents are allowed to choose points halfway between numbered intervals. Comparison can also be made with the clinician's rating.

Part IV: General Development and Health History

20. Were there physical illnesses or emotional problems that the mother experienced during pregnancy that caused concern or required treatment?

    _____

    _____

21. What medications, drugs, and other medical treatments did the mother have during pregnancy with this child? _____

22. Were there any problems related to delivery?

    No _____   Yes _____   Explain _____

23. Did the child require special medical attention at or immediately after birth?

    No _____   Yes _____   Explain _____

24. Were there any medical problems noted in the child, at birth or shortly after, at a level to cause concern?

    No _____   Yes _____   Explain _____

25. Has the child had any serious health problems since birth?

    No _____   Yes _____   Explain _____

26. Has the child ever had any facial tics, jerks of other body parts, or any other type of involuntary muscle movements?

    No _____   Yes _____   Explain _____

27. Is the child on any medication now?

    No _____   Yes _____   Explain _____

28. In general do you regard the child's health now as:

    _____ Good   _____ Fair   _____ Poor

29. Has the child ever had a behavioral or psychological problem? (ADHD, ADD, depression, BD, others)

    No _____   Yes _____   Explain _____

30. Indicate age in months when the child acquired the following skills:

    Sat without support _____   Crawled _____   Walked without support _____

31. Overall, how do you regard the child's motor development?

    Below Average_____   Average _____   Above Average _____

32. Child's handedness:

   Right _____   Left _____   Mixed _____   Undetermined _____

33. In terms of speech, at what age did the following occur?

   Babbling _____   First word _____   Combined 2 or 3 words _____

34. Overall, would you say that the child's speech development was:

   Below Average _____   Average _____   Above Average _____

35. Aside from stuttering, has the child ever had any speech/language problem? If so, describe.

   No _____   Yes _____   Explain _____

36. Has the child ever had hearing problems? If yes, describe.

   No _____   Yes _____   Explain _____

37. Has the child ever received any treatment for speech, language, or hearing disorders?

   No _____   Yes _____   Explain _____

38. Has the child ever exhibited any of the following at a level to cause concern, or at age-inappropriate levels?

   _____ Sleeping problems   _____ Separation anxiety
   _____ Eating difficulties   _____ Excessive crying
   _____ Unusual fears   _____ Refusal to talk
   _____ Destructiveness   _____ Withdrawn behavior
   _____ Temper tantrums   _____ Restlessness
   _____ Excessive shyness   _____ None of the above

38. In comparison to other children, how much energy does the child have?

   _____ Below average   _____ Average   _____ Above Average

39. In terms of overall maturity is this child:

   _____ Below Average   _____ Average   _____ Above Average

Comments on Part IV

Research has not found any consistent factors, or a tendency for medical factors in general, to be present in the health histories of children who stutter. Yairi and Ambrose (2005) reported that only 14% of cases reported any physical stress associated with stuttering onset. Sometimes stuttering does coexist with other developmental or health problems that should be considered in the clinical recommendations and intervention planning. The clinician, therefore, must discuss and take into consideration the medical and health history. But clinicians should realize there are many variations in pregnancy, delivery, and health histories that occur in the general population without any resultant stuttering. If, in one case, a mother had 2 weeks of confinement to bed rest during pregnancy, or, in another case, there was jaundice at delivery, there should be no assumption these were causes of the child's speech problem. The health history helps the clinician understand the client and the speech difficulty in the larger context of the whole person's individual issues and needs.

Collecting Clinical Data

Obtaining Speech Samples

After obtaining a comprehensive case history of the onset and development of stuttering, as well parental description of the stuttering and judgment of its severity, the clinician proceeds to observe and test the child to obtain more objective as well as quantifiable data. A considerable portion of this part of the evaluation is similar to typical speech-language-hearing evaluations of preschool children seen for other communication problems. The standard tests of phonology, language skills, hearing, motor, and other domains are administered. The main difference is the need to obtain recorded speech samples that will be used to quantify the stuttered speech. A few opportunities to observe the child talking may arise in the waiting room and hallways when the child talks to the parents or responds to the clinician's greetings. Hence having a small handheld tape recorder is advisable to secure these brief moments of spontaneous speech before entering the examination facility. Permissions for audiovisual recording are obtained beforehand.

The more formal recording procedures for young children require similar equipment as specified in Chapter 10 for adults but call for extra flexibility. For example, some children may respond well when sitting at a small table in the recording room; others do better sitting on the floor, interacting with the clinician or parent. This condition, however, makes it difficult to adapt video recordings, resulting in a loss of useful information. To be effective, the camera should be focused on the child's head and upper body. We have had excellent experience obtaining speech samples with the child "confined" to a chair-table setting in a small test room yielding both good speech output and high-quality video and audio recordings. A small tie-tack microphone attached to the child's shirt is ideal. But if the child will be free to move, an inexpensive, omnidirectional microphone can detect speech quite well.

Quiet play materials, such as plastic clay or interesting action pictures, are preferable. Plastic and wooden toys generate noise that interferes with the quality of the recording. The clinician or parent initiates conversation about what the child is making with clay, then moves on to open-ended questions regarding the child's favorite toys or TV shows. Find out from parents about topics that particularly excite the child, such as particular pets, toys, TV programs, or events. Stuttering increases with heightening emotion, such as excitement or frustration. These topics often stimulate longer responses that are also more likely to trigger stuttering. Avoid and minimize questions that invite "yes" or "no" because they stop the conversation and typically are not stuttered as often as words in phrases. After the child says something, questions such as "What happened next?" and prompts such as "Tell me more about it" are quite useful to get the child going. Additionally, single-word responses are less desirable for analysis.

Preschool age children who stutter, especially in early stages of the disorder, tend to exhibit considerable fluctuations in their stuttering (Yaruss, 1997b). An evaluation that happens to be conducted on a "good day" could underestimate the magnitude of the problem. Therefore, two or three speech samples recorded over different days should be the target, especially when the stuttering is seen as mild. If the child exhibits severe stuttering, a single sample provides much of the needed information because there is more interest in the potential severity than in how mild it may be at times. Also, due to expected fluctuations, home speech samples are particularly desired for the young child who stutters. We provide parents with a handheld recorder and ask for 15 to 20 minutes of speech recorded in three to four brief (e.g., 5-minute) segments.

Recording in the clinical setting, the goal is to obtain at least 500 to 600 syllables and ideally close to 1000 syllables of conversational speech. The higher figure can often be achieved over two recording sessions, 15 to 20 minutes each, separated by a few days.

As indicated in Chapter 9, data by Sawyer and Yairi (2006) show that in four consecutive 300-syllable segments taken from continuous 1200-syllable speech samples of 20 children who stutter, the greatest amount of disfluency tended to occur in the last two segments, especially the fourth one. Had they used only the first 300 syllables, some or much of the children's disfluency would not have been reflected in the data. Several disfluency types, such as sound prolongations/blocks or complex disfluent events (e.g., those containing four or more repetition units), might occur in low frequency and cannot be adequately tapped in short samples, if at all. In other words, the validity and reliability of the data may be questioned. The risk with short speech samples is greater when the stuttering appears to be mild or mild to moderate.

It is desirable to record one of the sessions when the child interacts with a parent and another one with the clinician. Of course, the interaction during the recording of longer samples also provides more time to observe the child's behavior, reaction, and interaction.

Other Related Assessments

Two other aspects of stuttering: secondary body movement and tensions involved with disfluencies, and the child's awareness and emotional reactions should be included in the direct initial evaluation of preschool children. In our experience, too often these do not receive sufficient attention. The child should also be assessed for the possibility of other concomitant speech, language, or hearing problems.

Secondary Characteristics

For a long time these were regarded as late phenomena, emerging in late developmental stages of stuttering. During the past 20 years, however, research that employed videotape analyses of young stuttering children's speech demonstrated head and neck movements near the onset of stuttering (Conture & Kelly, 1991; Throneburg, 1997; Yairi, Ambrose, & Niermann, 1993). Additionally, direct observation of nearly 150 children near stuttering onset revealed secondary characteristics, such as head turn, lip pursing, and eye blinking, in 75% of the children (Yairi & Ambrose, 2005). Hence clinicians should look for, and note, the type and severity of secondary characteristics. The same list of secondary characteristics that appears in Chapter 9 is reproduced below. The clinician indicates which ones are observed. At the end, assign a severity rating based on the global impression of these secondary behaviors (mild, moderate, or severe).

Awareness and Emotional Reactions

This aspect of the initial evaluation of preschool-age children who stutter is quite different than it is with older children or adults. As we discussed in Chapter 3, recent experimental data, as well as clinical observations and parental report, have indicated that some children do project various levels of awareness. Thus it may be possible to obtain important information for those children. Toward this end, we suggest three potential procedures.

First is *parental report*. Simply ask parents if they have noticed any indication that the child is aware of the stuttering and/or visibly reacting to it emotionally. If the answer is positive, pursue in more detail: What is the evidence for it? Let the parents

---

Secondary Characteristics Checklist

____ Head jerks	____ Head turns (side; up; down)
____ Forehead tension	____ Nostrils flaring/constricted
____ Eyes closed; squinting	____ Eyes widely open
____ Facial contortions	____ Lips pressured
____ Lip tremor	____ Jaw tremor
____ Jaw closed tightly	____ Teeth grinding
____ Jaw wide open	____ Rotational or sideways jaw movement
____ Tongue protrusion	____ Throat tightened
____ Body swaying	____ Hand and/or arm movements

Estimated Severity: ____

respond first, and note whether they refer to a clear verbal expression, such as "I cannot talk," or a nonverbal display of frustration during moments of stuttering. Also, ask them to evaluate the frequency and strength of the child's expressions of awareness and affective reactions. Second is *direct questioning.* Ask the child if he or she is a good talker or ever makes mistakes when talking. Perhaps better, the clinician may stutter on purpose (e.g., " Do you like i-i-i-i-ice cream?") and then proceed to ask the child, "Who else talk likes that?" and "Do you sometimes talk like that?" Note the verbal reply and other possible reactions. The third procedure is the *puppet test* (see Ambrose & Yairi, 1994). The clinician holds two identical puppets, one on each hand. Each puppet says an identical sentence, with one speaking fluently and the second one stuttering. The child is asked which puppet talks the way she or he talks. This should be repeated several times, changing the order and hand of the stuttering and the fluent puppets. The level of accuracy and consistency provides some information. A discussion of the methods with the parents beforehand may be helpful to ensure that they will be comfortable with the method used by the clinician to explore awareness.

Anxiety, Temperament, and Personality

Recent research by Conture and colleagues (Karass et al., 2006) has implicated a role for temperament in the disorder of stuttering (see discussion in Seery et al., 2007). They found that compared to nonstuttering children, a significant proportion of preschool children who stutter tended to (1) become more emotionally aroused, (2) settle down less easily after arousal, and (3) show less emotional control during everyday stressful and challenging situations. If these initial observations are valid, then an evaluation of temperament may aid intervention planning. Instruments of assessment include the Children's Behavior Questionnaire (CBQ; Rothbart, Ahadi, Hershey, & Fisher, 2001) and the Behavioral Style Questionnaire (BSQ; McDevitt & Carey, 1978), which have been used in research with children who stutter (Anderson, Pellowski, Conture, & Kelly, 2003). Considering typical results of a temperament assessment, clinicians might work together with parents to discourage overly exciting environmental conditions for their child to talk in, provide more reassurances and calming encouragements to their child, and/or make a special point of preparing the child for what to expect before new or potentially fear-evoking situations (e.g., medical exams, fire drills, sitters, travel, etc.).

Language, Phonology, Motor, and Hearing

The initial evaluation of children who stutter, like that of other children, should include comprehensive testing of the speech mechanism, phonology, language, and hearing domains. Motor and other skills may be added according to case needs. Standard tests or tape-recorded conversational speech samples can be used for phonological and language analyses. Because deficits in these domains may impact decisions of whether to initiate therapy, and what approach is selected (Byrd, Wolk, & Lockett Davis, 2007), careful assessment must be pursued in addition to the primary focus on stuttering. These aspects of the evaluation, however, are not discussed in this book.

Analyzing Clinical Data

Disfluency Frequency and Types

After securing a tape-recorded speech sample, the next task is to identify and quantify the characteristics of stuttering. In most respects, the procedures and parameters involved are identical to those employed in the initial evaluation of adults as described in Chapter 9. Again, clinicians are faced with the choice of metric. Some clinicians prefer making categorical judgments of each word or syllable as either stuttered or not, and then calculate the percentage of stuttered words or syllables. This is the easiest method of quantifying stuttering that provides general information. It is also the method used in the Stuttering Severity Instrument (SSI-3; Riley, 1994). As we already explained, however, this metric does not yield specific descriptive data about the characteristics of the person's stuttering: How did he or she stutter? Did the stuttering contain repetitions, prolonged sounds, blocks, or other behaviors? If the client repeated a word, how many times was the word repeated: one, four, or seven times? Measures of percentage of stuttered words or syllables simply do not address such questions because they report a single number of "stutterings." Because there is a growing body of information showing the significance of specific disfluency types, as well as the length of disfluency in terms of the range and mean number of repetition units[1] in differential diagnosis and prognosis of stuttering (e.g., Ambrose & Yairi, 1999; Schwartz & Conture, 1988; Throneburg & Yairi, 2001), we believe that reporting the frequency-type-length of disfluency is a preferred method even though it requires more analysis time. Furthermore, changes over time in the specific disfluency types and their extent or length, rather than just changes in the percent of stuttering events, is of great value in monitoring important aspects of the child's progress.

The importance of specific disfluency data is illustrated with the following example. Suppose one clinician counted 15% stuttered syllables at the initial evaluation of a child. Three months later, the child again scored 15% stuttered syllables, leading to the conclusion that no change had occurred. Consider a second clinician who saw the same child at each of those same times but analyzed sample data differently. She noted 20 stuttering-like disfluencies (SLD) per 100 syllables at the initial evaluation (more than one disfluency, e.g., repetition flowing by prolongation, may occur on the same syllable). Among these, 5 were sound prolongations and 15 were part-word or word repetitions. The mean number of repetition units was two (e.g., bu-bu-but). At the 3-month follow-up, the child again scored 20 SLDs per 100 syllables, however, 15 were sound prolongations and only 5 were part-word repetitions. Furthermore, the mean

---

[1] As we discussed in Chapter 12, repetition units refer to the number of extra productions of a syllable or a word. For example, in "bu-but," the number of repetition units is 1. In "bu-bu-but" there are 2 units, and in "bu-bu-bu-bu-but" there are 4. To calculate the range and mean of the number of repetition units, data for monosyllabic part-word and whole word repetitions are combined.

number of repetition units was four (bu-bu-bu-bu-but). In contrast with the first clinician, she infers that the child's speech is worsening, not stable. In conclusion, when total SLD or overall disfluency remains constant, there may still be significant changes in the stuttering characteristics both in type and length of the disfluent events. These could show a significant worsening or improvement of the problem. Such information is missed by the methods of counting employed by the first clinician.

The same procedures for disfluency analysis described in Chapter 9 for adult speech samples should be followed when analyzing the samples of little children. These procedures involve careful transcription, replaying the video-recorded speech phrase by phrase or word by word, identifying and classifying each disfluent event according to the six disfluency types listed here, then calculating the respective frequencies as guided by the following chart.

Disfluency Type	Number in Sample	Per 100 Syllables
Part-Word Repetition	____	____
Monosyllabic Word Repetition	____	____
Disrhythmic Phonation	____	____
SLD Subtotal	____	____
Interjection	____	____
Revision	____	____
Phrase Repetition	____	____
Other Disfluency Subtotal	____	____
Overall Disfluency Total	____	____

Disfluency Length

The following three measures of the extent, or length, of disfluencies are worth consideration for inclusion.

Repetition Units

In addition to estimating the mean repetition unit, it is quite important to keep track of the number of word or part-word repetitions (per 100 words or syllables) that contain three or more units. It is perhaps the most powerful information for differentiating early stuttering from normal disfluency (Ambrose & Yairi, 1995, 1999). Repetitions of this size are extremely rare in the speech of normally fluent children. In fact, even instances of two repetition units are infrequent in normally fluent children as reported by Ambrose and Yairi (1999) and by Yairi and Lewis (1984). Hence their conspicuous presence in a speech sample is a strong diagnostic sign of stuttering.

Rate of Repetitions

The temporal characteristics of the child's repetitions also provide diagnostic clues because children who stutter tend to repeat syllables and words considerably faster than normally fluent children. The repetitions are faster because the intervals between the iterations are shorter. Conversely, the repetitions of normally fluent children are slower because the intervals between their iterations are about twice as long as those of children who stutter. Investigators have reported that interval duration alone was sufficient to differentiate children who stutter from normally fluent peers with 72% to 87% accuracy (Throneburg & Yairi, 1994; Yairi & Hall, 1993). Such measurements may be too difficult to execute in a clinical setting. Nevertheless, clinicians should make a point to note the tempo with informal observation.

Sound Prolongations

The length of sound prolongations is measured in terms of time duration. Because most of these disfluencies are sustained only up to 1 second (Bloodstein, 1995), it is useful to obtain and document the mean of only the three longest prolongations. The presence of prolongations longer than 1 second is also a strong sign of stuttering (Zebrowski & Conture, 1989). A few such events can easily increase the overall severity rating.

Speech Rate

Speaking rate is of diagnostic interest because of its negative correlation with the amount of disfluent speech. It is, however, often difficult to assess with reasonable accuracy in young children in the clinical setting because of their high frequency of both short utterances and long silences. Thus some clinicians may opt to spend more of their assessment time on other measures. Regardless, if deemed desirable, speech rate data can be extracted from the spontaneous speech sample. Reasonable estimates of *overall speech rate* can be obtained by measuring several minutes of conversational speech using a stopwatch. As explained in Chapter 9, it is considerably more complicated to accurately measure *articulatory rate*, which is based only on fluent portions of the speech sample, and it is more reliably obtained with sophisticated equipment for acoustic analysis. The limited research with preschool children has shown that close to stuttering onset, children who stutter tend to exhibit somewhat slower articulatory rates than normally fluent peers. The respective means were 8.43 and 11.42 phones per second and standard deviations (SD) were 1.16 and 2.77 (Hall, Amir, & Yairi, 1999) for children 3 and 4 years of age. In another study conducted by Meyers and Freeman (1985), 4- and 5-year-old children who stutter had mean articulatory rates of 3.5 syllables per second compared to nonstuttering controls who had rates of 4.04 syllables per second.

Interpreting Clinical Data

Although a subjective determination that the child presents with stuttering can probably be made during the examination, and although it will most likely be correct and in agreement with the parents' diagnosis, the clinician should continue to apply a careful evaluation of all the information gathered, starting with the speech data, comparing the client with other children who stutter and with normally fluent children. As we stated earlier, in most cases of stuttering, the purpose of the initial evaluation is to describe the problem and understand all contributing and complicating factors. Hence, after the formal evaluation, the clinician should be able to provide a rather comprehensive description of the problem, determine its severity, assess prognosis, formulate recommendations, and inform the parents.

Disfluency Status

As in other standard speech-language evaluations, the client's performance is compared against available data starting with those pertaining specifically to stuttering: percentage of stuttered words or syllables, or the type/frequency of disfluency, the extent and/or duration of disfluency, and secondary characteristics. Table 13.1 displays disfluency data for large groups of stuttering and normally fluent preschoolers.

As you can see, there are large differences between children who stutter and normally fluent children both in absolute and relative measures of each of the three SLD components. It is very important to examine the total SLD. Note that it is almost 10 times larger for CWS than for CWNS. Also note that whereas the total SLD constitutes approximately two thirds, or 66%, of the CWS's *overall disfluency* (10.37/15.78), it is only a quarter, or 24% (1.33/5.65), for CWNS. Although the standard deviations indicate a wide range for all but one item in the table, the data do

Table 13.1: **Mean and Standard Deviations of Stuttering-Like Disfluencies, Other Disfluencies, and Number of Repetition Units per Repetition per 100 Syllables***

	CWS		CWNS	
Type	Mean (SD)	Proportion	Mean (SD)	Proportion
SLD				
Part-word repetition	5.29 (4.20)	0.34	0.56 (0.40)	.10
Single-syllable word repetition	3.34 (2.14)	0.21	0.69 (0.60)	.12
Disrhythmic phonation	1.75 (2.00)	0.11	0.09 (0.12)	.02
Total SLD	**10.37 (6.42)**	**0.66**	**1.33 (0.83)**	**.24**
Repetition units	1.54 (0.39)		1.10 (0.12)	
OD				
Interjection	2.55 (2.20)	0.16	2.08 (1.89)	0.37
Revision	1.97 (1.09)	0.12	1.80 (0.85)	0.32
Multisyllable/Phrase Repetition	0.89 (0.63)	0.06	0.44 (0.44)	0.08
Total OD	**5.41 (2.75)**	**0.34**	**4.32 (2.28)**	**0.76**
Overall disfluency	**15.78**			**5.65**

* Also, the proportion of each disfluency type in the overall number of disfluencies for children who stutter and normally fluent children ages 2 to 4. CWS, children who stutter; CWNS, children who do not stutter; OD, other disfluencies; SD, standard deviation; SLD, stuttering-like disfluencies.

Source: Reprinted with permission from "Normative Disfluency Data for Early Childhood Stuttering," by N. Ambrose and E. Yairi. *Journal of Speech, Language, and Hearing Research, 42,* 895–909. Copyright 1999 by American Speech-Language-Hearing Association. All rights reserved.

provide meaningful guidelines. Next, look at the line for repetition units. Although the numbers are small, they are extremely revealing. The mean of 1.10 for the CWNS tell us that these children mostly repeat once per instance (bu-but). By contrast, the mean of 1.54 tells us that most repetitions by CWS contain two or more units (bu-bu-but). Matching the client's data against these published normative values and by adding observations on the presence of secondary characteristics, the disfluency analysis provides an anchor for the diagnosis and offers a clear picture of the essential features of the child's stuttering. The clinician is then in a position to also estimate the severity of the stuttering.

Stuttering Severity

Having observed, recorded, quantified, and described the child's speech and associated behaviors, a general overall rating of the severity of stuttering is in order. As we discussed in Chapter 9, there are several ways to arrive at such a rating, the simplest one by means of a perceptual rating scale spreads over a range of intervals. This may be the same 8-point scale used earlier to obtain the parent's rating and is displayed here again. Or, it may be another scale with a different interval range, such as those discussed in relation to the evaluation of adults and school-age children who stutter. When a perceptual scale is employed for assigning a global severity rating, the rater presumably takes into account all the parameters that are typically analyzed in the evaluation of stuttering: frequency and length of disfluent events, the degree of muscular tension and effort involved, and the type and number of secondary characteristics. Either a specific scale number or an in between number (e.g., 4.5) may be selected. Using the identical scale and method as the parent has the advantage of allowing direct comparison between the clinician's and the parent's perception.

Rating Scale of Stuttering Severity

0	1	2	3	4	5	6	7
Normal		Mild		Moderate		Very Severe	

A subjective severity rating can be made online, that is, while the clinician watches and listens to the child talking with the parent. Severity can also be evaluated during the face-to-face interaction by the clinician with the child. It would be wise to assign a separate rating for the two speaking situations. Another option is to delay the rating until after completing the quantified analysis of the recorded speech sample. If desired, a formal instrument can be used, such as the Stuttering Severity Instrument-3 (Riley, 1994) or the University of Illinois Stuttering Severity Scale (Yairi & Ambrose, 2005). The Illinois scale scores four components of disfluency. The first three, frequency, duration, and tension, are rated from 0 to 6 where 0 = normal, 1 = borderline, 2 = mild stuttering, and 6 = severe stuttering. These three scores are added and averaged (a maximal mean of 6). The fourth component, accessory characteristics, is rated only from 0 to 1, and this number is added to the mean of the first three. Thus, in total, the maximum score is 7 (very severe stuttering).

Borderline Cases

The real diagnostic challenge in terms of identifying the problem are those children, a very small number in our extensive experience, who present clinicians with some difficulties in determining their fluency status, stuttering or normal, because too few disfluencies occurred in their speech sample. Group means and standard deviations are not too useful in such cases. The clinician should review again parents' detailed descriptions and their imitations of the child's stuttering at home that can provide very useful hints. If parents report and imitate occasional daily stuttering such as "whe-whe-when," or /a-a-ai/ ("I"), the case should not be dismissed even if the speech sample recorded in the clinic contained only isolated disfluent events that could have been perceived as stuttering. As stated earlier, the extra repetition units are perhaps the most powerful sign. The clinician must consider what constitutes minimally sufficient criteria for classifying the child as exhibiting stuttering.

The differential diagnosis of stuttering from normal disfluency requires familiarity with the nature of speech characteristics at the margins of both. No single speech characteristic, observed only once, is sufficient to confirm stuttering. Such a basis could cause mistakes of overdiagnosis. Requiring validation from too many instances or types of speech characteristics, however, could lead to an underidentification of cases. Adopting a careful approach, clinicians should look for data at the very low end of the range of children who stutter where there is still no, or only minimal, overlap with normally fluent children. There are two questions: (1) What are the minimal disfluent speech characteristics associated with very mild stuttering? and (2) What are the upper limits for normal?

Several differentiating protocols (i.e., Adams, 1977; Pindzola & White, 1986; Van Riper, 1971) are, for the most part, outdated. They do contain a few worthwhile hints, however. For example, among the few quantified items listed by Van Riper (1971), he required at least (1) two syllable repetitions and/or (2) one sound prolongation of 1 second or longer per 100 words. Van Riper's concept of minimal three stutterings appears to be nearly equal to what, in our terminology, would be 3 SLDs per 100 words except that we believe the measure should be derived per 100 syllables. This figure seems to be consistent with what is widely accepted in clinical and research matters (Conture 2001; Ingham, 1999; Webster, 1980b). Yairi and Ambrose (2005, p. 114) reported that mean SLD (core) disfluency per 100 syllables for 103 preschool children who stutter, ages 23 to 59 months, was 11.30 (SD = 6.64). Calculation of 1 SD below the mean yields a value of 4.6. Data for normally fluent children, ages 27 to 58 months (N = 52) revealed a mean SLD disfluency frequency per 100 syllables of 4.48 (SD = 2.41). That is, the 4.6 SLD for children who stutter mentioned above just exceeds the average range for their normally fluent peers.

A set of seven minimal diagnostic criteria specifically for young children (ages 2 to 5 years) who appear to be borderline cases was reported by Yairi and Ambrose (2005,

p. 338) based on a careful analysis of their data. Each of the following is assessed at a minimal occurrence per 100 syllables:

- Part-word repetition (PW)   1.5
- Single–syllable word repetition (SSW)   2.5
- Disrhythmic phonation   0.5
- Total SLD   3.0
- Weighted SLD[2]   4.0
- Mean repetition units   1.5
- PW + SSW with 2 or more extra units   2.0

It was concluded that the presence of *at least three* of the seven features on the list is necessary to establish stuttering. Finally, the parents' description and rating of stuttering severity should be considered. If the child does not exhibit stuttering in the clinic but parents describe speech characteristics at home that raise suspicion of stuttering, home speech samples should be secured for further analysis.

Making Prognosis

Having completed the data-gathering, analysis, and diagnosis stages of the initial evaluation, the clinician is faced with the challenge of assessing the likely future development of the child's stuttering, that is, making a prognosis. It should first be understood that a diagnosis of stuttering based on the characteristics described previously does not imply an unfavorable prognosis, particularly when the identification is made soon after stuttering onset. Thus the initial severity of stuttering observed does not predict the outcome for the child (Yairi & Ambrose, 2005). However, when a child has been stuttering without any indication of a decline for at least a year, the chances for recovery without treatment are substantially reduced, and prognosis becomes more guarded or negative. Once a child has stuttered for 3 or 4 years, the prognosis is "persistent" or "chronic" stuttering. With strong evidence that approximately 75% or more of children who begin stuttering can be expected to exhibit natural recovery (e.g., Andrews & Harris, 1964; Ryan, 2001; Yairi & Ambrose, 2005), the ability to make early predictions as to who will recover and who will develop persistent stuttering could be a tremendous asset to clinicians and a major factor in the clinical strategy recommended to parents. It also raises several serious ethical and practical issues.

The challenge of prognosis is highlighted by the example of a clinician who assesses a child as having good chances for natural recovery and recommends a waiting period rather than immediate intervention. What level of accuracy in prediction should be acceptable, and how long should the waiting period be, if the child continues to stutter

---

[2] Weighted SLD is a measure that reflects three dimensions of disfluency—frequency, type, and extent—in a single score. It is calculated by adding together the frequency of part- and single-syllable word repetitions per 100 syllables (PW + SS) and multiplying that sum by the mean number of repetition units (RU), and then adding twice the frequency of disrhythmic phonation (DP) (blocks and prolongations) per 100 syllables. See Ambrose and Yairi (1999, 2005).

3, 6, 9, 12 months, or even longer? Placing a child in unnecessary therapy poses a burden to the family, in terms of time, cost, and concern. Additionally, it unjustifiably places a strain on professional and public resources while children with other pressing needs compete for the same opportunity. It should be obvious that if all 5% of preschool children who begin stuttering are in line for treatment, resources could quickly be exhausted. Health insurance companies, too, would probably resist footing the bill for this high proportion of controversial cases.

> Some have argued that unnecessary treatment may be ethically questionable as seen in the following quotation: "[W]e should candidly entertain the proposition that it might be ethically *inappropriate* to categorically direct all cases of early childhood stuttering for treatment, as has been advocated by other clinicians. It seems that, intentionally or unintentionally, clinicians do tend to scare parents into submitting their child to treatment by presenting a bleak picture of what might happen to the child and his/her speech if therapy is not immediately initiated. Typically, they press the point that, if left untreated, stuttering will grow in severity and will acquire many additional unpleasant characteristics, such as strong fears of talking, social withdrawal, etc. Statistically, however, the reverse is true." (Yairi & Ambrose, 2005, p. 416)

Past Prediction Guidelines

Over the years, several clinicians have offered lists of danger signs and criteria for predicting persistent (chronic) stuttering in children; others published more elaborated guidelines and formal instruments. These are listed here to familiarize you with the variety of characteristics that have been proposed.

> **Stromsta (1965)**: Acoustic traces of the second formant transition were explored among the early attempts to identify predictors of persistent and recovered stuttering. In 1965, Stromsta analyzed the acoustic waveforms of disfluencies recorded from young children after they began stuttering. He reported that 89% of children whose disfluencies lacked F2 transition and/or showed irregular termination of phonations were still stuttering 10 years later. Conversely, 91% of children whose disfluencies contained normal transitions and terminations of phonation were deemed recovered 10 years later. Unfortunately, vague and unreported aspects of the procedures rendered these findings useless. Indeed, Yaruss and Conture (1993) failed to corroborate them. More recently, other investigators analyzed the *fluent* speech of children near stuttering onset and reported that those who eventually persisted demonstrated significantly smaller change in their F2 transitions than those who recovered. This implied that their oral movements, especially of the tongue, were more restricted (Subramanian, Yairi, & Amir, 2003). Thus the clinical application of acoustic data must wait for much more research.
>
> **Van Riper (1971)**: Four subgroups (tracks) were distinguished by Van Riper that, among other characteristics, also varied in their tendency to recover or persist.

Extracting criteria from his scheme, the danger signs for persistence include (1) blocks as the early dominant disfluency, (2) late onset, (3) sudden onset, (4) a lack of episodic cycles of stuttering, and (5) poor articulation skills.

Curlee (1980): The risk of chronic stuttering increases for cases that evidence (1) part-word repetition of two or more units on 2% or more of the words, (2) prolongations longer than 1 second, (3) involuntary blocks longer than 2 seconds, (4) secondary characteristics, (5) noticeable emotional reaction, (6) complaints of not being able to function satisfactorily, and (7) marked variation in frequency and severity of stuttering.

Conture (1990): At least two of the following characterize persistent stuttering: (1) sound prolongations or blocks that constitute more than 25% of the total disfluencies produced by the child, (2) lack of eye contact during more than 50% of conversations, (3) frequent and/or unusual use of phonological processes, (4) prolongations, blocks, or part-word repetitions on the first production of diadochokinetic tasks, and (5) oral motor or neurological screening scores indicating delayed neuromotor development.[3]

Riley (1981): Based on this author's *Stuttering Prediction Instrument for Young Children—SPI*: (1) presence of secondary characteristics, (2) the child's frustration with disfluencies, (3) parents' reactions to disfluencies, (4) more than three repeated units in part-word repetitions, (5) part-word repetitions repeated "abnormally," (6) presence of prolongations and blocks, and (7) frequency of disfluencies per 100 words. Information is gathered from the parents and observation of the child's speech. In this instrument, each item is scored within a range of possible points (e.g., 0 to 4). Combining all item scores, the total score ranges from 0 to 40. A score of 10 or greater suggests a risk for chronic stuttering.

Cooper and Cooper (1985): Based on the author's Chronicity Prediction Checklist, the child exhibits any of the following: (1) 5% of words are disfluent for over 6 months, (2) the average duration of disfluencies is greater than 2 seconds, (3) struggling articulatory gestures or blocks, (4) the presence of secondary characteristics, (5) the child has negative feelings about disfluencies, or (6) the parents have negative feelings about disfluencies that may be detrimental to the child. These are the most important items in the instrument that also generates scores from 0 to 27. A score from 7 to 15 indicates a need for vigilant observation; a score from 16 to 27 is predictive of chronic stuttering.

***Yaruss, LaSalle, and Conture* (1998)**: Several of the following: (1) more than 10% total disfluency, (2) larger than 30% ratio of sound prolongation to repetition, (3) a score higher than 3 on the Iowa Scale of stuttering severity, (4) a score higher than 18 on the Stuttering Severity Instrument, (4) a score higher than 16 on the Stuttering Prediction Instrument.

---

[3] Conture also believed that the use of fast speaking rate or complex vocabulary by the parents might aggravate the child's stuttering, making it more difficult to become fluent.

Review and Summary

We note with interest that the top criteria listed in these sources refer to stuttered speech: type or frequency of disfluency, acoustic features, or secondary characteristics. Overall, the main focus is on the severity of overt stuttering with some consideration of the emotional reaction to it. Van Riper also considered some information regarding onset. Unfortunately, these and other past ideas on the subject were not accompanied by scientific data sufficient to support them. For example, in the Stuttering Prediction Instrument (SPI) (Riley, 1981) some data were collected from children who were nearly 9 years old. Hence their predictive value for children near the onset of stuttering, typically between the ages of 2 and 4, when the prognosis is most needed and meaningful, is substantially diminished. Also, the sample consisted of 75% persisting and 25% recovered children, just the reverse of the expected proportion, raising more questions about the instrument. Similarly, several items on the Chronicity Prediction Checklist (Cooper & Cooper, 1985) assume the child has already stuttered for 2 years, much too long for "early" prediction.

> In reviewing past criteria and the way they were derived, Yairi and Ambrose (2005) pointed out two fundamental requirements essential for establishing criteria for early prediction of the course of stuttering. First, data should be collected from *unbiased, representative samples* of many stuttering children over several years. Second, children must be observed and followed from a time as *close* to *onset* as possible, so that those who exhibit early natural recovery are taken into account. They emphasized the second point, stating, "It goes without saying that the longer the stuttering history is at the point when data are collected, the less applicable they are to predicting the course of very early stuttering, when prognosis is needed the most" (Yairi & Ambrose, 2005, p. 346).

Recent Developments: The Illinois Prediction Criteria

The large scale longitudinal study conducted at the University of Illinois mentioned in Chapter 3 identified a substantial number of children close to the time of stuttering onset and followed them for several years. A wide range of aspects of the disorder were examined, such as type of onset, characteristics of early stuttering, language and phonology, motor skills, cognition, affective reactions, genetics, and many others (Yairi & Ambrose, 2005). Because changes over time were measured for children who eventually recovered without treatment, as well as for those who persisted in stuttering, the study is unique in its wealth of information pertaining to clinical assessment of a child's risks for persistent stuttering or the chance for natural recovery. These authors distinguished three levels of prognostic criteria according to their strength. These are listed here followed by explanations. Also, see Chapter 3, the section on predictive factors, for additional information.

Predictive Factors

Primary Factors	Secondary Factors	Tertiary Factors
Family history	Stuttering severity	Concomitant disorders
Gender	Head and neck movement	Awareness and affective reactions
Stuttering (SLD) trends	Phonological skills	
Duration of stuttering	Expressive language	
Age at onset	Acoustic features	
Disfluency length		
Sound prolongations/blocks		

Comments on Primary Factors

Familial History.   At the present this appears to be the strongest as well as earliest predictor. A history of familial stuttering, however, is not sufficient information. What counts is the specific *pattern* of the history. If the child has relatives who recovered from stuttering, as stated earlier, he or she has a 65% chance for natural recovery. Conversely, a familial history of persistent stuttering gives the child a similar chance for developing persistent stuttering. A pattern of familial persistence is apt to reduce the amount of waiting time prior to intervention.

Gender.   If the child is a boy, the risk for persistency is greater than if the child is a girl. Not only do girls have better prognosis for recovery, they also tend to recover sooner. When a girl fails to improve within a year, her risk for persistent stuttering increases.

Age at Onset.   Late age at onset, for example, 50 to 60 months (4 to 5 years), tends to be associated with persistency. Age also presents another risk because the older the child is at the time of onset, the higher is the awareness of stuttering and the consequent emotional reactions. Additionally, the child's friends are older, and they too are more likely to react negatively to the stuttering.

Duration of Stuttering History.   If stuttering has continued for 1 year, the risk for persistency increases. The longer the history, the higher is the risk. When other information is unavailable, this factor becomes more critical. Soon after onset, a child's chance for recovery is at least 75%. A year later, the chance for recovery is down to 63%, declining to 47% at 2 years post-onset, dropping to 16% at 3 years, and to only 5% at 4 years after onset. Unfortunately, except for the Yairi and Ambrose (2005) source, this critical information has been overlooked in the various prognostic schemes reviewed previously. For example, if the prognostic criteria include a certain level of stuttering as a risk factor, it has no practical meaning without reference to the duration of the stuttering history.

SLD Trends.   The frequency and severity of stuttering during the first year post-onset provide important clues. It is not the specific number of stuttering (or SLD) which is critical but its trend over time. A *downward* trend during the first year, even if the frequency remains high, is a strong sign for eventual recovery. A decline from 20 to 12 SLDs over 3 months is a good sign. A stable number of 12 SLDs over the same period is not. For the majority of children who show such decline, however, full recovery will take 2 or 3 years postonset. However, a child who exhibits a flat or an upward trend of stuttering by the end of 1 year should be regarded as being at risk. Ideally, children should be recorded every 3 months to obtain data. Severity ratings made by the parents may also be used to analyze the trend.

Disfluency Length and Tempo.   During the first year of stuttering, the *continuing* presence of disfluencies with more than one repetition unit, especially those containing three or more units (e.g., bu-bu-bu-but) is a sign of risk. Reduction of the repetition units typically coincides with a diminution in the frequency of stuttering. If repetitions become shorter in number of units, prognosis is more positive. Slower tempo of repetitions is also a positive sign for recovery. However, the length (duration) of blocks and prolongations early on is *not* a predictive factor. (At the early stage, however, blocks or prolongations are relevant for differential diagnosis.)

Sound Prolongation/Blocks.   A substantial number of sound prolongations or blocks poses a possible risk, although *not* during the first few months of the disorder. When the percentage of sound prolongations in the total disfluency declines over time, it signals recovery. Conversely, when the percentage grows, so does the risk for persistency.

Comments on Secondary and Tertiary Factors

Stuttering Severity.   Stuttering severity during the early stage of the disorder (6 months or so) is *not* a predictive sign. One year after onset, however, severe stuttering does become a risk signal.

Head and Neck Movement.   Secondary characteristics are *not* an early danger sign. They become a sign of risk if, after 1 year, there is no substantial decline in their number and severity.

Phonology.   During the early phase of stuttering, phonology skills below norms might be a risk. In isolation, however, it is not a strong factor. But if other signs for persistency are present, the phonology status serves to reinforce them. Poor phonology, however, should alert the clinician to look for other possible risk signs. During the second year, phonological skills lose their predictive power.

Expressive Language.   The power of the child's language skills in the prediction of stuttering pathways is not clear. If at all, advanced skills may be a danger sign, especially if they remain ahead of normative expectations across time (Watkins, 2005). Delayed language, however, may complicate stuttering.

Acoustic Features.   Current F2 transition data present an insufficient basis for early prediction of the course of stuttering.

Concomitant Disorders.   The prognostic power of other disorders associated with stuttering, not including language and phonology discussed earlier, is unknown. The presence of concomitant disorders and medications used for treatment (particularly theophylline) may exacerbate stuttering. Thus the additional complication of various disorders or health-related problems may increase risk for persistency.

Awareness and Affective Reactions.   Thus far, there is no evidence from research that a young child's awareness of, and emotional reaction to, stuttering, predict persistency. Yet it is possible that either the child's or a parent's strong reaction to stuttering might complicate the speech difficulty and negate potential recovery if other factors were favorable.

Case Studies

The predictive power of the Illinois criteria varies greatly, and no single characteristic is sufficient for valid estimates of the chances for persistence or recovery. It is the converging of several factors that clinicians must look for. A few cases will illustrate the point.

Julie was first evaluated at 29 months of age, 4 months after onset. At the time she exhibited severe stuttering, about 18 SLD per 100 syllables, mostly repetitions of two to four units with moderate tension. Being so young with a brief stuttering history and no apparent danger signs, waiting and reevaluation in 3 months was recommended in spite of the severe stuttering. At the second visit, the frequency of SLD dropped to 13 per 100 syllables and repetition units to only 2 per instance. Her mother reported similar observations. Although the stuttering was still moderate in severity, being a girl, the clear decline in frequency and length of disfluency, and the continuing lack of other danger signs indicated high chances for recovery. Again, a waiting period and another reevaluation was recommended. Three months later, stuttering was mild. By 1 year post-onset, she displayed completely normally fluent speech without intervention.

Matthew was evaluated at 34 months of age, 2 months post stuttering onset. He exhibited low-moderate stuttering, about 8 SLD per 100 syllables that composed mainly of repetitions of two extra units. The boy's father had a history of stuttering and still exhibited mild-to-moderate stuttering. No other danger signs were identified. In spite of the family history of persistent stuttering, because of the very short history of the problem and the moderate stuttering, it was decided to recommend a 3-month waiting period under close monitoring. At the reevaluation, the frequency of SLD rose to 11 SLD per 100 syllables, and a few sound prolongations were observed. Hence because of the three danger signs: being a boy, family history of persistent stuttering, and the increase in the level of stuttering over time, immediate therapy was recommended.

Todd was evaluated at 58 months of age, 6 months after a sudden onset. At that time he exhibited moderate stuttering, about 12 SLD per 100 syllables, consisting of about 50% sound prolongations and 50% repetitions, mostly of two to three units, all associated with moderate tension and some secondary characteristics. Language tests revealed indicated precocious skills, but a few age-inappropriate phonological errors were noticed. There were also indications of frustration associated with stuttering episodes. No history of stuttering was recalled by parents. The mother reported essentially consistent amount and pattern of stuttering over the past several months. In view of the multiple danger signs: being a boy, sudden and late onset, a large percentage of sound prolongations, precocious language, phonological delay, and apparently consistent, unabated stuttering patterns, Todd was viewed as having a high risk for persistent stuttering. Therapy was recommended.

Concluding Parent Conference

Having taken part in providing the background information at the beginning of the evaluation, the parents, most often only the mother, are brought back into the process for the conclusion that includes two distinct parts: (1) receiving feedback about the clinician's findings and recommendations, and (2) having an opportunity to ask questions and receive information and guidance regarding stuttering.

Diagnosis, Prognosis, and Recommendations

As in any other speech-language evaluation, the clinician should state the main finding, most often confirming the parent's diagnosis of stuttering, as well findings concerning additional problems in other areas covered in the evaluation. The clinician then outlines the main characteristics of the stuttering, such as the dominant disfluency type(s), typical length of the disfluencies, e.g., three repetition units, secondary characteristics, tension, variations in the frequency of stuttering when talking to parent and clinician, the overall level of stuttering severity, indications of awareness or emotional reactions, and whether the stuttering seems to be at an early or a more advanced stage. Of course, when warranted, parents might instead be informed that the child exhibits normal disfluency. Next, specific results of language, phonology, motor, hearing, and any other tests and observations are presented with explanations and comparisons to the normative range.

The focus then shifts to discussion of the possible future course (prognosis) of the disorder. The clinician points out to parents the fact that about 5% of all children experience stuttering for some period during the preschool years but that at least 75% of them stop stuttering on their own, a phenomenon referred to as *natural recovery*. Some experience natural recovery rather quickly, within a few months to 1 year after onset; most take 2 to 3 years. Although the outlook for positive development is statistically good, parents should keep in mind that some children do not recover and develop chronic stuttering that lasts for several or many years.

The clinician should clearly caution parents that, at the present state of knowledge, it is not possible to make an accurate prediction about a specific child's eventual course of stuttering. Nevertheless, given what we do know, reasonable estimates of the relative chances of change in the near future are possible and can be helpful in making clinical recommendations and decisions. Therefore the clinician proceeds to review for the parents their child's standing in relation to the various risk factors listed and discussed earlier.

This example reviews some relevant prognostic factors as may be discussed with the parents during postassessment counseling. "The child is a boy. Boys have a poorer chance for recovery than girls, which is a negative point. Your son's grandfather, however, stuttered when he was very young but stopped after 3 years. This is a favorable sign because your son has a good chance to follow the same pattern. Still, many of the child's disfluencies are sound prolongations at half a year post-onset, another negative point. But although you have expressed concerns that the boy has stuttered for 6 months, you have noticed an overall improvement during the last 2 months from a stuttering severity rating of 6 (severe) to a rating of 4 (moderate). This is a positive point." Given the family history and the signs of improvement, the clinician would be in a position to support an additional waiting period with continued monitoring over the next 2 to 3 months. A decision to initiate intervention is appropriate, however, when the parents prefer it.

Having considered all factors with due regard to their importance, the clinician has the responsibility of either recommending a waiting period of 2 to 3 months followed by reevaluation or urging the parents to seek an immediate intervention program. When a waiting period is recommended, the child can be monitored for the prescribed duration, allowing the clinician to compare her own data over that time period. If the improvement endures, the monitoring will continue. If the stuttering is not improved, intervention options will be considered in due time. If therapy is recommended, parents should be provided with a list of local providers. The clinician may explain that whereas in the past, intervention was conducted mostly in the form of parent counseling, the past 25 years have seen a growing trend of providing direct therapy to the child while keeping the parents in the picture too. Now the clinician can proceed by pointing out the rationale for the traditional and the current approaches, explaining essential features of the major current types of therapies, as follows:

1. Practice the child in slow speech or other voluntary speech movement.
2. Reinforce fluency and discourage speech behavior that triggers disfluencies.
3. Improve parent-child relation and child's interpersonal skills.
4. Psychological play therapy.

A review of several specific therapy programs representing these approaches is presented in Chapter 14. The clinician explains that practitioners use different specific techniques under each of the categories just listed. For example, slow speech may be practiced using stretched speech or a metronome-paced speech. Reinforcing fluency can be done by praising each instance of fluent speech (e.g., the Lidcombe method; Harrison, Onslow, & Rousseau, 2007) or by reinforcing a gradually increased length of fluent utterances (e.g., the ELU; J. Ingham, 1999). Parents, however, should be informed that although therapies sometimes appear to help either directly to reduce stuttering or indirectly to create a more favorable home environment for fluency, there are still very few strong, well-controlled research studies confirming the clinical effectiveness for most treatment programs and strategies.

Parent Counseling

Limited immediate parent counseling in conjunction with the initial evaluation of the preschool child who stutters has been a standard practice for a long time. Already several decades ago, many authors wrote on this subject, offering general and specific advice (e.g., Brown, 1949; Johnson, 1961b; Sander, 1959; Schuell, 1949; Zwitman, 1978). Their ideas are reflected in more recent sources (see review by Yairi & Ambrose, 2005, Chapter 11). Not knowing what action parents will take or when, or in response to their queries about stuttering, the clinician should impart (1) essential information about the disorder, (2) advice about the desired home environment, (3) advice concerning responding to the child's stuttering, and (4) follow-ups. It is important, however, for the clinician and parents to understand that much of the commonly given advice lacks sufficient scientific evidence for the sake of realistic expectations. Nevertheless, much of it reflects common sense and clinical experience. A special visit without the child affords a more relaxed and open discussion. Yairi and Ambrose (2005) provide a verbatim text as an example of typical feedback and advice given to parents. Their main points, based on a review of the rich literature, are summarized here by providing answers to four questions.

What Causes Stuttering?

Parents are briefly informed of the diverse ideas regarding the cause of stuttering, representing four theoretical orientations: psychological, learning, organic, and multiple causation. Research data do not support the first two categories. For example, it has been found that people who stutter, as a group, are not emotionally maladjusted. Although it is still not known what makes a child stutter, there is evidence implicating neurological and motor components. Also, whatever is the cause, it is genetically transmitted. Once the stuttering begins, however, environmental factors come into play, shaping its features and development. Parents can contribute to improving the child's stuttering by creating a favorable home environment that might facilitate natural recovery, or, if the child develops chronic stuttering, help him or her become a well-adjusted person.

What Can Be Done at Home?

Four points of advice are presented to parents:

1. Decrease undue pressures. Knowing that stuttering tends to increase under various pressures, parents are to identify and reduce the various sources. Some are common, such as excessive demands, rules, or high expectations. Others are unique to the family.
2. Create a more relaxed home atmosphere. Physical and emotional stimulation, excitability, being in a hurry, or fatigue all tend to increase stuttering.

Parents should strive to create a more relaxed home atmosphere, avoid rushing, minimize excitement, and select slow-paced activities.

3. Slow speech and conversational exchanges. Slow speaking rate has been known to increase fluency. To this end, parents do best by slowing down their own speech, providing a model. Parents need some practice in slow speech. Hence experiment first in selected brief situations, such as telling a story when alone with the child. Then expand to other situations when possible. In particular, slow down the pace of conversational turn-taking by having a slight delay before responding to the child's statement or question (see Bernstein Ratner, 2004).

4. Build self-confidence. Stuttering has the potential to impair the child's self-image and self-confidence. This may be as handicapping as the stuttering. Simple parental behaviors, such as giving praise for performing small jobs, are suggested. Parents are also encouraged to make sure the child's communicated messages are valued even if he or she stutters.

What to Do When the Child Stutters?

After a comprehensive review of the rich literature on this topic, Yairi and Ambrose (2005) settled on four suggestions that represent a passive-active mixture:

1. When stuttering is mild or moderate, wait patiently. Allow the child to finish without comments or help. Acceptance is implied and pressure is avoided.

2. When the stutter event is moderate to severe or worse, use echoing: Parent is to repeat the stuttered word in an easy, somewhat prolonged but fluent manner. This provides a model for self-correcting without applying direct pressure.

3. When severe stuttering occurs, parents may take a more direct approach, suggesting to the child to say the word again slowly and easily. Sometimes the parent may offer to say the word in unison and then let the child repeat alone. Such suggestions must be made very calmly.

4. Parents should respond with empathy and encouragement when the child is frustrated during or after stuttering (e.g., by stating, "Sometimes talking is hard, but that's okay, you will be fine"). Such attitude may help create open communication about the problem.

Clinicians may explain to parents that children often react to stuttering in whatever way listeners/parents react. If listeners are worried/concerned, or if the child's speech is interrupted or cut short frequently because of stuttering, the child will soon learn that it is not okay to say something if it might come out with "bumpy" stuttering. This can lead to more hesitation over talking and interfere with the learning process for smoothing out speech. Listeners need to show they are comfortable and patient with all the bumpy, stuck, or struggled speech, so that the child does not get upset when doing it. The listener needs to convey that there is time for the child to work it out. This means

> waiting neutrally for the child to finish, with a mind focused on the child's message. Remaining neutral and comfortable, however, can be difficult when the child's struggle is particularly severe. The clinician should help parents understand that getting upset is not helpful either to the child or for themselves.

What's Next?

Regardless of the clinical recommendations, whether immediate therapy or a waiting period, parents are instructed to closely monitor their child's speech, other behaviors, and reactions. Schedule a follow-up visit within a few weeks. If possible, parents should obtain audio or video speech samples and keep detailed notes concerning variations in the features and severity of the stuttering. These will be very helpful in assessing the child's progress and in making changes regarding treatment decisions. Parents are also encouraged to secure missing background details, such as the family history of stuttering.

Summary

The initial evaluation of the preschool-age child who stutters is typically initiated by concerned parents. In the great majority of cases, the evaluation ends up as a systematic process of information gathering about the various aspects or dimensions of the disorder rather than a classic diagnostic search for an unknown condition. This is so because most often parental diagnosis of the child's speech impediment as "stuttering" is shared by the speech-language clinician who backs up his or her subjective perception with objective data. Questionable, borderline cases in the gray area between normal disfluency and stuttering are few. We have provided finer diagnostic procedures and criteria for such cases.

The major parts of the evaluation include an extensive parent interview; audiovisual recording of speech; analyses of disfluency and secondary characteristics; probing into awareness, emotional reactions, and temperament; and testing for language, phonology, hearing, and motor skills. Interview materials, normative disfluency data, and stuttering severity scales were offered, as well as suggestions for additional instruments. The evaluation concludes with parent counseling, which, among other objectives, focuses on providing information about stuttering, suggestions for modifying general home environment, and advice concerning handling stuttering.

Overall, the young age of the child necessitates greater involvement of the parents at several points throughout the evaluation. The brief history of the disorder in young children allows for the collection of more reliable information, some of which, such as the familial history of stuttering, may be particularly useful for prognosis and clinical recommendations. Furthermore, because at this early stage of the disorder children have a good chance for natural recovery, the weighing of these chances for prediction purposes is an important element of the evaluation. The knowledge that most children will outgrow the disorder without intervention presents clinicians with questions: Should children who are good candidates for recovery be directed to receive therapy or wait awhile? If waiting is recommended, for how long? Clinicians, and parents, should bear in mind that the prognostic criteria reviewed here are tools for making reasonable risk assessments. They are not, however, powerful enough for making accurate predictions. Their review is a matter of assessing probabilities and risks. Children who appear to be at low risk and are recommended for waiting should continue to be closely monitored.

STUDY QUESTIONS AND DISCUSSION TOPICS

1. What are the main differences between the initial evaluation of preschool children and adult or school-age children who stutter?
2. Why it is important to determine accurately the time of stuttering onset?
3. Why it is important to ask parents to compare the various characteristics and severity of stuttering at the time of onset and at the time of the evaluation.
4. What are the minimally sufficient disfluent speech characteristics required for the classification of a child as exhibiting mild stuttering?

5. What dimension and characteristics of stuttered speech are typically used in rating its overall severity?
6. Is it necessary to include speech and nonspeech domains other than fluency in the evaluation of stuttering in preschool children? Defend your answer.
7. What are the main criteria for assessing a child's chance for natural recovery or persistent stuttering? Briefly explain each one.
8. What are the main objectives of parent counseling at the conclusion of the initial evaluation? Explain.

SUGGESTED READINGS

Dillolo, A., & Manning, W. (2007). Counseling children who stutter and their children. In E. Conture & R. Curlee (Eds.), *Stuttering and related disorders* (3rd ed., Chapter 7). New York: Thieme.

Gordon, P., & Luper, H. (1992a). The early identification of beginning stuttering I: Protocols. *American Journal of Speech-Language Pathology, 1*, 43–53.

Gordon, P., & Luper, H. (1992b). The early identification of beginning stuttering II: Problems. *American Journal of Speech-Language Pathology, 1*, 49–55.

Gregory, H., & Hill, D. (1999) Differential evaluation—differential therapy for stuttering children. In R. Curlee (Ed.), *Stuttering and related disorders of fluency* (2nd ed.). New York: Thieme.

Riley, G. (1984). *Stuttering prediction instrument for young children*. Austin, TX: Pro-Ed.

Yairi, E., & Ambrose, N. (2005). *Early childhood stuttering: For clinicians by clinicians*. Austin, TX: Pro-Ed. See Chapters 10 and 11.

Chapter 14: Treatment of Preschool-Age Children Who Stutter

LEARNER OBJECTIVES

Readers of this chapter will understand:

- Factors related to intervention for preschool children who stutter.
- The historical background of therapy for early stuttering.
- The range of treatment objectives for preschool children who stutter.
- Clinical programs representing the major treatment approaches to early stuttering.
- Research issues concerned with treatment of preschool who stutter.

General Considerations

Having reviewed and discussed the treatment of stuttering in adults and school-age children, we now shift attention to general approaches, specific techniques, and programs that have been offered for the treatment of preschool-age children. Chapter 2, which focused on the distribution of the stuttering population, established that the overwhelming majority of people who stutter experience the onset of the disorder (incidence) during the preschool period, ages 2 to 5, mostly before age 3. Additionally, the data show that the prevalence of stuttering (the percentage of people who exhibit active stuttering) is also the largest in this age group.[1]

In spite of these indisputable facts, systematic clinical intervention programs aimed specifically for preschool-age children who stutter have been relatively late to appear, and for a long time they lacked the breadth of treatment methods offered to adults who stutter. This trend paralleled the one seen in the research domain that, for many years, favored adults who stutter. It probably reflects several realities. First has been the lingering "hands off the child" attitude toward treatment of early stuttering that was promoted especially in the United States. Second may have been a tendency toward thinking that stuttering in children and adults was all the same. Third, university laboratories and clinics were mainly accessible to college students. Fortunately, the trend has been reversed, and the

---

[1] One study (Craig et al., 2002), however, suggested a peak prevalence in the 6- to 10-year age group.

past three decades have seen a substantial increase both in research activity and clinical programs pertaining to preschool-age children who stutter. The following brief historical account of past therapies for this age group is intended to provide a broadened perspective on current clinical issues and therapy programs.

A Brief Historical Review

Therapeutic interventions for early childhood stuttering have operated with different philosophies that have alternated over the years, reflecting changes in the dominant thinking of mainstream speech pathology in respect to direct and indirect intervention modes. The distinction between direct and indirect therapies for stuttering is not clear. Some clinicians, for example Conture (2001), make the distinction primarily in the approach taken to change the child's speech. Hence an indirect approach does *not* explicitly, overtly, or directly change the child's speech fluency. Rather, the focus is on changing the child's environment, especially parents' behavior. Direct approaches, however, involve explicit attempts to modify the child's speech. Our interpretation, by contrast, encompasses a wider context of what is considered direct therapy.

The term *direct therapy* applies to methods in which the clients themselves are subjected to treatment. In addition to methods in which the child who stutters receives guidance for making speech changes (speech therapy), psychologically oriented therapy and/or physical stimulation of parts of the body (e.g., oral structures) are viewed as direct. For example, play therapy with the child as a participant in a process aimed at altering his or emotionality and behavior is direct therapy. Although play therapy does not deal with speech modification, it is a method that requires a very direct contact between clinician and child. A therapy that is limited to physical stimulation of oral muscles (not speech therapy) is also viewed as direct.

In view of the constraints placed on early intervention, particularly by the client's age and the nature of the early stuttering, discussed later, it is interesting to note the diversity of treatments that have been applied. In that light it also is surprising that many share a fair number of objectives with the major therapeutic approaches listed in Chapter 9 for older children and adults. The procedures, however, have been adapted to suit young children.

Direct Treatments

Toward the end of the 19th century and the first decades of the 20th century, the most frequently advocated types of programs involved direct therapy in which the child was the main recipient of the treatment. They leaned toward what we have referred to as *fluency enhancement*, that is, the elicitation and subsequent practice of talking patterns that produce fluent speech, rather than modification of instances of stuttering. Such philosophy was particularly dominant in Europe.

European Methods

According to Pay and Sirotkina (1955), Russian clinicians devised intensive programs, including all-day clinics, that required children as young as 2 years of age to memorize and repeat sentences, tell picture stories, rehearse questions and answers, and drill rhythmic activities. These activities perhaps reflected a strong view, held in eastern Europe, that stuttering is also a disorder of language. Hence enriching the child's vocabulary and expressive language were important therapeutic objectives (Daskalov, 1962). Others focused on developing speech breathing and easy phonation to facilitate fluency. Music and singing were also favored because they introduced rhythm into the speech pattern, a condition that yields fluency. In one program, the children practiced coordinating speech utterances with body movements and music to facilitate speech rhythm. Although some attention was given to modification of emotional reactions, there was more emphasis on regimented rest and sleep to achieve relaxation, which, in turn, was supposed to facilitate fluency. Even sedation was sometimes used for this purpose (Vlasova, 1962).

By contrast, linguistically oriented therapies were not practiced in western Europe. There, some clinicians employed motorically oriented techniques. These included having children say phrases that were timed with body movements (Pichon & Borel-Maisonny, 1937), teaching them to speak slowly and practice coordination of speech with breathing (Emil-Behnke, 1947), or talking in unison (Kingdon-Ward, 1941). Others devised therapies based on the conception of stuttering as a perceptual disorder that disrupted auditory feedback. Consequently, children were asked to talk while shadowing the clinician's speech so as to not depend on their own feedback (Marland, 1957).

American Methods

A different direct therapy was employed by a few clinicians in the United States who viewed stuttering as a neurological problem affecting muscle coordination. They opted for a nonspeech approach, working with the child to manipulate neurological and muscular functions. For example, based on Lee Travis's (1931) theory that stuttering results from lack of cerebral dominance, Johnson (1934) thought it was possible to eliminate early stuttering by retraining the child's handedness, shifting it from left to right. Supposedly, it should have helped the child establish left cerebral dominance. Other clinicians who adhered to the moto-kinesthetic method stimulated the child's speech muscles (e.g., touching the lips or tongue), instructed the correct placement of the speech organs, as well as drilling children in specific speech movement sequences (Young & Hawk, 1955).

A third direct approach reflected psychogenic perspectives of stuttering that relegated the blame for stuttering to the child's neurotic parents. Although some clinicians coming from this orientation directed considerable therapeutic attention to the parents (indirect therapy), the child too was suspected of harboring neurotic reactions that warranted therapy. This gave rise to diverse psychotherapeutic programs, especially play therapy that focused directly on the child (e.g., Harle, 1946). Perhaps the most notable effort was Murphy and Fitzsimmons's (1960) extensive play therapy that sought to help the child project deep feelings through the highly symbolic medium of play. As we discuss later, the belief was that play serves to bring emotions to the child's awareness, emotions accepted with impunity by the clinician.

Indirect Treatments

As explained earlier, direct treatments are methods in which the child is the primary recipient of clinical instruction. Indirect treatments, by contrast, are methods in which those who interact with the child (i.e., parents, teachers, and clinicians) are recipients of instructions to create conditions believed or expected to promote fluency. Whereas direct treatments are based on an assumption that the child's actions should be changed, indirect treatments are based on an assumption that the child's environment (i.e., listener actions) should be changed. Indirect approaches became popular in the United States for several decades. There has been a common misperception that the latest trend back to direct treatments represents a bold and revolutionary approach to early childhood stuttering when, in fact, such interventions have existed for long time, having a prominent influence in other countries. This misperception came about because in the United States during the mid-20th century, there was a popular belief in parental responsibility for stuttering.

A 180-degree shift in philosophy occurred in the late 1930s when direct speech and nonspeech therapies were largely abandoned for 30 to 40 years in favor of indirect therapies that focused on the child's parents, leaving the child out of the therapeutic contact (hence the expression "indirect"). This has been referred to often as the "hands off the child" philosophy. Typical of the voluminous literature of that period is Schuell's (1949) statement that "it is impossible to escape the need for working with the parents of the young child who stutters" (p. 251). This change occurred for several reasons, mostly because of the combined effects of the diagnosogenic theory and certain aspects of psychogenic theories of stuttering.

Psychotherapy for Parents

As we discussed in Chapter 6, psychogenic theories traced stuttering to parents, mainly mothers, having neurotic personalities. A pathological mother-child relationship, it was postulated, encumbered the child with deep emotional conflicts, eventually expressed as stuttering. Hence the neurotic parent(s) became an important target of intervention, calling for psychotherapies to help them achieve emotional adjustment and insight into their unhealthy relations with the child. Glauber (1958) prescribed traditional psycho-analysis, primarily for the mother, viewed as the main source of conflict and anxiety. Other members of the nuclear family also received therapy as deemed necessary. Glasner (1949) was another clinician to include extensive psychiatric guidance for the child's family members, although not in the form of psychoanalysis. The underlying assumption was that to alleviate the child's neurotic behaviors, parents had to recognize their own problems and redirect their relationships with the child. Psychotherapy for parents of children who stutter, however, was practiced only by a few psychiatrists and psychologists. This form of intervention never became commonplace, probably because the vast majority of parents of children who stutter are not, in fact, neurotic or in need of psychotherapy.

Parent Counseling

In a very different vein, the diagnosogenic theory (Johnson et al., 1959), a learning theory, also placed the blame for stuttering on parents, especially their child-rearing practices and overreaction to the child's normal disfluency. This view gained support from several studies that found parents of children who stutter to be more demanding, or to exert more pressure on their children as compared with parents of normally fluent children (see the review by Yairi, 1997). These impressions emanated the logic that intervention should target the parents, not the child, with counseling geared toward changing the pressure behaviors employed in routines of childrearing. Note this is very different from psychotherapies aimed at correcting a parental personality disorder. Another rationale for keeping the child out of active participation in therapy was the strong belief that an awareness of disfluent speech would be instrumental in transforming it into full-fledged stuttering (e.g., Bluemel, 1932).

> Many speech-language clinicians adopted parent counseling as the preferred form of intervention for early childhood stuttering. Most programs were mounted to instruct parents in what was regarded as "good parenthood" as well as providing them with guidance related to handling stuttering. The typical advice of how to respond and how not to respond to the child's stuttering rendered this counseling with a directive-authoritarian character.

Johnson's approach (1948) emphasized parent education about speech development, the normalcy of disfluencies, and his contention that overreactions of overanxious parents to normal disfluency were the cause of stuttering. Parents were told that they should not feel and show any concern about stuttering, and that they should avoid any negative responses to it, be patient listeners when the child stutters, and avoid giving suggestions to help the child through a moment of stuttering. Clinicians often prescribed specific details of planned parent-child activities. Similar counseling approaches were offered by Schuell (1949) and by Brown (1949).

Winds of Change

After more than three decades dominated by the philosophy of indirect treatment for early childhood stuttering, winds of change eventually altered the clinical landscape of the field. An important reason for this was the decline of Johnson's diagnosogenic theory, a central foundation of the therapeutic approach. Among contrary evidence were data showing that the speech of children who stutter was substantially different from the speech of normally disfluent children, indicating that stuttering was fundamentally different from normal disfluency rather than an outgrowth of it (Throneburg & Yairi, 1994; Yairi & Lewis, 1984). Additionally, studies inspired by operant conditioning theories demonstrated that stuttering, instead of being increased, could actually be reduced by calling attention to it (Martin, Kuhl, & Haroldson, 1972; Reed & Godden, 1977), and there was growing evidence for genetic factors underlying stuttering (Kidd, 1977). At the same time, a new, much larger, generation of speech-language clinicians was more willing to recognize insufficiencies of the limited indirect intervention reflected in many cases that persisted in stuttering in spite of all the counseling and advice given to their parents. Hence renewed interest in direct treatment, either speech or more psychologically oriented, emerged by the 1980s. Parental involvement, however, has continued, and, in some programs, maintained a prominent feature.

Current Issues Concerning Early Intervention

Prior to presenting current approaches to clinical management for preschool children who stutter, it is important to keep in mind a few facts and factors that influence general clinical considerations for this age group. Several of these pertain to the characteristics of stuttering, whereas others pertain to the preschool age itself.

Factors Pertaining to Stuttering

The most notable factor is the strong prospects for natural recovery. That is, inasmuch as stuttering is expected to improve or expire on its own accord, a logical question to be asked is whether intervention should be pursued for every child. Treatment is expensive and presents a burden to the family in several other respects. If the clinician shares our view that not all children who begin stuttering require intervention, the next question becomes, *Who* should receive it and *when*? Some of the answers may be found in the information about chances for natural recovery or risks for developing chronic stuttering, as well as other considerations (e.g., parents' reactions) presented in Chapters 3 and 13. This issue is further discussed in a later section.

Another factor is awareness of stuttering. Although some indications of awareness are seen in a good number of children under age 4, they tend to be unstable, perhaps because the history of the disorder is too short to trigger complex emotional or social reactions. It is uncommon, for example, for a preschool-age child who stutters to be teased by peers. In light of this, we believe a third significant factor should be recognized: In its early stages, stuttering is primarily a disorder of speech difficulty. The intensive attention to emotionality, emphasized by many clinicians in the treatment of adults, becomes secondary in the treatment of most cases of early childhood stuttering where the focus is on changing speech patterns and the child's environment.

Factors Pertaining to Age

There are three important factors in this category. First, preschoolers who stutter, like most of their peers, function with limited cognitive and language skills. The child who stutters has limited, if any, comprehension of the stuttering problem as understood by adults or of the nature of therapy goals, or similar considerations. Therefore, speech therapy with young children should be conducted with minimal instruction or expla-nation. Instead, it should be rich with demonstrations, and the clinician should use simple language. Modeling (e.g., slow speech) and simple feedback to reinforce (increase) or punish (decrease) certain behaviors become prominent. Second, preschoolers who stutter do not ask for therapy but are brought in by worried parents. Hence therapy should also focus in some way on the parents' feelings, reactions to, and interactions with the child. Third, home and the immediate family constitute an overwhelming portion of the child's world. Therefore, it would be wise, as well as pro-ductive, to have the parents involved in the child's therapy so that they can cooperate and carry on some of the procedures at home (e.g., model slow speech).

Who Should Be Treated? When?

During the historical period when indirect treatment of early childhood stuttering was popular among speech clinicians, especially in the United States, the prevailing view was that no child should be provided with therapy. As described, intervention was focused on their parents, primarily in the form of standard counseling and some-times in the form of psychotherapy. As direct therapies were revived and more widely practiced during the past 30 years, an opposing view was voiced: Every child should be treated as soon as possible (e.g., Starkweather, Gottwald, & M. Halfond, 1990). In between these two extremes, a third view also emerged: Therapy should be offered selectively, primarily to those with high risk for developing persistent stuttering (Andrews, 1984; Curlee, 1993; Curlee & Yairi, 1997; Ryan, 2001a; Yairi & Ambrose, 2005). Other children should be monitored during a waiting period. We agree with this view and submit that it is supported by current scientific information, by well-grounded practical concerns, and by ethical considerations.

From objective scientific perspectives, the documented high percentage of natu-ral recovery (see Chapter 3) implies that it is not necessary to provide therapy to all children who begin stuttering because most of them will recover on their own accord. Furthermore, although information necessary to make precise predictions of which children will recover and which will continue to stutter is incomplete, the cur-rent research does permit identification of those children with the highest risk for persistent stuttering. Certainly, these children should be recommended for therapy. More detailed considerations of pertinent risk factors were discussed in Chapter 13.

From a practical perspective, treating a group of children, 75% to 80% of whom will do well on their own, might be a questionable use of professional and budgetary resources, diverting them from those who need them most. At least one health insurance com-pany, to our knowledge, has questioned paying for therapy for early stuttering in view of natural recovery prospects. Quite likely, there are not enough clinicians in this country, let alone the many countries outside the United States, to do the job if every child who begins stuttering is referred for treatment. Additionally, bringing a child for therapy can

(continued)

be a significant burden on the family, for example, availability of working parents, cost, time (driving to and from the clinic), lack of insurance participation, impact on the rest of the family, and more. Should the family and the child go through all these inconveniences if they are not needed? Clinicians should exercise their best judgment based on research evidence and participate in decisions with parents weighing the costs/benefits for individual cases.

Finally, there is the issue of ethics. Some clinicians have posited that delaying therapy is unethical because it places the child at unnecessary risk and because delay reduces the success of therapy in older ages (Ingham & Cordes, 1998). Another surprising argument has been that therapy should be provided to all children because it will not hurt (Bernstein Ratner, 1997b). We, however, agree with Yairi and Ambrose (2005) who countered by suggesting that providing *unnecessary* treatment might be considered unethical. Unfortunately, when clinicians counsel parents, they often exaggerate the urgency for immediate therapy, painting a dark, less than objective possible prognosis. These two authors also argued that therapy should be given on a positive basis: Because it is necessary and helps, not because it would not hurt.

So what general clinical strategy for preschool children who just began stuttering is to be pursued? The answer is that therapy should be delivered selectively. For most of these children a waiting period is our preferred option. Even proponents of early intervention suggest flexibility in regard to when treatment should begin (Packman & Onslow, 1999). Ingham and Cordes (1998) indicated waiting up to 6 months from the time of onset before initiating intervention. Yairi and Ambrose (1999b, 2005) suggested that a longer waiting period, 9 to 12 months, to observe a shift toward recovery is justified by data from their longitudinal study. At that point in time, those who will recover become more identifiable. Given that some high-risk children are easily identified for immediate intervention, for example, boys whose fathers also stutter, disagreement among scholars and clinicians about the timing of intervention for those who fail to show signs of early recovery is primarily in regard to the specific length of the waiting, not to the wisdom of the decision to wait.

Concerns that delayed intervention will harm future therapy, if it becomes necessary, should be alleviated in view of findings of no significant relation between the length of the interval (even 1 year) from stuttering onset to the beginning of therapy or with the amount of therapy required for a desired outcome (Jones, Onslow, Harrison, & Packman, 2000; Kingston, Huber, Onslow, & Jones, 2003). The attribution of low therapeutic success rates in school-age children to long delays of treatment in early stages of the disorder (Ingham & Cordes, 1998) does not hold water for another reason. This is because school-age children who stutter are in the small minority who resisted natural recovery, a tendency shown to be determined, at least in part, by genetic factors. They may not respond well to therapy primarily because they have a more resistant type of stuttering (Ambrose, Cox, & Yairi, 1997). Thus decisions regarding the timing for intervention are based on each child's combination of risk factors, indication of progress or lack of it, and unique circumstances. In short, at the present, there are general guidelines (see Chapter 13) but not definite rules as to when intervention should begin.

Current Therapies

As we pointed out earlier, direct treatments for early childhood stuttering, common during the first few decades of the 20th century, were overtaken by indirect therapies from about the late 1930s. The wheel, however, kept on turning. The years since the mid-1970s have witnessed the reemergence of direct treatment programs where the child's speech is at the center. Parent counseling, though, has remained an integral part of most therapies. Furthermore, there has also been a tendency to have parents participate in the therapy sessions and assume an active role in its administration at home. To help clinicians and students better comprehend the sometimes confusing pool of current therapies for preschool-age children, we have organized them in four classes according to their main procedural focus: therapies that focus on (1) modifying speech motor patterns, (2) reinforcing fluency and punishing stuttering via operant conditioning, (3) altering parent-child interaction, and (4) modifying the emotional domain. We also make reference to another class, integrated therapies, in which attempts are made to incorporate several of these in a single program. Finally, parent counseling, which is included, one way or another, in most therapy programs was already covered in the previous chapter. The purpose of the following is to offer an overview of sample programs for each of the therapy classes.

Focus on Speech/Motor Patterns

Therapies in this class geared toward preschool children reflect some differences in theoretical frame of reference and vary in specific procedures compared to those applied with adolescents or adults. They are similar in principle, however, to the parallel class of adult therapies in that they rely primarily on fluency-generating techniques. Although stuttered speech and emotional aspects may receive some attention, these are secondary and do not constitute a central part of the main therapy. Four program types are presented here as examples:[2] Shine's Easy Speaking Voice, Pindzola's Stuttering Intervention Program (SIP), the Illinois program, and Riley and Riley's Speech Motor Training.

The Shine and Pindzola Programs

The underlying assumption of Shine's (1980) *Easy Speaking Voice* program, one of the first in this group, is that physiologic and aerodynamic factors, such as laryngeal tension and airflow rate, result in stuttering and should be altered. Its stated objective is to have the child understand and incorporate the concept of an "easy speaking voice." The twice-weekly sessions present a mixture of training in two skills: gentle voice and

---

[2] Among other programs are those suggested by Meyers Fosnot and Woodford (1992) and Bøstrup and Møller (1990).

slow speaking rate. The program begins with drills in saying single-syllable words using a whispered voice and "stretched" speech. Picture stimuli for words the child can speak fluently are used to facilitate practice. An extremely soft voice (whisper is encouraged) is practiced initially and gradually altered into a more normal speaking voice. Activities are highly structured to minimize stuttered conversational speech. From fluently spoken single-syllable words, the child progresses to practice of longer speech segments, up to the conversation level. Some speaking activities other than structured drills on words and sentences are included in each session to facilitate transfer. A story book and a surprise box afford opportunities to practice different standard phrases, and a language lotto game allows for the practice of asking and answering questions. All speech is executed with a soft voice and slow rate. Generalization activities are incorporated at each intermediate level of speech size segment when the criterion for fluency (0.5 or fewer stuttered words per minute) is reached at that level. When generalization is successful at the conversation level, the therapy shifts into a 1-year maintenance schedule as the frequency of clinical visits is gradually diminished.

A rather similar therapy can be seen in Pindzola's (1987) *Stuttering Intervention Program* (SIP), which, she claims, is rooted in the demands and capacities model discussed in Chapter 6. Inasmuch as stuttering results from the child's insufficient capacities (not specified) to cope with demands placed on the speech system, SIP strives to increase those capacities so that fluent speech can be produced. Children are drilled intensively with three speech patterns (targets) that promote fluency: slow-stretched speech, soft speaking voice, and smooth flow of speech. These motoric strategies are enhanced by control of linguistic content, which at the beginning permits only short, simple utterances (e.g., single-syllable words) and progresses to longer complex utterances. Soft voice, especially on the first syllable of an utterance, and smoothly connected speech are introduced and practiced. The target of smooth flow of speech means blending of syllables and words within a breath group to maintain continuous movement. To facilitate pacing and blending, the child moves the index finger from side to side while talking. Practice takes place in the clinical setting and at home under parental supervision.

The Illinois Program

In the late 1970s, one of us (EY), at the University of Illinois Stuttering Research Program, independently developed a therapy regimen similar in several fundamental aspects to the two therapies just described with an emphasis on slow-stretched speech. It emerged after several years during which we experimented with rhythmic speech therapy. To us, both methods, slow rate and rhythmic speech, were summed up in the theoretical notion espoused by Van Riper (1971, 1982) and others that stuttering is a disorder of mistiming of speech movement associated with difficulties in planning upcoming speech sequences. These result in articulatory discoordination.[3]

---

[3] It is interesting to note here the phenomenon of coarticulation, which involves a "looking ahead" in the execution of speech sequences. For example, research has shown that lip rounding for the vowel 'u' in "*construe*" can already be detected four sounds earlier, during the formation of the 'n' (Daniloff & Moll, 1968).

Such difficulties, we hypothesized, are particularly pronounced during the second and third years of life, a period of accelerated speech development and the time most typical for the onset of stuttering. Hence slow, regulated speech should allow the child more time for the planning and execution of the required coordination of movements. Although the therapies focus on speech manipulation, parent counseling has remained an integral aspect of the two programs.

Rhythmic Speech.   Our experimentation with direct speech therapy began with metronomic-paced speech that forces the speaker into monotonous rhythm and a highly controlled speaking rate. Van Riper (1973) employed rhythmic speech (although not metronome paced), such as rhymes and "Indian talk" in his therapeutic regimen for preschoolers who stutter. The technique, however, did not attract much interest, and there has been but a single published study of metronome-paced speech applied to this age group (Copolla & Yairi, 1982). We demonstrated that even 2-year-old children can master the technique and attend to the task.

Our therapy began with practice of saying bisyllabic words (e.g., baseball, hotdog) paced by a desk metronome. This was enhanced by a stimulus picture for each word and a clinician's model for each word, starting at 80 beats per minute (bpm), gradually progressing to 120 bpm. Next, a similar progression from 80 to 120 bpm was completed with two- to three-word utterances, such as "ride school bus." Abundant reinforcement was applied, and there were periodic diversions to other activities as necessary if the child became tired. After several sessions, the most comfortable metronomic rate for each child, typically 104 to 112 bpm, was determined and used through the rest of the program as the children advanced to practice phrases, sentences, questions, storytelling, and conversational speech. The last few sessions were devoted to practicing rhythmic speech without metronomic pacing. Brief meetings with parents were held throughout the program to assess progress at home and answer questions. If parents were reluctant to model rhythmic speech at home, they still were advised to slow down their own speech when talking to the child.

Coppola and Yairi (1982) reported moderate success in decreasing stuttering frequency and generalization at home. The children actually appeared to have fun with the robotic-type speech. We concluded that rhythmic speech practice can enhance the fluency of young children who stutter and should be considered an option in conjunction with other techniques, or as the main technique in selected cases.

Slow-Stretched Speech.   As our experimentation with intervention methods for early childhood stuttering progressed, we eventually adopted slow-stretched speech as the preferred technique because it sounds more acceptable to parents who were more willing to model it for their children than rhythmic speech. In this program, the three general objectives are (1) to provide children and their parents with intensive exposure to slow speech, (2) to provide the child with ample practice of slow speech, and (3) to provide parents with practice of slow speech as well as to prepare them to carry on with it at home. Broadly speaking, the program combines structured and unstructured speech activities where the clinician always provides the child and parents with extensive modeling of slow speech. Parent counseling sessions were held periodically to deal with their concerns, provide specific advice when called for, and to obtain progress reports.

In the beginning, the clinician models slow speech in unstructured play activities. This is followed by drills in structured activities, starting with slow speech in short segments enhanced by visual stimuli and verbal modeling, progressing to speaking slowly without external cues. The complexity and length of the speaking materials are gradually increased along with the speaking rate. To minimize children's loss of interest, structured drills are alternated with unstructured free play. Parents first observe and later assume more active roles in the sessions, learning to speak slowly and gaining experience of doing so while interacting with the child. To provide a better sense of constructing a therapy program, the 12-session 6-week sequence, 45 to 50 minutes per session, twice per week, is outlined here on a week-by-week basis.

Speech Rate Therapy for Preschoolers Who Stutter: An Outline
Week 1: Sessions 1–2
This period is dedicated to establishing a positive relationship between the child and clinician, introducing the main technique of slow speech, and assessing the child's reaction to it. Parents do not observe. The session structure for this week has three parts.

1. The first 15 to 20 minutes of the session are dedicated to free play and conversation to provide a comfortable atmosphere for the child. The clinician (a) engages the child in unstructured slow-paced play activities conducive to slow speech (e.g., making forms with plastic clay), (b) bombarding the child with a model of slow speech at a rate of about 1 word per second while playing and interacting, and (c) echoing in a slow easy manner the child's stuttered or fast speech. That is, if the child stutters, or says a sentence fast even if it is fluent, the clinician repeats (echoes) the word or the phrase in a slow-stretched manner.
2. The next 10- to 15-minute period involves structured practice. The clinician models single words containing one or two syllables, using slow-stretched speech at 1 word per second while presenting 20 to 30 picture cards, one at a time, saying the word for each picture. For example: "school bus," "hotdog," "chair," "table." The clinician instructs the child to "Say it like I say it." The child is to repeat the word following the clinician model. Each word is repeated three consecutive times. Simple verbal reinforcements, for example, "good" or "good, this was slow," are applied when responses are uttered slowly (words are almost never stuttered). Initially, reinforcement is frequent, becoming more random as the program progresses.
3. The last 15 to 20 minutes of the session repeat the unstructured, slow-paced play/conversation activities described in part 1.

Week 2: Sessions 3–4
During week 2, the format is slightly modified by dividing the session into four parts, 10 to 12 minutes each, adding some more time for structured practice. Additionally,

the child is encouraged to perform some of the practice tasks without the clinician's prior modeling. The goal is to have the child initiate slow speech on his or her own. Parents begin to observe behind the mirror.

1. The first part is spent in unstructured free-play/conversation. The clinician affords slow-paced play to enhance the modeling of slow speech at the 1 word per second rate. These procedures are also aimed at demonstrating a quiet, relaxed interaction with the child for the parents. The clinician continues echoing the child's stuttered or fast speech, repeating in a slow, easy manner. Brief, frequent verbal reinforcement (e.g., "good") for slow fluent speech is applied also in this context, becoming more random as the program progresses.

2. The second part is devoted to structured drills, beginning with simply saying single words in naming 20 to 30 pictures after the clinician's slow speech model. Upon completion, a new procedure is introduced. Now, the clinician presents the picture series again and the child is instructed to say each word slowly when a picture is shown. Each word is repeated three consecutive times, but there is no immediate clinician modeling unless the child speaks faster than desired. In addition to verbal reinforcement, tokens (e.g., stickers) are given for every several words uttered fluently.

3. The third part is a return to unstructured free-play/conversation with the clinician's modeling and echoing. The clinician begins to intentionally include the phrase "slow, easy speech" in the verbal reinforcement (e.g., "Good, this was slow easy speech").

4. The fourth part is devoted to additional structured drills as described in number 2 for this week.

During sessions 3 and 4, parents are introduced to the therapy as observers behind a two-way mirror. They are counseled to (1) observe how the clinician engages the child in slow-paced activities that facilitate slow speech, (2) become familiar with our notion of slow speech and how to model it, and (3) begin thinking about when/how they might use slow speech and slower paced movements and activities at home,

Week 3: Sessions 5–6

The overall format is very similar to that of sessions 3 and 4, but the length of the utterances used in structured practice increases to two- to three-word phrases with words containing one or two syllables. Like before, sessions are composed of four parts. The clinician, however, should be flexible in the time distribution among the four periods. Verbal and token reinforcement continue as before. Parents observe behind the mirror.

1. The first period is again spent in free-play/conversation with slow-paced activities and clinician modeling of slow speech at the 1 word per second level. As before, the clinician corrects the child's stuttered or fast speech by repeating ("echoing") the utterance in the desired fashion. The play includes

more themes that parents can easily adopt at home (e.g., making cookies out of clay, folding clothes, etc.).

2. The second period is devoted to structured drills. The clinician models slow speech using two- to three-word phrases in describing each of 20 to 30 picture cards. For example, "Ride school bus," "Eat hotdog." The child is to repeat the clinician's utterance three times in slow speech at about the same rate. Next, the child repeats the same series of short utterances when each card is presented, this time without the clinician's model. If the child fails to speak within the desired rate, a model is provided.

3. The third period is another brief unstructured free-play/conversation during slow-paced activities. Slow speech and echoing dominate. When the child speaks slowly the clinician introduces reinforcing comments, such as "Nice slow and easy talking."

4. The fourth period is a repeat of the structured drill described in number 2 for this week.

Week 4: Sessions 7–8

Three significant changes take place: (1) the length of the utterances increases to four to six words, (2) the structured practice progresses to a series of meaningful sentence sequences, and (3) the parents move from the observation station into the therapy room. The speaking rate remains at 1 word per second.

1. In session 7, the parent(s) are seated in the room, just observing. The session begins with free-play/conversation with the additional objective of making the parents more comfortable with modeling slow speech. The procedures are similar to those described in earlier sessions. Echoing is employed, and the clinician draws the parent's attention to the manner in which it is done. She also attempts to use and model short sentences of four to six words appropriate for the situation (e.g., "Let's make some cookies" or "Can you also make bread?"). The child is requested to tell what he or she is making, or, if necessary, repeat after the clinician's model: "I am making cookies." The parents' presence helps the child in generalizing slow speech to home. During session 8, parents are invited to participate in the free activities using slow speech themselves under the clinician's monitoring.

2. Switching to structured practice, the clinician uses four- to six-word sentences to model slow speech. Now, the stimuli used are sequenced picture cards that present a short story or description of a simple event. Each sequence contains four to five cards. For example, "the boy wakes up; he is getting dressed; boy and Mom eat breakfast together; they go to the grocery store." The child is requested to repeat each sentence after the clinician, maintaining the slow speech rate. Upon completion of each sequence, the child retells the story alone as the clinician points to one picture at a time. A model is provided when the child's speech does not fall within the desired range. Token reinforcement is administered.

3. The last part of the session is a return to unstructured activities, again with the parents' participation.

4. At the end of session 7, parents are asked to begin using the slow speech to the extent that they feel comfortable. Consultation with parents at the end of following sessions assesses their success in implementing slow-paced play activities at home and increasing awareness of their own speaking rate, attempting to slow down.

Week 5: Sessions 9–10

Three changes occur during this week: (1) the speaking rate is increased to about 1.5 words per second (90 words per minute), (2) the speaking content includes questions and answers, and (3) parents participate in the structured drills as well as the unstructured free play.

1. The first part, about 10 minutes, is free-play/conversation time involving parent participation.

2. In the second part, structured drills, up to 20 minutes, are carried on with a focus on short stories aided by several series of sequence cards. The practice proceeds as follows: First, the clinician uses four- to six-word sentences to model slow speech in telling the brief story depicted in a picture sequence. Second, the parent repeats, sentence by sentence, after the clinician, pointing to the appropriate picture in the series. Third, the parent asks the child to repeat the same sequence following the modeling. Fourth, the child is directed to tell the sentence sequence without a model. Of course, the clinician intervenes when needed. The entire procedure is then practiced again with another picture sequence.

3. The third part of the session, approximately 15 minutes, is a somewhat different structured activity, steered into the direction of a simple dialogue. The parents are advised about the purpose of this procedure. The clinician, using the slow speaking rate, asks the child questions about the sequenced stories used in activity 2. The child is requested to respond, using four- to six-word sentences while maintaining the slow speech rate practiced earlier. A model is provided at the beginning and as needed as the practice progresses.

4. The session is concluded with a few minutes of free-play activities.

Week 6: Sessions 11–12

The main changes for the week are seen in (1) progression to longer speaking tasks, (2) a greater role for the parents, and (3) increased speaking rate to 2 words per second (about 120 words per minute).

1. Unstructured free-play/conversation with the clinician introducing the faster speaking rate (which is still slower than normal). Echoing continues when needed with occasional reminders to use "slow, easy speech" or the feedback "this was slow and easy."

2. Proceeding to a more structured activity, the clinician tells a story, some-what longer than in the previous card sequence materials. Short sentences, at the new rate, are used. The child is to repeat the story or tell one of his or her own, maintaining slow speech. Verbal and token reinforcement are applied. Parents obtain ideas as to how to do similar activities at home.

3. The third part of the session is a return to free play/conversation. Now, however, the parent takes the sole role in modeling slow speech, monitoring, and echoing the child.

4. The fourth part is similar to part 2, that is, practice during storytelling. Also for this task the parent takes over as the teller and model. The child repeats and practices with the parent.

We feel that 6 weeks is sufficient for the first round of therapy for both child and parents. The program may be repeated or continued if necessary after a few weeks interval, allowing for assessment of child progress and parental reactions. Regarding effectiveness, data were analyzed for six children who exhibited moderate-to-severe stuttering from 13 to 29 months after onset at the time therapy began. Changes in the frequency of stuttering-like disfluency were compared for two pre-therapy testing periods and two post-therapy follow-up periods. Four of the children demonstrated substantial improvement between the pre- and initial posttherapy testing. Six months later, three of the six children exhibited substantial improvement, two showed modest or minimal improvement, and one had a substantial increase in stuttering (Yairi & Ambrose, 2005, p. 453). Perhaps aspects such as the chronic nature or the initial severity of the stuttering may explain the variable levels of improvement in spite of the intensive treatment. But, as explained, the purpose of presenting the program in a step-by-step fashion is to provide clinicians with concrete ideas about how to plan and execute a therapy program that addresses the child's stuttering and also guides parents in cooperating, thus increasing potential attainment. Clinicians, however, should be flexible, for example, selecting other speaking rates, altering order of progress or time distribution among activities, or making other adjustments. The point is that if there are good reasons to believe that slow speech is helpful for the child, this could be a reasonable approach to pursue in a systematic manner. Interestingly, some elements of the therapy, such as modeling slow easy speech, having parents practicing the new speaking pattern and applying it at home, are also found in a Danish program developed independently by Bøstrup and Møller (1990).

Speech Motor Training

A unique current treatment for early childhood stuttering that belongs in this class of therapies is the *Speech Motor Training* program (Riley & Riley, 1985, 1999). It was motivated by data interpreted to show that children who stutter exhibit reduced integration of the speech motor system. Hence its goal is to develop, or strengthen, speech motor control by correcting the deficient oral speech movement sequences necessary for normal production of syllables by means of extensive drill. The target is uninterrupted production of multiple iterations of nonsense syllable sequences at the fastest rate possible while maintaining accuracy.

The 14-stage program begins with the child practicing sequences of meaningless syllables, such as /vami/. The reason behind the meaningless content is to minimize cognitive self-monitoring. Also, nonwords may pose less risk of triggering stuttering than real words (Eisenson & Horowitz, 1945). Gradually, the number of syllables increases from 1 to 4, the speaking rate from 1 to 3 syllables per second, and unvoiced consonants from 0 to 2. The complexity is also increased from the CV structure at level 1 to the CVCVCCVVC structure at level 14. In Riley and Riley's (1999) view, the extensive drill in the speech motor skills is a contributing factor to successful long-term maintenance of fluency gains because, as they rationalize, overlearned motor skills tend to remain stable. Their reported data for six children who underwent 24 therapy sessions indicated that stuttering frequency was diminished by 49% and its severity by 46%. One of us (CS) has had modest experience with this technique and found it supportive toward fluency gains in conjunction with other strategies (e.g., slower easier speech) in the case of a young school-age child who had relatively weak diadochokinetic syllable sequencing skills.

Focus on Operant Conditioning

In Chapter 6, stuttering was discussed within the framework of operant learning theory with an underlying assumption that stuttering is a behavioral response that may be modified by its consequences. Research has supported this view by showing that stuttering can be diminished through punishment, withdrawal of reinforcement, and withdrawal of aversive stimuli. A well-known, although small, controlled laboratory study by Martin, Kuhl, and Haroldson (1972) demonstrated the power of operant conditioning also on the diminution of stuttering in preschool children. They had two preschool-age children converse with a lighted puppet. Each time the child stuttered, the puppet stopped talking and the light was turned off for 10 seconds. At the end of the program, stuttering was reduced in the clinic and home.

Actually, however, operant-based stuttering therapy for young children already flourished as seen, for example, in the clinical programs developed by Bar (1971) and Ryan (1971). Although some forms of punishment and withdrawal of reinforcement have been incorporated in therapeutic regimens for children, it appears that positive reinforcement of fluent speech, rather than punishment of stuttering, has received greater emphasis. Bar (1971) applied positive reinforcement, whereas Van Riper (1973) used both. Describing his early clinical programs he wrote, "by intermittently and casually showing more attention and appreciation of the child's fluent communication but only ordinary acceptance of his stuttering speech, we have been able to get marked gain in fluency by this simple procedure and without the child's conscious awareness of the contingency" (cf. p. 409). Two programs applied to preschool children are described here to represent the approach.

Extended Length of Utterance

The Extended Length of Utterance (ELU) program was devised by Janis Costello Ingham (Costello, 1983; J. Ingham, 1999) for young children who stutter and bears similarities to the GILCU program for school-age children described in Chapter 11.

Primarily achieved through positive reinforcement of fluent speech, it seeks to gradually increase the length of fluently produced speech segments, as well as the length of time during which fluency can be maintained. With contingent feedback and following a stepwise progression, the child learns to produce the desired speech more frequently. The main speaking contexts of the ELU program (e.g., picture naming) make it particularly suitable for preschool children. The clinician reinforces fluency with verbal feedback, such as "Good talking!" or "Excellent speech!" while the contingent instruction "Stop" is made after moments of stuttering. Token reinforcements may also be administered. The objective is to maintain fluency throughout the elicited speech responses.

The ELU is a highly structured 20-step program where the target utterances progress through a sequence from monosyllabic words to longer utterances and up to 5 minutes connected speech. Table 14.1 describes the target contexts for fluent speech associated with the 20 steps grouped into four sets.

To conduct the therapy, the clinician needs the following stimulus materials: 50 picture cards to elicit monosyllabic words, a list of 50 two-syllable words, a list of 50 two-syllable phrases, and 50 each of 3-, 4-, 5-, 6-syllable words and phrases. Progress is monitored by measuring the percentage of correct utterances, numbers of syllables spoken, and numbers of trials to reach criterion. Stage advancement requires a certain number of consecutive fluent trials. Another feature of the program is that when the simple contingencies are insufficient, other "additives" may be targeted, such as reduced speaking rate, gentle voice onset, reduced linguistic complexity, and/or modification of attitudes.

The ELU program received support in two very small studies. Riley and Ingham (2000) treated six children and reported 63.5% median reduction in stuttering frequency from pre- to posttherapy. Onslow (1996) reported on one child who produced less than 0.5% syllables stuttered at follow-up assessment. Still unknown is the extent to which all 20 steps are needed and how many children need "additives" and altering for various aspects of the program. Another program of interest in which reinforcement is applied to increasingly longer fluent speech segments is the *Stocker Probe Technique* (Stocker, 1976; Stocker & Goldfarb, 1995). Its special feature is the heavy emphasis placed on a systematic increase in linguistic complexity of the verbal content practiced at each progressive level of difficulty.

Table 14.1: Target Responses Corresponding to the Sets of Steps in the ELU Program

Set	ELU Target Responses
Steps 1–6	Monosyllabic to 6-syllable utterances
Steps 7–10	3- to 60-s monologues
Steps 11–16	75-s to 3-min monologues
Steps 17–20	2-min to 5-min conversations

The Lidcombe Program

Among pioneers in the application of operant conditioning techniques to treatment of preschool children was Bar (1971). He reported on a program in which parents of 59 stuttering preschoolers were trained in reinforcing fluent utterances in their child's speech using verbal contingencies such as "I like the way you said this word." Perhaps Bar's (1971) heavy reliance on parent-administered conditioning therapy had a substantial influence on the later to appear Lidcombe program (Harrison, Onslow, & Rousseau, 2007; Onslow, Costa, & Rue, 1990; Onslow, Packman, & Harrison, 2003) that was developed in Australia and has gained considerable popularity. It, too, delivers direct speech therapy for the child and rests heavily on parents' active participation in carrying out the therapy at home. The therapy program is tied to operant learning principles: contingent verbal positive reinforcement of the child's fluent speech and contingent verbal mild disapproval ("punishment" in operant conditioning terminology) of stuttered speech. Still, it is not as rigid as the typical operant program in terms of progressive stage, criteria for progress, and tight contingency schedules.

The best age for children to receive this program may be from 4 to 6 years. Data showed that younger children (e.g., ages 2 to 3) took a much longer time to respond to the therapy (Rousseau, Packman, Onslow, Harrison, & Jones, 2007). According to Onslow and colleagues, when a child is older than 6 years, stuttering tends to already be more complicated and less responsive to parental response. Other eligibility criteria for this program are that the child must exhibit "unambiguous stuttering" and more than 6% syllables stuttered. Children should be at least 6 months post-onset and have no other cognitive or linguistic disorders.

The objective of the program's first phase is to achieve near zero stuttering. Treatment begins with several 1-hour weekly sessions conducted by the clinician with the parents initially observing but quickly learning the principles and administration of verbal contingencies to their child's stutter-free as well as stuttered speech. The child is encouraged to speak during play or other activities, and the clinician is keen on providing praise or acknowledgment when the child is fluent by saying, "That was smooth speech" and similar reinforcing praises. But when the child stutters, the clinician responds with mild corrective feedback in the form of acknowledgment of stuttering (e.g., "That was bumpy speech"). An overall 5:1 ratio of praises to corrections is maintained. No particular speaking rate or pattern is targeted. There are, however, additional important features to the program that expand it outside the parameters of operant procedures, for example, self-evaluation. At times, after either fluent or stuttered speech, the child is requested to evaluate his or her own speech with a question such as "Was that smooth speech?" There are also requests for self-correction. After stuttering had occurred, instead of the usual acknowledgment, the clinician may say, "Can you fix that bump?" or combines an acknowledgment with self-correction: "That was bumpy. Say it again to smooth it out." The program, however, does not include practice in modifying instances of stuttering. The child is left to experiment on his or her own.

Parental involvement is an essential part of the whole program. As mentioned, they attend all early sessions together with their child and are trained to deliver the therapy at home. The parent demonstrates the ability to administer the procedures in the clinic, and the speech-language pathologist (SLP) gives feedback to ensure that the treatment is appropriate. The SLP demonstrates necessary adjustments to be made in the coming week, taking into account how the child is responding to the therapy. As parents become more proficient, they apply contingencies at home, starting with two 10-minute talking session to increase stutter-free speech at home, first applying positive reinforcement, and then adding corrective feedback for stuttered speech. Gradually, the structured home sessions are reduced and contingencies are applied in unstructured life routines. A 5:1 ratio of praises to corrections is maintained. The contingency schedule is intermittent rather than after every utterance. Parents must not feel uncomfortable or judgmental of stuttering when they apply the contingencies.

The practice sessions in the clinic are gradually reduced after the child has been stutter-free at home for a sufficient time (3 consecutive weeks). Parents use a 10-point stuttering severity rating scale (1 = no stuttering, 2 = extremely mild stuttering, and 10 = extremely severe stuttering) to indicate daily fluctuations. Progress is also monitored by the clinician's measurement of percentage of stuttered syllables (%SS) taken at the start of each visit to the clinic.

When stuttering levels reach program criteria on both these measures (absence or very low level of stuttering both within and beyond the clinic) for 3 consecutive weeks, the program continues with maintenance. Parents and child visit the clinic a few times for monitoring changes in the stuttering and making adjustments in parents' handling of the stuttering. Follow-up continues for a while to ensure long-term gains. The goal of stage 2 is to maintain the fluency criteria while the parental verbal contingencies are withdrawn and the frequency of clinic visits decreases. Research indicates that the treatment time to complete stage 1 varies around a median of 11 clinic visits, with 90% of children completing stage 1 in 22 clinic visits (Jones, Onslow, Harrison, & Packman, 2000; Kingston, Huber, Onslow, Jones, & Packman, 2003). The Lidcombe program has been subjected to considerable clinical effectiveness research with encouraging published findings. Among the more recent ones are Jones et al. (2005), Miller and Guitar (2009), and Woods, Shearsby, Onslow, and Burnham (2002).

The Lidcombe program has several strengths. It is administered in natural settings so that no generalization targets are necessary. Children enjoy the talking activities that always involve connected speech. The program is not too complicated to implement, and parents and children do not find themselves uncertain about how to respond to stuttering. There are several limitations to the program, however. It is not easily altered for children with cognitive or language delays. Minor deviations in the regimen can compromise its effects, and not all parents are prepared to be consistent in carrying it out. The approach does not address disfluency that may be ambiguous with respect to stuttering. Finally research by Bonelli, Dixon, Bernstein Ratner, and Onslow (2000) suggested that children may be responding to the intervention by simplifying their language to stay within fluency capacities and possibly pushing their stuttering under the surface.

Focus on Altering Parent-Child Interaction

Indirect therapies, alluded to earlier in the chapter, were initially driven by theories that parents are the major cause of stuttering. Hence it was quite logical to conclude that parents should be the main target for clinical intervention. Although these ideas have been substantially diminished over the years, they have been replaced by strong beliefs that, regardless of whether or not parents are the cause of stuttering, they exert powerful influences on the characteristics the disorder takes on throughout its developmental course, including the child's emotional adjustment and ways of coping. Thus various degrees of traditional, individual, face-to-face parent counseling aimed at altering behaviors with, and attitudes toward, the child have remained an important component in many current therapy programs for young children. Furthermore, as seen in the Onslow program, parents are sometimes recruited to actually deliver speech therapy at home.

Several clinicians, however, have opted to focus on changing home environment, especially the nature of the parent-child interaction, by having parents participate in programs that actively engage them in the activities, not just providing standard advice, in examining and altering behaviors. Simultaneously, these programs also involve the child in various ways, such as teaching better interpersonal communication skills. They do not, however, exclude more direct speech therapy. Sometimes it is employed as a secondary procedure. In this section, we review a few programs in which modifying home environment is either *the* focus or one of a few major foci of therapy.

Interaction Therapy

The main objectives of *Interaction Therapy* are to involve both parents, if possible, in an active process of helping them develop and refine constructive behaviors that support the child's fluency through their interaction style. It also aims at dealing with parental anxiety, as well as with the child's self-confidence and behavior.

The *Parent Child Interaction* program, developed by clinicians in the United Kingdom (Rustin, Botterill, & Kelman, 1996), exemplifies this approach. The therapy is anchored in the assumption that stuttering, as a multifactorial disorder, can be improved through manipulating the child's environment, an important contributing factor. Nevertheless, direct speech therapy may be implemented as necessary. At an earlier time, the program emphasized teaching parents what *not* to do in order to reduce their child's stuttering. This was done by analyzing videotaped parent-child interactions for potential parental behaviour that could undermine fluent speech. In a recent development (Kelman & Nicholas, 2008), the therapy took on a more positive approach, building on parents' intuitive understanding of what their child needs to be more fluent, increasing and reinforcing their ability for helpful interactions in the home environment.

Following a thorough assessment of the child and the home environment, the program proceeds in four phases:

1. *Establishing talking time.* Therapy begins with instructing parents to establish at home a brief *talking time* or *special time* where each parent makes a commitment to spend 5 minutes, three to six times per week,

playing and talking with the child. It is an opportunity for quality time for the child and parent to spend together, a feature that is the foundation of the therapy. During these periods, the parents are encouraged to implement their chosen interaction strategies. They are to listen carefully to what is being said, acknowledge the child's speaking difficulty, and maintain an open dialogue with the child about it.

2. *Weekly clinical sessions.* Typically, parents learn to master the routine of Special Times within a few days. These are set up during the initial therapy session, leading to the next phase, which involves six weekly sessions held in the clinic. Therapy sessions begin with feedback concerning the previous weeks' Special Times. Then, a few minutes of child-parent interaction are video recorded. The parents and clinician review the video together. This allows parents to take a step back, consider what they are already doing to help their child's fluency, based on what they already know about their child as well as what they have learned from the assessment about what may affect the child's fluency. From this discussion, a target behavior for the parents to employ in the forthcoming week is agreed on. Examples of typical interaction targets are following the child's lead, slowing down speech rate, listening attentively, conversational turn-taking, having a balance of questions and comments, extending response time latency (giving the child time to initiate, respond, and finish his or her talking), and using language that is appropriate to the child's level. Parents are encouraged to think about why that interaction target may be helpful for the child's fluency. The interaction target is first practiced in the clinic before being applied at home during the Special Times.

3. *Consolidation Period.* The six weekly clinical sessions are followed by a 6-week consolidation period during which the behaviors targeted for change are implemented at home. The clinician monitors the case weekly through parent-written progress reports.

4. *Follow-up.* The last phase consists of 3-month follow-ups for at least a year. If the child persists in stuttering, further sessions to work on interaction strategies or family strategies may be carried out. If needed, direct therapy is implemented and the child is taught a variety of strategies for managing speech.

To date, research evidence for the effectiveness of the Interaction Therapy method has been reported in two studies. A significant reduction in stuttering after therapy, sustained during the consolidation period, was reported for one child by Matthews, Williams, and Pring (1997). A recent single-subject design study that included six preschool-age children, ages 3 years 3 months to 4 years 10 months, indicated that, by the end of the follow-up phase of the program, four exhibited statistically significant reduction in stuttering frequency with both parents and one child improved only with one parent. The sixth child required direct speech therapy in order to improve (Millard, Nicholas, & Cook, 2008).

Parent-Child Groups

The *Parent-Child Groups* program (Conture, 2001; Conture & Melnick, 1999) is another example of current intervention in early childhood stuttering that places priority on improving home environment and interpersonal communication skills rather than on achieving perfect fluency. It has three foci: communication *interaction*, child and parent *attitudes* toward speech, and speech production *behavior*. Delivery is in the format of two small groups: one for children within a limited age range (e.g., 3 to 5 years old) and one for their parents. Both meet once per week over a 12-week period.

Through modeling and direct instruction, children improve interaction skills with rules such as listen when another person speaks, refrain from talking when someone else talks, and wait patiently for your turn to talk. Direct speech therapy is administered only occasionally, mainly when progress is slow or when the excessive overt stuttering calls for it. In that case, the child is taught through modeling and direct instruction to make the stuttering easy. Parents, in their group, are educated about the possible negative effects on the child's stuttering of frequent interruptions, talking for him, talking in long complex utterances, talking with excessively rapid rate, and frequent correction of stuttering. Desired behaviors are suggested and/or modeled for the parents. Parents are encouraged to use normally slow speech, as well as short, simple sentences. Also, they either observe part of the child's sessions and/or participate in them. An update of the program, attempting to rationalize it by research data in several domains related to early childhood stuttering, was published more recently (Richels & Conture, 2007).

The procedures used in the Parent-Child Groups bear similarity to those employed by Wyatt and Herzen (1962) and Egolf, Shames, Johnson, and Kaprisin-Burrelli (1972). Among other clinicians whose programs included a focus on home environment as one of several alternative strategies are Gregory and Hill (1984) in the United States and Lundstrom and Garsten (2000) in Sweden. One option in the Swedish program is intensive therapy with the child and one parent in a 3-week clinical camp that offers daily group and individual therapy for the child and a daily parent support group meeting.

Differential Strategies

One program that clearly attempts differential treatment based on the developmental status of the stuttering was offered by Gregory and Hill in 1984 (also described in Gregory, 1999). The first strategy, *preventive parent counseling*, is selected for a child who mostly exhibits disfluencies typical of normally speaking children but parents are concerned. Parents receive one or two counseling sessions concerning speech development and styles of communication and interaction that may increase or decrease disfluency. Some follow-up takes place too. The second strategy, *prescriptive parent counseling*, is aimed at children with mild stuttering. In addition to the counseling already described, parents are taught to keep daily charts of the child's stuttering behaviors, awareness, and reactions. This information is used in the counseling. The program also includes four to six therapy sessions with the child, emphasizing modeling of easy, relaxed speech, first by the clinician and then the parent. The third strategy, a *comprehensive therapy program*, is applied to children whose speech contains many stuttering instances and perhaps also concomitant disorders in speech, language, and/or behavior. This program includes the counseling and charting techniques employed in the first two strategies. This is an intensive program in which parents receive weekly counseling and the child is seen two to four times weekly for approximately 6 to 12 months. The child program may include desensitization, modeling of slow, easy fluent speech in increasingly longer and more complicated speech segments, and language structure.

Focus on Emotionality

As previously discussed, the past 30 years have seen a strong trend of returning to direct therapy where modification of the child's speech has been the most popular approach. Still, within the overall trend, there have been a few attempts to include psychologically oriented therapies in which the child is the focus and immediate recipient of, the treatment. Hence these too are classified as "direct." Their objectives and methods varied widely. Van Riper (1973) had in mind the prevention of future development of negative emotionality (e.g., avoidance of talking). To increase the child's interest in talking as well as verbal output, Van Riper advocated "fun" activities that elicited more speech. Hence speech becomes associated with joyful experiences.

Other methods bear greater similarities to psychotherapy with objectives that vary from resolving the child's emotional conflicts and resolving difficulties in mother-child emotional ties to increasing the child's self-confidence and interpersonal skills. Although most speech-language clinicians have not received training in this area, we feel it is useful to be aware of and perhaps apply the techniques to selected clients as needed by referral to a trained professional. We also believe it wise to gain information and experience through continuing education. The two therapies presented here reflect this approach.

Psychotherapeutic Play

Play has long been viewed as an essential component of healthy child development, both emotionally and cognitively. There are many forms and variations of play therapy. It may be directive and structured, even geared toward specific trauma by presenting play materials relevant to the child's stressful experiences, thus facilitating release of the associated emotions. The technique, originally offered by Levy (1938), is known as *release therapy*.

> Psychologists believe that play provides a vehicle to express experiences and feelings in the most natural way available to children and also allows them to work through inner anxieties. Froebel (1903, p. 22) asserted that play alone "is the free expression of what is in the child's soul." Play therapy is built on these assumptions by helping children communicate what they cannot verbalize. The play is seen as having therapeutic value similar to free association for adult psychoanalysis because it leads to the child's unconscious (Klein, 1932, 1955; A. Freud, 1946).

A different technique is nondirective play, developed by Carl Rogers, which later became known as *client-centered therapy* (Rogers, 1951). Its objective is to provide a secure relationship between the child and an adult, the clinician, and help the child resolve emotional problems. Virginia Axline (1947) expanded on Rogers's work, and her approach to nondirective child play therapy has been among the most widely practiced. These are the main principles:

- The clinician does not direct the child's actions or conversations. The child plays, or behaves otherwise, as he or she wishes. Only minimal limitations are established (e.g., the child cannot hurt self or others).
- The clinician develops a warm relationship with the child, accepting him or her as is. A permissive atmosphere must be created that allows the child complete freedom to express feelings.
- The clinician should be able to recognize those feelings during play and reflects them back so to help the child gain insight into his or her behavior.
- The child should be given ample opportunities to solve problems and make choices and changes.

As the child plays, the clinician reflects on the activity (e.g., "Johnny tore down the block tower. Johnny is angry."). The clinician is careful to state observations without making interpretations. Nonetheless, there may be times when the clinician reflects back in such a manner that she or he becomes directive in interpreting the child's inner world (e.g., is the emotion anger or frustration? Was the tower knocked down partly by accident before it was on purpose?). Hence the concept of *nondirective therapy* should be understood as a relative one.

According to Kenjo (2005, p. 9), "In Japan, the primary treatments with younger children, including those with severe stuttering, have for a long time been play therapy and modification of the environment." Wakaba (1983, 1999), also in Japan, posited that a good number of preschool children who stutter experienced insufficient maternal attachment in infancy and, therefore, she has preferred psychotherapeutic play. Her treatment was strongly influenced by the Axline (1947) approach. In addition to the common focus on accepting and reflecting the child's emotions, thoughts, and aggressive behaviors, special attention is given to the child's stuttering experience and its impact. Of course, the clinician must accept the stuttering. Therapy varies from two or three sessions for a child exhibiting mild stuttering to long-term (several years) for a child with a severe, complicated problem. Small group therapy conducted with the same method of free play is warranted when social interaction emerges as a problem. In weekly parent counseling, the clinician discusses with the mother any changes in the child's stuttering, positive social and aggressive behaviors, or regression to seeking attachment to the mother.

Drama Therapy

Another form of psychotherapy, drama therapy, is very different in concept and procedures than those based in free play. It employs theater techniques to promote the psychological health of individuals, couples, families, and groups. Drama therapy appears to be an outgrowth of psychodrama (Moreno, 1946) and role play. Rather than aiming at treating deeply seated emotional conflicts rooted in infancy, the objectives are to reduce fear, increase self-confidence, stimulate positive attitudes toward communication, and explore and resolve unhealthy patterns of personal relations. So far, drama therapy has been practiced at a rather modest level in the treatment of stuttering. Its main advocates have been Tomaiuoli et al. (2007) in Italy.

Applied to young children who stutter, the technique uses stories that are played on a stage by a group. Stories are selected in consideration of the characters, the reality problems they present, and suitability to the clients' needs. Children's complex problems and concerns, for example, being isolated, clumsy, or mocked, are simplified and projected through the story's characters that the children assume. The clinician participates in the play, serving as a verbal and behavioral model for the child and parents.

> Through acting, the child moves closer to experiencing real-world situations. Because the play, however, is somewhat removed from reality, those situations become less stressful. The play also teaches the child to figure out solutions, adopt optimal behavior, and change habitual responses. Although not dealing directly with speech modification, the play acting does help the child cope better with the stuttering, improve self-confidence, and function well in various educational programs and society. Greater fluency is a by-product.

At the end of a typical 6-month program, the children put on a show in a real theater where the audience is composed of families and friends. EY had several opportunities to attend this theater while visiting the Rome center. Seeing the stuttering children put up an hour-long play on the stage and display courage in spite of some stuttering is an uplifting emotional experience.

Tomaiuoli et al. (2007) reported results for 10 preschool children without histories of treatment who completed the entire therapy program. Their data indicated statistically significant reduction in typical and atypical speech disfluency in several speaking situations. Additional data showed improvement in the children's withdrawal behavior and their difficulties with problem solving.

Integrated Therapies

In Chapter 12 we discussed attempts to combine several approaches to therapy for adults who stutter into a single program. A range of integrated alternatives is also seen in many treatment programs for preschool children who stutter. For example, various methods of working with the child on changing speech include at least some form of parent counseling as well. A rather inclusive integration was described by Guitar (1998) in which fluency shaping, modification of stuttering, and addressing emotional reactions were all included.

Using slow speech and clinician modeling, fluency is established in single words, then, in 13 steps, is expanded to sentences and conversations. At each step, the clinician and parent take turns as the leading speaking partner. As the child progresses through the phases, modeling is faded, the speaking rate returns to normal, and fluency is generalized to the home. This is the time when the element of desensitization is introduced into the treatment for beginning children who continue to exhibit stuttering and signs of tension and may need help to prevent feelings of frustration. The clinician introduces play with deliberate stuttering. This, according to Guitar, makes the children feel all right about their stutters. This also helps desensitize the parents so they do not become uptight and radiate their uncomfortable feelings to the child. Desensitization aimed to increase tolerance of disruptors is also pursued. The child is encouraged to continue with smooth speech in the face of disruptors injected by the clinician. Children who continue to exhibit tense stuttering are then taught modification techniques to make their stuttering easier (e.g., contrasting "hard speech" with "easy speech), reminiscent of Van Riper's techniques described earlier. More recently, Guitar (2006) has preferred to employ the Lidcombe program instead of this integrated program.

Clinical Research

Past and Current Research

Research has been slow to take place concerning the effectiveness and efficacy of therapy for stuttering in preschool-age children; that is, does a specific therapy work, and is it better than other therapies? Until the early 1990s, only six relevant studies, with a total of 14 subjects, were identified (Yairi, 1993). More than 15 years later, with a few exceptions, published therapy programs have not undergone even remotely appropriate controlled research to document either effectiveness or efficacy. For example, seven different therapies published in a compendium edited by Fosnot (1995) were not accompanied with supporting data, and even claims of 100% therapeutic success were made without scientific backing (e.g., Starkweather, Gottwald, & Halfond, 1990). Some critics argued that several clinicians advocate techniques that research has actually shown ineffective (Ingham & Cordes, 1999).

In view of scant past research, it is encouraging to note a more recent trend for a substantial increase in clinical research activities that have included more children and encompassed a wide range of therapies. Among other studies, overall success in reducing the frequency of stuttering was reported for a group of 5 children using the ELU method (Riley & J. Ingham, 1995), 6 children using speech motor training (Riley & Riley, 1999), 19 children using play therapy (Wakaba, 1999), 88 children using mainly parent counseling (Lundstrom & Garsten, 2000), 32 children using child-parent therapy groups (Richels & Conture, 2007), 6 children using slow speech (Yairi & Ambrose, 2005), 10 children using the drama therapy (Tomaiuoli et al., 2007), 6 children using parent-child interaction therapy (Millard, Nicholas, & Cook, 2008), and more.

A related research direction has been pursued to study the effect of parents' speaking rate on the child's disfluency, motivated by the fact that a number of therapies and parent counseling programs encourage parents to speak slowly, hoping to influence the child into adopting slower speech that, in turn, should reduce disfluency. Three small studies with a total of 13 mother-child pairs revealed that that when mothers slowed down their speaking rate, the children's fluency improved, although children's speaking rate was not lowered (Guitar, Schaefer, Donahue-Kilburg, & Bond, 1992; Starkweather & Gottwald, 1984; Stephanson-Opsal & Bernstein Ratner, 1988). Little effect of parent's slowing down their speech on the children's speaking rate was also reported for 20 normally speaking children and their mothers (Bernstein Ratner, 1992). The length of the exposure to slow speech, however, was short, and there were individual variations. Similar findings with five parent-child dyads were reported by Zebrowski, Weiss, Savelkoul, and Hammer (1996), although in their study there was a uniform trend toward reduction in the children's speaking rate. Most recently, Guitar and Marchinkoski (2001) studied six mother-child dyads employing improved procedures that included a substantially reduced (50%) parent speech rate. These investigators were the first to report statistically significantly reduced rate in five children. Clearly, much more research of this critical issue is required, paying attention to the length of exposure and the specific speaking rate required of parents.

A promising, more systematic, clinical research program concerned with young children who stutter has been carried on by a team of speech-language clinicians in Australia that provided better baseline data, clearer procedures, and follow-up data. Starting with a small preliminary study of four children who received a few hours of therapy with the Lidcombe technique described earlier, it was reported that none of them exhibited stuttering 9 months after treatment. Subsequent studies were larger in scope (Onslow, Costa, & Rue, 1990). One study included 47 children who were followed up from 2 to 7 years. Speech samples recorded at home by parents indicated that near zero stuttering was maintained (Lincoln & Onslow, 1997). Another study reported on 250 participants (Jones, Onslow, Harrison, & Packman, 2000) who completed the program. It was reported that the median number of 11 clinical visits was sufficient to achieve zero or near stuttering and that some waiting period between stuttering onset and the initiation of therapy did not necessitate increase treatment time.

Weaknesses and Other Issues in Research

In spite of the welcome progress, the state of the art of clinical research for early childhood stuttering is afflicted by one, or several, experimental flaws that impede their credibility. One such failing has been an absent or vague definition of stuttering. If the definition of stuttering employed in a study, for example, "unambiguous stuttering" (Harrison, Onslow, & Rousseau, 2007), is actually a bit ambiguous, the clinician/investigator may discount instances of stuttering and thus bias the data in a particular direction. Another problem has been the period of baseline measures prior to treatment. If baseline measures are not collected over a sufficient time, children in the midst of natural recovery will not be identified, and the rest of their progress will be erroneously assigned to the effect of therapy. Other issues arise from an uncontrolled time period following the onset of the disorder. If children in a clinical study have stuttered for 3 months or a shorter duration prior to the beginning of treatment, as in the Reed and Godden (1977) study, the likelihood for contaminated data is high because at this early stage of stuttering the chance for natural recovery is nearly 80%. It should be noted that selecting children who have stuttered for twice as long, at least 6 months, does not improve the situation much. Even 2 years after onset, a child still has a 47% chance for natural recovery (Yairi & Ambrose, 2005). A similar problem is presented when control children who did not receive treatment are not included. When such studies report successful therapy, the findings should be suspected for contamination by failing to separate the effect of the treatment from that of natural processes. If family history is not controlled, genetic research has shown that children coming from families with histories of recovered stuttering would also tend to recover on their own (Ambrose et al., 1997).

Clinical studies in stuttering have suffered from a number of shortcomings. There have been weaknesses related to participant recruitment, such as small numbers of participants, an age range that is too wide or too limited, and inadequate attention to gender distribution. Procedural drawbacks have included (1) too small or unspecified speech sample size, (2) limited types of measures, and (3) insufficient or no treatment follow-up. Finally, there has been an absence of several elements regarded as critical in the general field of human health research:

- Random assignment of participants into various treatment groups
- Administration of the treatment in several sites by different clinicians
- Data analyses in locations and by people not involved in the data collection
- Comparing different treatments instead of investigating just one treatment

Fortunately, most recent research has attempted to accommodate at least some of the previously mentioned concerns. A clinical study regarding the effectiveness of the Lidcombe program carried out in New Zealand was careful to employ a no-treatment control group (Jones et al., 2005). Of the 54 stuttering children, ages 3 to 6, enrolled in the study, 47 remained for the 9-month follow-up. Of these, 27 were randomly assigned to the treatment group and 20 to the nontreatment group. Children had to be at least 6 months post-onset and have not received therapy during 1 year prior to start of the study. The results indicated that children in both groups improved substantially by the follow-up. Those receiving therapy, however, made better progress found to be statistically and clinically significant. We note, however, that the seven children who did not complete the study were 9 months older, on average, than the rest of the group. It is important to point out, that the older the child (and 9 months is a big difference at this age), the less they are likely to recover. Had these participants continued with the study, somewhat different findings could have been resulted. Another study conducted in the Netherlands by Franken, Kielstra-Van der Schalk, and Boelens (2005) compared two very different therapies: the Lidcombe program and a treatment based on the demands and capacities model (Gottwald & Starkweather, 1999). Here, 32 children were randomly assigned to their two treatment groups, and each child received 12 therapy sessions. No statistically significant differences were revealed between the two treatments in the decrease of stuttering frequency, and parents evaluated the two treatments as equal.

In addition to conducting more, larger, and better controlled studies, future research should attempt to separate the multiple aspects of therapy programs to find out which ones do, or do not, contribute to their outcomes (Yairi & Ambrose, 2005). For example, what are the relative contributions of the parents' group versus the children's group in the Conture (2001) program? Or which of the various elements in the Lidcombe program are essential versus extraneous?

General Reflections

Earlier in the chapter, a background discussion of therapy for preschool-age children who stutter pointed out two main sources of constraints on treatment for this sub-population: age and the characteristics of the problem. In spite of these, the review has revealed a broad range of major treatment approaches. As is the case with adults who stutter, no consensus has been reached concerning best practices of treatment with young children who stutter. Most of the general approaches are based on the same, or similar, principles to those used with adults. Clinicians, however, had to sometimes employ or devise procedures that were more suitable to a child's level. Hence, inasmuch as 3-year-olds are not capable of verbalizing complicated emotions in ways that many adult clients can, clinicians electing to focus on the general approach of modifying emotional reactions have employed play therapy as the vehicle for the children to vent feelings. If children cannot comprehend or follow direct instructions to change their speaking patterns, clinicians who prefer the general approach of fluency shaping have adapted by applying modeling as an alternative procedure to accommodate the approach. Those clinicians whose general approach involves operant conditioning methods to reinforce fluency or extinguish stuttering, have not had to adapt procedures too drastically from those used for adults.

Overall, it appears that the most unique therapeutic approach for preschool children in contrast to adult intervention has been the indirect modification of the environment via various modes, be it psychotherapy for the parents (Glauber, 1958), direct parent counseling (Johnson, 1948; Johnson, 1961a; Sander, 1959), interaction therapy (Kelman & Nicholas, 2008), or others. Another relatively unique therapy for children is the *speech motor training* program (Riley & Riley, 1999), which has not been practiced widely. This evaluation, however, does not mean that modifying the child's environment has been the most effective among other approaches. Unfortunately, clinical research has been late to arrive on the scene and has mostly been focused on the effectiveness of a single therapy. Comparative clinical treatment has been minimal. Still, it has been encouraging to witness growing clinical research activities concerned with the preschool age who stutter. Future research should strive to follow more careful methodologies in terms of controlling various parameters of subject selection, employing control groups, and using multiple sites and separate data collection and data analysis teams and sites. A major question that deserves more discussion, and certainly much more research, is which children require immediate intervention and which ones can be left to recover on their own.

As stated earlier in the chapter, declarations of apparent "consensus" in favor of early intervention for all children (e.g., Jones et al., 2005) are less than accurate, desire much stronger scientific basis, and certainly do not consider the reality of the ratio between available services and the population in need.

Summary

Historically, systematic clinical programs for early childhood stuttering were late to develop as compared to those for advanced stuttering in adults. During the early part of the 20th century, therapies focused directly on the child were employed. At the time, the number of clinicians was small. A shift toward indirect therapy, targeting the parents of the stuttering child, occurred early in 1940s, reflecting the rise of the diagnosogenic theory. Another reversed shift—a renewed interest in bringing the child closer to the therapeutic focus—began surfacing in the mid-1970s.

Several critical considerations concerning treatment of stuttering in preschool-age children were highlighted. Among them are special characteristics of early childhood stuttering, the factor of awareness (or lack of) of the stuttering, natural recovery, cognitive and emotional limits in young children, the need to adjust therapeutic technique to children's age, the great influence of home environment, and more. Current major therapy approaches for preschoolers who stutter can be distinguished according to their focus on (1) speech/motor patterns, (2) operant conditioning, (3) altering parent-child interaction, (4) emotionality, and (5) integrated therapies. Each of these approaches has been pursued by several different programs and techniques, making the overall field quite rich. These were briefly described. Finally, past and present clinical research pertaining to the treatment of this age group was discussed.

STUDY QUESTIONS AND DISCUSSION TOPICS

1. Compare the general objectives and procedures of direct and indirect therapy approaches for early childhood stuttering. What have been the theoretical rationales for the two?

2. What special issues, in terms of age and the characteristics of the stuttering disorder, should be considered regarding therapy for preschool children who stutter? List and explain.

3. Describe the differences in the nature of parental involvement in the following programs discussed in the chapter: (a) the authors' speech rate therapy, (b) Lidcombe, (c) parent-child interaction, and (d) parent-child groups.

4. What are the principles and procedures employed in psychotherapeutic play methods?

5. What are the principles and procedure employed in the extended length of utterance program?

6. Discuss the methodological issues faced in pursuing clinical efficacy research regarding stuttering therapy in preschool-age children.

SUGGESTED READINGS

Axline, V. (1947). *Play therapy*. New York: Ballantine Books.

Harrison, E., Onslow, M., & Rousseau, I. (2007). Lidcombe program 2007: Clinical tales and clinical trials. In E. Conture & R. Curlee (Eds.), *Stuttering and related disorders* (3rd ed.). New York: Thieme.

Ingham, J. C. (1999). Behavioral treatment of young children who stutter: An extended length of utterance method. In R. F. Curlee (Ed.), *Stuttering and related disorders of fluency* (2nd ed., pp. 80–100). New York: Thieme.

Kelman, E., & Nicholas, A. (2008). *Practical intervention for early childhood stammering: Palin PCI approach*. Milton Keynes, UK: Speechmark.

Riley, G., & Riley, J. (1999). Speech motor training. In M. Onslow & A. Packman (Eds.), *The handbook of early stuttering intervention* (pp. 139–158). San Diego, CA: Singular.

Yairi, E., & Ambrose, N. (2005). *Early childhood stuttering*. Austin, TX: Pro-Ed. See Chapters 3, 12, and 13.

Chapter 15: Other Fluency Disorders and Multicultural/Bilingual Issues

LEARNER OBJECTIVES

Readers of this chapter will understand:

- The distinction between stuttering and other fluency disorders.
- Principles of diagnosis, evaluation, and treatment of cluttering.
- Principles of diagnosis, evaluation, and treatment of neurogenic stuttering.
- Principles of diagnosis, evaluation, and treatment of psychogenic stuttering.
- Stuttering and fluency issues for those with multiple languages and cultures.

Introduction

If we accept the definition of stuttering, proposed in Chapter 1, as *speech that is disrupted by one or all of the following: sound/syllable repetitions, sound/postural prolongations, and complete blockages of the vocal tract*, then it follows that when other forms of disfluency are disruptive to speech, these may represent other fluency disorders. Further, suppose a disorder is characterized by one or all of the stuttering characteristics just listed but also by different features, for example, a sudden acquired onset at adulthood following a head injury. This too may be classified as an "other fluency disorder," even though the speech characteristics may meet criteria for "stuttering."

Examples of other fluency disorders cases include the child with impairment of language formulation that causes excessive disfluency *not* characterized as stuttering-like (SLD), or the child whose speech fluency is solely affected by an irregular pattern of pauses and breaths mid-utterance. It is important for speech-language clinicians to consider the other fluency disorders that may be encountered because not all disfluent speech is regarded as stuttering.

In addition to childhood forms of other fluency disorders, there are some "acquired" adult-onset forms of stuttering. In these disorders, several of the disfluency types observed in the classical developmental stuttering disorder may be seen, but the etiology, other speech characteristics, and phenomena surrounding the speech problem tend to be different. Psychogenic stuttering and neurogenic

Table 15.1: **Other Disfluency Disorders in Children and Adults**

Age Group	Fluency Disorder
Childhood	**Developed:** Unusual breathing patterns Word-final disfluency Language disorders Cluttering
Adulthood	**Acquired:** Neurogenic stuttering Psychogenic stuttering

stuttering are examples of these other types of fluency disorders. Table 15.1 outlines the set of other fluency disorders addressed in this chapter.

Other Childhood Fluency Disorders

The speech-language clinician who engages in a fluency evaluation needs to be aware that sometimes speech is excessively disfluent but not stuttered. The following examples are not meant to be exhaustive but represent typical clinical encounters. They include (1) unusual pausing/breathing patterns, (2) word-final disfluencies, (3) disfluency secondary to language disorders, and (4) cluttering.

Unusual Breathing Patterns

Like stuttering, the cause of other childhood fluency problems is not well understood. Why does a child who previously spoke with no noticeable problem of smoothness suddenly one day adopt an unusual pattern of inhaling in the middle of words? Was it a physical immaturity in respiratory capacity that failed to sustain utterances to completion without interruption? Were there hormonal changes that led to shallow breathing? Did situational pressures and heightened emotions cause muscular tensions and rigid postures leading to insufficient breath support? Or was it merely a compensatory solution to timing turned into a habit, for example, secondary to an attempt to say more words than the airstream would carry?

Published literature suggests that abnormal breathing patterns, both nonspeech and speech, at any age, can be observed secondary to a variety of physical impairments, including but not limited to asthma, dysarthrias, traumatic brain injury (Murdoch, Pitt, Theodoros, & Ward, 1999), deafness (Waltzman & Cohen, 2000), and Tourette's syndrome (Jagger et al., 1982). Usually the abnormal breathing of these populations is accompanied by disruptions to dimensions of vocal quality and intelligibility as well. A pattern of pausing or breathing mid-word without any other physical, speech or language impairments represents an isolated fluency disorder with an unknown origin. No specific literature on this speech problem was found at the time of this writing. Nonetheless, CS has observed three such cases in elementary school age children, who demonstrated only unusual patterns of pausing/breathing interrupting the flow of speech. The particular patterns of pausing or breathing in these fluency disorders vary with the individual child, just as they do for stuttering, but here is a potential example characterizing this type of problem:

Unusual Breathing: A Sample Case

Description: CS was asked by a second-grade teacher to evaluate a child for a stuttering/fluency problem. She said that for the past few weeks the child had been talking with an odd pattern that seemed like a kind of stuttering. When assessed, the boy's only disfluent speech behavior was his propensity to breathe in the middle of words. These occurred at the noticeable frequency of every few sentences. The boy exhibited no physical tension or effortful struggle to speak and had never had a history of any other fluency or stuttering problems. He was not aware of the disrupted speech or embarrassed by it. He did not have any unusual speaking rate, articulation, voice features, or hearing problems. Although noticeably distracting, the etiology appeared to be a superficial matter of mismanaged speech production. Because his speech pattern was not a form of stuttering, he readily responded to systematic instruction for breathing in appropriate locations.

Intervention: The intervention for the boy just described did not need to address reduction of any physical tension or emotional reaction during speech because such features were absent. Inasmuch as the problem was determined to be mismanaged speech execution, an approach similar to that used with a traditional articulation disorder was applied. That is, the boy was taught to change his habit of breathing mid-words. Ear training served as the starting point. He learned to identify and contrast the inappropriate breathing behavior with appropriate breathing behavior, listening to these models in the clinician's speech. Next, skills of accurate detection of the inappropriate versus appropriate breathing pattern in audio recordings of his own speech were developed. In the third step, he was taught to plan breath locations appropriately for oral reading and for scripts of conversational speech. These planned speech tasks were then produced for audio recordings. After each segment of several utterances or longer segments, the child was asked to self-evaluate his breathing behavior. The recordings were reviewed together to check on how well he had self-evaluated. When consistent and independent ability to produce speech segments with appropriate breathing patterns was demonstrated in the therapy room, the teacher reported carryover into the classroom speaking activities. Finally, the child had learned where breaths should take place and had developed the ability to self-monitor and use his own judgment to generate appropriate breathing behavior when he talked. The therapy and the remediation process were completed in only a handful of sessions.

Word-Final Disfluency

People who stutter rarely do so on the final syllables of words. The research literature includes just a few accounts of people with disfluency patterns consisting of sound or syllable repetitions occurring at the ends of words (McAllister & Kingston, 2005; Stansfield, 1995; Van Borsel, Van Coster, & Van Lierde, 1996). Sometimes a language learning deficiency or brain injury were involved as etiological factors, but others were found to be completely normal. For example, two school-age boys, who were described as having no other known impairments, produced mainly word-final part-word repetitions (McAllister & Kingston, 2005). It was noted that these disruptions occurred at all positions within the sentence (initial, medial, final) but primarily at sentence-medial locations. An example is *"I don't think – nk we got the whole way through those"* (McAllister & Kingston, 2005, p. 261). No tension, awareness, avoidance or negative reaction, or secondary behaviors were displayed, similar to the breathing/pausing cases described by CS previously. McAllister and Kingston (2005) argue that because words affected by this form of disruption have already been spoken prior to the repeated final segment/s, these disfluencies minimally impact listener comprehension and likely raise little concern by anyone. They suggest the possibility that such disfluencies, as the only pattern, should not be viewed as constituting a communicative disorder. When the disruptions are sufficiently frequent, however, they may distract and/or bother both teachers and parents alike, resulting in a referral to a speech-language clinician. Again, CS has encountered two or three such cases.

Cognitive-linguistic processing appears to be the most probable etiology, but it is still uncertain what factors lead to this less typical form of disfluent behavior. Although most speakers mark a delay in an upcoming decision of what words to say next by uttering the neutral syllables of "uh" or "um" or a silent pause, reiterations of the word ending may serve as the holding pattern to mark where a speaker has left off until ready to complete the rest of the utterance. Of course these questions then arise: Why is the latter method used as the holding pattern rather than the more common methods of interjecting syllables or pausing? And why are speakers so remarkably unaware of such features having occurred? Motoric perseveration, palilalia, and behavioral compulsion have been conjectured as other possible explanations, but these types of repetitive acts tend to have different features[1] and are diagnosed in association with neurogenic or psychogenic causes. Further research is necessary to confirm whether the proposed underlying etiology applies or whether some other conditions are involved. The following case example illustrates an approach to this kind of fluency problem:

Word-Final Disfluency: A Sample Case

Description: Another speech-language clinician referred a 10-year-old who was "stuttering." The child displayed chiefly word-final repetitions; other forms of disfluency were at normal, rarely occurring levels. No tension, awareness, or negative reaction were evident. Language testing revealed within average to above-average range receptive vocabulary and receptive/expressive abilities. The early adolescent

---

[1] In palilalia, the word repetitions become progressively faster and less audible in loudness (Duffy, 1995).

temperament questionnaire completed by the boy revealed no remarkable issues. He was reportedly well adjusted psychologically and had an unremarkable medical history. During both oral reading and conversation, the boy displayed frequent repetitions of sounds or syllables at the ends of words, such as "We left Saturday-ay-ay morning," "There was a hole-ole in the side of it," and "It took a good-ood four hours." The word-final repetitions occurred on 56% (28 of 50) of utterances. Other forms of disfluency occurred at minimal frequencies. There was no apparent emotional reaction to the disfluency, nor other atypical speech, voice, or language behaviors. The boy passed hearing and oral mechanism screenings. His academic performance was reported to be typical for his age.

Intervention: A traditional approach to speech production training was adopted, starting with sensory/perceptual training and progressing to production training following a hierarchy from phrase level, to sentence level, and finally to a conversational context. Enhanced awareness and self-monitoring of speech began with an initial exercise in perceptual awareness in which the child was asked to identify same-different phrase pairs produced by the clinician (e.g., *"Are these two sentences exactly the same or are they said in some way that is different?: It was four months ago. It was four-our months ago."* After a consistent detection of the target behavior was established in the clinician's speech, the child was asked to review and listen to audio-recorded segments of his own speech to detect whether they were said smoothly or with the repeated word ending. When detection and description of his own productions was at least 90% (more than 45 of 50), he was to engage in a kind of "cancellation" in which he repeated the utterance smoothly after the detection of the atypical repetitions. Verbal encouragement and positive reinforcement of accurate detection and smooth reproduction were generously applied. As the child increased his awareness and practice of speech in various activities, occurrences of the behavior progressively decreased both in and out of the clinic.

Language Disorders

Disfluent Speech in Disordered Language

The nature of disfluent speech typical of language disorders has been documented in several scientific sources (Boscolo, Bernstein Ratner, & Rescorla, 2002; Hall, Yamashita, & Aram, 1993). The children with specific language impairment (SLI) produce a preponderance of maze revisions, phrase repetitions, and circumlocutions compared to children with normal language matched for mean length of utterance (MLU) (Thordardottir & Weismer, 2002). Surprisingly, interjections are used with lower frequency among children with SLI compared to those with normal language (Thordardottir & Weismer, 2002).

It is reasonable to expect that children with language disorders may tend to be more disfluent because when a person struggles with formulating a message, it is often evident in hesitations and disruptions to the flow of talking. An investigation of the speech of children with SLI in story narratives revealed significantly greater levels of both SLD and other disfluencies (Boscolo, Bernstein Ratner, & Rescorla, 2002) than in normally fluent children. The 1% SLD level, however, is still considerably lower than the 3% or greater SLD levels typical of children who stutter.

Several other studies have not found differences in disfluency frequencies between children with SLI and those with normally developing language (Lees, Anderson, & Martin, 1999; Miranda, McCabe, & Bliss, 1998; Scott & Windsor, 2000). The absence of differences in these cases could have been because the language difficulty tends to affect phrase-level rather than word-level speech fluency. It has been shown that as language (syntactic) complexity increases, the number of disfluent utterances increases rather than the number of disfluencies altogether (Bernstein Ratner & Sih, 1987).

In addition to observations of phrase-level disfluency, formal and informal language assessment of disfluent children with SLI may reveal weaknesses in word-finding skills, short-term memory, expressive semantic and syntactic abilities, and pragmatic skills (Miller, Long, McKinley, Thormann, Jones, & Nockerts, 2005). Thus their disfluencies arise because of delays and difficulties generating the language forms needed to express ideas. Emotionally, they may tend to feel frustration with the communication failure they experience more generally rather than embarrassed or disturbed by the disfluency specifically.

Stuttering and Concomitant Language Disorders

As we discussed in Chapters 3 and 4, there are children for whom stuttering and language disorders coexist. Research has suggested a higher prevalence of other communication disorders in children who stutter than in the general population, with concomitant language disorders ranking second behind articulation/phonology disorders (Arndt & Healey, 2001; Blood et al., 2003; Hall, Wagovitch, & Bernstein Ratner, 2007). As we have previously stated, however, the extent of such coexisting disorders in different age groups is controversial. It is currently not known why there is this tendency for coexisting disorders. Perhaps children who stutter are at higher risk for developing other problems, or alternatively, children with other problems may be at greater risk to develop stuttering. Perhaps stuttering and other communication disorders are both related to a common underlying problem, or perhaps the treatment for communication disorders raises a child's risk for stuttering somehow. J. Riley (1971) actually proposed two subtypes that rest on a language-physiology distinction: children exhibiting concomitant language deficits only, and those exhibiting inferior motor skills. Nippold (1990) questioned whether the tendency for co-occurring communication disorders actually exists. She reasoned that children who stutter who have additional disorders are more often referred for services and identified for intervention. Indeed, many stuttering prevalence studies used data gathered from school clinician caseloads, which perhaps were not representative of the population of children who stutter.

The presence of multiple disorders creates a need for additional remediation decisions. The clinician must decide whether to treat the multiple problems sequentially or concurrently. If sequential treatment is selected, then which disorder will be treated first? Will the first target be the stuttering or the other disorder/s? Several factors may enter into the decision of order, for example, relative severity of each problem, relative ease of expected success remediating each problem, and relative concern or distress experienced related to each problem.

Alternatively, if concurrent treatment is selected (instead of sequential), then other decisions will have to be made about the implementation of the therapeutic approaches. Options may include (1) a simultaneous blending of strategies or approaches to the two disorders, (2) cycling or rotating between the treatments of the two disorders within each session, or (3) simultaneous but adapted or altered approaches to the disorders (e.g., no direct corrections, no imitation demands, etc.). Arndt and Healey (2001) surveyed 241 speech clinicians from a variety of U.S. states and found that the order of most to least preferred options was simultaneous approach, other approach, cycling approach, concurrent but without calling attention to errors, treating fluency first. Of course, preferences are not evidence for what is best practice, but these findings do tell us what clinicians may generally be doing.

Other research evidence tends to support a simultaneous but adapted approach. More specifically, an indirect approach to phonological disorders is recommended in children who stutter due to concern that direct speech correction may adversely affect stuttering (Bernstein Ratner, 1995; Conture, 2001; Louko, 1995). For example, a fluency-shaping protocol would be combined with focused speech models for phonology without direct feedback on the speech (i.e., giving no attention to errors). Altered approaches to articulation or language targets may involve their practice in simultaneous conditions of speaking slowly, monitored rate/rhythm, smooth transitions between words, reduced interruptions in group situations, longer turn-taking latencies, and use of an easy, relaxed speaking manner (Byrd, Wolk, & Lockett Davis, 2007; Conture, Louko, & Edwards, 1993). Progressive speaking contexts related to utterance length and complexity should be carefully controlled to ensure success in both areas. If a direct approach to correction is applied, then it is advised that the phonological targets be practiced in a relaxed, unhurried manner, avoiding excessive motoric/linguistic demands (Conture, 2001).

The two advantages of treating the two disorders concurrently are (1) progress may be made in both areas without delaying attention to one of the problems, and (2) a broad versus narrow focus on communication effectiveness is more holistic. The disadvantage is that it can be difficult to select an optimal speaking context. For example, the child might benefit most from a conversational context for fluency but need phrase-level practice for the articulation or language problem. Stuttering frequency and severity should be monitored during treatment for other speech/language targets, so that if fluency worsens, appropriate adjustments are made such as easing production accuracy demands, slowing pace of production or activity demands, or reducing linguistic context demands (Conture, 2001).

When children are being treated for multiple communication problems, parents need to be informed that progress may need more time. They need to be counseled in employing support strategies for the fluency (slower pace, longer turn-taking latencies, not correcting errors, etc.) and understand that although these strategies optimize the potential for fluency, they are not directly related to the cause of either stuttering or fluency. Note, however, when parents are asked to provide some sort of home practice for two behaviors at the same time (e.g., stuttering and language), it may be too overwhelming for both the parent and child.

Language and Disfluency: Other Considerations

Several investigators have revealed that disfluent speech may arise secondary to language therapy (Hall, 1977; Merits-Patterson & Reed, 1981). It was proposed that perhaps therapy promotes uncertainty with language formulation that leads to greater disfluency (Hall, 1977). Another hypothesis is that the demands of producing sentences of greater length and complexity may be exceeding the child's fluency capacities (Hall, Yamashita, & Aram, 1993), in keeping with a demands-capacities model (Adams, 1990). A further possibility that has not received much attention is that greater speech disruptions arise from more frequent attempts to self-monitor ongoing speech (Ratner & Healey, 1999). In contrast to precipitating disfluent speech, speech and language therapy can decrease disfluency as was shown in the case of one child following language therapy for narrative organization (Sieff & Hooyman, 2006). Improved fluency may be expected if the disfluency is primarily based on language formulation impairment. Clinicians should be reminded that if the correct focus in therapy is chosen, then the treatment progresses, but focusing on stuttering when the problem is in language formulation could lead to a lack of progress.

Following is a brief description of a school-age child who presented a fluency problem (not stuttering) associated with a language disorder.

Language Disorders: A Sample Case

Description: An 11-year-old boy was referred for an assessment by his parents, who reported concern about his poor communication abilities. His story explanations were disorganized and disfluent with many revisions and restarts (phrase repetitions). He passed hearing and oral mechanism screenings but scored below age level on formal tests of expressive language. His difficulties with word-finding were evident in his over-use of empty words such as "thing," "stuff," "like that," and a below-average score on a formal test of word-finding. He was performing below age/grade level in both reading and writing.

Intervention: The approach in therapy to this fluency issue may be indirectly addressed through strengthening the child's language skills. The speech clinician col-laborated with the special education specialist and classroom teacher to identify and select a target vocabulary and concepts to incorporate into therapy activities. Word-finding ability was improved by boosting semantic associations through elaboration training and categorical organization tasks (Owens, 2010; Wallach & Butler, 1994), as well as phonological awareness (e.g., rhyming and phoneme segmentation). These involved the targeted classroom-related vocabulary. Concepts were strengthened with description tasks involving use of terminology to compare/contrast characteristics

(Owens, 2010). For example, for geography concepts, he was prompted to compare/contrast vocabulary pairs such as "plain versus plateau," "cape versus peninsula," and more. With each pair, he was prompted with questions of "How are they alike? How are they different?" Language organization and sequencing was improved through activities involving narrative schemes. For example, the child had to develop scripts for a variety of his daily routines, practice with sequenced pictures, and drill with story grammars (e.g., telling and retelling the stories of his vacation trips, field trips, holiday events, etc.). Although some difficulties persisted, his fluency improved as he developed more consistent strategies for telling about objects and events.

Cluttering

Cluttering is a disorder of speech and language formulation resulting in a rapid, imprecise, dysrhythmic, disorganized production of speech (Daly, 1996). The nature of cluttering has been controversial. Whereas it was previously described as an impairment of central language processes (Weiss, 1967), more recently it has been viewed as a problem involving central speech processes (St. Louis, Raphael, Myers, & Bakker, 2003).

The following list provides examples of characteristics that may be observed in children who clutter (Daly, 1996; St. Louis, Myers, Bakker, & Raphael, 2007):

- Excessive repetitions of all kinds (part word, whole word, phrase)
- Fast bursts of speech; choppy rhythm
- Imprecise, slurred articulation; sound transpositions
- Short attention span and poor concentration
- Lack of awareness of disfluency (poor self-monitoring)
- Deficits in expressive language, reading, writing skills

It has been opined that cluttering begins during childhood, but, unlike stuttering, the problem does not cause sufficient concern to bring it to the attention of the clinician for differential diagnosis (Daly & Burnett, 1999; St. Louis et al., 2007). This is why school-age and adults are those who are seen for therapy. In our opinion, there is no evidence for an observable "cluttering onset," that is, that the child's speech was initially normal, then, either gradually or suddenly, cluttering appeared. Perhaps, like some cases of language delay, the difficulties that are present even from the beginning do not resolve when expected with maturation. Thus it takes more time to raise parents' and other people's attention.

The tendency for its later identification as compared with developmental stuttering could be related to (1) the typical lack of awareness or concern by the speaker, and/or (2) the tendency for other accompanying impairments to overshadow the problem of disfluent speech. Aspects of the development of cluttering have also been underresearched. This may be one reason why there are no data on either the incidence or the prevalence of cluttering in the population. Daly (1996) reported that, based on his own caseload, those who purely clutter were far fewer (about 5%) than those who purely stutter (about 55%), but that those with a mix of cluttering and stuttering were fairly common (about 40%). Because over the years many clinicians and researchers alike have not differentially diagnosed cluttering from stuttering, Daly's estimates may hint that a number of research studies of stuttering could have been conducted with participants who also cluttered. Some inconsistent findings among studies may have resulted from an imprecise identification of participants.

Children who clutter present a wide variety of characteristics and ability sets. Currently, there is considerable controversy over the features that should comprise the obligatory symptoms of cluttering. For example, some scholars include excessively fast speaking rate as essential (St. Louis et al., 2007); others argue that excessively fast speech rate should not be a key feature (Daly & Burnett, 1999). Research is needed to reveal the nature of factors leading to an impression of faster than normal speech rate for those who clutter. It is possible that they do not pause appropriately at clause or sentence boundaries, whereas those who stutter, even if their overall rates may prove similar, may pause more appropriately. Also, excessive rate may be perceived when a speaker does not observe the temporal relationships typically associated with word and syllable composition. For example, a speaker may collapse and combine the gestures for a three-word (and three-syllable) utterance: "Did you eat?" into an utterance that sounds like one syllable: "Jeet?" or the two-syllable remark "Let's go!" may be shortened to "Sko!"

The characteristics that distinguish the disfluencies of cluttering from those of language learning disabilities are ambiguous. It has been suggested that the disfluencies of cluttering are almost exclusively an excess of "other" or "normal" disfluencies rather than SLD types that would be characteristic of stuttering (Conture & Curlee, 2007). They further state that the disfluency excess is not the principal symptom of cluttering. In contrast, another source describes cluttering as characterized primarily by excessive repetitions (Daly, 1996). Although the repetitions may be of all kinds, there might be overlap with SLD types.[2] The lack of self-awareness of speech difficulty appears to be particularly distinctive between stuttering and cluttering because individuals who stutter are usually keenly aware they have a speech problem, presenting with embarrassment and fear about speaking.

Assessment of Cluttering

The assessment of cluttering involves the standard components of obtaining case history and background information, a description of the client's speech characteristics, and observing the conditions and variables affecting the client's speech (e.g., imitation, rote or automatic speech tasks, oral reading, utterance length and linguistic complexity, etc.). Beyond the usual disfluency frequency and type analysis obtained from the speech sample, measures of speech rate and temporal features

---

[2] Although word-final disfluency did not share features in common with palilalia, cluttering might. Daly and Burnett (1996) describe the tendency for the speaker to finish utterances with decreased loudness in their case example.

(e.g., pause locations and timing) will be informative. Consideration of personal factors related to the client's home, school, social and/or work environment and the impact of the communication disorder on the individual's life should be included. Finally, it is important to assess speech and language abilities thoroughly, including articulation in both word and connected speech contexts, language skills (i.e., receptive and expressive vocabulary, semantics, syntax, pragmatics), and academic reading and writing abilities. The clinician should be sure to note the client's speech-language error awareness and self-monitoring skills. How frequently are self-corrections attempted?

Methods of cluttering assessment may include formal norm-referenced tests, informal tests, or checklists of characteristics, such as the one here based on information provided in both Daly (1996) and St. Louis et al. (2007):

Cluttering Characteristics Checklist
- Excessive other disfluencies
- Excessive repetitions (all types)
- Excessive speech rate
- Poor use of pauses during speech
- Articulatory imprecision
- Short attention span and poor concentration
- Poorly organized thinking
- Lack of awareness of cluttering problem

Other Common Characteristics:
- Atypical grammatical errors
- Atypical speech sound errors
- Poor auditory awareness
- Reading problems
- Writing problems
- Unregulated vocal quality
- Impulsive, forceful personality

Literature is lacking with regard to evidence-based treatment of cluttering. A single case study was reported by Daly and Burnett (1996) including only broad treatment goals and description of the implementation in the schools. Emphasis was placed on description of evaluation methods.

Cluttering: A Sample Case

Description: A 9-year-old boy was referred by parents for a fluency evaluation. He previously received speech therapy for several years through a birth-to-3 program due to late speech and language development. His mother reported he had frequent ear infections until the age of 7 years. He had begun to stutter at approximately age 4 when he was

(continued)

putting longer sentences together. Formal tests of his language revealed average receptive vocabulary and language skills, but expressive language skills placed him at near the 15th percentile for his age. Stuttering severity was mild, with 3% of syllables characterized by SLD, primarily part-word and whole-word repetitions. His frequency of other disfluencies was 7% and consisted mainly of interjections ("um, uh") and revisions. Speech imprecision was noted in the form of sound transpositions (e.g., "aminal" for animal) and syllable elisions (e.g., "pop-lar" for popular and "cuppla" for couple of). An oral motor assessment of diadochokinesis (DDK) revealed that he reached typical speeds of repetitive syllables but produced irregular rhythms and inaccurate targets, mainly sound transpositions ("pakata" for pataka). The clinician had a subjective impression of a fast rate of speech, with frequent rushing into his utterances. Both the parent and clinician observed that the child did not appear concerned or aware of speech disfluencies.

Intervention: A three-pronged treatment approach to improve temporal aspects (slower rate and phrasing), increased self-monitoring, and phonological awareness was pursued. To modify speed of talking, the clinician modeled a slow-natural rate while continuously sliding her finger across the table to cue the start and end points of the spoken utterance. The child was to imitate both the finger sliding and the slow manner of speaking while repeating the utterance. The hierarchy of speaking tasks progressed from short multisyllable words and phrases to longer sentences, and finally to conversation. The modeling hierarchy progressed from imitation to indirect model (clinician models the manner of speaking but not using the same words), and eventually to no model. On the longer sentences, the clinician modeled pauses and phrasing, along with appropriate breath support. Pausing and phrasing were addressed in both spontaneous speech and oral reading. To prepare for oral reading, the child and clinician searched the passage for the commas and sentences to mark them in big red circles as a sign of where to stop. At first the clinician modeled how to read and follow the stop signs; later the child engaged in locating as well as observing the stop signs. Because the perception of fast rate was often due to insufficient pauses, during talking activities the clinician would instruct, "Tell me one thing and stop." "Now tell me one more thing and stop." To address self-monitoring, the child and clinician observed a videotape of the child talking and together engaged in finding segments when the child's speech was hard to follow either due to disfluencies, imprecise articulation, or irregular rate and rhythm. The clinician and child came up with three terms to label the targets of concern: "smooth," "clear," and "restful." Thus, on an almost utterance-by-utterance basis, they would evaluate "How smooth (connected)?" "How clear (articulated)?" and/or "How restful (not rushed)?" In early stages, the clinician would attempt to exactly imitate the child's utterance with the manner of talking, and then offer a contrasting production of the same sentence improved on one of the target parameters, and ask, "Which sentence sounded clearer?" (or smoother, or more restful, depending on the parameter targeted). Later on, after many examples had been reviewed, the child was asked to produce the contrasting productions, such as "Say that sentence for me in a way that is more restful." Clarity was also addressed by activities to improve phonological awareness by, together, analyzing the multisyllabic words the child produced. For example, the clinician might say "stadium." Let's listen to its parts: "sta- dee- um." How many parts are there?" Or, sometimes, "Say each part one at a time with me." (or in imitation, or independently, depending on the readiness of the child). "What sound does each part start with?" "What sound does 'sta' start with?" "What does 'dee' start with?" "Now I will make each part longer and connect them to say: staaaay-deeee-uuuumm (no breaks between syllables); now you say it that way." Eventually, it continued with, "Now I will put that word in a sentence (said at a slow-natural rate). The stadium was crowded." "Say that sentence the way I did." "Is there another sentence you could make with that word?"

Acquired Stuttering

Neurogenic Stuttering

Adults and, less frequently children, who suffered one or several of a wide range of brain injuries or other neurological diseases occasionally exhibit, among other problems, disfluent speech that shares similarities with stuttering. Usually there is a history of normal speech prior to the injury or disease. Those more commonly affected are in the geriatric subpopulation, although stroke-related stuttering has been documented in a 2-year-old (Nass, Sclireler, & Heier, 2008). It is remarkable that lesions of many different areas of the brain are associated with an increase in disfluent or stuttered speech: left hemisphere, right hemisphere, frontal, parietal, and temporal cortical regions, corpus callosum, basal ganglia, brainstem, and cerebellum (Van Borsel, Van Lierde, Van Cauweberge, Guldemont, & Van Orshoven, 1998). That is, pyramidal, extrapyramidal, and corticobulbar motor systems have been implicated separately.

A neurogenic disorder of any type by definition results from an impairment of the nervous system. Thus the term *neurogenic stuttering* is applied when there is clear evidence that the speaker's disfluent speech was acquired in connection with a neurological lesion (Duffy, 1995; Helm-Estabrooks, 1999). The term, however, should be applied with caution because much of the disfluent speech of brain-damaged people cannot be regarded as stuttering, and most brain-damaged people do not exhibit neurogenic stuttering. In a study comparing the disfluent speech of 15 individuals with Broca's aphasia and right hemiplegia, 15 nonaphasics with left hemiplegia, and 15 normally speaking people, the frequency of disfluency in the aphasic group was three times greater than that of either control group. Most of the disfluencies uttered by those with aphasia, however, were of the type commonly found in the speech of normal speakers (Yairi, Gintautas, & Avent, 1981). Although many challenges are related to the issue of what to refer to as "neurogenic stuttering" (Helm-Estabrooks, 1999), there are times when the speech disruptions observed in neurogenic stuttering are indistinguishable from characteristic of developmental stuttering (Van Borsel & Tailleau, 2001). In some cases disfluent speech becomes chronic; in other cases it is transient (Jokel, De Nil, & Sharpe, 2007).

Another type of neurogenically based disfluent speech pattern is *palilalia*, in which the same word or phrase is repeated over and over. Palilalia must also be differentiated from stuttering. Although often palilalia has been characterized as diminishing in loudness and increasing in rate with each successive iteration, this may not always be the case (Kent & Lapointe, 1982). Another potential source of repetitive speech behavior is Tourette's syndrome (TS). TS is an inherited neurological disorder named for the French neurologist Gilles de la Tourette, who in 1885 first described this condition primarily characterized by motor tics. In some cases, stuttering and TS may co-occur, but there is also evidence to suggest that the disfluencies of TS are distinctive from those of stuttering, cluttering, and palilalia (Van Borsel, Goethals, & Vanryckeghem, 2004).

Characteristics and Differential Diagnosis

As in developmental stuttering, there is great diversity in the symptoms and characteristics of acquired neurogenic stuttering. A variety of core and accessory disfluency types have been described: sound prolongations, part-word repetitions, tonic blocks, hesitation pauses, interjections, and word prolongations (Helm-Estabrooks & Hotz, 1998). In many cases SLD types of disfluencies are the main speech characteristic (e.g., Ackermann, Hertrich, Ziegler, Bitzer, & Bien, 1996; Helm-Estabrooks & Hotz, 1998; Lebrun & Leleux, 1985). For some, the speech disruptions occur in the absence of any symptoms of aphasia or cognitive disability (Ciabarra, Elkind, Roberts, & Marshall, 2000; Hamano et al., 2005). More commonly, however, the fluency disruptions are accompanied by other neurologically based speech problems, such as slurred articulation resulting from dysarthria, halted speech resulting from apraxia, as well as voice disorders, cognitive disturbances impairing memory, and language disorders such as aphasia (Attanasio, 1987; Ardila & Lopez, 1986; Ciabarra et al., 2000). Some patients also exhibit emotional tension, depression, or anxiety (Roth, Aronson, & Davis, 1989), whereas others have relatively little concomitant affective reactions (Market, Montague, Buffalo, & Drummond, 1990). As stated, only a few brain-damaged individuals exhibit what can be diagnosed as neurogenic stuttering, and they too reveal several important differences from the much more common developmental stuttering.

The following list offers several examples of features that may contrast neurogenic stuttering from developmental stuttering (Helm-Estabrooks, 1999):

- The onset is acquired, usually in adulthood.
- A neurological impairment has been confirmed.
- Speech disfluency is less variable across situations.
- Stuttering occurs across all the words of an utterance, not mainly on initial words.
- Content and function words are stuttered equally.
- The person may be frustrated but not usually embarrassed by stuttering.
- Secondary behaviors are less likely.
- An adaptation effect is less likely.
- Stuttering also occurs on highly automatic speech tasks.

Concerning the adaptation effect listed, although most reports have indicated that no adaptation effect occurred in their neurogenic stuttering patients (e.g., Ardila & Lopez, 1986; Nowack & Stone, 1987), at least one case did present adaptation (Hamano et al., 2005). No reports have been found pertaining to the consistency effect in neurogenic stuttering. Also, note in the preceding list that the distribution of stuttered events in the speech stream is wider than it is in developmental stuttering. Given this reduced predictability regarding locations, it is tempting to hypothesize that the consistency effect as well may be smaller than the 69% reported by Johnson and Leutenegger (1955, p. 211). A low consistency effect supports the impression that neurogenic stuttering represents a separate form of fluency disorder. For further explanations of the adaptation and consistency effects, see Chapter 4.

A more recent survey of speech clinicians regarding 58 Dutch-speaking individuals with neurogenic stuttering revealed some interesting results. Theys, Wieringen, and De Nil (2008) observed that more than one-fourth (27%) of the 164 clinicians who were serving populations with neurological disorders had worked with one or more patients with neurogenic stuttering. These results suggested that it is a more common problem than previously thought. In addition, patient characteristics contrasted with the previously listed criteria in a few ways. A larger proportion than expected, 39% of patients, displayed an adaptation effect. Secondary characteristics, also supposedly rare, were noted among 40%. A remarkable majority (64%) of patients were reported to have emotional reactions to their stuttering, but data upheld the impression that irritation rather than anxiety is a more common response.

Assessment and Treatment of Neurogenic Stuttering

The assessment of neurogenic stuttering includes areas very similar to those of cluttering, but the expected findings differ. In addition to the standard components, such as case history, description of speech characteristics, speaking rate and other temporal features, emotional and social impact, it is important to assess other dimensions of speech and language that may have been affected by the neurological disorder. In this case, however, the types of problems with articulation, language, cognition and memory, and capacities to self-correct errors will all be evaluated relative to the client's premorbid abilities. The potential for spontaneous recovery following the injury and the medical prognosis will also be important.

Treatments of neurogenic stuttering have included a variety of approaches: traditional therapies of stuttering modification and/or fluency shaping, biofeedback, speech rate changes, pacing, delayed auditory feedback, cognitive therapy, voice therapy techniques, respiration training, relaxation exercises, and similar techniques toward an easier approach to speech movements. Medical interventions have included surgery, thalamic stimulation, subcutaneous nerve stimulation, and prescription drugs.

Neurogenic Stuttering: A Sample Case

Description: A 55-year-old woman was referred for a speech-language evaluation secondary to a brain hemorrhage. Medical scans revealed diffuse injury to the right temporal lobe. Speech characteristics included sound/syllable repetitions and postural fixations in all positions of words and utterances. Content and function words were stuttered with proportionately the same frequency. Stuttering occurred during both conversational and oral reading speech samples. No adaptation effect was observed. Although she was also disfluent on automatic speech tasks (e.g., counting, swearing, saying the alphabet), her language skills, both receptive and expressive, were normal. Only mild signs of frustration with speech disruptions were observed.

Intervention: Therapeutic probes revealed improved fluency when speaking each syllable while tapping the beat and when slowing the initiation and connectedness across words in sentences. A pacing board was introduced to facilitate the client's self-monitoring of rhythm and slow speaking rate. The clinician demonstrated the use of the board by pointing to a space for each syllable as she talked, and the client then imitated. Independent use of the board was targeted in a hierarchy of speaking tasks progressing from short phrases to longer sentences. A drawing of a simple pacing board is seen in Figure 15.1. When the client was consistently successful with the pacing board, she was instructed to look up from the board and make eye contact with the clinician while talking, maintaining a similar rate/rhythm. After consistently fluent speech was maintained in the therapy room, transfer of fluency in multiple outside settings was accomplished after developing an individualized situation hierarchy, starting with easier settings and progressing to more difficult.

Psychogenic Stuttering

Psychogenic stuttering occurs when there is a sudden onset of chronic abnormal disfluency following a psychoemotional trauma, and the speech disorder is not found to be associated with an organic etiology (Baumgartner, 1999). It is a rare condition and should not be confused with cases of adults with previously existing developmental stuttering who experience a new episode of stuttering triggered by psychoemotional factors. The term *psychogenic disorder* is also sometimes used interchangeably with "functional disorder" and "somatic disorder." The original

Figure 15.1: Pacing Board

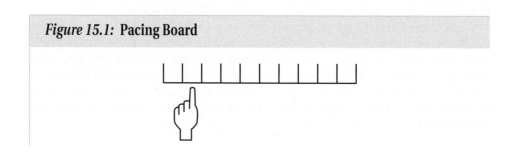

cause of this form of stuttering is emotional breakdown or psychological trauma, such as firsthand views of the tragedies of war. Its core symptomatology includes the essential disfluency features included in our definition of stuttering (see Chapter 1). A variety of disfluency types have been observed among individuals with psychogenic stuttering, although repetitions are frequently cited (Mahr & Leith, 1992). The dynamics of psychogenic stuttering are similar to that of other psychogenic speech disorders, such as functional aphonia and functional dysphonia. Instead of a loss of voice or hoarseness secondary to an emotional trauma, however, dysfluent speech is the symptom of what the psychopathological literature refers to as a *conversion reaction* (Breuer & Freud, 1936). As we discussed in Chapter 6, a conversion reaction occurs when there is an impairment of physical action or sensation that cannot be explained by organic disease or a medical condition, and it arises following deep unconscious conflict. More than one psychosomatic illness sometimes arises in the same individual, but a person who has had another form of conversion reaction is not necessarily inclined to develop psychogenic stuttering. In one person a conversion reaction results in a paralyzed limb; in another it causes loss of speech. Why the symptoms vary across individuals remains unknown. Possible reasons for the variation, however, include the potential of secondary gains from the particular symptom (e.g., being excused from responsibility for a communication role) or a symbolic expression of the psychological conflict (e.g., being blocked from expressing one's opinions). The person typically has no awareness of the nature of the problem or the secondary gain that it may have. In contrast to developmental stuttering, they often are emotionally apathetic toward the stuttering, a response that has been termed *la belle indifférence* (Roth, Aronson, & Davis, 1989).

In a retrospective examination of 184 cases of sudden onset of adult stuttering, Roth et al. (1989) found that 100 had suspected psychogenic components. Diagnoses included neurogenic stuttering, psychogenic stuttering, a mixed diagnosis (psychogenic + neurogenic), or undetermined origin. Among the 100 with psychogenic stuttering, 12 met criteria for closer scrutiny. Six men and six women, ages 21 to 79 years, with no childhood history of stuttering, all underwent psychiatric, medical, and speech pathology examinations, and for whom neurological diagnoses had been ruled out. The characteristics of their psychogenic stuttering cases were in turn described. Their stuttering problem had lasted anywhere from 1.5 to 4 years. Speech characteristics included repetitions, prolongations, and blocks that ranged in severity from mild to severe. Nine had some episodes of normal speech. Eleven were classified as "conversion reaction." Psychologically, six experienced acute stress, four chronic stress, and one with undetermined stress. All had associated somatic complaints as well, such as headache, backache, leg pain, chest pain, numbness or tingling of an extremity, staring spells, fatigue, fainting, panic attacks, choking sensation, hyperventilation, memory loss, or ringing in the ears. Muscle contractions or twitches occurred among six of them. Eleven experienced a recovery of some fluent speech: five from individual speech therapy, one from group therapy, one from the evaluation processes, and four from spontaneous recovery.

Depression appears to be a common diagnosis among individuals with psychogenic stuttering (Roth, Aronson & Davis, 1989). Other potential psychological conditions that may be present include schizophrenia, neurosis, and psychosis. Assessment and diagnosis by a licensed psychiatric or psychotherapy professional is warranted. It is important that health-care professionals maintain a respectful stance toward the client because it is vital to the process of healing. When a client believes his or her symptoms represent a physical ailment, recovery is not aided by being told that the symptoms are psychological. Instead, improvement is based in the client's acquisition of skills and strategies. Similar to conventional stuttering treatment, as the speaker gains self-confidence in his or her own capacities to manage the speech symptoms with new behavioral responses, the problem weakens and progressively recedes.

The onset of psychogenic stuttering typically occurs in adulthood and is sudden and rare. It is different from developmental stuttering because the disfluencies usually persist even in typically fluency-inducing conditions such as singing, unison, and delayed auditory feedback (Mahr & Leith, 1992). Also unlike developmental stuttering, the stuttering symptoms have the potential to go into remission rapidly, especially when the period of acute psychological stress has passed and the individual had no issues premorbidly. Concurrent psychological counseling can aid holistic recovery. Caring support and skilled intervention by multiple professionals can be instrumental to facilitate progress. Although the following case description depicts the potential outcome of an improvement, published reports suggest psychogenic stuttering may continue for months or years (Roth, Aronson, & Davis, 1989) and in some cases does not resolve (Mahr & Leith, 1992).

Psychogenic Stuttering: A Sample Case

Description: The SLP was contacted by a woman looking for help for her husband, age 38, who suddenly began stuttering for no apparent reason. His speech is characterized by frequent stereotypic repetitions of initial syllables: "Whi-whi-which one do you want?" "I-I-I like that one." "Let-let-let's get it." He looks people in the eyes, does not avoid speaking situations, and is not particularly bothered by the speech pattern. He has never stuttered before. He is unmotivated to seek help, but his wife encourages him to do just that. The client also has had some unexplained episodes of neck and back pain, for which several medical professionals have been consulted, who found no physical problems. The client has been in good physical health throughout most of his life. The couple's physician suggested they contact the speech-language pathologist for a consultation. Further discussion reveals the client has been seriously depressed and dealing with some stressful interpersonal conflicts within the family. He has recently begun sessions of psychological therapy.

Intervention: The speech clinician began by educating the client about the vocal tract structures and their function for speech production. Then strategies for slow, easy initiation of speech were taught via modeling and instruction. The client achieved targeted objectives of describing his speech movements accurately and modifying moments of simulated stuttering (particularly syllable repetitions). Skills were practiced in multiple speaking tasks and situational contexts. The client simultaneously gained cognitive-emotional coping skills through the psychological therapy, and one day the client came to therapy reporting that his stuttering had disappeared and that his attitudes and adjustment with life more generally had improved.

Malingering

On occasion, a family member or professional may wonder whether the symptoms of stuttering are faked behavior. Malingering, or faking the presence of a disorder, is a remote possibility when a speaker has something to gain from the diagnosis, especially for financial, legal, or vocational gains (Seery, 2005). Although parents sometimes suspect a child is stuttering out of a motive to annoy or gain attention, these are not typical of malingering. Especially if other characteristics of the developmental disorder fit diagnostic criteria, such as early stuttering onset, SLD, progression, emotional responses, and fluency-inducing situations, these should outweigh the suspicions of underlying motives. A child who shows signs that she or he does *not* want to be stuttering should not be suspected of malingering.

However, a person who malingers is more apt to show signs that it is favorable to be acknowledged for stuttering and would be motivated to want to be identified as someone who stutters. Typically, there is an underlying gainful motivation. For example, on the basis of stuttered speech, criminal identification could be ruled out, a release from military service granted, and so on. Faked stuttering is apt to lack variability and take on a stereotypical form. The diagnosis of malingering is aided by the tendency for the faker's profile and characteristics to be consistent only with what the individual knows about stuttering. The areas where a malingerer's knowledge is weak, or incompatible with what we know about stuttering, are apt to give away the charade. Differential diagnosis in the case of a man suspected of a crime who partially malingered stuttering is described by Seery (2005).

Stuttering in Bilingual/Multicultural Populations

Large waves of immigrants across continents and countries, as well as the ease of transportation for various purposes, have led to societies with far greater numbers of bilingual/multilingual speakers than ever before. There are millions of multilingual people worldwide, including in the United States (Tucker, 1998). It is therefore likely that speech-language clinicians will examine and deliver clinical services to people who stutter who speak more than one language or stutter in more than one language. Such encounters raise the possibility of misinterpretation of data, resulting in possible misdiagnosis of speech and/or language disorders (e.g., Finn & Cordes, 1997).

Recently, several scholars stated that examiners' lack of familiarity with African American English (AAE), a dialect spoken by a large number of African Americans, might have led to an erroneous overestimate of stuttering prevalence among African Americans because normal disfluencies, such as revisions, repetitions, filled pauses, and prosodic features, denote various meanings in AAE. The presence of some or all of these linguistic features in a speaker may be mistaken for stuttering by individuals unfamiliar with AAE (Proctor, Yairi, & Duff, 2008).

General Considerations

Whether familiarity with the client's language influences identification of stuttering, however, has not been yet determined. One study investigated whether bilingual English-Spanish speaking judges are better at making disfluency judgments in Spanish than monolingual English-speaking judges. No statistically differences between the two groups of judges were found (Humphrey, 2004). Other investigators, however, reported contradictory findings, showing that language familiarity does influence stuttering judgment. In a series of listener judgment experiments, native speakers of Brazilian Portuguese identified and judged stuttering in Dutch speakers and in Portuguese speakers while native speakers of Dutch identified and judged stuttering in Brazilian Portuguese speakers and in Dutch speakers. Both panels found identification of stuttering more difficult in the foreign language than in the native language (Van Borsel & Britto Pereira, 2005). The investigators suggested that their results might have been different if the judgment had involved languages that are less remote from each other.

Three main questions should be addressed relative to stuttering, multilingualism, and cultural background: (1) Are those who speak more than one language more apt to be disfluent? (2) Are there distinctive stuttering speech characteristics among those who speak more than one language? and (3) Does cultural background affect beliefs and attitudes about the disorder and should it be considered in the therapeutic approach?

Bilingualism is a not a singular characteristic. There can be differences among individuals based on the timing of their acquisition of the second language. Some children are exposed to two languages essentially from birth on. Others may have been exposed to just one language in the home until they started attending a pre-school, day-care, or school program where they became exposed to the second language from that point on. In the latter situation, there may be many varied schedules of exposure to the second language (e.g., daily versus two mornings per week, etc.) that contribute to differences among children in the developmental progress of their second-language learning. Yet another situation arises when there are two languages spoken in a home since birth, and a third or additional languages are introduced through other settings.

One of the primary concerns in the assessment of bilingual speakers who stutter is the examiner's capacity to recognize the occurrence, location, and nature of disfluent behaviors in another language (Finn & Cordes, 1997). A recent study by Einarsdottir and Ingham (2009) showed that experienced speech clinicians were fairly reliable at identifying stuttered intervals in video-recorded samples of preschool children speaking in an unfamiliar language. It is, however, appropriate for clinicians to be cautious about their identification of stuttering and disfluency in bilingual speakers. It can be difficult even when listening to young monolingual children to distinguish a doubling pattern (e.g., "car-car," "bye-bye") from a whole-word repetition. When a young child is speaking in an unfamiliar language with different patterns of prosody, the clinician would do well to make sure that the listeners who are familiar with the child's language would similarly detect speech disruptions. The clinician may need to include a translator, a parent, or another person proficient in the language for assistance and confirmation. A recent review of the literature on stuttering and bilingualism can be found in Roberts and Shenker (2007).

Disfluencies in the speech of those who are learning to speak a second language are a potential distraction for listeners (Corley, MacGregor, & Donaldson, 2007). Distracting behaviors can include unfilled pauses, self-repetitions, inappropriate rate, and fillers/interjections (Rossiter, 2009). Their speech, however, is usually not stuttered, as suggested by the observation that there has been no concern found in published literature about the frequency of SLD being greater than that of other normally fluent speakers. This inference is preliminary, however, and research should be conducted to test whether SLD might be more frequent among second-language learners. Investigations have reported that second-language learners (i.e., those who have only been learning to speak a language for a few years) produce a preponderance of various forms of hesitation (e.g., silent and filled pauses, self-repairs, etc.) that typify language formulation and working memory overload compared to native speakers. The frequency of these behaviors significantly exceeds those produced by monolingual speakers (Temple, 2000).

Cultural and Ethnic Considerations

In discussing the incidence and prevalence of stuttering (see Chapter 2), we pointed out that stuttering has been identified in most parts of the world in many societies and cultures. Possible variation in incidence in a few societies has been attributed in the past to cultural factors. For certain societies, a link was proposed between high incidence and excessive pressure on children's achievements and ability to speak well and between low incidence and society's tolerant attitudes in these matters (Lemert, 1962). Even if the incidence/prevalence data are valid, which we doubt, the research data to support the causative relations are weak. Also, you should keep in mind that either high or low incidence might reflect genetic factors, especially in societies that were not open to outside blood lines.

Of more relevance to clinicians are the effects of cultural background on the characteristics of stuttering, cultural beliefs about the cause of the disorder, attitudes toward the person who stutters, attitudes toward treatment in general, acceptability of specific therapeutic approaches, reactions to specific techniques, and who should be the provider of treatment. For example, peoples from some cultures may not react well to certain advice typically given in the United States in parent counseling, or they may not be open to requests that parents participate in the therapy sessions, especially not both parents. In some cultures, adults may not be willing to openly express deep feelings or emotional problems in group therapy. Clinical assignments, such as stuttering on purpose to strangers, may be unacceptable; so is maintaining eye contact with listeners older in age or superior in status, and so on. Roberts and Shenker (2007) list other examples of interest. Keep in mind that cultural influences include many factors. For example, religious beliefs and social class are relevant in addition to ethnicity, race, and geographic locale. EY encountered some people who stutter who believed they were afflicted by God and that a minister should provide the counseling. Differences in overt stuttering patterns between African Americans and whites were tied to cultural background, according to Leith and Mims (1975). They concluded that forces within the African American culture actually negate certain common clinical approaches. Still, Roberts and Shenker (2007) have cautioned against stereotypes based on cultural background, explaining that a middle-age lawyer from Hong Kong would have more in common with an Anglo architect from the United States than with a young adult street vendor from his own city of Hong Kong. Robinson and Crowe (1998) offer a model of service delivery to be followed when offering services to multicultural populations. They also offer examples of etiological and remediation myths that clinicians may encounter in their work with African American populations.

Several suggestions may help to improve services provided to culturally and linguistically diverse populations (Santos & Reese, 1999):

1. Understand and learn about the aspects of your cultural practices that may differ from others from other ethnic backgrounds.
2. Learn as much as you can about the culture of those people you serve. What kinds of accomplishments are respected within their community? What do they believe their children should be learning and doing? How do they view the roles of family members (parents, grandparents, aunts/uncles, siblings, etc.)? What elements of their culture are treated as public versus private? What is their history with educational, health-care, and social services, and does that history affect their outlook regarding these services?
3. Is the literature that I am sharing going to be appropriate, or might there be implicit or explicit assumptions, beliefs, or values that could be potentially problematic, disrespectful, or confusing? Is the mode of presentation (oral, visual, auditory) going to best facilitate their understanding of information? Is the literacy level appropriate and technical/jargon terms kept to a minimum or explained sufficiently? If material is translated, is it appropriate given their particular dialect and community? Clinicians may want to find someone to review material beforehand to prevent potential misunderstandings.

4. Does the program of services assume that family members will take an "active role" in treatment that is not customary in their culture? Care must be taken that professionals do not presume that parents or family who do not take on "active" roles do not care, when in fact they do but show concern in other ways. The clinician may need to adapt the level of family participation to their culture and/or discuss with the family possible options related to their role in treatment.

Summary

Although classic developmental stuttering is clearly the largest in incidence and most known within the group of fluency disorders, clinicians must be aware of, and familiar with, other fluency disorders in this group, both in regard to differential diagnosis and treatment. As the chapter showed, these vary from peculiarities, such as word-final disfluencies, to cluttering, to stuttering associated with other disorders of adult onset, and more. Potential overlap in symptomatology can be confusing, masking very different etiologies and the need for different counseling and treatment regimens. Clinicians must carefully evaluate differential diagnostic criteria as they consider neurogenic, psychogenic, or malingering as possible sources of stuttering and disfluent behaviors. In regard to treatment, there has been minimal research published to reveal how individuals with other fluency disorders are best served. Case samples and potential considerations were discussed that may be useful in clinical decision making. There has been a growing interest in bilingualism in relation to stuttering. It is still unclear if bilingualism influences the incidence of stuttering and whether characteristics of stuttering vary across languages spoken by the same individual. Finally, examples were given of possible cultural values to consider when therapy is provided to clients of diverse backgrounds.

STUDY QUESTIONS AND DISCUSSION TOPICS

1. What characteristics of neurogenic stuttering differ from those of developmental stuttering?

2. How is treatment of neurogenic stuttering similar to and/or different from that of developmental stuttering?

3. What would lead you to suspect that a client presents psychogenic stuttering?

4. What would be your approaches to treatment of psychogenic stuttering, and why?

5. What characteristics aid the identification of cluttering? What are some reasons why differential diagnosis of cluttering from stuttering may be beneficial?

6. What special considerations need to be made in the treatment of speakers who clutter?

7. What can you do to help ensure your services are culturally appropriate for your clients?

WEB SITES

Brochures by the Stuttering Foundation of America
Neurogenic stuttering: www.stutteringhelp.org/Portals/english/0111neur.pdf
Cluttering: www.stutteringhelp.org/Portals/english/0065C.pdf

Tourette's syndrome: www.stutteringhelp.org/portals/english/tourettes.pdf
Bilingual child: www.stutteringhelp.org/Portals/english/0110bilc.pdf

SUGGESTED READINGS

Boscolo, B., Bernstein Ratner, N., & Rescorla, L. (2002). Fluency of school-aged children with a history of specific expressive language impairment: An exploratory study. *American Journal of Speech-Language Pathology, 11*, 41–49.

De Nil, L., Jokel, R., & Rochon, E. (2007). Etiology, symptomatology, and treatment of neurogenic stuttering. In E. Conture & R. Curlee (Eds.), *Stuttering and related disorders of fluency* (3rd ed., pp. 326–343). New York: Thieme.

Roberts, P., & Shenker, R. (2007). Assessment and treatment of stuttering in bilingual speakers. In E. Conture & R. Curlee (Eds.), *Stuttering and related disorders of fluency* (3rd ed., pp. 183–206). New York: Thieme.

Van Borsel, J., Maes, E., & Foulon, K. (2001). Stuttering and bilingualism: A review. *Journal of Fluency Disorders, 26*, 179–205.

References

Ackermann, H., Hertrich, I., Ziegler, W., Bitzer, M., & Bien, S. (1996). Acquired dysfluencies following infarction of left mesiofrontal cortex. *Aphasiology, 10,* 409–417.

Adams, M. R. (1977). A clinical strategy for differentiating the normally nonfluent child and the incipient stutterer. *Journal of Fluency Disorders, 2,* 141–148.

Adams, M. (1987). Voice onsets and segment durations of normal speakers and beginning stutterers. *Journal of Fluency Disorders, 12,* 133–139.

Adams, M. R. (1990). The demands and capacities model: I. Theoretical elaborations. *Journal of Fluency Disorders, 15,* 135–141.

Agnello, J., & Wingate, M. (1972). Some acoustic aspects of stuttered speech. *Journal of Acoustical Society of America, 52,* 159.

Alm, P. (2004a). Stuttering, emotions, and heart rate during anticipatory anxiety: A critical review. *Journal of Fluency Disorders, 29,* 123–133.

Alm, P. (2004b). Stuttering and basal ganglia circuits: A critical review of possible relations. *Journal of Communication Disorders, 37,* 325–369.

Ambrose, N., Cox, N., & Yairi, E. (1997). The genetic basis of persistence and recovery in stuttering. *Journal of Speech, Language, and Hearing Research, 40*(3), 567–580.

Ambrose, N., & Yairi, E. (1994). The development of awareness of stuttering in preschool children. *Journal of Fluency Disorders, 19,* 229–245.

Ambrose, N., & Yairi, E. (1995). The role of repetition units in the differential diagnosis of early childhood incipient stuttering. *American Journal of Speech-Language Pathology, 4*(3), 82–88.

Ambrose, N., & Yairi, E. (1999). Normative disfluency data for early childhood stuttering. *Journal of Speech, Language, and Hearing Research, 42,* 895–909.

Ambrose, N., & Yairi, E. (2001). Perspectives on stuttering: Response to Onslow & Packman (2001). *Journal of Speech, Language, and Hearing Research, 44,* 595–597.

Ambrose, N., & Yairi, E. (2002). The Tudor study: Data and ethics. *American Journal of Speech-Language Pathology, 11,* 190–203.

Ambrose, N., Yairi, E., & Cox, N. (1993). Genetic aspects of early childhood stuttering. *Journal of Speech and Hearing Research, 36,* 701–706.

American Speech-Language-Hearing Association. (1995, March). Guidelines for practice in stuttering treatment. *ASHA, 37* (Suppl. 14), 26–35.

American Speech-Language-Hearing Association Special Interest Division 4: Fluency and Fluency Disorders.

(1999, March). Terminology pertaining to fluency and fluency disorders: Guidelines. *ASHA, 41* (Suppl. 19), 29–36.

Anderson, J., & Conture, E. (2000). Language abilities of children who stutter: A preliminary study. *Journal of Fluency Disorders, 25,* 283–304.

Anderson, J., & Conture, E. (2004). Sentence structure priming in young children who do and do not stutter. *Journal of Speech, Language, and Hearing Research, 47,* 552–571.

Anderson, J. D., Pellowski, M. W., Conture, E. G., & Kelly, E. M. (2003). Temperamental characteristics of young children who stutter. *Journal of Speech, Language, and Hearing Research, 46,* 1221–1233.

Anderson, J., Wagovich, S., & Hall, N. (2006). Nonword repetition skills in young children who do and do not stutter. *Journal of Fluency Disorders, 31,* 177–199.

Andrews, G. (1984). The epidemiology of stuttering. In R. F. Curlee & W. H. Perkins (Eds.), *Nature and treatment of stuttering: New Directions* (pp. 1–12). San Diego, CA: College-Hill.

Andrews, G., & Craig, A. (1988). Prediction of outcome after treatment for stuttering. *The British Journal of Psychiatry, 153,* 236–240.

Andrews, G., Craig, A., Feyer, A., Hoddinott, S., Howie, P., & Neilson, M. (1983). Stuttering: A review of research findings and theories circa 1982. *Journal of Speech and Hearing Disorders, 48,* 226–246.

Andrews, G., & Cutler, J. (1974). Stuttering therapy: The relation between changes in symptom level and attitudes. *Journal of Speech and Hearing Disorders, 39,* 312–319.

Andrews, G., & Dozsa, M. (1977). Haloperidol and the treatment of stuttering. *Journal of Fluency Disorders, 2,* 217–224.

Andrews, G., Guitar, B., & Howie, P. (1980). Meta-analysis of the effects of stuttering treatment. *Journal of Speech and Hearing Disorders, 45,* 287–307.

Andrews, G., & Harris, M. (1964). *The syndrome of stuttering: Clinics in developmental medicine,* No. 17. London: Spastics Society Medical Education and Information Unit in association with Wm. Heinemann Medical Books.

Andrews, G., Harris, M., Garside, R., & Kay, D. (1964). The inhibition of stuttering by syllable-timed speech. *The syndrome of stuttering.* The Spastic Society Medical and Educational Unit. London: Heineman.

Andrews, G., Howie, P., Dozsa, M., & Guitar, B. (1982). Stuttering: Speech pattern characteristics under fluency-inducing conditions. *Journal of Speech and Hearing Research, 25,* 208–216.

Andrews, G., & Ingham, R. (1972). Stuttering: An evaluation of follow-up procedures for syllable-timed speech/token system therapy. *Journal of Communication Disorders, 5*(4), 307–319.

Andrews, G., & Ingham, R. (1973). An analysis of a token economy in stuttering therapy. *Journal of Applied Behavior Analysis, 6*(2), 219–229.

Andrews, G., Morris-Yates, A., Howie, P., & Martin, N. G. (1991). Genetic factors in stuttering confirmed. *Archives of General Psychiatry, 48*, 1034–1035.

Antipova, E., Purdy, S., Blakeley, M. & Williams, S. (2008). Effects of altered auditory feedback (AAF) on stuttering frequency during monologue speech production. *Journal of Fluency Disorders, 33*, 274–290.

Archibald, L., & De Nil, L. (1999). The relationship between stuttering severity and kinesthetic acuity for jaw movements in adults who stutter. *Journal of Fluency Disorders, 24*, 25–42.

Ardila, A., Bateman, J., & Niño, C. (1994). An epidemiologic study of stuttering. *Journal of Communication Disorders, 27*(1), 37–48.

Ardila, A., & Lopez, M. V. (1986). Severe stuttering associated with right hemisphere lesion. *Brain & Language, 27*, 239–246.

Arias-Carrión, O., & Pöppel, E. (2007). Dopamine, learning and reward-seeking behavior. *Acta Neurobiological Experimental, 67*, 481–488.

Arndt, J., & Healey, E. C. (2001). Concomitant disorders in school-age children who stutter. *Language, Speech, and Hearing Services in Schools, 32*, 68–78.

Arnott, N. (1928). *Elements of physics.* Edinburgh.

Aron, M. (1962). The nature and incidence of stuttering among a Bantu group of school-going children. *Journal of Speech and Hearing Disorders, 27*(2), 116–128.

Aron, M. (1967). The relationships between measurements of stuttering behavior. *Journal of the South African Logopedic Society, 14*, 15–34.

ASHA. (1997–2007a). Incidence and prevalence of communication disorders and hearing loss in Children—2008 edition. Retrieved from www.asha.org/members/research/reports/children.htm

ASHA (1997–2007b). Introduction to evidence-based practice. Retrieved from www.asha.org/members/ebp/intro.htm

ASHA. (2008a). *Membership and certification handbook of the American-Speech-Language-Hearing Association.* Retrieved from www.asha.org/about/membership-certification/handbooks/slp/slp_standards.htm

ASHA. (2008b). *Speech and language disorders and diseases.* Retrieved from www.asha.org/public/speech/disorders/default.htm

Atack, J. (2003). Anxioselective compounds acting at the GABA(A) receptor benzodiazepine binding site. *Current Drug Targets. CNS and Neurological Disorders, 2*, 213–232.

Attanasio, J. (1987). A case of late-onset or acquired stuttering in adult life. *Journal of Fluency Disorders, 12*, 287–290.

Au-Yeung, J., Gomez, I., & Howell, P. (2003). Exchange of disfluency with age from function words to content words in Spanish speakers who stutter. *Journal of Speech, Language, and Hearing Research, 46*, 754–765.

Au-Yeung, J., Howell, P., Charles, N., & Sackin, S. (2000). UCL survey of bilingualism and stuttering. In *Proceedings of the 3rd World Congress on Fluency Disorders,* pp. 129–132. H-G.G. Bosshardt, J. S. Yaruss, & H. Peters (Eds). Nijmegen University Press.

Avari, D., & Bloodstein, O. (1974). Adjacency and prediction in school-age stutterers. *Journal of Speech and Hearing Research, 17*, 33–40.

Axline, V. M. (1947). *Play therapy.* London: Methuen.

Backus, O. (1938). Incidence of stuttering among the deaf. *Annals of Otology, Rhinology, and Laryngology, 47*, 632–635.

Baken, R. (1987). *Clinical measurement of speech and voice.* Boston: College-Hill.

Bar, A. (1971). The shaping of fluency not the modification of stuttering. *Journal of Communication Disorders, 4*, 1–8.

Barbara, D. (1954). *Stuttering: A psychodynamic approach to its understanding and treatment.* New York: Julian Press.

Barbara, D. (1962). *The psychotherapy of stuttering.* Springfield, IL: Charles C. Thomas.

Barlow, D., Hayes, S., & Nelson, R. (1984). *The scientist practitioner: Research and accountability in clinical and educational settings.* New York: Pergamon.

Barr, H. (1940). A quantitative study of specific phenomena observed in stuttering. *Journal of Speech Disorders, 5*, 277–280.

Baumgartner, J. M. (1999). Acquired psychogenic stuttering. In R. F. Curlee (Ed.), *Stuttering and Related Disorders of Fluency* (2nd ed.). New York: Thieme.

Beal, D., Gracco, V., Lafaille, S., & De Nil, L. (2007). Voxel-based morphometry of auditory and speech-related cortex in stutterers. *Neuroreport, 18*(12), 1257–1260.

Beitchman, J. H., Nair, R., Clegg, M., & Patel, P. G. (1986). Prevalence of speech and language disorders in 5-year-old kindergarten children in the Ottawa-Carleton Region. *Journal of Speech and Hearing Disorders, 51*, 98–110.

Bender, J. (1943). The prophylaxis of stuttering. *Nervous Child, 2*, 181–198.

Berlin, A. (1954). *An exploratory attempt to isolate types of stuttering* (Unpublished doctoral dissertation). Northwestern University, Evanston, IL.

Bernstein Ratner, N. (1992). Measurable outcomes in instructions to modify normal parent-child verbal interactions: Implications for indirect stuttering therapy. *Journal of Speech and Hearing Research, 35*, 14–20.

Bernstein Ratner, N. (1995). Treating the child who stutters with concomitant language or phonological impairment. *Language, Speech, and Hearing Services in Schools, 26*, 180–186.

Bernstein Ratner, N. (1997a). Stuttering: A psycholinguistic perspective. In R. F. Curlee & G. M. Siegel (Eds.), *Nature and treatment of stuttering: New directions* (2nd ed., pp. 99–127). Boston: Allyn & Bacon.

Bernstein Ratner, N. (1997b). Leaving Las Vegas: Clinical odds and individual outcomes *American Journal of Speech-Language Pathology, 6*, 29–33.

Bernstein Ratner, N. (2004). Caregiver-child interactions and their impact on children's fluency: Implications for treatment. *Language, Speech, and Hearing Services in Schools, 35*, 46–56.

Bernstein Ratner, N. (2005). Evidence-based practice in stuttering: Some questions to consider. *Journal of Fluency Disorders, 30*, 163–188.

Bernstein Ratner, N., & Healey, E. C. (1999). *Stuttering research and practice*. Mahwah, NJ: Erlbaum.

Bernstein Ratner, N., & Sih, C. (1987). The effects of gradual increases in sentence length and complexity on children's dysfluency. *Journal of Speech and Hearing Disorders, 52*, 278–287.

Blanton, S. (1916). A survey of speech defects. *Journal of Educational Psychology, 7*(10), 581–592.

Block, S., Onslow, M., Roberts, R., & White S. (2004). Control of stuttering with EMG feedback. *Advances in Speech-Language Pathology, 6*, 100–106.

Blomgren, M., Roy, N., Callister, T., & Merrill, R. M. (2005). Intensive stuttering modification therapy: A multidimensional assessment of treatment outcomes. *Journal of Speech, Language, and Hearing Research, 48*(3), 509–523.

Blood, G. (1995). Power: Relapse management with adolescents who stutter. *Language, Speech, and Hearing Services in Schools, 26*, 169–179.

Blood, G., & Conture, E. (1998). Outcome measurements issues in fluency disorders. In C. Frattali (Ed.), *Measuring outcomes in speech-language pathology* (pp. 387–405). New York: Thieme.

Blood, G., Ridenour, V., Qualls, C., & Scheffner Hammer (2003). Co-occurring disorders in children who stutter. *Journal of Communication Disorders, 36*, 427–448.

Blood, G., & Seider, R. (1981). The concomitant problems of young stutterers. *Journal of Speech and Hearing Disorders, 46*, 31–33.

Blood, I., Wertz, H., Blood, G., Bennett, S., & Simpson, K. (1997). The effects of life stressors and daily stressors on stuttering. *Journal of Speech, Language, and Hearing Research, 40*, 134–143.

Bloodstein, O. (1944). Studies in the psychology of stuttering: XIX. The relationship between oral reading rate and severity of stuttering. *Journal of Speech Disorders, 9*, 161–173.

Bloodstein, O. (1950). A rating scale study of conditions under which stuttering is reduced or absent. *Journal of Speech and Hearing Disorders, 15*, 29–36.

Bloodstein, O. (1960a). The development of stuttering: I. Changes in nine basic features. *Journal of Speech and Hearing Disorders, 25*, 219–237.

Bloodstein, O. (1960b). The development of stuttering: II. Developmental phases. *Journal of Speech and Hearing Disorders, 25*, 366–376.

Bloodstein, O. (1961). The development of stuttering: III. Theoretical and clinical implications. *Journal of Speech and Hearing Disorders, 26*, 67–82.

Bloodstein, O. (1970). Stuttering and normal disfluency: A continuity hypothesis. *British Journal of Disorders of Communication, 5*, 30–39.

Bloodstein, O. (1981). *A handbook on stuttering*. Chicago: National Easter Seal Society.

Bloodstein, O. (1987). *A handbook on stuttering* (4th ed.). Chicago: National Easter Seal Society.

Bloodstein, O. (1990). On pluttering, skivering, and floggering: A commentary. *Journal of Speech and Hearing Disorders, 55*, 392–393.

Bloodstein, O. (1995). *A handbook on stuttering* (5th ed.). San Diego, CA: Singular.

Bloodstein, O. (1997). Stuttering as an anticipatory struggle reaction. In R. Curlee and W. Perkins (Eds.), *Nature and treatment of stuttering: New directions* (2nd ed.) Needham Heights, MA: Allyn & Bacon.

Bloodstein, O. (2002). Early stuttering as a type of language difficulty. *Journal of Fluency Disorders, 27*, 163–167.

Bloodstein, O., & Bernstein Ratner, N. (2008). *A handbook on stuttering* (6th ed.). Clifton Park, NY: Delmar.

Bloodstein, O., & Gantwerk, B. (1967). Grammatical function in relation to stuttering in young children. *Journal of Speech and Hearing Research, 10*, 786–789.

Bloodstein, O., & Grossman, M. (1981). Early stutterings: Some aspects of their form and distribution. *Journal of Speech and Hearing Research, 24*, 298–302.

Bluemel, C. (1913). *Stammering and cognate defects of speech* (Vol. 1). New York: Stechert.

Bluemel, C. (1932). Primary and secondary stammering. *Quarterly Journal of Speech, 18*, 187–200.

Boberg, E., Ewart, B., Mason, G., Lindsay, K., & Wynn, S. (1978). Stuttering in the retarded: II. Prevalence of stuttering in EMR and TMR children. *Mental Retardation Bulletin, 6*(2), 67–76.

Boberg, E., & Kully, D. (1985). *Comprehensive stuttering program*. San Diego, CA: College-Hill Press.

Boberg, E., & Kully, D. (1994). Long-term results of an intensive treatment program for adults and adolescents who stutter. *Journal of Speech and Hearing Research, 37*, 1050–1059.

Boberg, E., Yeudall, L., Schopflocher, D., & Bo-Lassen, P. (1983). The effect of an intensive behavioral program on the distribution of EEG alpha power in stutterers during the processing of verbal visuospatial information. *Journal of Fluency Disorders, 8*, 245–263.

Bohannon, R. W. (1995). Stopwatch for measuring thumb-movement time. *Perceptual and Motor Skills, 81*, 211–216.

Bohme, E. (1977). *Das stotter-syndrome: Aetiologi, dignose, und therapie*. Bern, Switzerland: Verlag Hans Ruber.

Boldon, A. (1955). *The co-existence of, and certain relationship between diabetes and stuttering* (master's thesis). University of Wisconsin.

Bonelli, P., Dixon, M., Bernstein Ratner, N., & Onslow, M. (2000). Child and parent speech and language following the Lidcombe programme of early stuttering intervention. *Clinical Linguistics and Phonetics, 14*, 427–446.

Boome, E. & Richardson, M. (1932). *The nature and treatment of stuttering*. New York: Dutton.

Boome, E., & Richardson, M. (1947). *The nature and treatment of stammering* (2nd ed.). London: Methuen.

Bornstein, M., Bellack, A., & Hersen, M. (1977). Social skill training for unassertive children: A multiple baseline analysis. *Journal of Applied Behavior Analysis, 10,* 183–195.

Bortfeld, H., Leon, S., Bloom, J., Schober, M., & Brennan, S. (2001). Disfluency rates in conversation: Effects of age, relationship, topic, role, and gender. *Language and Speech, 44*(2), 123–147.

Boscolo, B., Bernstein Ratner, N., & Rescorla, L. (2002). Fluency of school-aged children with a history of specific expressive language impairment: An exploratory study. *American Journal of Speech-Language Pathology, 11,* 41–49.

Bosshardt, H. G. (2002). Effects of concurrent cognitive processing on the fluency of word repetition: Comparison between persons who do and do not stutter. *Journal of Fluency Disorders, 27,* 93–114.

Bøstrup, B., & Møller, B. (1990). Småbørnsstammegrupper. *Dansk Audiologopædi, 1,* 21–25.

Bothe, A. (2004). *Evidence-based treatment of stuttering: Empirical bases and clinical applications.* Mahwah, NJ: Erlbaum.

Bothe, A., Davidow, J., Bramlett, R., & Ingham, R. (2006). Stuttering treatment research 1970–2005: I. Systematic review incorporating trail quality assessment of behavioral, cognitive, and related approaches. *American Journal of Speech-Language Pathology, 15,* 321–341.

Bothe, A., Davidow, J., Bramlett, R., Franic, D., & Ingham, R. (2006). Stuttering treatment research 1970–2005: II. Systematic review incorporating trial quality assessment of pharmacological approaches. *American Journal of Speech-Language Pathology, 15,* 342–352.

Boutsen, F. R., & Hood, S. B. (1997). Determinants of speech rate and fluency in fast and slow speaking normally fluent children. In W. Hulstijn, H. F. M. Peters, & P. H. M. Van Leishout (Eds.), *Speech production: Motor control, brain research, and fluency disorders* (pp. 557–564). Amsterdam: Elsevier.

Brady, G. (1971). Metronome-conditioned speech training for stuttering. *Behavior Therapy, 2,* 129–150.

Brady, J. (1991). The pharmacology of stuttering: A critical review. *American Journal of Psychiatry, 1448,* 1309–1316.

Brady, J., & Ali, Z. (2000). Alprazolam, citalopram and clomipramine for stuttering. *Journal of Clinical Psychopharmacology, 20,* 287.

Brady, J., & Ryan, M. (1994). Stuttering: Current pharmacological options. *CNS Drugs, 1,* 261–268.

Brady, P. (1968). A behavioral approach to the treatment of stuttering. *American Journal of Psychiatry, 125,* 843–848.

Brady, W. A., & Hall, D. E. (1976). The prevalence of stuttering among school-age children. *Language, Speech, and Hearing Services in Schools, 7*(2), 75–81.

Branscom, M. (1942). The construction and statistical evaluation of a speech fluency test for young children (master's thesis). University of Iowa.

Branscom, M., Hughes, J., & Oxtoby, E., (1955). Studies of non-fluency in the speech of preschool children. In W. Johnson & R. Leutenegger (Eds.) *Stuttering in Children and Adults* (pp. 157–180). Minneapolis: University of Minnesota Press.

Bray, M., Kehle, T., Lawless, K., & Theodore, L. (2003). The relationship between self-efficacy and depression to stuttering. *American Journal of Speech-Language Pathology, 12,* 425–431.

Brenner, N., Perkins, W., & Soderberg, G. (1972). The effect of rehearsal on frequency of stuttering. *Journal of Speech and Hearing Research, 15,* 483–486.

Breuer, J., & Freud, S. (1936). Studies in hysteria. *Nervous and Mental Disease Monograph Series, No. 61.* New York: Nervous and Mental Disease Publishing.

Brill, A. (1923). Speech disturbances in nervous mental diseases. *Quarterly Journal of Speech, 9,* 129–135.

Brody, M., & Harrison, S. (1954). Group psychotherapy with male stutterers. *International Journal of Group Psychotherapy, 14,* 154–162.

Broomfield, J., & Dodd, B. (2004). Children with speech and language disability: Caseload characteristics. *International Journal of Language & Communication Disorders, 39*(3), 303–324.

Brosch, S., & Pirsig, W. (2001). Stuttering in history and culture. *International Journal of Pediatric Otorhinolaryngology, 59*(2), 81–87.

Brown, R. (1973). *A first language: The early stages.* Cambridge, MA: Harvard.

Brown, S. (1945). The locus of stuttering in the speech sequence. *Journal of Speech Disorders, 10,* 181–192.

Brown, S. (1949). Advising parents of early stutterers. *Pediatrics, 4,* 170–175.

Brown, S., Ingham, R., Ingham, J., Laird, A., & Fox, P. (2005). Stuttered and fluent speech production: An ALE meta-analysis of functional neuroimaging studies. *Human Brain Mapping, 25,* 105–117.

Bruce, M., & Adams, M. (1978). Effects of two types of motor practice on stuttering adaptation. *Journal of Speech and Hearing Research, 21,* 421–428.

Brutten, G. (1985). *Communication Attitude Test Form A.* Revised 1997.

Brutten, E. J., & Shoemaker, D. (1967). *The modification of stuttering.* Englewood Cliffs, NJ: Prentice-Hall.

Brutten, G., & Dancer, J. (1980). Stuttering adaptation under distributed and massed conditions. *Journal of Fluency Disorders, 5,* 1–10.

Brutten, G. & Dunham, S. (1989). The communication attitude test. A normative study of grade school children. *Journal of Fluency Disorders, 14,* 371–377.

Bryngelson, B. (1931). Treatment of stuttering. *Journal of Expression, 5,* 19–26.

Bryngelson, B. (1932). A photo-phonographic analysis of the vocal disturbances in stuttering. *Psychological Monograph, 43,* 1–30.

Bryngelson, B. (1938). Prognosis of stuttering. *Journal of Speech Disorders, 3,* 121–123.

Bryngelson, B., & Rutherford, B. (1937). A comparative study of laterality of stutterers and non-stutterers. *Journal of Speech Disorders, 2,* 15–16.

Buchel, C., Raedler, T., Sommer, M., Sach, M., Weiller, C., Koch, M. A. (2004). White matter asymmetry in the human brain: A diffusion tensor MRI study. *Cerebral Cortex, 14*, 945–951.

Buck, S., Lees, R., & Cook, F. (2002). The influence of family history of stuttering on the onset of stuttering in young children. *Folia Phoniatrica et Logopaedica, 54*, 117–124.

Bullen, A. (1945). A cross-cultural approach to the problem of stuttering. *Child Development, 16*, 1–88.

Burdin, G. (1940). The surgical treatment of stuttering, 1840–1842. *Journal of Speech Disorders, 5*, 43–64.

Burns, D., Brady, J. P., & Kuruvilla, K. (1978). The acute effect of haloperidol and apomorphine on the severity of stuttering. *Biological Psychiatry, 13*, 255–264.

Byrd, C., Conture, E., & Ohde, R. (2007). Phonological priming in young children who stutter: Holistic versus incremental processing. *American Journal of Speech-Language Pathology, 16*, 43–53.

Byrd, C. T., Wolk, L., & Lockett Davis, B. (2007). Role of phonology in childhood stuttering and its treatment. In E. Conture & R. Curlee (Eds.), *Stuttering and related disorders* (3rd ed.) (pp. 168–182). New York: Thieme.

Campbell, J., & Hill, D. (1987). *Systematic disfluency analysis.* Unpublished manuscript. Evanston, IL: Northwestern University.

Canter, G. (1971). Observations on neurogenic stuttering: A contribution to differential diagnosis. *British Journal of Disorders of Communication, 6*, 139–143.

Caprara, G., & Cervone, D. (2000). *Personality: Determinants, dynamics and potentials.* Cambridge: University Press.

Carp, F. (1962). Psychosexual development of stutterers. *Journal of Projective Techniques, 26*, 388–391.

Carson, C., & Kanter, C. E. (1945). Incidence of stuttering among white and colored school children. *Southern Speech Journal, 10*, 57–59.

Caruso, A., Chodzko-Zajko, W., Bidinger, D., & Sommers, R. (1994). Adults who stutter: Responses to cognitive stress. *Journal of Speech and Hearing Research, 37*, 746–754.

Caruso, A., Max, L., & McClowry, M. T. (1999). Perspectives on stuttering as a motor speech disorder. In A. Caruso & E. Strand (Eds.), *Clinical management of motor speech disorders in children.* New York: Thieme.

Caruso, A. J., & Max, L. (1997). Applications of motor learning theory of stuttering research. In W. Hulstijn, H. F. M. Peters, & P. H. H. M. Van Lieshout (Eds.), *Speech production: Motor control, brain research and fluency disorder* (pp. 213–220). Amsterdam: Elsevier.

Chang, S., Erickson, K., Ambrose, N., Hasegawa-Johnson, M., & Ludlow, C. (2008). Brain anatomy differences in childhood stuttering. *Neuroimage, 39*, 1333–1344.

Chapman, A., & Cooper, E. (1973). Nature of stuttering in a mentally retarded population. *American Journal of Mental Deficiency, 78*(2), 153–157.

Cherry, C., & Sayers, B. (1956). Experiments upon the total inhibition of stammering by external control and some clinical results. *Journal of Psychosomatic Research, 1*, 233–246.

Cherry, C., Sayers, B., & Marland, P. (1955). Experiments on the complete suppression of stammering. *Nature, 176*, 874–875.

Chevekeva, N. A. (1967). About methods of overcoming stuttering: A survey of the literature. *Spetsial Shkola, 3*, 9–15.

Chmela, K. (2006). *The Fluency Tool Kit.* Greenville, SC: Super Duper Publications.

Chmela, K., & Reardon, N. (2001). *The school-age child who stutters: Working effectively with attitudes and emotions.* Memphis, TN: Stuttering Foundation of America.

Ciabarra, A. M., Elkind, M. S., Roberts, J. K., & Marshall, R. S. (2000). Subcortical infarction resulting in acquired stuttering. *Journal of Neurology, Neurosurgery, Psychiatry, 69*, 546–549.

Clark, R., & Snyder, M. (1955). Group therapy for parents of preadolescent stutterers. *Group Psychology, 8*, 226–232.

Conradi, E. (1904). Psychology and pathology of speech development in the child. *Pedagogical Seminary, 11*, 328–380.

Conture, E. G. (1982). *Stuttering* (1st ed.). Englewood Cliffs, NJ: Prentice-Hall.

Conture, E. G. (1990). *Stuttering* (2nd ed.). Englewood Cliffs, NJ: Prentice Hall.

Conture, E. G. (1991). Young stutterers' speech production: A critical review. In H. F. M. Peters, W. Hulstijn, & C. W. Starkweather (Eds.), *Speech motor control and stuttering: Proceedings of the 2nd international conference on speech motor control and stuttering* (pp. 365–384). New York: Elsevier.

Conture, E. G. (2001). *Stuttering: Its nature, diagnosis, and treatment.* Boston: Allyn & Bacon.

Conture, E. G., & Brayton, E. (1975). The influence of noise on stutterers' different disfluency types. *Journal of Speech and Hearing Research, 18*, 381–384.

Conture, E. G., & Curlee, R. (2007). *Stuttering and related disorders of fluency* (3rd ed.). New York: Thieme.

Conture, E. G., & Kelly, E. M. (1991). Young stutterers' non-speech behaviors during stuttering. *Journal of Speech and Hearing Research, 34*, 1041–1056.

Conture, E. G., Louko, L., & Edwards, M. (1993). Simultaneously treating stuttering and disordered phonology in children: Experimental therapy, preliminary findings. *American Journal of Speech-Language Pathology, 2*, 72–81.

Conture, E. G., McCall, G., & Brewer, D. (1977). Laryngeal behavior during stuttering. *Journal of Speech and Hearing Research, 20*, 661–668.

Conture, E. G., & Melnick, K. (1999). Parent-child group approach to stuttering in preschool and school-age children. In M. Onslow & A. Packman (Eds.), *Early stuttering: A handbook of intervention strategies* (pp. 17–51). San Diego, CA: Singular.

Conture, E. Schwartz, H., & Brewer, D. (1985). Laryngeal behavior during stuttering: A further study. *Journal of Speech and Hearing Research, 28*, 233–240.

Cooper, E., & Cooper, C. (1985). *Cooper personalized fluency control therapy* (revised). Allen, TX: DLM Teaching Resources.

Cooper, E. B., & Cooper, C. S. (1998). Multicultural considerations in the assessment and treatment of stuttering. In

D. Battle (Ed.), *Communication disorders in multicultural populations* (2nd ed., pp. 247–274). Boston: Butterworth-Heinemann.

Coppola, V. A., & Yairi, E. (1982). Rhythmic speech training with preschool stuttering children: An experimental study. *Journal of Fluency Disorders, 7*, 447–457.

Cordes, A. (1998). Current status of stuttering treatment literature. In A. Cordes & R. Ingham (Eds.), *Treatment efficacy for stuttering: A search for empirical bases* (pp. 117–144). San Diego, CA: Singular.

Cordes, A., & Ingham, R. (1994). Time-interval measurement of stuttering: Effects of interval duration. *Journal of Speech and Hearing Research, 37*, 779–788.

Cordes, A., & Ingham, R. (1999). Effects of time-interval judgment training on real-time measurement of stuttering. *Journal of Speech, Language, and Hearing Research, 42*, 862–879.

Coriat, I. (1928). Stammering. A psychoanalytic interpretation. *Nervous Mental Disorder Monographs, Ser. No. 47*, 1–68.

Coriat, I. (1943a). Theory. In E. F. Hahn (Ed.), *Stuttering: Significant theories and therapies* (pp. 28–30). Stanford, CA: Stanford University Press.

Coriat, I. (1943b). The psychoanalytic conception of stammering. *Nervous Child, 2*, 167–171.

Corley, M., MacGregor, L., & Donaldson, D. (2007). It's the way that you, er, say it: Hesitations in speech affect language comprehension. *Cognition, 105*, 658–668.

Costa, D. (1992). Antidepressants and the treatment of stuttering [Letter to the editor]. *The American Journal of Psychiatry, 149*, 1281.

Costello, J. (1977). Programmed instruction. *Journal of Speech and Hearing Disorders, 42*, 3–28.

Costello, J. (1980). Operant conditioning and the treatment of stuttering. In W. H. Perkins (Ed.), Strategies in Stuttering Therapy. In J. L. Northern (Series Ed.) *Seminars in Speech, Language and Hearing*. New York: Thieme-Stratton.

Costello, J. (1983). Current behavioral treatments for children. In D. Prins & R. Ingham (Eds.), *Treatment of stuttering in early childhood* (pp. 69–112), San Diego, CA: College-Hill.

Costello, J., & Ingham, R. (1984). Assessment strategies for stuttering. In R. Curlee & W. Perkins (Eds.), *Nature and treatment of stuttering: New directions*. Boston: College-Hill.

Cox, N., Cook, E., Ambrose, N., Yairi, E., Rydmarker, S., Lundstrom, C., et al. (2000). *The Illinois-Sweden-Israel genetics of stuttering project*. Paper presented at the Third World Congress on Fluency Disorders, Nyborg, Denmark.

Craig, A. (1990). An investigation into the relationship between anxiety and stuttering. *Journal of Speech and Hearing Disorders, 55*, 290–294.

Craig, A. (1998). Relapse following treatment of stuttering: A critical review and correlative data. *Journal of Fluency Disorders, 23*, 1–30.

Craig, A., Franklin, J., & Andrews, G. (1984). A scale to measure locus of control of behaviour. *British Journal of Medical Psychology, 57*, 173–180.

Craig, A., Hancock K., Chang, E., McCready, C., Shepley, A., McCaul, A., et al. (1996). A controlled clinical trial for stuttering in persons aged 9 to 14 years. *Journal of Speech and Hearing Research, 39*, 808–826.

Craig, A., Hancock, K., Tran, Y., & Craig, M. (2003). Anxiety levels in people who stutter: A randomized population study. *Journal of Speech, Language, and Hearing Research, 46*, 1197–1206.

Craig, A., Hancock, K., Tran, Y., Craig, M., & Peters, K. (2002). Epidemiology of stuttering in the community across the entire life span. *Journal of Speech, Language, and Hearing Research, 45*, 1097–1105.

Craig, A., & Tran, Y. (2005). The epidemiology of stuttering: The need for reliable estimates of prevalence and anxiety levels over the lifespan. *Advances in Speech Language Pathology, 7*(1), 41–46.

Cross, D., & Cooke, P. (1979). Vocal and manual reaction times of adult stutterers and nonstutterers. *ASHA, 21*, 693.

Cross, H. (1936). The motor capacities of stutterers. *Archives of Speech, 7*, 112–132.

Curlee, R. (1980). A case selection strategy for young disfluent children. *Seminars in Speech, Language, and Hearing, 1*(4), 277–287.

Curlee, R.(1981). Observer agreement on disfluency and stuttering. *Journal of Speech and Hearing Research, 24*, 595–600.

Curlee, R.(1993). Identification and management of beginning stuttering. In R. F. Curlee (Ed.), *Stuttering and related disorders of fluency* (pp. 1–22). New York: Thieme.

Curlee, R. (1999). *Stuttering and related disorders of fluency* (2nd ed.). New York: Thieme.

Curlee, R., & Perkins, W. (1969). Conversational rate control therapy for stuttering. *Journal of Speech and hearing Disorders, 34*, 245–250.

Curlee, R., & Perkins, W. (1973). Effectiveness of a DAF conditioning program for adolescent and adult stutterers. *Behaviour Research and Therapy, 11*(4), 395–401.

Curlee, R., & Yairi, E. (1997). Early intervention with early childhood stuttering: A critical examination of the data. *American Journal of Speech-Language Pathology, 6*, 8–18.

Curlee, R. & Yairi, E. (1998). Treatment of early childhood stuttering: Advances and research needs. *American Journal of Speech-Language Pathology, 7*, 20–26.

Cypreansen, L. (1948). Group therapy for adult stutterers. *Journal of Speech and Hearing Disorders, 13*, 313–319.

Dalston, R., Martinkosky, S., & Hinton, V. (1987). Stuttering prevalence among patients at risk for velopharyngeal inadequacy: A preliminary investigation. *Cleft Palate Journal, 24*, 233–239.

Daly, D. (1996). *The source for stuttering and cluttering*. East Moline, IL: Linguisystems.

Daly, D., & Burnett, M. (1996). Cluttering: Assessment, treatment planning and case study illustration. *Journal of Fluency Disorders, 21,* 239–248.

Daly, D., & Burnett, M. (1999). Cluttering: Traditional views and new perspectives. In R. Curlee (Ed.), *Stuttering and related disorders of fluency* (2nd ed.). New York: Thieme.

Daniels, E. (1940). An analysis of the relation between handedness and stuttering with special reference to the Orton-Travis theory of cerebral dominance. *Journal of Speech Disorders, 5,* 309–326.

Daniloff, R., & Moll, K. (1968). Coarticulation of lip rounding. *Journal of Speech and Hearing Research, 11,* 707–721.

Dantzig, M. (1940). Syllable-tapping, a new method of the help of stammerers. *Journal of Speech Disorders, 5,* 209–210.

Darley, F. (1955). The relationship of parental attitudes and adjustment to the development of stuttering. In W. Johnson & R. R. Leutenegger (Eds.), *Stuttering in children and adults: Thirty years of research at the University of Iowa* (pp. 74–156). Minneapolis: University of Minnesota.

Darley, F., & Spriestersbach, D. C. (1978). *Diagnostic methods in speech pathology* (2nd ed.). New York: Harper & Row.

Daskalov, D. (1962). Kvoprosu ob osnovnikh printsipakh I metodakh preduprezhdenia lechenia zaikania. *Zhurnal Nevropatologii Psikhiatrii, 62,* 1047–1052.

Davis, D. (1939). The relation of repetitions in the speech of young children to certain measures of language maturity and situational factors: Part I. *Journal of Speech Disorders, 4,* 303–318.

Davis, M., Robbins-Eshelman, E., & McKay, M. (1988). *The relaxation and stress reduction workbook.* Oakland, CA: New Harbinger Publications.

Davis, S., Howell, P., & Cook, F. (2002). Sociodynamic relationships between children who stutter and their nonstuttering classmates. *Journal of Child Psychology and Psychiatry, 43,* 939–947.

De Ajuriaguerra, J., De Gobineau, D., Narlian, S., & Stambak, M. (1958). Stuttering. *Press Medicale Disorders, 48,* 171–177.

Deal, J. (1982). Sudden onset of stuttering: A case report. *Journal of Speech and Hearing Disorders, 47,* 301–304.

Dell, C. (1980). *Treating the school-age stutterer: A guide for clinicians.* Memphis, TN: Speech Foundation of America.

De Nil, L. (1997). Stuttering: A neurophysiological perspective. In N. Bernstein Ratner & E. C. Healey (Eds.), *Current perspective in stuttering: Nature and treatment.* Hillsdale, NJ: Erlbaum.

De Nil, L., & Brutten, G. (1991). Speech-associated attitudes of stuttering and normally fluent children. *Journal of Speech and Hearing Research, 34,* 60–66.

De Nil, L., Jokel, R., & Rochon, E. (2007). Etiology, symptomatology, and treatment of neurogenic stuttering. In E. Conture & R. Curlee (Eds.), *Stuttering and related disorders of fluency* (3rd ed., pp. 326–343). New York: Thieme.

De Nil, L., Kroll, R., & Houle, S. (2001). Functional neuroimaging of cerebellar activation during single word reading and verb generation in stuttering and nonstuttering adults. *Neuroscience Letters, 302*(2–3), 77–80.

De Nil, L., Kroll, R., Kapur, S., & Houle, S. (2000). A positron emission tomography study of silent oral single word reading in stuttering and nonstuttering adults. *Journal of Speech, Language, Hearing Research, 43,* 1038–1053.

De Nil, L., Kroll, R., Lafaille, S., & Houle, S. (2003). A positron emission tomography study of short- and long-term treatment effects on functional brain activation in adults who stutter. *Journal of Fluency Disorders, 28,* 357–380.

Denny, M., & Smith, A. (2000). Respiratory control in stuttering speakers: Evidence from respiratory high-frequency oscillations. *Journal of Speech, Language, and Hearing Research, 43,* 1024–1037.

De Oliveira Martins, V., & Furquim de Andrade, C. (2008). Speech fluency developmental profile in Brazilian Portuguese speakers. *Pró-Fono Revista de Atualização Científica, 20,* 7–13.

Derazne, J. (1966). Speech pathology in the U.S.S.R. In R.W. Rieber & R. S. Brubaker, (Eds.), *Speech Pathology.* Amsterdam: North Holland.

Dewar, A., Dewar, A. D., Austin, W., & Brash, H. (1979). The long term use of an automatically triggered auditory feedback masking device in the treatment of stammering. *British Journal of Disorders of Communication, 14,* 219–229.

Di Carlo, L., Katz, J., & Batkin, S. (1959). An exploratory investigation of the effect of meprobamate on stuttering behavior. *Journal of Nervous and Mental Disorders, 128,* 558–561.

Dickson, S. (1971). Incipient stuttering and spontaneous remission of stuttered speech. *Journal of Communication Disorders, 4*(2), 99–110.

DiLollo, A., & Manning, W. (2007). Counseling children who stutter and their parents. In E. Conture & R. Curlee (Eds.), *Stuttering and related disorders* (3rd ed., pp. 115–130). New York: Thieme.

Donovan, G. E. (1971). A new device for the treatment of stuttering. *British Journal of Disorders of Communication, 6,* 86–88.

Dowden, P., Stone-Goldman, J., & Olswang, L. (2006). *Course glossary, SPHSC 500 fall quarter 2006.* Retrieved from University of Washington, http://faculty.washington.edu/lolswang/html/500/glossary2006.pdf

Duchin, S., & Mysak, E. (1987). Disfluency and rate characteristics of young adult, middle-aged, and older males. *Journal of Communication Disorders, 20,* 245–257.

Duffy, J. (1995). *Motor speech disorders.* St. Louis, MO: Mosby.

Dunlap, K. (1932). *Habits: Their making and unmaking.* New York: Liveright.

Dunlap, K. (1944). Stammering: Its nature, etiology, and therapy. *Journal of Comparative Psychology, 37,* 187–202.

Egolf, D. B., Shames, G. H., Johnson, P. R., & Kasprisin-Burelli, A. (1972). The use of parent-child interaction patterns in therapy for young stutterers. *Journal of Speech and Hearing Disorders, 37,* 222–232.

Einarsdottir, J., & Ingham, R. (2009). Does language influence the accuracy of judgments of stuttering in children? *Journal of Speech, Language, and Hearing Research, 52,* 766–779.

Eisenson, J. (1958). A perseverative theory of stuttering. In J. Eisenson (Ed.), *Stuttering: A symposium* (pp. 223–271). New York: Harper & Row.

Eisenson, J., & Horowitz, E. (1945). The influence of propositionality on stuttering. *Journal of Speech and Hearing Disorders, 10,* 193–197.

Ellis, A. (1973). *Humanistic psychotherapy: The rational-emotive approach.* New York: McGraw-Hill.

Embrechts, M., Ebben, H., Franke, P., & vandePoel, C. (2000). Temperament: A comparison between children who stutter and children who do not stutter. In H. Bosshardt, J. S. Yaruss, & H. F. M. Peters, (Eds.), *Proceedings of the Third World Congress on Fluency Disorders: Theory, research, treatment and self-help* (pp. 557–562). Nijmegen, Netherlands: University of Nijmegen Press.

Emerick, L. (1965). Therapy for young stutterers. *Exceptional Children, 3,* 398–402.

Emerick, L. (1970). *Therapy for young stutterers.* Danville, IL: Interstate.

Emil-Behnke, K. (1947). *Stammering: Its nature, causes, and treatment.* London: Williams & Norgate.

Erickson, R. (1969). Assessing communication attitudes among stutterers. *Journal of Speech and Hearing Research, 12,* 711–724.

Ezrati-Vinacour, R., & Levin, I. (2004). The relationship between anxiety and stuttering: A multidimensional approach. *Journal of Fluency Disorders, 29,* 135–148.

Ezrati-Vinacour, R., Platzky, R., & Yairi, E. (2001). The young child's awareness of stuttering-like disfluency. *Journal of Speech, Language, and Hearing Research, 44,* 368–380.

Fagan, J. (1984). The relationship of novelty preferences during infancy to later intelligence and later recognition memory. *Intelligence, 8,* 339–346.

Fagan, L. (1931). The relation of dextral training to the onset of stuttering. *Quarterly Journal of Speech, 17,* 73–76.

Fairbanks, G. (1960). *Voice and articulation drillbook* (2nd ed.). New York: Harper & Row.

Fein, L. (1970). Stuttering as a cue related to the precipitation of moments of stuttering [Abstract]. *ASHA, 12,* 456.

Feinberg, A., Griffen, B., & Levey, M. (2000). Psychological aspects of chronic tonic and clonic stuttering: Suggested therapeutic approaches. *American Journal of Orthopsychiatry, 70*(4), 465–473.

Felsenfeld, S., Kirk, M., Zhu, G., Statham, D., Neale, M., & Martin, N. (2000). A study of the genetic and environmental etiology of stuttering in a selected twin sample. *Behavioral Genetics, 30,* 359–366.

Fenichel, O. (1945). *The psychoanalytic theory of neurosis.* New York: Norton.

Fieser, J. (2006). *Ethics.* Retrieved from The Internet Encyclopedia of Philosophy, www.iep.utm.edu/e/ethics.htm

Finn, P. (2003a). Addressing generalization and maintenance of stuttering treatment in the schools: A critical look. *Journal of Communication Disorders, 36,* 153–164.

Finn, P. (2003b). Evidence-based treatment of stuttering: II. Clinical significance of behavioral stuttering treatments. *Journal of Fluency Disorders, 28,* 209–218.

Finn, P. (2003c). Self-regulation and the management of stuttering. *Seminars in Speech and Language, 24,* 27–32.

Finn, P., & Cordes, A. K. (1997). Multicultural identification and treatment of stuttering: A continuing need for research. *Journal of Fluency Disorders, 22,* 219–236.

Finn, P., Ingham, R., Ambrose, N., & Yairi, E. (1997). Children recovered from stuttering without formal treatment: Perceptual assessment of speech normalcy. *Journal of Speech, Language, and Hearing Research, 40,* 867–876.

Fisher. M. (1970). Stuttering: a psychoanalytic view. *Journal of Contemporary Psychotherapy, 2,* 124–127.

Fitzgerald, H., Djurdjic, S., & Maguin, E. (1992). Assessment of sensitivity to interpersonal stress in stutterers. *Journal of Communication Disorders, 25,* 31–42.

Fivush, R., Gray, J. T., & Fromhoff, F. A. (1987). Two-year-olds talk about the past. *Cognitive Development, 2,* 393–409.

Flanagan, B., Goldiamond, I., & Azrin, N. (1958). Operant stuttering: The control of stuttering behavior through response-contingent consequences. *Journal of the Experimental Analysis of Behavior, 1,* 173–177.

Fletcher, J. (1914). An experimental study of stuttering. *American Journal of Psychology, 25,* 201–255.

Fletcher, J. (1928). *The problem of stuttering.* New York: Longmans, Green.

Fogerty, E. (1930). *Stammering.* New York: Dutton.

Fosnot, S. M. (1993). Research design for examining treatment efficacy in fluency disorders. *Journal of Fluency Disorders, 18,* 221–251.

Fosnot, S. M. (1995). Some contemporary approaches in treating fluency disorders in preschool-age, and adolescent children. *Language, Speech, and Hearing Services in Schools, 26,* 115–116.

Fossler, H. (1930). Disturbances in breathing during stuttering. *Psychological Monographs, 40,* 1–32.

Foundas, A., Bollich A., Corey, D., Hurley, M., & Heilman, K. (2001). Anomalous anatomy of speech-language areas in adults with persistent developmental stuttering. *Neurology, 57,* 207–215.

Foundas, A., Bollich, A., Feldman, J., Corey, D., Hurley, M., Lemen, L., & Heilman, K. (2004). Aberrant auditory processing and atypical planum temporale in developmental stuttering. *Neurology, 63,* 1640–1646.

Foundas, A., Corey, D., Angeles, V., Bollich, A., Crabtree-Hartman, E., & Heilman, K. (2003). Atypical cerebral laterality in adults with persistent developmental stuttering. *Neurology, 61,* 1378–1385.

Fox, P., Ingham, R., Ingham, J., Hirsch, T., unter Downs, J., Martin, C., Jerabek, P., Glass, P., & Lancaster, J. (1996). A PET study of the neural systems of stuttering. *Nature, 382,* 158–162.

Fox, P., Ingham, R., Ingham, J., Zamarripa, F., Xiong, J., & Lancaster, J. (2000). Brain correlates of stuttering and syllable production: A PET performance-correlation analysis. *Brain, 123*, 1985–2004.

Fraiser, J. (1955). An exploration of stutterers' theories of their own stuttering. In W. Johnson & R. Leutenegger (Eds.), *Stuttering in children and adults* (pp. 317–324). Minneapolis: University of Minnesota Press.

Franic, D., & Bothe, A. (2008). Psychometric evaluation of condition-specific instruments used to assess health-related quality of life, attitudes and related constructs in stuttering. *American Journal of Speech-Language Pathology, 17*, 60–80.

Frankel, V. (1963). *Man's search for meaning.* Boston: Beacon Press.

Franken, M., Kielstra-Van der Schalk, C., & Boelens, H. (2005). Experimental treatment of early stuttering: A preliminary study. *Journal of Fluency Disorders, 30*, 189–199.

Freeman, F. J., & Ushijima, T. (1978). Laryngeal muscle activity during stuttering. *Journal of Speech and Hearing Research, 21*, 538–562.

Freud, A. (1946). *The psycho-analytic treatment of children.* London: Imago.

Freud, A. (1965). Normality and pathology in childhood. In P. L. Adams & I. Fras (Eds.), *Beginning child psychiatry.* New York: Brunner/Mazel.

Freud, S. (1899). *Die Traumdeutung [The interpretation of dreams].* Adamant Media.

Freud, S. (1901). *Psychopathology of everyday life* (translated by A. A. Brill), London: T. Fisher Unwin.

Freund, H. (1955). Psychosis and stuttering. *Journal of Nervous and Mental Diseases, 122*, 161–172.

Fried, C. (1972). Behavior therapy and psychoanalysis in the treatment of a severe chronic stutterer. *Journal of Speech and Hearing Disorders, 37*, 347–372.

Fritzell, B. (1976). The prognosis of stuttering in school-children: A 10-year longitudinal study. In *Proceedings of the XVI Congress of the International society of Logopedics and Phoniatrics* (pp. 186–187). Basel, Switzerland: Karger.

Froebel, F. (1903). The education of man. In G. L. Landreth (Ed.), *Play therapy: The art of the relationship.* Muncie, IN: Accelerated Development.

Froeschels, E. (1921). Beitrage zur symptomatologie des stotterns. *Monatsschrift fur Ohren-heilkunde, 55*, 1109–1112.

Froeschels, E. (1943). Pathology and therapy of stuttering. *Nervous Child, 2*, 148–161.

Furquim de Andrade, C., & De Oliveira Martins, V. (2007). Fluency variation in adolescents. *Clinical Linguistics & Phonetics, 21*, 771–782.

Gathercole, S. E., & Baddeley, A. D. (1990). The role of phonological memory in vocabulary acquisition: A study of young children learning arbitrary names of toys. *British Journal of Psychology, 81*, 439–454.

Gathercole, S. E., Willis, C. S., Baddeley, A. D., & Emslie, H. (1994). The children's test of nonword repetition: A test of phonological working memory. *Memory, 2*, 103–127.

Gathercole, S. E., Willis, C. S., Emslie, H., & Baddeley, A. D. (1991). The influences of number of syllables and word-likeness on children's repetition of nonwords. *Applied Psycholinguistics, 12*, 349–367.

Gendelman, E. (1977). Confrontation in the treatment of stuttering. *Journal of Speech and Hearing Disorders, 42*, 85–89.

Gens, G. (1951). The speech pathologist looks at the mentally deficient child. *Training School Bulletin, 48*, 19–27.

Gillespie, S., & Cooper, E. (1973). Prevalence of speech problems in junior and senior high schools. *Journal of Speech and Hearing Research, 16*, 739–743.

Gilman, M., & Yaruss, J. S. (2000). Stuttering and relaxation: Applications for somatic education in stuttering treatment. *Journal of Fluency Disorders, 25*, 59–76.

Glasner, P. J. (1949). Personality characteristics and emotional problems in stutterers under the age of five. *Journal of Speech and Hearing Disorders, 14*, 135–138.

Glasner, P. J., & Rosenthal, D. (1957). Parental diagnosis of stuttering in young children. *Journal of Speech and Hearing Disorders, 22*, 288–295.

Glauber, P. (1958). Stuttering and personality dynamics. In J. Eisenson (Ed.), *Stuttering: A symposium* (pp. 71–120). New York: Harper & Row.

Glogowski, K. (1976). Is stuttering inherited? *Folia Phoniatrica, 28*, 235–236.

Godai, U., Tatarelli, R., & Bonanni, G. (1976). Stuttering and tics in twins. *Acta Geneticae Medicae et Gemellologiae, 25*, 369–375.

Goldiamond, I. (1965). Stuttering and fluency as manipulatable operant response classes. In L. Krasner and L. Ullman (Eds.), *Research in behavior modification.* New York: Holt, Rinehart and Winston.

Goldman, R. (1967). Cultural influences on the sex ratio in the incidence of stuttering. *American Anthropologist, 69*, 78–81.

Goldman, R., & Taylor, F. (1966). Coloured immigrant children: A survey of research, studies and literature on their educational problems and potential: In the U.S.A. *Educational Research, 9*(1), 22–43.

Goldman-Eisler, F. (1961). The significance of changes in the rate of articulation. *Language and Speech, 4*, 171–174.

Goldstein, J. A. (1987). Carbamazepine treatment for stuttering [Letter to the editor]. *Journal of Clinical Psychiatry, 48*, 39.

Good, R. H., & Kaminski, R. A. (Eds.). (2002). *Dynamic indicators of basic early literacy skills, DIBELS, 6th edition.* Eugene, OR: Institute for the Development of Educational Achievement.

Goodstein, L. (1958). Functional speech disorders and personality: A survey of the research. *Journal of Speech and Hearing Research, 1*(4), 359–376.

Gordon, P., & Luper, H. (1992a). The early identification of beginning stuttering I: Protocols. *American Journal of Speech and Language Pathology, 1*(3), 43–53.

Gordon, P., & Luper, H. (1992b). The early identification of beginning stuttering II: Problems. *American Journal of Speech-Language Pathology, 1*(4), 49–55.

Gottsleben, R. H. (1955). The incident of stuttering in a group of mongoloid. *Training School Bulletin, 51*, 209–218.

Gottwald, S., & Starkweather, C. (1999). Stuttering prevention and early intervention: A multiprocess approach.

In M. Onslow & A. Packman (Eds.), *The handbook of early stuttering intervention.* San Diego, CA: Singular.

Gray, B. (1965a). Theoretical approximations of stuttering adaptation. *Behavior Research and Therapy, 3,* 171–185.

Gray, B. (1965b). Theoretical approximations of stuttering adaptation: Statement of predictive accuracy. *Behavior Research and Therapy, 3,* 221–227.

Gray, B., & England, G. (1972). Some effects of anxiety deconditioning upon stuttering frequency. *Journal of Speech and Hearing Research, 15,* 114–122.

Gregg, B., & Yairi, E. (2007). Phonological skills and disfluency levels in preschool children who stutter. *Journal of Communication Disorders, 40,* 97–115.

Gregory, H. (1968). Applications of learning theory concepts in the management of stuttering. In H. Gregory (Ed.), *Learning theory and stuttering therapy.* Evanston, IL: Northwestern University Press.

Gregory, H. (1999). Developmental intervention: Differential strategies. In M. Onslow & A. Packman (Eds.), *The handbook of early stuttering intervention* (pp. 83–102). San Diego, CA: Singular.

Gregory, H. (2003). *Stuttering therapy: Rationale and procedures.* Boston: Allyn & Bacon.

Gregory, H., & Hill, D. (1984). Stuttering therapy for children. In W. H. Perkins (Ed.), *Stuttering disorders* (pp. 351–364). New York: Thieme-Stratton.

Gregory, H., & Hill, D. (1999). Differential evaluation—differential therapy for stuttering children. In R. Curlee (Ed.), *Stuttering and related disorders of fluency* (2nd ed.). New York: Thieme.

Greiner, J., Fitzgerald, H., Cooke, P., & Djurdjic, S. (1985). Assessment of sensitivity to interpersonal stress in stutterers and nonstutterers. *Journal of Communication Disorders, 18,* 215–225.

Guitar, B. (1975). Reduction of stuttering frequency using analog electromyographic feedback. *Journal of Speech and Hearing Research, 18,* 672–685.

Guitar, B. (1976). Pretreatment factors associated with the outcome of stuttering therapy. *Journal of Speech and Hearing Research, 19,* 590–600.

Guitar, B. (1998). *Stuttering: An integrated approach to its nature and treatment* (2nd ed.). Baltimore: Williams and Wilkins.

Guitar, B. (2006). *Stuttering: An integrated approach to its nature and treatment* (3rd ed.). Baltimore: Lippincott Williams & Wilkins.

Guitar, B., Guitar, C., Neilson, P., O'Dwyer, N., & Andrews, G. (1988). Onset sequencing of selected lip muscles in stutterers and nonstutterers. *Journal of Speech and Hearing Research, 31,* 28–35.

Guitar, B., & Marchinkoski, L. (2001). Influence of mothers' slower speech on their children's speech rate. *Journal of Speech, Language, and Hearing Research, 44,* 853–861.

Guitar, B., & Reville, J. (1997). *Easy talker.* Austin, TX: Pro-Ed.

Guitar, B., Schaefer, H., Donahue-Kilburg, G., & Bond, L. (1992). Parent verbal interactions and speech rate: A case study in stuttering. *Journal of Speech and Hearing Research, 35,* 742–754.

Gutzmann, H. (1912). *Sprachheilkunde. Das stottern und seine grundliche beseitigung.* Berlin: Weber.

Häge, A. (2001). Können kognitive und linguistische Fähigkeiten zur Verlaufsprognose kindlichen Stotterns beitragen? [Cognitive and linguistic abilities in young children: Are they able to predict the further development of stuttering?]. *Sprache Stimme Gehör, 25,* 20–24.

Hahn, E. (1956). *Stuttering: Significant theories and therapies* (2nd ed.). Stanford, CA: Stanford University Press.

Hakim, H. B., & Bernstein Ratner, N. (2004). Nonword repetition abilities in children who stutter: An exploratory study. *Journal of Fluency Disorders, 29,* 179–199.

Hall, F., Mielke, P., Willeford, J., & Timmons, R. (1976). *National speech & hearing survey.* [Final report, project No. 50978, grant No. OE-32-15-0050-5010 (607)]

Hall, K., Amir, O., & Yairi, E. (1999). A longitudinal investigation of speaking rate in preschool children who stutter. *Journal of Speech, Language, and Hearing Research, 42,* 1367–1377.

Hall, K., & Yairi, E. (1992). Fundamental frequency, jitter, and shimmer in preschoolers who stutter. *Journal of Speech and Hearing Research, 35,* 1002–1008.

Hall, N., Wagovitch, S., & Bernstein Ratner, N. (2007). Language considerations in childhood stuttering. In E. Conture & R. Curlee (Eds.), *Stuttering and related disorders* (3rd ed., pp. 153–167). New York: Thieme.

Hall, N., Yamashita, T., & Aram, D. (1993). Relationship between language and fluency in children with developmental language disorders. *Journal of Speech and Hearing Research, 36,* 568–579.

Hall, P. (1977). The occurrence of disfluencies in language-disordered school-age children. *Journal of Speech and Hearing Disorders, 42,* 364–370.

Ham, R. (1990). *Therapy of stuttering: Preschool through adolescence.* Englewood Cliffs, NJ: Prentice Hall.

Hamano, T., Hirajcj, S., Kawamura, Y., Hirayama, M., Mutoh, T., & Kuriyama, M. (2005). Acquired stuttering secondary to callosal infarction. *Neurology, 64,* 1092–1093.

Hancock, K., Craig, A., McCready, C., McCaul, A., Costello, D., Campbell, K., et al. (1998). Two- to six-year controlled-trail stuttering outcomes for children and adolescents. *Journal of Speech, Language, and Hearing Research, 41,* 1242–1252.

Hanson, B., Gronhovd, K., & Rice, P. (1981). A shortened version of the Southern Illinois University Speech Situation Checklist for the identification of speech-related anxiety. *Journal of Fluency Disorders, 6,* 351–360.

Harasty, J., & Reed, V. (1994). The prevalence of speech and language impairment in two Sydney metropolitan schools. *Australian Journal of Human Communication Disorders, 22*(1), 1–23.

Harle, M. (1946). Dynamic interpretation and treatment of acute stuttering in a young child. *American Journal of Orthopsychiatry, 16,* 156–162.

Harms, M., & Malone, J. (1939). The relationship of hearing acuity to stammering. *Journal of Speech and Hearing Disorder, 4,* 363–370.

Haroldson, S., Martin, R., & Starr, C. (1968). Time-out as a punishment for stuttering. *Journal of Speech and Hearing Research, 11,* 560–566.

Harrington, J. (1988). Stuttering, delayed auditory feedback and linguistic rhythm. *Journal of Speech and Hearing Research, 31,* 36–47.

Harrison, E., Onslow, M., & Rousseau, I. (2007). Lidcombe Program 2007: Clinical tales and clinical trials. In E. Conture & R. Curlee (Eds.), *Stuttering and related disorders* (3rd ed.). New York: Thieme.

Hartwell, E. M. (1895). Application of the laws of physical training for the prevention and cure of stuttering. *Proceedings of the International Congress of Education* (2nd ed.). New York: J. J. Little & Co.

Hauner, K., Shriberg, L., Kwiatkowski, J., & Allen, C. (2005). A subtype of speech delay associated with developmental psychosocial involvement. *Journal of Speech, Language, and Hearing Research, 48,* 635–650.

Healey, E. C. & Bernstein B. (1991). Acoustic analysis of young stutterers' and nonstutterers' disfluencies. In H. Peters, W. Hulstijn, & C.W. Starkweather (Eds.). *Speech motor control and stuttering* (pp. 401–407). New York: Elsevier Science.

Healey, E. C., Scott Trautman, L., & Susca, M. (2004). Clinical application of a multidimensional approach to the assessment and treatment of stuttering. *Contemporary Issues in Communication Science and Disorders, 31,* 40–48.

Hearne, A., Packman, A., Onslow, M., & Quine, S. (2008). Stuttering and its treatment in adolescence: The perceptions of people who stutter. *Journal of Fluency Disorders, 33,* 81–98.

Helm-Estabrooks, N. (1999). Stuttering associated with acquired neurological disorders. In R. Curlee (Ed.), *Stuttering and related disorders of fluency* (2nd ed.). New York: Thieme.

Helm-Estabrooks, N., & Hotz, G. (1998). Sudden onset of "stuttering" in an adult: Neurogenic or psychogenic? *Seminars in Speech and Language, 19,* 23–29.

Hewat, S., Onslow, M., Packman, A., & O'Brian, S. (2006). A Phase II clinical trial of self-imposed time-out treatment for stuttering in adults and adolescents. *Disability and Rehabilitation, 28*(1), 33–42.

Hillman, R., & Gilbert, H. (1977). Voice onset time for voiceless stop consonants in the fluent reading of stutterers and nonstutterers. *Journal of the Acoustical Society of America, 61,* 610–611.

Hinkle, W. (1971). *A study of subgroups within the stuttering population* (Unpublished doctoral dissertation). Purdue University.

Hogewind, F. (1940). Medical treatment of stuttering. *Journal of Speech Disorders, 5,* 203–208.

Holzman, A. (Co-Producer & Director), & Amick, R. (Co-Producer). (1988). *No words to say* [VHS video]. Available from Amick/Holzman Company, 10061 Riverside Drive, Toluca Lake, CA 91602–2560.

Honig, P. (1947). The stutterer acts it out. *Journal of Speech Disorders, 12,* 105–109.

Howell, P. (2002). The EXPLAN theory of fluency control applied to the treatment of stuttering by altered feedback and operant procedures. In E. Fava (Ed.), *Current Issues in Linguistic Theory series: Pathology and Therapy of Speech Disorders* (pp. 95–118). Amsterdam: John Benjamins.

Howell, P., & Au-Yeung, J. (1995). The association between stuttering, brown factors, and phonological categories in child stuttering ranging in aged between 2 and 12 years. *Journal of Fluency Disorders, 20,* 331–344.

Howell, P., Au-Yeung, J., & Sackin, S. (1999). Exchange of stuttering from function words to content words with age. *Journal of Speech, Language, and Hearing Research, 42,* 345–354.

Howell, P., Davis, S., Patel, H., Cuniffe, P., Downing-Wilson, D., Au-Yeung, J., & Williams, R. (2004). Fluency development and temperament in fluent children and children who stutter. In A. Packman, A. Meltzer, H. F. M. Peters (Eds.), *Theory, research and therapy in fluency disorders. Proceedings of the 4th World Congress on Fluency Disorders,* IFA Montreal, 250–256.

Howell, P., Davis, S., & Williams, R. (2009). The effects of bilingualism on stuttering during late childhood. *Archives of Disease in Childhood, 94,* 42–46.

Howell, P., Sackin, S., & Williams, R. (1999). Differential effects of frequency shifted feedback between child and adult stutterers. *Journal of Fluency Disorders, 24,* 127–136.

Howie, P. (1981). Concordance for stuttering in monozygotic and dizygotic twin pairs. *Journal of Speech and Hearing Research, 24,* 317–321.

Howie, P., & Andrews, G. (1984). Treatment of adult stutterers: Managing fluency. In R. Curlee & W. Perkins (Eds.), *Nature and treatment of stuttering: New directions* (pp. 245–445). San Diego, CA: College-Hill Press.

Howie, P., & Woods, C. (1982). Token reinforcement during the instatement and shaping of fluency in the treatment of stuttering. *Journal of Applied Behavior Analysis, 15,* 55–64.

Hubbard, C., & Yairi, E. (1988). Clustering of disfluencies in the speech of stuttering and nonstuttering preschool children. *Journal of Speech and Hearing Research, 31,* 228–233.

Hubbard, C. & Prins, D. (1994). Word familiarity, syllabic stress pattern, and stuttering. *Journal of Speech and Hearing Research, 37,* 564–571.

Hubbard, C., & Yairi, E. (1988). Clustering of disfluencies in the speech of stuttering and nonstuttering preschool children. *Journal of Speech and Hearing Research, 31,* 228–233.

Hull, C. (1943). *Principles of behavior.* New York: Appleton-Century.

Hull, F., Mielke, P., Willeford, J., & Timmons, R. (1976). *National speech and hearing survey: Final report.* Project No. 50987. Washington, DC: Office of Education, Department of Health, Education and Welfare.

Humphrey, B. D. (2004). Judgments of disfluency in a familiar vs. an unfamiliar language. In A. Packman,

A. Meltzer, & H. F. M. Peters (Eds.), *Theory, research and therapy. Proceedings of the Fourth World Congress on Fluency Disorders* (pp. 423–427). Nijmegen, Netherlands: Nijmegen University Press.

IDEA (1997). Individuals with Disabilities Education Act (IDEA '97). Retrieved from www.ed.gov/offices/OSERS/Policy/IDEA/index.html

Indevus. (2006). www.indevus.com/site/index.php?Intemid=45& id=31&option=comcontent&task=view

Ingham, J. (1999). Behavioral treatment for young children who stutter: An extended length of utterance method. In R. F. Curlee (Ed.), *Stuttering and related disorders of fluency* (2nd ed., pp. 80–109). New York: Thieme.

Ingham, J. (2003). Evidence-based treatment of stuttering: I. Definition and application. *Journal of Fluency Disorders, 28,* 197–208.

Ingham, J., & Riley, G. (1998). Guidelines for documentation of treatment efficacy for young children who stutter. *Journal of Speech, Language, and Hearing Research, 41,* 753–770.

Ingham, R. (1984). *Stuttering and behavior therapy.* San Diego, CA: College-Hill Press.

Ingham, R. (1990). Commentary on Perkins (1990) and Moore and Perkins (1990): On the valid role of reliability in identifying "What is stuttering?" *Journal of Speech and Hearing Disorders, 55,* 394–397.

Ingham, R. (1999). Performance contingent management of stuttering in adolescents and adults. In R. Curlee (Ed.), *Stuttering and related disorders of fluency* (2nd ed., pp. 200–221). New York: Thieme.

Ingham, R., Andrews, G., & Winkler, R. (1972). Stuttering: A comparative evaluation of the short term effectiveness of four treatment techniques. *Journal of Communication Disorders, 5*(1), 91–117.

Ingham, R., & Bothe, A. K. (2001). Recovery from early stuttering: Additional issues within the Onslow & Packman-Yairi & Ambrose (1999) exchange. *Journal of Speech, Language, and Hearing Research, 44,* 862–867.

Ingham, R., & Cordes, A. (1998). Treatment decisions for young children who stutter: Further concerns and complexities. *American Journal of Speech-Language Pathology, 7*(3), 10–19.

Ingham, R., & Cordes, A. (1999). On watching a discipline shoot itself in the foot: Some observations on current trends in stuttering treatment research. In N. Bernstein Ratner & E. C. Healey (Eds.), *Stuttering research and treatment: Bridging the gap* (pp. 211–230). Mahwah, NJ: Erlbaum.

Ingham, R., Fox, P., Ingham, J., Xiong, J., Zamarripa, F., Hardies, L., & Lancaster, J. (2004). Brain correlates of stuttering and syllable production: Gender comparison and replication. *Journal of Speech Language Hearing Research, 47*(2), 321–341.

Ingham, R., Ingham, J., Onslow, M., & Finn, P. (1989). Stutterers' self-ratings of speech naturalness: Assessing effects and reliability. *Journal of Speech, Language, and Hearing Research, 32,* 419–431.

Ingham, R., Warner, A., Byrd, A., & Cotton, J. (2006). Speech effort measurement and stuttering: Investigating the chorus reading effect. *Journal of Speech, Language, and Hearing Research, 49,* 660–670.

Iowa Department of Education. (2008). Iowa core curriculum. Retrieved from www.iowacorecurriculum.iowa.gov.

Jacobson, E. (1938). *Progressive relaxation.* Chicago: University of Chicago Press.

Jagger, J., Prusoff, B., Cohen, D., Kidd, K., Carbonari, C., & John, K. (1982). The epidemiology of Tourette's syndrome: A pilot study. *Schizophrenia Bulletin, 8,* 257–278.

James, J. (1981). Behavioral self-control of stuttering using time-out from speaking. *Journal of Applied Behavior Analysis, 14*(1), 25–37.

James, J., Ricciardelli, L., Hunter, C., & Rogers, P. (1989). Relative efficacy of intensive and spaced behavioral treatment of stuttering. *Behavior Modification, 13*(3), 376–395.

Jancke, L. (1994). Variability and duration of voice onset time in stuttering and nonstuttering adults. *Journal of Fluency Disorders, 19,* 21–37.

Jancke, L., Hanggi, J., Steinmetz, H. (2004). Morphological brain differences between adult stutterers and non-stutterers. *BMC Neurology, 4,* 23.

Jayaram, M. (1984). Distribution of stuttering in sentences: Relationship to sentence length and clause position. *Journal of Speech and Hearing Research, 27,* 338–341.

Jewell, E., & Abate, F. (Eds.). (2001). *The new Oxford American dictionary.* New York: Oxford University Press.

Johnson, W. (1934). Stuttering in the preschool child. *Child Welfare Pamphlets No. 37.* Iowa City: University of Iowa.

Johnson, W. (1942). A study of the onset and development of stuttering. *Journal of Speech Disorders, 7,* 251–257.

Johnson, W. (1944a). The Indians have no word for it: Stuttering in children. *Quarterly Journal of Speech, 30,* 330–337.

Johnson, W. (1944b). The Indians have no word for it: Stuttering in adults. *Quarterly Journal of Speech, 30,* 456–465.

Johnson, W. (1946). *People in quandaries: The semantics of personal adjustment.* New York: Harper and Bros.

Johnson, W. (1948). Stuttering. In W. Johnson, S. Brown, J. Curtis, C. Edney, & J. Keaster (Eds.), *Speech handicapped school children.* New York: Harper & Row.

Johnson, W. (1955a). The time, the place, and the problem. In W. Johnson & R. Leutenegger (Eds.), *Stuttering in children and adults.* Minneapolis: University of Minnesota Press.

Johnson, W. (1955b). A study of the onset and development of stuttering. In W. Johnson and R. Leutenegger (Eds.), *Stuttering in children and adults.* Minneapolis: University of Minnesota Press.

Johnson, W. (1958). Introduction: The six men and the stuttering. In J. Eisenson (Ed.), *Stuttering: A symposium* (pp. 123–166). New York: Harper & Row.

Johnson, W. (1961a). Measurements of oral reading and speaking rate and disfluency of adult male and female stutterers and nonstutterers. *Journal of Speech and Hearing Disorders, Monograph Supplement 7,* 1–20.

Johnson, W. (1961b). *Stuttering and what you can do about it.* Minneapolis: University of Minnesota.

Johnson, W., & Associates. (1959). *The onset of stuttering: Research findings and implications.* Minneapolis: University of Minnesota.

Johnson, W., & Colley, W. H. (1945). The relationship between frequency and duration of moments of stuttering. *Journal of Speech Disorders, 10,* 35–38.

Johnson, W., Darley, F., & Spriesterbach, D. (1963). *Diagnostic methods in speech pathology.* New York: Harper & Row.

Johnson, W., & Inness, M. (1939). Studies in the psychology of stuttering: XIII. A statistical analysis of the adaptation and consistency effects in relation to stuttering. *Journal of Speech Disorders, 10,* 35–38.

Johnson, W., & Knott, J. (1937). Studies in the psychology of stuttering: I. The distribution of moments of stuttering in successive readings of the same material. *Journal of Speech Disorders, 2,* 17–19.

Johnson, W., & Leutenegger, R. (1955). *Stuttering in children and adults.* Minneapolis: University of Minnesota Press.

Johnson, W., & Millsapps, L. (1937). Studies in the psychology of stuttering: VI. The role of cues representative of stuttering moments during oral reading. *Journal of Speech Disorders, 2,* 101–104.

Johnson, W., & Rosen, L. (1937). Studies in the psychology of stuttering. VII. Effect of certain changes in speech pattern upon frequency of stuttering. *Journal of Speech Disorders, 2,* 195–209.

Johnston, S., Watkin, L., & Macklem, P. (1993). Lung volume changes during relatively fluent speech in stutterers. *Journal of Applied Physiology, 75,* 696–703.

Jokel, R., De Nil, L., & Sharpe, A. (2007). Speech disfluencies in adults with neurogenic stuttering associated with stroke and traumatic brain injury. *Journal of Medical Speech-Language Pathology, 15*(3), 243–261.

Jones, E. (1955). Explorations of experimental extinction and spontaneous recovery in stuttering. In W. Johnson & R. Leutenegger (Eds.), *Stuttering in Children and Adults.* (pp. 226–231). Minneapolis: University of Minnesota Press.

Jones, J. A., & Striemer, D. (2007). Speech disruption during delayed auditory feedback with simultaneous visual feedback. *The Journal of the Acoustical Society of America, 122,* EL135–EL141.

Jones, M., Onslow, M., Harrison, E., & Packman, A. (2000). Treating stuttering in young children: Predicting treatment time in the Lidcombe program. *Journal of Speech, Language, and Hearing Research, 43,* 1440–1450.

Jones, M., Onslow, M., Packman, A., Williams, S., Ormond, T., Schwartz, I., et al. (2005). Randomized controlled trial of the Lidcombe programme of early stuttering intervention. *British Medical Journal, 331,* 659–661.

Kalinowski, J., Guntupalli, V., Stuart, A., & Saltuklaroglu, T. (2004). Self-reported efficacy of an ear-level prosthetic device that delivers altered auditory feedback for the management of stuttering. *International Journal of Rehabilitation Research, 27,* 167–170.

Kamhi, A. (2006). Treatment decisions for children with speech–sound disorders. *Language, Speech and Hearing Services in Schools, 37,* 271–279.

Karass, J., Walden, T., Conture, E., Graham, C., Arnold, H., Hartfield, K., et al. (2006). Relation of emotional reactivity and regulation to childhood stuttering. *Journal of Communication Disorders, 39,* 402–423.

Katsovaskaia, I. (1962). The problems of children stuttering. *Deafness, Speech, and Hearing Abstracts, 2,* 296.

Kawai, N., Healey, E. C., & Carrell, T. (2007). Listeners' identification and discrimination of digitally manipulated sounds as prolongations. *Journal of the Acoustical Society of America, 122,* 1102–1110.

Kelly, E., Smith, A., & Goffman, L. (1995). Orofacial muscle activity of children who stutter: A preliminary study. *Journal of Speech and Hearing Research, 38,* 1025–1036.

Kelly, G. (1963). *A theory of personality: The psychology of personal constructs.* New York: Norton.

Kelman, E., & Nicholas, A. (2008). *Practical intervention for early childhood stammering: Palin PCI approach.* Milton Keynes, UK: Speechmark.

Kempen, G., & Huijbers, P. (1983). The lexicalization process in sentence production and naming: Indirect election of words. *Cognition, 14,* 185–209.

Kenjo, M. (2005). Stuttering research and treatment around the world: Japan. *The ASHA Leader, 36,* 9.

Kent, L. (1961). Carbon dioxide therapy as a medical treatment for stuttering. *Journal of Speech Disorders, 26,* 268–271.

Kent, R., & Lapointe, L. (1982). Acoustic properties of pathologic reiterative utterances: A case study of palilalia. *Journal of Speech and Hearing Research, 25,* 95–99.

Kent, R. D. (2000). Research on speech motor control and its disorders: A review and prospective. *Journal of Communication Disorders, 33*(5), 391–428.

Kidd, K. K. (1977). A genetic perspective on stuttering. *Journal of Fluency Disorders, 2,* 259–269.

Kidd, K. K. (1984). Stuttering as a genetic disorder. In R. F. Curlee & W. H. Perkins (Eds.), *Nature and treatment of stuttering: New directions* (pp.149–169). San Diego, CA: College-Hill.

Kidd, K. K., Kidd, J. R., & Records, M. A. (1978). The possible causes of the sex ratio in stuttering and its implications. *Journal of Fluency Disorders, 3,* 13–23.

Kingdon-Ward, W. (1941). *Stammering.* London: Hamilton.

Kingston, M., Huber, A., Onslow, M., Jones, M., & Packman, A. (2003). Predicting treatment time with the Lidcombe program: Replication and meta-analysis. *International Journal of Language and Communication Disorders, 38,* 165–177.

Klein, J., & Hood, S. (2004). The impact the stuttering on employment opportunities and job performance. *Journal of Fluency Disorders, 29,* 255–273.

Klein, M. (1932). *The psycho-analysis of children.* London: Hogarth Press.

Klein, M. (1955). The psychoanalytic play technique. *American Journal of Orthopsychiatry, 25,* 223–237.

Klein, M. (1967). U.S. Patent No. 3,349,179. Washington, DC: U.S. Patent and Trademark Office.

Kleinow, J., & Smith, A. (2000). Influences of length and syntactic complexity on the speech motor stability of the fluent speech of adults who stutter. *Journal of Speech, Language, and Hearing Research, 43,* 548–559.

Klingbell, G. (1939). The historical background of the modern speech clinic. *Journal of Speech Disorders, 4,* 115–132.

Kloth, S. A. M., Janssen, P., Kraaimaat, F. W., & Brutten, G. J. (1995). Speech-motor and linguistic skills of young stutterers prior to onset. *Journal of Fluency Disorders, 20*, 157–170.

Koenisberger, R. (Ed.). (1989). *Churchill's illustrated medical dictionary*. New York: Churchill Livingstone.

Kormos, J., & Denes, M. (2004). Exploring measures and perceptions of fluency in the speech of second language learners. *System: An International Journal of Educational Technology and Applied Linguistics, 32*, 145–164.

Kraaimaat, F., Vanryckeghem, M., & Van Dam-Baggen, R. (2002). Stuttering and social anxiety. *Journal of Fluency Disorders, 27*, 319–331.

Kroll, R., De Nil, L., Kapur, S., & Houle, S. (1997). A positron emission tomography investigation of post-treatment brain activation in stutterers. In W. Hulstijn, H. F. M. Peters, P. H. H. M. Van Lieshout (Eds.), *Speech production: Motor control, brain research and fluency disorders*. Amsterdam: Elsevier.

Kroll, R., & Hood, S. (1976). The influence of task presentation and information load on the adaptation effect in stutterers and normal speakers, *Journal of Communication Disorders, 9*, 95–110.

Kully, D. (2002). Venturing into telehealth: Applying interactive technologies to stuttering treatment. *The ASHA Leader, 7*(1), 6–7, 15.

Kully, D., & Boberg, E. (1988). An investigation of inter-clinic agreement in the identification of fluent and stuttered syllables. *Journal of Fluency Disorders, 13*, 309–318.

Kully, D., & Boberg, E. (1991). Therapy for school aged-children. In W. Perkins (Ed.), *Seminars in speech and language, 12* (pp. 291–300). New York: Thieme.

Kully, D., Langevin, M., & Lomheim, H. (2007). Intensive treatment of stuttering in adolescent and adult. In E. Conture & R. Curlee (Eds.), *Stuttering and related disorders of fluency* (3rd ed.). New York: Thieme.

Landers, D., & Landers, D. (1973). Teacher versus peer models: Effect of model's presence and performance level on motor behavior. *Journal of Motor Behavior, 5*, 129–139.

Langevin, M., Huinck, W. J., Kully, D., Peters, H. F. M., Lomheim, H., & Tellers, M. (2006). A cross-cultural, long-term outcome evaluation of the ISTAR comprehensive stuttering program across Dutch and Canadian adults who stutter. *Journal of Fluency Disorders, 31*(4), 229–256.

Langevin, M., Kully, D., & Ross-Harold, B. (2007). A comprehensive stuttering program for school age children with strategies for managing teasing and bullying. In E. Conture & R. Curlee (Eds.), *Stuttering and related disorders* (3rd ed., pp. 131–150). New York: Thieme.

Lanyon, R. (1965). The relationship of adaptation and consistency to improvement in stuttering therapy. *Journal of Speech and Hearing Research, 8*, 263–269.

Lanyon, R. (1969). Behavior change in stuttering through systematic desensitization. *Journal of Speech and Hearing Disorders, 34*, 253–260.

Lanyon, R., & Barocas, V. (1975). Effects of contingent events on stuttering and fluency. *Journal of Consulting and Clinical Psychology, 43*, 786–793.

Lanyon, R., & Duprez, D. (1970). Nonfluency, information, and word length. *Journal of Abnormal Psychology, 76*, 93–97.

LaSalle, L., & Conture, E. (1995). Disfluency clusters of children who stutter: Relation of stutterings to self-repairs. *Journal of Speech and Hearing Research, 38*, 965–977.

Lass, N., Ruscello, D., Schmitt, J., Pannbacker, M., Orlando M., Dean, K., & Ruziska, J. (1992). Teachers' perception of stutterers. *Language, Speech, and Hearing Services in Schools, 23*, 78–81.

Law, J., Boyle, J., & Harris, F. (2000). Prevalence and natural history of primary speech and language delay: Findings from a systematic review of the literature. *International Journal of Language & Communication Disorders, 35*, 165–188.

Leadholm, B., & Miller, J. (1992). *Language sample analysis: The Wisconsin guide* (Bulletin No. 92424). Madison: Wisconsin Department of Public Instruction.

Leath, W. (1984). *Handbook of stuttering therapy for the school clinician*. San Diego, CA: College-Hill Press.

Leath, W., & Mims, H. (1975). Cultural influences in the development and treatment of stuttering: A preliminary report on the black stutterer. *Journal of Speech and Hearing Disorders, 40*, 459–466.

Leavitt, R. (1974). *The Puerto Ricans: Culture change and language deviance*. Oxford, UK: University of Arizona Press.

Lebrun, Y., & Leleux, C. (1985). Acquired stuttering following right brain damage in dextrals. *Journal of Fluency Disorders, 10*, 137–141.

Lee, B. S. (1950). Some effects of side-tone delay. *Journal of the Acoustical Society of America, 22*, 639–640.

Lees, R., Anderson, H., & Martin, P. (1999). The influence of language disorder on fluency: A pilot study. *Journal of Fluency Disorders, 24*, 227–238.

Lehiste, I. (1972). The timing of utterances and linguistic boundaries. *Journal of the Acoustical Society of America, 51*, 2018–2024.

Leith, W. (1986). Treating the stutterer with atypical cultural influences. In K. O. St. Louis, (Ed.), *The atypical stutterer*. San Diego, CA: Academic Press.

Leith, W., & Mims, H. (1975). Cultural influences in the development and treatment of stuttering: A preliminary report on the Black stutterer. *Journal of Speech and Hearing Disorders, 40*, 459–466.

Lemert, E. M. (1953). Some Indians who stutter. *Journal of Speech and Hearing Disorders, 18*, 168–174.

Lemert, E. M. (1962). Stuttering and social structure in two pacific societies. *Journal of Speech and Hearing Disorders, 27*, 3–10.

Leutenegger, R. R. (1957). Adaptation and recovery in the oral reading of stutterers. *Journal of Speech and Hearing Disorders, 22*, 276–287.

Levelt, W. J. M. (1989). *Speaking: From intention to articulation*. Cambridge, MA: MIT Press.

Levelt, W., Roelofs, A., & Meyer, A. (1999). A theory of lexical access in speech production. *Behavioral and Brain Sciences, 22*, 1–75.

Levy, D. (1938). Release therapy in young children. In G. L. Landreth (Ed.), *Play therapy: The art of the relationship.* Muncie, IN: Accelerated Development.

Lewis, K. (1991). The structure of disfluency behaviors in the speech of stutterers. *Journal of Speech and Hearing Research, 34*(3), 492–500.

Lewis, K., & Golberg, L. (1997). Measurements of temperament in the identification of children who stutter. *European Journal of Disorders of Communication, 32,* 441–448.

Lilienfeld, S. (Ed.). (2003). *Science and pseudoscience in clinical psychology.* New York: Guilford.

Lincoln, M., & Onslow, M. (1997). Long-term outcome of early intervention for stuttering. *American Journal of Speech-Language Pathology, 6,* 51–58.

Lincoln, M., Onslow, M., Lewis, C., & Wilson, L. (1996). A clinical trial of operant treatment for school-age children who stutter. *American Journal of Speech-Language Pathology, 5,* 73–85.

Lincoln, M., Packman, A., & Onslow, M. (2006.) Altered auditory feedback and the treatment of stuttering. *Journal of Fluency Disorders, 31,* 71–89.

Lindberg, K. (1900). Zur Haufigkeit des Stotterns bei Schulkindern. *Medizinisch-padagogische Monatsschrift fur die gesamte Sprachheilkunde,* 281–286.

Lindblom, B. (1963). Spectrographic study of vowel reduction. *Journal of the Acoustical Society of America, 35,* 1773–1781.

Lingwall, J., & Bergstrand, G. (1979, November). *Perceptual boundaries for judgment of "normal," "abnormal," and "stuttered" prolongations.* Paper presented at the convention of the American Speech-Language-Hearing Association, Atlanta, GA.

Logan, K., & Haj Tas, M. (2007). Effect of sample size on the measurement of stutter-like disfluencies. *Perspectives on Fluency and Fluency Disorders, 17*(3), ASHA SID 4, 3–6.

Logan, K., Roberts, R., Pretto, A., & Morey, M. (2002). Speaking slowly: Effects of four self-guided training approaches on adults' speech rate and naturalness. *American Journal of Speech Language Pathology, 11,* 163–174.

Long, N., & Dalston, R. (1983). Comprehension abilities of one-year-old infants with cleft lip and palate. *Cleft Palate Journal, 20,* 300.

Louko, L. (1995). Phonological characteristics of young children who stutter. *Topics in Language Disorders, 15,* 48–59.

Louko, L., Edwards, C., & Conture, E. (1990). Phonological characteristics of young stutterers and their normally fluent peers: Preliminary observations. *Journal of Fluency Disorders, 15,* 191–210.

Louttit, C. M., & Halls, E. C. (1936). Surveys of speech defects among public school children of Indiana. *Journal of Speech Disorders, 1,* 73–80.

Lowinger, L. (1952). The psychodynamics of stuttering: An evaluation of the factors of aggression and guilt feelings in a group of institutionalized children. *Dissertation Abstracts, 12,* 725.

Lubker, B. B. (1997). Epidemiology: An essential science for speech-language pathology and audiology. *Journal of Communication Disorders, 30*(4), 251–267.

Luchsinger, R., & Arnold, G. (1965). *Voice-speech-language.* Belmont, CA: Wadsworth.

Ludlow, C. (2000). Stuttering: Dysfunction in a complex and dynamic system. *Brain, 123,* 1983–1984.

Ludlow, C., & Loucks, T. (2003). Stuttering: A dynamic motor control disorder. *Journal of Fluency Disorders, 28,* 273–295.

Lund, N., & Duchan, J. F. (1993). *Assessing children's language in naturalistic contexts* (3rd ed.). Englewood Cliffs, NJ: Prentice Hall.

Lundstrom, C., & Garsten, M. (2000). A model for intervention with childhood stuttering. In *Proceedings of the 3rd World Congress of Fluency Disorders* (pp. 335–340). Nijmigen, Netherlands: Nijmigen University.

Luterman, D. (1991). *Counseling the communicatively disordered and their families* (2nd ed.). Austin, TX: Pro-Ed.

MacCulloch, M., Eaton, R., & Long, E. (1970). The long term effect of auditory masking on young stutterers. *British Journal of Disorders of Communication, 5,* 165–173.

MacKay, D. (1970). Spoonerisms: The structure of errors in the serial order of speech. *Neuropsychologia, 8,* 323–350.

Madding, C. C. (1995). *The stuttering syndrome: Feelings and attitudes of stutterers and non-stutterers among four cultural groups* (Unpublished doctoral dissertation). Claremont Graduate School.

Maguire, G., Riley, G., Franklin, D., & Gottschalk, L. (2000). Risperidone for the treatment of stuttering. *Journal of Clinical Psychopharmacology, 20,* 479–482.

Maguire, G., Riley, G., Franklin, D., Maguire, M., Nguyen, C., & Brojeni, P. (2004). Olanzapine in the treatment of developmental stuttering: A double-blind, placebo-controlled trial. *Annals of Clinical Psychiatry, 16,* 63–67.

Maguire, G., Riley, G., Wu, J., Franklin, D., & Potkin, S. (1997). Effects of risperidone in the treatment of stuttering. In W. Hulstijn, H. F. M. Peters, & P. H. H. M. Van Lieshout (Eds.), *Speech production: Motor control, brain research and fluency disorder.* Amsterdam: Elsevier.

Maguire, G., Yu, B., Franklin, D., & Riley, G. (2004). Alleviating stuttering with pharmacological intervention. *Expert Opinion on Pharmacotherapy, 5,* 1565–1571.

Mahr, G., & Leith, W. (1992). Psychogenic stuttering of adult onset. *Journal of Speech and Hearing Research, 35,* 283–286.

Mahr, G. C., & Torosian, T. (1999). Anxiety and social phobia in stuttering. *Journal of Fluency Disorders 24,* 119–126.

Makuen, G. (1914). A study of 1,000 cases of stammering with special reference to the etiology and treatment of the affliction. *Therapeutic Gazette, 38,* 385–390.

Makuen, G. (1941). Psychology of stuttering. *Journal of Nervous and Mental Disorders, 43,* 68–72.

Mallard, A.R. (1991). Using families to help the school-age stutterer: A case study. In L. Rustin (Ed.), *Parents, families, and the stuttering child* (pp. 72–87). San Diego, CA: Singular.

Mallard, A. R. (1998). Using problem solving procedures in family management of stuttering. *Journal of Fluency Disorders, 23*, 127–135.

Manning, W. (1994). *The SEA scale: Self-efficacy scaling for adolescents who stutter.* Paper presented at the annual meeting of the American Speech-Language-Hearing Association convention, New Orleans, LA.

Manning, W. (2001). C*linical decision making in fluency disorders* (2nd ed.). San Diego, CA: Singular.

Manning, W. (2006). Therapeutic change and the nature of our evidence: Improving our ability to help. In N. Bernstein Ratner & J. Tetnowski (Eds.), *Current issues in stuttering research and practice.* Mahwah, NJ: Erlbaum.

Månsson, H. (2000). Childhood stuttering: Incidence and development. *Journal of Fluency Disorders, 25*, 47–57.

Månsson, H. (2006). *Complexity and diversity in early childhood stuttering.* Paper presented at the 5th International Congress of Fluency Disorders, Dublin, Ireland.

Market, K. E., Montague, J. C., Buffalo, M. D., & Drummond, S. S. (1990). Acquired stuttering: Descriptive data and treatment outcome. *Journal of Fluency Disorders, 15*, 21–33.

Marland, P. M. (1957). Shadowing: A contribution to the treatment of stuttering. *Folia Phoniatrica, 9*, 242–245.

Martin, R., & Haroldson, S. (1971). Time-out as a punishment for stuttering during conversation. *Journal of Communication Disorders, 4*, 15–19.

Martin, R., & Haroldson, S. (1981). Stuttering identification: Standard definition and moment of stuttering. *Journal of Speech and Hearing Research, 24*(1), 59–63.

Martin, R., & Haroldson, S. (1982). Contingent self-stimulation for stuttering. *Journal of Speech and Hearing Disorders, 47*, 407–413.

Martin, R., Haroldson, S., & Triden, K. (1984). Stuttering and speech naturalness. *Journal of Speech and Hearing Disorders, 49*, 53–58.

Martin, R. R., Kuhl, P., & Haroldson, S. (1972). An experimental treatment with two preschool stuttering children. *Journal of Speech and Hearing Research, 15*, 743–752.

Martin, R., & Siegel, G. (1966). The effects of simultaneously punishing stuttering and rewarding fluency. *Journal of Speech and Hearing Research, 9*, 466–475.

Matthews, S., Williams, R., & Pring, T. (1997). Parent-child interaction therapy and dysfluency: A single case study. *European Journal of Disorders of Communication 32*, 1244–1259.

Max, L., & Caruso, A. (1998). Adaptation of stuttering frequency during repeated readings. *Journal of Speech, Language, and Hearing Research, 41*, 1265–1281.

Max, L., Caruso, A., & Gracco, V. (2003). Kinematic analyses of speech, orofacial nonspeech, and finger movements in stuttering and nonstuttering adults. *Journal of Speech, Language, and Hearing Research, 46*, 215–232.

Max, L., & Gracco. V., (2005). Coordination of oral and laryngeal movements in the perceptually fluent speech of adults who stutter. *Journal of Speech, Language, and Hearing Research, 48*, 524–542.

Max, L., Guenther, F., Gracco, V., Ghosh, S., & Wallace, M. (2004). Unstable or insufficiently activated internal models and feedback-biased motor control as sources of dysfluency: A theoretical model of stuttering. *Contemporary Issues in Communication Science and Disorders, 31*, 105–122.

McAllister, J., & Kingston, M. (2005). Final part-word repetitions in school-age children: Two case studies. *Journal of Fluency Disorders, 30*, 255–267.

McClean, M., & Runyan, C. (2000). Variations in the relative speeds of orofacial structures with stuttering severity. *Journal of Speech, Language and Hearing Research, 43*, 1524–1531.

McDevitt, S. C., & Carey, W. B. (1978). The measurement of temperament in 3–7 year-old children. *Journal of Child Psychology and Psychiatry and Allied Disciplines, 19*, 245–253.

McKinnon, D., McLeod, S., & Reilly, S. (2007). The prevalence of stuttering, voice, and speech-sound disorders in primary school students in Australia. *Language, Speech, and Hearing Services in Schools, 38*, 5–15.

McMillan, J. (2004). *Educational research: Fundamentals for the consumer* (4th ed., pp. 227–228). Boston: Allyn & Bacon.

Meltzer, H. (1935). Talkativeness in stuttering and nonstuttering children. *Journal of Genetic Psychology, 46*, 371–390.

Meltzoff, A. (1995). What infant memory tells us about amnesia: Long-term recall and deferred imitation. *Journal of Experimental Child Psychology, 59*, 497–515.

Merits-Patterson, R., & Reed, C. (1981). Disfluencies in the speech of language-delayed children. *Journal of Speech and Hearing Research, 46*, 55–58.

Meyer, V., & Mair, J. (1963). A new technique to control stammering: A preliminary report. *Behavioral Research and Therapy, 1*, 251–254.

Meyers, S. C., & Freeman, F. J. (1985). Mother and child speech rates as a variable in stuttering and disfluency. *Journal of Speech and Hearing Research, 28*, 436–444.

Meyers Fosnot, S., & Woodford, L. (1992). *The fluency development system for young children.* Buffalo, NY: United Educational Services.

Miles, S., & Ratner Bernstein, N. (2001). Parental language input to children at stuttering onset. *Journal of Speech, Language, and Hearing Research, 44*, 1116–1130.

Milisen, R., & Johnson, W. (1936). A comparative study of stutterers, former stutterers, and normal speakers whose handedness has been changed. *Archives of Speech, 1*, 61–86.

Millard, S., Nicholas, A., & Cook, F. (2008). Is parent-child interaction therapy effective in reducing stuttering? *Journal of Speech, Language, and Hearing Research, 51*, 636–650.

Miller, B., & Guitar, B. (2009). Long-term outcome of the Lidcombe program for early stuttering intervention. *American Journal of Speech-Language Pathology, 18*, 42–49.

Miller, J., Long, S., McKinley, N., Thormann, S., Jones, M., & Nockerts, A. (2005). *Language Sample Analysis II: The*

Wisconsin guide. Madison, WI: Wisconsin Department of Public Instruction.

Mills, A. W., & Streit, H. (1942). Report of a speech survey, Holyoke, Massachusetts. *Journal of Speech Disorders, 7*, 161–167.

Miranda, A., McCabe, A., & Bliss, L. (1998). Jumping around and leaving things out: A profile of the narrative abilities of children with specific language impairment. *Applied Psycholinguistics, 19*, 647–668.

Moleski, R., & Tosi, D. (1976). Comparative psychotherapy: Rational-emotive therapy versus systematic desensitization in the treatment of stuttering. *Journal of Consulting and Clinical Psychology, 44*(2), 309–311.

Montgomery, B., & Fitch, J. L. (1988). The prevalence of stuttering in the hearing-impaired school age population. *Journal of Speech & Hearing Disorders, 53*, 131–135.

Moore, W. (1946). Hypnosis in a system of therapies for stutterers. *Journal of Speech Disorders, 11*, 117–122.

Moore, W. (1959). A study of the blood chemistry of stutterers under two hypnotic conditions. *Speech Monographs, 26*, 64–68.

Moore, W. H., Jr., Flowers, P., & Cunko, C. (1981). Some relationships between adaptation and electromyographic activity at laryngeal and masseter sites in stutterers. *Journal of Fluency Disorders, 4*, 149–161.

Morely, A. (1937). An analysis of associated and predisposing factors in the symptomatology of stuttering. *Psychological Monographs, 49*, 50–107.

Moreno, J. (1946). *Psychodrama*. Beacon, NY: Beacon House.

Moreno, J. L. (1953). *Who shall survive? Foundations of sociometry, group psychotherapy and psychodrama* (2nd ed.). Beacon, NY: Beacon House.

Morgenstern, J. J. (1956). Socio-economic factors in stuttering. *Journal of Speech and Hearing Disorders, 21*, 25–33.

Morley, M. E. (1957). *The development and disorders of speech in childhood*. Edinburgh, UK: Livingstone.

Moscicki, E. (1993). Fundamental methodological considerations in controlled clinical trials. *Journal of Fluency Disorders, 18*, 183–196.

Moskowitz, H. (1941). Psychiatric factors in speech correction. *Quarterly Journal of Speech, 27*, 537–541.

Mowrer, D. E. (1998). Analysis of the sudden onset and disappearance of disfluencies in the speech of a $2\frac{1}{2}$-year-old boy. *Journal of Fluency Disorders, 23*, 103–118.

Murdoch, B., Pitt, G., Theodoros, D., & Ward, E. (1999). Real-time continuous visual biofeedback in the treatment of speech breathing disorders following childhood traumatic brain injury: Report of one case. *Developmental Neurorehabilitation, 3*(1), 5–20.

Murphy, A., & Fitzsimons, R. (1960). *Stuttering and personality dynamics: Play therapy, projective therapy, and counseling*. New York: Ronald.

Murphy, W., Yaruss, J. S., & Quesal, R. (2007a). Enhancing treatment for school-age children who stutter: I. Reducing negative reactions through desensitization and cognitive restructuring. *Journal of Fluency Disorders, 32*, 121–138.

Murphy, W., Yaruss, J. S., & Quesal, R. (2007b). Enhancing treatment for school-age children who stutter: II. Reducing bullying through role-playing and self-disclosure. *Journal of Fluency Disorders, 32*, 139–162.

Nao, C. (1964). The results of hypnosis as stuttering therapy. *Mental and Physical Medicine* (Japan), *4*, 176–177.

Nass, R., Sclireler, B., & Heier, L. (2008). Acquired stuttering after a second stroke in a two year old. *Developmental Medicine & Child Neurology, 36*, 73–78.

National Institutes of Health. (1997). NIH Publication 97–4232. Available at www.nidcd.nih.gov/health/voice/stutter.asp.

Natke, U., Sandrieser, P., van Ark, M., Pietrowsky, R., & Kalveram, K. (2004). Linguistic stress within-word position, and grammatical class in relation to early childhood stuttering. *Journal of Fluency Disorders, 29*, 109–122.

Neely, M. M. (1960). *An investigation of the incidence of stuttering among elementary school children in the parochial schools of Orleans Parish* (Unpublished master's thesis). Tulane University.

Neilson, M., & Andrews, G. (1992). Intensive fluency training of chronic stutterers. In R. Curlee (Ed.), *Stuttering and related disorders of fluency* (pp. 139–165). Thieme: New York.

Newman, L., & Smit, A. (1989). Some effects of variations in response time latency on speech rate, interruptions, and fluency in children's speech. *Journal of Speech and Hearing Research, 32*, 635–644.

Newman, P. (1963). Adaptation performances of individual stutterers: Implications for research. *Journal of Speech and Hearing Research, 6*, 293–294.

Nippold, M. (1990). Concomitant speech and language disorders in stuttering children: A critique of the literature. *Journal of Speech and Hearing Disorders, 55*, 51–60.

Nippold, M. A. (2001). Phonological disorders and stuttering in children: What is the frequency of co-occurrence? *Clinical Linguistics and Phonetics, 15*(3), 219–228.

Nippold, M. (2002). Stuttering and phonology: Is there an interaction? *American Journal of Speech-Language Pathology, 11*, 99–110.

Nippold, M. (2004). Phonological and language disorders in children who stutter: Impact on treatment recommendations. *Clinical Linguistics & Phonetics, 18*, 145–159.

North, M. M., North, S. M., & Coble, J. R. (1997). Virtual reality therapy: An effective treatment for psychological disorders. *Student Health Technology and Information, 44*, 59–70.

Nowack, W. J. & Stone, R. E. (1987). Acquired stuttering and bilateral cerebral disease. *Journal of Fluency Disorders, 12*, 141–146.

Nwokah, E. E. (1988). The imbalance of stuttering behavior in bilingual speakers. *Journal of Fluency Disorders, 13*, 357–373.

Ojemann, R. (1931). Studies in handedness: III. Relation of handedness to speech. *Journal of Educational Psychology, 22*, 120–126.

Okasha, A., Bishry, Z., Kamel, M., & Hassan, A. H. (1974). Psychosocial study of stammering in Egyptian children. *British Journal of Psychiatry, 124,* 531–533.

Olswang, L. (1993). Treatment efficacy research: A paradigm for investigating clinical practice and theory. *Journal of Fluency Disorders, 18,* 125–131.

Olswang, L. (1998). Treatment efficacy research. In C. Frattali (Ed.), *Measuring outcomes in speech-language pathology* (pp. 134–150). New York: Thieme.

Onslow, M. (1996). *Behavioral management of stuttering.* San Diego, CA: Singular.

Onslow, M., Andrews, C., & Lincoln, M. (1994). A control/experimental trial of an operant treatment for early stuttering. *Journal of Speech and Hearing Research, 37,* 1244–1259.

Onslow, M., Costa, L., & Rue, S. (1990). Direct early intervention with stuttering: Some preliminary data. *Journal of Speech and Hearing Disorders, 55,* 405–416.

Onslow, M., Costa, L., Andrews, C., Harrison, E., & Packman, A. (1996). Speech outcomes of a prolonged-speech treatment for stuttering. *Journal of Speech and Hearing Research, 39,* 734–749.

Onslow, M., Costa, L., & Rue, S. (1990). Direct early intervention with stuttering: Some preliminary data. *Journal of Speech and Hearing Disorders, 55,* 405–416.

Onslow, M., & Ingham, R. (1987). Speech quality measurement and the management of stuttering. *Journal of Speech and Hearing Disorders, 52,* 2–17.

Onslow, M., Packman, A., & Harrison, E. (Eds). (2003). *The Lidcombe program of early stuttering intervention: A clinician's guide.* Austin, TX: Pro-Ed.

Onslow, M., van Doorn, J., & Newman, D. (1992). Variability of acoustic segment durations after prolonged-speech treatment for stuttering. *Journal of Speech and Hearing Research, 35,* 529–536.

Ornstein, A., & Manning, W. (1985). Self-efficacy scaling by adult stutterers. *Journal of Communication Disorders, 18,* 313–320.

Otto, F., & Yairi, E. (1976). A disfluency analysis of Down's syndrome and normal subjects. *Journal of Fluency Disorders, 1,* 26–32.

Owens, R. (2010). *Language disorders: A functional approach to assessment and intervention.* Boston: Allyn & Bacon.

Oyler, M. (1996). Vulnerability in stuttering children. *Dissertation Abstracts International Section A: Humanities & Social Sciences, 56*(9-A), 3374.

Ozawa, Y. (1960). Studies of misarticulation in Wakayama district. *Journal of Medicine: University of Osaka, 5,* 319.

Packman, A., Code, C., & Onslow, M. (2007). On the cause of stuttering: Integrating theory with brain and behavioral research. *Journal of Neurolinguistics, 20,* 353–362.

Packman, A., & Onslow, M. (1999). Issues in the treatment of early stuttering. In M. Onslow & A. Packman (Eds.), *The handbook of early stuttering intervention* (pp.1–16). San Diego, CA: Singular.

Paden, E. (2005). Development of phonological abilities. In E. Yairi & N. Ambrose (Eds.), *Early childhood stuttering* (pp. 197–235). Austin, TX: Pro-Ed.

Paden, E., Ambrose N., & Yairi, E. (2002). Phonological progress during the first two years of stuttering. *Journal of Speech, Language, and Hearing Research, 44,* 256–267.

Paden, E., & Yairi, E. (1996). Phonological characteristics of young children with persistent and recovering stuttering. *Journal of Speech and Hearing Research, 39,* 981–990.

Paden, E. P., Yairi, E., & Ambrose, N. G. (1999). Early childhood stuttering: II. Initial status of phonological abilities. *Journal of Speech, Language, and Hearing Research, 42,* 1113–1124.

Parker, C., & Christopherson, F. (1963). Electronic aid in the treatment of stammer. *Medical Electronics and Biological Engineering, 1,* 121–125.

Patel, R., & Brayton, J. (2009). Identifying prosodic contrasts in utterances produced by 4-, 7-, and 11-year-old children. *Journal of Speech, Language, Hearing Research, 52,* 790–801.

Pavlov, I. P. (1927). *Conditioned reflexes: An investigation of the physiological activity of the cerebral cortex* (Trans. G. V. Anrep). London: Oxford University Press.

Pay, A., & Sirotkina, M. M. (1955). *My experience in logoped work.* Moscow: Academy of Education, Institute of Defectology.

Pellowski, M. W., & Conture, E. G. (2002). Characteristics of speech disfluency and stuttering behaviors in 3- and 4-year-old children. *Journal of Speech, Language, and Hearing Research, 45,* 20–34.

Perkins, W. (1973a). Replacement of stuttering with fluent speech: I. Rationale. *Journal of Speech and Hearing Disorders, 38,* 283–294.

Perkins, W. (1973b). Replacement of stuttering with normal speech: II. Clinical procedures. *Journal of Speech and Hearing Disorders, 38,* 295–303.

Perkins, W. (1990a). What is stuttering? *Journal of Speech and Hearing Disorders, 55,* 370–382.

Perkins, W. (1990b). Gratitude, good intentions, and red herrings: A response to commentaries. *Journal of Speech and Hearing Disorders, 55,* 402–404.

Perkins, W. (1992a). Fluency controls and automatic fluency. *American Journal of Speech-Language Pathology, 1*(2), 9–10.

Perkins, W. (1992b). *Stuttering prevented.* San Diego, CA: Singular.

Perkins, W. & Curlee, R. (1969). Clinical impressions of portable masking unit effects in stuttering. *Journal of Speech and Hearing Disorders, 34,* 360–362.

Perkins, W., Kent, R. D., & Curlee, R. F. (1991). A theory of neurolinguistic function in stuttering. *Journal of Speech and Hearing Research, 34*(4), 734–752.

Perkins, W., Rudas, J., Johnson, L., & Bell, J. (1976). Stuttering: Discoordination of phonation with articulation and respiration. *Journal of Speech and Hearing Research, 19,* 509–522.

Phares, E. (1979). *Clinical psychology: Concepts, methods, and profession.* Georgetown, Ontario, Canada: Dorsey Press.

Pichon, E., & Borel-Maisonny, S. (1937). *Le Bégaiement, sa nature, et son traitement.* Paris: Masson.

Pindzola, R. H. (1987). *Stuttering intervention program: Age 3 to grade 3.* Austin, TX: Pro-Ed.

Pindzola, R. H., Jenkins, M. M., & Lokken, K. J. (1989). Speaking rates of young children. *Language, Speech, and Hearing Services in Schools, 20,* 133–138.

Pindzola, R. H., & White, D. (1986). A protocol for differentiating the incipient stutterer. *Language, Speech, and Hearing Services in the Schools, 17,* 2–11.

Postma, A., Kolk, H., & Povel, D-J. (1991). Disfluencies as resulting from covert self-repairs applied to internal speech errors. In H. F. M. Peters, W. Hulstijn, & C. W. Starkweather (Eds.), *Speech motor control and stuttering.* Amsterdam: Elsevier Science.

Postma, A., & Kolk, H. (1992). Error monitoring in people who stutter: Evidence against auditory feedback deficit theories. *Journal of Speech and Hearing Research, 35,* 1024–1032.

Postma, A. & Kolk, H. (1993). The covert repair hypothesis: Prearticulatory repair processes in normal and stuttered disfluencies. *Journal of Speech and Hearing Research, 36,* 472–487.

Poulos, M. G., & Webster, W. G. (1991). Family history as a basis for subgrouping people who stutter. *Journal of Speech and Hearing Research, 34,* 5–10.

Preibisch, C., Neumann, K., Raab, P., Euler, H., von Gudenberg, A., Lanfermann, H., et al. (2003). Evidence for compensation for stuttering by the right frontal operculum. *Neuroimage 20,* 1356–1364.

Preus, A. (1973). Stuttering in Down's syndrome. In Y. LeBrun & R. Hoops (Eds.), *Neurolinguistic approaches to stuttering* (pp. 90–100). The Hague: Mouton.

Preus, A. (1981). *Identifying subgroups of stutterers.* Oslo, Norway: University of Oslo.

Preus, A. (1990). Treatment of mentally retarded stutterers. *Journal of Fluency Disorders, 15,* 223–234.

Prins, D. (1993). Management of stuttering: Treatment of adolescents and adults. In R. Curlee (Ed.), *Stuttering and related disorders of fluency.* New York: Thieme.

Prins, D., & Hubbard, C. (1988). Response contingent stimuli and stuttering: Issues and implications. *Journal of Speech and Hearing Research, 31,* 696–709.

Prins, D., & Hubbard, C. (1990). Acoustical durations of speech segments during stuttering adaptation. *Journal of Speech and Hearing Research, 33,* 494–504.

Prins, D., Hubbard, C., & Krause, M. (1991). Syllabic stress and the occurrence of stuttering. *Journal of Speech and Hearing Research, 34,* 1011–1016.

Prins, D., & Lohr, F. (1972). Behavioral dimensions of stuttered speech. *Journal of Speech and Hearing Research, 15*(1), 61–71.

Prins, D., Main, V., & Wampler, S. (1997). Lexicalization in adults who stutter. *Journal of Speech, Language, and Hearing Research, 40,* 373–384.

Prins, D., Mandelkorn, T., & Cerf, A. (1980). Principal and differential effects of Haloperidol and placebo treatments upon speech disfluencies in stutterers. *Journal of Speech, Language, and Hearing Research, 23,* 614–629.

Proctor, A., Yairi, E., Duff, M., & Zhang, J. (2008). Prevalence of stuttering in African American preschool children. *Journal of Speech, Language, and Hearing Research, 50,* 1465–1474.

Quarrington, B. (1965). Stuttering as a function of the information value and sentence position of words. *Journal of Abnormal Psychology, 70,* 221–224.

Quesal, R., Yaruss, J. S., & Molt, L. (2004). Many types of data: Stuttering treatment outcomes beyond fluency. In A. Packman, A. Meltzer, & H. Peters (Eds.), *Theory research and therapy in fluency disorders. Proceedings of the 4th World Congress on Fluency Disorders* (pp. 218–224). Nijmegen, Netherlands: Nijmegen University Press.

Quinn, P., & Preachy, E. (1973). Haloperidol in the treatment of stutterers. *British Journal of Psychiatry, 123,* 247–248.

Raczek, B., & Adamczyk, B. (2004). Concentration of carbon dioxide in exhaled air in fluent and non-fluent speech. *Folia Phoniatrica Logopedia, 56,* 75–82.

Ralston, L. D. (1981). Stammering: A stress index in Caribbean classrooms. *Journal of Fluency Disorders, 6*(2), 119–133.

Ramig, P., & Bennett, E. (1997). Clinical management of children: Direct management strategy. In R. F. Curlee & G. M. Siegel (Eds.), *Nature and treatment of stuttering: New Directions* (2nd ed., pp. 292–312. Boston: Allyn & Bacon.

Rantala, S. & Petri-Larmi, M. (1976). Haloperidol (serenase) in the treatment of stuttering. *Folia Phoniatrica, 28,* 354–361.

Reed, C. G., & Godden, A. L. (1977). An experimental treatment using verbal punishment with two preschool stutterers. *Journal of Fluency Disorders, 2,* 225–233.

Reilly, S., Onslow, M., Packman, A., Wake, M., Bavin, E., Prior, M., et al. (2009). Predicting stuttering onset by age of 3: A prospective, community cohort study. *Pediatrics, 123,* 270–277.

Retherford, K. (2000). *Guide to analysis of language transcripts* (3rd ed.). Eau Claire, WI: Thinking Publications.

Rheinberger, M., Karlin, I., & Berman, A. (1943). Electroencephalographic and laterality studies of stuttering and non-stuttering children. *Nervous Child, 2,* 117–133.

Riaz, N., Steinberg, S., Ahmad, J., Pluzhnikov, A., Riazuddin, S., Cox, N. J., et al. (2005). Genomewide significant linkage to stuttering on chromosome 12. *American Journal of Human Genetics, 76,* 647–651.

Richels, C., & Conture, E. G. (2007). An indirect treatment approach for early intervention for childhood stuttering. In E. Conture & R. Curlee (Eds.), *Stuttering and related disorders,* (3rd ed.). New York: Thieme.

Rickard, H., & Mundy, M. (1965). Direct manipulation of stuttering behavior in experimental-clinical approach. In L. Ulman & L. Krasner (Eds.), *Case studies in behavioral modification* (pp. 268–272). New York: Holt, Rinehart and Winston.

Riley, G. (1981). *Stuttering prediction instrument for young children.* Austin, TX: Pro-Ed.

Riley, G. (1994). *Stuttering severity instrument for children and adults* (3rd ed.). Austin, TX: Pro-Ed.

Riley, G. (2009). *SSI-4: Stuttering Severity Instrument* (4th ed.). Austin, TX: Pro-Ed.

Riley, G. & Ingham, J. C. (1995). Vocal response time changes associated with two types of treatment. In C. W. Starkweather & H. M. F. Peters (Eds.), *Stuttering: Proceedings of the First World Congress in Fluency Disorders* (pp. 470–474). New York: Elsevier.

Riley, G., & Ingham, J. C. (2000). Acoustic duration changes associated with two types of treatment for children who stutter. *Journal of Speech, Language, and Hearing Research, 43*, 965–978.

Riley, G., & Riley, J. (1985). *Oral motor assessment and treatment: Improving syllable production.* Austin, TX: Pro-Ed.

Riley, G., & Riley, J. (1999). Speech motor training. In M. Onslow & A. Packman (Eds.), *The handbook of early stuttering intervention* (pp. 139–158). San Diego, CA: Singular.

Riley, G., & Riley, J. (2000). A revised component model for diagnosing and treating children who stutter. *Contemporary Issues in Communication Sciences and Disorders, 27*, 188–199.

Riley, J. (1971). *Language profiles of thirty-nine children who stutter grouped by performance on a motor problems inventory* (Master's thesis). California State University, Fullerton.

Riley, J., Riley, G., & Maguire, G. (2004). Subjective screening of stuttering severity, locus of control and avoidance: research edition. *Journal of Fluency Disorders, 29*, 51–62.

Robb, M., & Blomgren, M. (1997). Analysis of F2 transition in the speech of stutterers and nonstutterers. *Journal of Fluency Disorders, 22*, 1–16.

Roberts, P., Meltzer, A., Wilding, J. (2009). Disfluencies in non-stuttering adults across sample lengths and topics. *Journal of Communication Disorders, 42*, 414–427.

Roberts, P., & Shenker, R. (2007). Assessment and treatment of stuttering in bilingual speakers. In E. Conture & R. Curlee (Eds.), *Stuttering and related disorders* (3rd ed., pp. 183–206). New York: Thieme.

Robinson, F. (1964). *Introduction to stuttering.* Englewood Cliffs, NJ: Prentice Hall.

Robinson, T., & Crowe, T. (1998). Culture-based considerations in programming for stuttering intervention with African-American clients and their families. *Language, Speech and Hearing Services in School, 29*, 172–179.

Rogers, C. (1951). *Client-centered therapy: Its current practice, implications, and theory.* Boston: Houghton Mifflin.

Rogers, C. (1957). The necessary and sufficient conditions of therapeutic personality change. *Journal of Consulting Psychology, 21*, 95–103.

Rommel, D., Hage, A., Kalehne, P., & Johannsen, H. (1999). Developmental, maintenance, and recovery of childhood stuttering: Prospective longitudinal data 3 years after first contact. In K. Baker, L. Rustin, & K. Baker (Eds.), *Proceedings of the Fifth Oxford Disfluency Conference* (pp. 168–182). Chappell Gardner, UK: Windsor, Berkshire.

Rosenbeck, T., Messert, B., Cillins, M., & Wertz, R. (1978). Stuttering following brain damage. *Brain and Language, 6*, 82–96.

Rossiter, M. (2009). Perceptions of L2 fluency by native and non-native speakers of English. *Canadian Modern Language Review, 65*, 395–412.

Roth, C., Aronson, A., & Davis, L. (1989). Clinical studies in psychogenic stuttering of adult onset. *Journal of Speech and Hearing Disorders, 54*, 634–646.

Rothbart, M. K., Ahadi, S. A., Hershey, K. L., & Fisher, P. (2001). Investigations of temperament at three to seven years: The Children's Behavior Questionnaire. *Child Development, 72*, 1394–1408.

Rothbaum, B., Hodges, L., Smith, S., Lee, J., & Price, L. (2000). A controlled study of virtual reality exposure therapy for the fear of flying. *Journal of Consulting and Clinical Psychology, 68*, 1020–1026.

Rousseau, I., Packman, A., Onslow, M., Harrison, E., & Jones, M. (2007). An investigation of language and phonological development and the responsiveness of preschool age children to the Lidcombe program. *Journal of Communication Disorders, 40*, 382–397.

Rubin, D., Wetzler, S., & Nebes, R. (1986). Autobiographical memory across the adult lifespan. In D. Rubin (Ed.), *Autobiographical memory* (pp. 202–221). Cambridge, MA: Cambridge University Press.

Runyan, C., & Runyan, S. (1986). A fluency rules therapy program for young children in the public schools. *Language, Speech, and Hearing Services in Schools, 17*, 276–284.

Runyan, C., & Runyan, S. (1993). Therapy for school-aged stutterers: An update on the fluency rules program. In R. Curlee (Ed.), *Stuttering and related disorders of fluency* (pp. 101–123). New York: Thieme.

Runyan, C., & Runyan, S. (2007). A fluency rules therapy program for young children in the public schools. In E. Conture & R. Curlee (Eds.), *Stuttering and related disorders* (3rd ed.). New York: Thieme.

Rustin, L., Botterill, W., & Kelman, E. (1996). *Assessment and therapy for young disfluent children: Family interaction.* London: Whurr.

Rustin, L., & Cook, F. (1983). Intervention procedures for the disfluent child. In P. Dalton (Ed.), *Approaches to the treatment of stuttering.* London: Croom Helm.

Rustin, L., Cook, F., & Spence, R. (1995). The management of stuttering in adolescence: A communication skills approach. London: Whurr.

Ryan, B. (1971). Operant procedures applied to stuttering therapy for children. *Journal of Speech and Hearing Disorders, 36*, 264–280.

Ryan, B. (1974). *Programmed therapy for stuttering in children and adults.* Springfield, IL: Charles C. Thomas.

Ryan, B. (1979). Stuttering therapy in a framework of operant conditioning and programmed learning. In H. Gregory (Ed.), *Controversies about Stuttering Therapy* (pp. 129–173). Baltimore: University Park Press.

Ryan, B. (1992). Articulation, language, rate, and fluency characteristics of stuttering and nonstuttering preschool children. *Journal of Speech and Hearing Research, 35,* 333–342.

Ryan, B. (1997). A reanalysis of the stuttering and syllable: Counting data in Kully and Boberg (1988). *Journal of Fluency Disorders, 22,* 331–338.

Ryan, B. (2001a). A longitudinal study of articulation, language, rate, and fluency of 22 preschool children who stutter. *Journal of Fluency Disorders, 26,* 107–127.

Ryan, B. (2001b). *Programmed therapy for stuttering in children and adults* (2nd ed.). Springfield, IL: Charles C. Thomas.

Ryan, B. P., & Ryan, B. V. (1995). Programmed stuttering treatment for children: Comparison of two establishment programs through transfer, maintenance, and follow-up. *Journal of Speech and Hearing Research, 38,* 61–75.

Sackett, D., Rosenberg, W. M. C., Gray, J. A. M., Haynes, R., & Richardson, W. (1996). Evidence based medicine: What it is and what it isn't. *British Medical Journal, 312,* 71–72.

Sackett, D., Straus, S., Richardson, W., Rosenberg, W., & Haynes, R. (2000). Evidence-based medicine: How to practice and teach EBM. Edinburgh, UK: Churchill Livingstone.

Sadoff, R., & Siegel, R. (1965). Group psychotherapy for stutterers. *International Journal of Group Psychotherapy, 15,* 72–80.

Sander, E. (1959). Counseling parents of stuttering children. *Journal of Speech and Hearing Disorders, 24,* 262–271.

Sander, E. (1961). Reliability of the Iowa Speech Disfluency Test. *Journal of Speech and Hearing Disorders, Monograph Supplement 7,* 21–30.

Sander, E. (1963). Frequency of syllable repetition and "stutter" judgments. *Journal of Speech and Hearing Disorders, 28,* 19–30.

Sander, E. (1968). Interrelations among the responses of mothers to a child's disfluencies. *Speech Monographs, 35,* 187–195.

Sandow, I. (1989). *Mechanik des Stotterns.* Nordhousen, Germany: Elder.

Santos, R., & Reese, D. (1999, June). Selecting culturally and linguistically appropriate materials: Suggestions for service providers. *ERIC Digest,* University of Illinois.

Sawyer, J. (2005). *Characteristics of disfluency clusters in stuttering and normally fluent preschool children: A longitudinal study* (Unpublished doctoral dissertation). University of Illinois, Urbana-Champaign.

Sawyer, J., & Yairi, E. (2006). The effect of sample size on the assessment of stuttering severity. *American Journal of Speech-Language Pathology, 15,* 36–44.

Sawyer, J., & Yairi, E. (in press). Characteristics of disfluency clusters over time in preschool children who stutter. *Journal of Speech, Language, and Hearing Research.*

Saxon, K., & Ludlow, C. (2007). A critical review of the effect of drug on stuttering. In E. Conture & R. Curlee (Eds.), *Stuttering and other fluency* disorders (3rd ed., pp. 277–294). Thieme: New York.

Scarbrough, H. (1943). A quantitative and qualitative of the electro electroencephalograms of stutterers and non-stutterers. *Journal of Experimental Psychology, 32,* 156–167.

Schindler, M. D. (1955). A study of educational adjustment of stuttering and nonstuttering children. In W. Johnson, & R. R. Leutenegger (Eds.), S*tuttering in children and adults.* Minneapolis: University of Minnesota Press.

Schlanger, B. B. (1953). Speech examination of a group of institutionalized mentally handicapped children. *Journal of Speech and Hearing Disorders, 18,* 339–349.

Schlanger, B. B., & Gottsleben, R. (1957). Analysis of speech defects among the institutionalized mentally retarded. *Journal of Speech and Hearing Disorders, 22,* 98–103.

Schmidt, R., & Lee, T. (2005). *Motor control and learning: A behavioral emphasis* (4th ed.) Champaign, IL: Human Kinetics.

Schubert, O. (1966). *The incidence rate of stuttering in a matched group of institutionalized mentally retarded.* Convention address at the American Association of Mental Deficiency, Chicago.

Schuell, H. (1947a). Sex differences in relation to stuttering: Part I. *Journal of Speech Disorders, 12,* 23–28.

Schuell, H. (1947b). Sex differences in relation to stuttering: Part II. *Journal of Speech Disorders, 12,* 421–427.

Schuell, H. (1949). Working with parents of stuttering children. *Journal of Speech and Hearing Disorders, 14,* 251–254.

Schwartz, H. (1999). *A primer for stuttering therapy.* Boston: Allyn & Bacon.

Schwartz, H., & Conture E. (1988). Subgrouping young stutterers. *Journal of Speech and Hearing Research, 31,* 62–71.

Schwartz, H., Zebrowski, P. M., & Conture, E. G. (1990). Behaviors at the onset of stuttering. *Journal of Fluency Disorders, 15,* 77–86.

Schwartz, M. (1976). *Stuttering solved.* Philadelphia: Lippincott.

Scott, C., & Windsor, J. (2000). General language performance measures in spoken and written narrative and expository discourse of school-age children with language learning disabilities. *Journal of Speech, Language, and Hearing Research, 43,* 324–339.

Scott Trautman, L., & Cairns, D. (2003). *Time pressure and disfluency: An empirical report.* Paper presented at the 4th World Congress on Fluency Disorders, Montreal, Canada.

Seery, C. (2005). Differential diagnosis of stuttering for forensic purposes. *American Journal of Speech-Language Pathology, 14,* 284–297.

Seery, C., Watkins, R., Ambrose, N., & Throneburg, R. (2006). *Non-word repetition by school age children who stutter.* Paper presented at the Annual Convention of the American Speech-Language-Hearing Association, Miami, FL.

Seery, C., Watkins, R., Mangelsdorf, S., & Shigeto, A. (2007). Subtyping stuttering II: Contributions from language and temperament. *Journal of Fluency Disorders, 32,* 197–217.

Seider, R. A., Gladstien, K. L., & Kidd, K. K. (1983). Recovery and persistence of stuttering among relatives of stutterers. *Journal of Speech and Hearing Disorders, 48,* 402–409.

Sermas, C., & Cox, M. (1982). The stutterer and stuttering: Personality correlates. *Journal of Fluency Disorders, 7,* 141–158.

Shames, G., & Florence,C. (1980). *Stutter free speech: A goal for therapy.* Columbus, Ohio: Charles E. Merrill.

Shames, G., & Sherrick, C. (1963). A discussion of nonfluency and stuttering as operant behavior. *Journal of Speech and Hearing Disorders, 28,* 3–18.

Shane, M. (1955). Effect on stuttering of alteration in auditory feedback. In W. Johnson & R. Leutenegger (Eds.), *Stuttering in children and adults.* Minneapolis: University of Minnesota Press.

Shapiro, A. (1980). An electromyographic analysis of the fluent and disfluent utterances of several types of stutterers. *Journal of Fluency Disorders, 5,* 203–231.

Shapiro, D. (1999). *Stuttering intervention: A collaborative journey to fluency freedom.* Austin, TX: Pro-Ed.

Sheehan, J. (1958). Conflict theory of stuttering. In J. Eisenson (Ed.), *Stuttering: A symposium* (pp. 123–166). New York: Harper & Row.

Sheehan, J. (1970). *Stuttering: Research and therapy.* New York: Harper & Row.

Sheehan, J. (1980). Problems in the evaluation of progress and outcome. In W. H. Perkins (Ed.), *Seminars in speech, language, and hearing* (pp. 389–401). New York: Thieme.

Sheehan, J., & Costley, M. S. (1977). A reexamination of the role of heredity in stuttering. *Journal of Speech and Hearing Disorders, 42,* 47–59.

Sheehan, J., & Martyn, M. (1966). Spontaneous recovery from stuttering. *Journal of Speech and Hearing Research, 9,* 121–135.

Sheehan, J., & Martyn, M. M. (1970). Stuttering and its disappearance. *Journal of Speech and Hearing Research, 13,* 279–289.

Sherman, D. (1952). Clinical and experimental use of the Iowa Scale of Severity of Stuttering. *Journal of Speech and Hearing Disorders, 17,* 316–320.

Shine, R. (1980). Direct management of the beginning stutterer. In W. Perkins (Ed.), *Strategies in stuttering therapy* (pp. 339–350). An issue of *Seminars in Speech, Language, and Hearing.* New York: Thieme.

Shriberg, L., Tomblin, J., & McSweeny, J. (1999). Prevalence of speech delay in 6-year-old children and comorbidity with language impairment. *Journal of Speech, Language, and Hearing Research, 42*(6), 1461–1481.

Shugart, Y., Mundorff, J., Kilshaw, J., Doheny, K., Doan, B., Wanyee, J., et al. (2004). Results of a genome-wide linkage scan for stuttering. *American Journal of Medical Genetics, 124,* 133–135.

Sieff, S., & Hooyman, B. (2006). *Language-based disfluency: A child case study.* Paper presented at the convention of the American Speech-Language-Hearing Association, Miami Beach, FL.

Siegel, G. (1998). Stuttering: Theory, research, and therapy. In A. Cordes and R. J. Ingham (Eds.), *Treatment efficacy for stuttering: A search for empirical bases.* San Diego, CA: Singular.

Silverman, E., & Zimmer, C. (1979). Women who stutter: Personality and speech characteristics. *Journal of Speech and Hearing Research, 22,* 553–564.

Silverman, F. (1974). Disfluency behavior of elementary-school stutterers and nonstutterers. *Language, Speech and Hearing Services in Schools, 5,* 32–37.

Silverman, F. (1988). The monster study. *Journal of Fluency Disorders, 13,* 225–231.

Silverman, F. (2004). *Stuttering and other fluency disorders* (3rd ed.). Long Grove, IL: Waveland Press.

Silverman, F., & Silverman, E. (1971). Stuttering-like behavior in manual communication of the deaf. *Perceptual and Motor Skills, 33,* 45–46.

Skinner, B. (1953). *Science and human behavior.* New York: Macmillan.

Smith, A. (1989). Neural drive to muscles in stuttering. *Journal of Speech and Hearing Research, 32,* 252–264.

Smith, A. (1990). Toward a comprehensive theory of stuttering: A commentary. *Journal of Speech and Hearing Disorders, 55,* 398–401.

Smith, A. (1999). Stuttering: A unified approach to a multifactorial, dynamic disorder. In N. B. Ratner and E. C. Healey (Eds.), *Stuttering research and practice: Bridging the gap.* Mahwah, NJ: Erlbaum.

Smith, A., Denny, M., Shaffer, L., Kelly, E., & Hirano, M. (1996). Activity of intrinsic laryngeal muscles in fluent and disfluent speech. *Journal of Speech and Hearing Research, 39,* 329–348.

Smith, A., Goffman, L., Zelaznik, H. N., Ying, G., & McGillem, C. (1995). Spatiotemporal stability and patterning of speech movement sequences. *Experimental Brain Research, 104,* 493–501.

Smith, A., & Kelly, E. (1997). Stuttering: A dynamic, multifactorial model. In R. Curlee & G. Siegel (Eds.), *Nature and treatment of stuttering: New directions* (2nd ed.). Boston: Allyn & Bacon.

Smith, A., & Kleinow, J. (2000). Kinematic correlates of speaking rate changes in stuttering and normally fluent adults. *Journal of Speech, Language, and Hearing Research, 43,* 521–536.

Smith, M. (1975). *When I say no, I feel guilty.* New York: Dial Press.

Smits-Bandstra, S., & DeNil, L. (2009). Speech skill learning of persons who stutter and fluent speakers under single and dual task conditions. *Clinical Linguistics & Phonetics, 23,* 38–57.

Snidecor, J. (1947). Why the Indian does not stutter. *Quarterly Journal of Speech, 33,* 493–495.

Snow, D. (1994). Phrase-final syllable lengthening and intonation in early child speech. *Journal of Speech and Hearing Research, 37,* 831–840.

Snowling, M., Goulandris, N., Bowlby, M., & Howell, P. (1986). Segmentation and speech perception in relation to reading skill: A developmental analysis. In S. E. Gathercole, C. S. Willis, A. D. Baddeley, & H. Emslie (1994), The children's test of nonword repetition: A test of phonological working memory. *Memory, 2,* 103–127.

Soderberg, G. (1967). Linguistic factors in stuttering. *Journal of Speech and Hearing Research, 10,* 801–810.

Soderberg, G. (1971). Relations of word information and word length to stuttering disfluencies. *Journal of Communication Disorders, 4,* 9–14.

Sommer, M., Koch, M. A., Paulus, W., Weiller, C., & Buchel, C. (2002). Disconnection of speech-relevant brain areas in persistent developmental stuttering. *Lancet, 360,* 380–383.

Sparks, G., Grant, D., Millay, K., Walker-Batson, D., & Hynan, L. (2002). The effect of fast speech rate on stuttering frequency during delayed auditory feedback. *Journal of Fluency Disorders, 27,* 187–201.

Spielberger, C., Gorsuch, R., Luschene, R., Vagg, P., & Jacobs, G. (1983). *Manual for the state-trait anxiety inventory.* Palo Alto: Consulting Psychologists Press.

Ssikorski, J. (1981). *Uber das stottern.* Berlin, Germany: Hirschwald.

Stager, S., Calis, K., Grothe, D., Block, M., Berensen, N., Smith, P., et al. (2005). Treatment with medications affecting dopaminergic and serotonergic mechanisms: Effects on fluency and anxiety in persons who stutter. *Journal of Fluency Disorders, 30,* 319–335.

Stager, S., Jeffries, K., & Braun, A. (2003). Common features of fluency-evoking conditions studied in stuttering subjects and controls: An H(2)15O PET study. *Journal of Fluency Disorders, 28,* 319–335.

Stansfield, J. (1995). Word-final disfluencies in adults with learning difficulties. *Journal of Fluency Disorders, 20,* 1–10.

Starkweather, C. W. (1987). *Fluency and stuttering.* Englewood Cliffs, NJ: Prentice-Hall.

Starkweather, C. W., & Givens-Ackerman, J. (1997). *Stuttering.* Austin, TX: Pro-Ed.

Starkweather, C. W., & Gottwald, S. (1984, November). *Children's stuttering and parents' speech rate.* Paper presented at the convention of the American Speech-Language-Hearing Association, San Francisco, CA.

Starkweather, C. W., & Gottwald, S. (1990). The demands and capacities model: II. Clinical implications. *Journal of Fluency Disorders, 15,* 143–157.

Starkweather, C. W., Gottwald, S., & Halfond, M. (1990). *Stuttering prevention: A clinical method.* Englewood Cliffs, NJ: Prentice Hall.

Stephanson-Opsal, D., & Bernstein Ratner, N. (1988). Maternal speech rate modification and childhood stuttering. *Journal of Fluency Disorders, 13,* 49–56.

Stern, E. (1948). A preliminary study of bilingualism and stuttering in four Johannesburg schools. *Journal of Logopaedics, 1,* 15–25.

Stevens, T. (2005). Assertion training. Retrieved from www.csulb.edu/~tstevens/assertion_training.htm

Stewart, J. L. (1960). The problem of stuttering in certain North American Indians societies. *Journal of Speech and Hearing Disorders, Monograph Supplement No. 6,* 1–87.

Still, A., & Griggs, S. (1979). Changes in the probability of stuttering following a stutter: A test of some recent models. *Journal of Speech and Hearing Research, 22,* 565–571.

Still, A., & Sherrard, C. (1976). Formalizing theories of stuttering. *The British Journal of Mathematical and Statistical Psychology, 29,* 129–138.

St. Louis, K. (1986). *The atypical stutterer.* San Diego, CA: Academic Press.

St. Louis, K. (2007). A group therapy model for adults who stutter. 10th International Stuttering Awareness Day On-Line Conference. www.mnsu.edu/comdis/isad10/papers/therapy10/stlouis10.htm

St. Louis, K., & Myers, F. (1995). Clinical management of cluttering. *Language, Speech, and Hearing Services in Schools, 26,* 187–195.

St. Louis, K., Myers, F., Bakker, K., & Raphael, L. (2007). Understanding and treating cluttering. In E. Conture & R. Curlee (Eds.), *Stuttering and related disorders of fluency* (3rd ed., pp. 297–325. New York: Thieme.

St. Louis, K., Myers, F., Faragasso, K., Townsend, P., & Gallagher, A. (2004). Perceptual aspects of cluttered speech. *Journal of Fluency Disorders, 29,* 213–235.

St. Louis, K., Raphael, L. J., Myers, F. L., & Bakker, K. (2003, November 18). Cluttering updated. *The ASHA Leader,* pp. 4–5, 20–22.

Stocker, B. (1976). *The Stocker probe technique for diagnosis and treatment of stuttering in young children.* Tulsa, OK: Modern Education Corporation.

Stocker, B., & Goldfarb, R. (1995). *The Stocker probe for fluency and language* (3rd ed.). Vero Beach, FL: The Speech Bin.

St. Onge, K., & Calvert, J. (1964). Stuttering research. *Quarterly Journal of Speech, 50,* 159–165.

Stromsta, C. (1965). A spectrographic study of disfluencies labeled as stuttering by parents. *De Therapia Vocis et Loquelae, 1,* 317–318.

Stuart, A., Kalinowski, J., Rastatter, M., Saltuklaroglu, T., & Dayalu, V. (2004). Investigations of the impact of altered auditory feedback in-the-ear devices on the speech of people who stutter: Initial fitting and 4-month follow-up. *International Journal of Language and Communication Disorders, 39,* 93–119.

Stuart, G. L., Treat, T. A., & Wade, W. A. (2000). Effectiveness of an empirically based treatment for panic disorder delivered in a service clinic setting. *Journal of Consulting and Clinical Psychology, 68*(3), 506–512.

Stunden, A. (1965). The effects of time pressure as a variable in the verbal behavior of stuttering. *Dissertation Abstracts, 26,* 1784–1785.

Sturm, J., & Seery, C. (2007). Speech and articulatory rates of school-age children in conversation and narrative contexts. *Language, Speech, and Hearing Services in Schools, 38,* 47–59.

Subramanian, A., & Yairi, E. (2006). Identification of traits transmitted in association with stuttering. *Journal of Communication Disorders, 39,* 200–216.

Subramanian, A., Yairi, E., & Amir, O. (2003). Second formant transitions in fluent speech of persistent and recovered preschool children who stutter. *Journal of Communication Disorders, 36,* 59–75.

Suresh, R., Ambrose, N., Roe, C., Pluzhnikov, A., Wittke-Thompson, J., C-Y Ng, M., et al. (2006). New complexities in the genetics of stuttering: Significant sex-specific linkage signals. *American Journal of Human Genetics, 78*, 554–563.

Susca, M., & Healey, E. C. (2001). Perceptions of simulated stuttering and fluency. *Journal of Speech, Language and Hearing Research, 44*, 61–73.

Sutton, S., & Chase, R. (1961). White noise and stuttering. *Journal of Speech and Hearing Research, 4*, 72.

Taylor, G. (1937). *An observational study of the nature of stuttering at its onset* (Unpublished master's thesis). State University of Iowa, Iowa City.

Taylor, I., & Taylor, M. (1967). Test of predictions from the conflict hypothesis of stuttering. *Journal of Abnormal Psychology, 72*, 431–433.

Temple, L. (2000). Second language learner speech production. *Studia Linguistica, 54*, 288–297.

Theys, C., Van Wieringen, A., and DeNil, L. (2008). A clinician survey of speech and non-speech characteristics of neurogenic stuttering. *Journal of Fluency Disorders, 33*, 1–23.

Thomas, C., & Howell, P. (2001). Assessing efficacy in stuttering treatment. *Journal of Fluency Disorder, 26*, 311–333.

Thompson, C., Wolk, L., & Lockett Davis, B. (2007). Role of phonology in childhood stuttering and its treatment. In E. Conture & R. Curlee (Eds.), *Stuttering and related disorders* (3rd ed., pp. 168–182). New York: Thieme.

Thordardottir, E., & Weismer, E. (2002). Content mazes and filled pauses in the spontaneous speech of school-aged children with specific language impairment. *Brain and Cognition, 48*, 587–592.

Throneburg, R. (1997). *Temporal characteristics of disfluencies as predictors of persistency and recovery in early childhood stuttering* (Unpublished doctoral dissertation). University of Illinois.

Throneburg, R., & Yairi, E. (1994). Temporal dynamics of repetitions during the early stage of childhood stuttering: An acoustic study. *Journal of Speech and Hearing Research, 37*, 1067–1075.

Throneburg, R., & Yairi, E. (2001). Durational, proportionate, and absolute frequency characteristics of disfluencies: A longitudinal study regarding persistence and recovery. *Journal of Speech, Language, and Hearing Research, 44*, 38–51.

Throneburg, R., Yairi, E., & Paden, E. (1994). The relation between phonologic difficulty and the occurrence of disfluencies in the early stage of stuttering. *Journal of Speech and Hearing Research, 37*, 504–509.

Till, J., Goldsmith, H., & Reich, A. (1981). Laryngeal and manual reaction times of stuttering and nonstuttering adults. *Journal of Speech and Hearing Research, 24*, 192–196.

Tomaiuoli, D., Del Gado, F., Falcone, P., Marchese, C., Pasqua, E., & Grazia Spinetti, M. (2007). The use of drama-therapy in the rehabilitation of stuttering patients. Retrieved from www.mnsu.edu/comdis/isad10/papers/tomaiuoli10.html

Tomblin, J. B., Morris, H. L., & Spriestersbach, D. C. (2000). *Diagnosis in speech-language pathology* (2nd ed.). San Diego, CA: Singular.

Toomey, G., & Sidman, M. (1970). An experimental analogue of the anxiety-stuttering relationship. *Journal of Speech and Hearing Research, 13*, 122–129.

Toyoda, B. (1959). A statistical report. *Clinical Paediatrica, 12*, 788.

Travis, L. (1927). Studies in stuttering: I. Dysintegration of the breathing movements during stuttering. *Archives of Neurology & Psychiatry, 18*, 673–690.

Travis, L. (1931). *Speech Pathology*. New York: Appleton-Century-Crofts.

Travis, L. (1934). Dissociation of the homologous muscle function in stuttering. *Archives of Neurological Psychiatry, 31*, 127–133.

Travis, L. (1957). The unspeakable feelings of people, with special reference to stuttering. In L. Travis (Ed.), *Handbook of speech pathology* (Chapter 29). New York: Appleton-Century-Crofts.

Travis, L. (1971). The unspeakable feelings of people, with special reference to stuttering. In L. Travis (Ed.), *Handbook of speech pathology* (2nd ed.). New York: Appleton-Century-Crofts.

Travis, L. (1978a). Neurophysiological dominance. *Journal of Speech and Hearing Disorders, 43*, 275–277.

Travis, L. (1978b). The cerebral dominance theory of stuttering, 1931–1978. *Journal of Speech and Hearing Disorders, 43*, 278–281.

Travis, L., Johnson, W., & Shover, J. (1937). The relation of bilingualism to stuttering. *Journal of Speech Disorders, 2*, 185–189.

Travis, L., & Knott, J. (1936). Brain potential from normal speakers and stutterers. *Journal of Psychology, 2*, 137–150.

Travis, L., & Malamud, W. (1937). Brain potential from normal subjects, stutterers, and schizophrenic patients. *American Journal of Psychiatry, 93*, 929–936.

Trotter, W. (1955). The severity of stuttering during successive readings of the same material. *Journal of Speech and Hearing Disorders, 20*, 17–25.

Trotter, W., & Lesch, M. (1967). Personal experience with a stutter-aid. *Journal of Speech and Hearing Disorders, 32*, 270–272.

Tsao, Y.-C., & Weismer, G. (1997). Inter-speaker variation in habitual speaking rate: Evidence of a neuromuscular component. *Journal of Speech, Language and Hearing Research, 40*, 858–866.

Tucker, G. (1998). A global perspective on multilingualism and multilingual education. In J. Cenos & F. Genese (Eds.), *Beyond bilingualism: Multilingualism and multilingualism education* (pp. 3–15). Clevendon, UK: Multilingual Matters.

Tudor, M. (1939). An experimental study of the effect of evaluative labeling on speech fluency (Unpublished master's thesis). University of Iowa, Iowa City.

Tuthill, C. (1946). A quantitative study of extensional meaning with special refernce to stuttering. *Speech Monograph, 13*, 81–98.

Tyre, T., Maisto, S., & Companik, P. (1973). The use of systematic desensitization in the treatment of chronic stuttering behavior. *Journal of Speech and Hearing Disorders, 38*, 514–519.

Ulliana, L., & Ingham, R. J. (1984). Behavioral and nonbehavioral variables in the measurement of stutterers' communication attitudes. *Journal of Speech and Hearing Disorders, 49*, 83–89.

Van Borsel, J., Beck, C., & Delanghe, J. (2003). *Stuttering and medication: A look at the symptoms*. Poster session presented at the 4th World Congress on Fluency Disorders, Montreal, Quebec, Canada.

Van Borsel, J., & Britto Pereira, M. M. (2005). Assessment of stuttering in a familiar versus an unfamiliar language. *Journal of Fluency Disorders, 30*, 109–124.

Van Borsel, J., Goethals, L., & Vanryckeghem, M. (2004). Disfluency in Tourette Syndrome: Observational study in three cases. *Folia Phoniatrica et Logopaedica, 56*, 358–366.

Van Borsel, J., Maes, E., & Foulon, K. (2001). Stuttering and bilingualism: A review. *Journal of Fluency Disorders, 26*, 179–205.

Van Borsel, J., Moeyaert, E., Rosseel, M., Van Loo, E., & Van Renterghem, L. (2006). Prevalence of stuttering in regular and special school population in Belgium based on teacher perception. *Folia Phoniatrica et Logopaedica, 58*, 289–302.

Van Borsel, J., Sunaert, R., & Engelen, S. (2005). Speech disruption under delayed auditory feedback in multilingual speakers. *Journal of Fluency Disorders, 30*, 201–217.

Van Borsel, J., & Taillieu, C. (2001). Neurogenic stuttering versus developmental stuttering: An observer judgment study. *Journal of Communication Disorders, 34*, 385–395.

Van Borsel, J., Van Coster, R., & Van Lierde, K. (1996). Repetitions in final position in a nine-year-old boy with focal brain damage. *Journal of Fluency Disorders, 21*, 137–146.

Van Borsel, J., Van Lierde, K., Van Cauweberge, P., Guldemont, I., & Van Orshoven, M. (1998). Severe acquired stuttering following injury of the left supplementary motor region: A case report. *Journal of Fluency Disorders, 23*, 49–58.

van Lieshout, P. H., Peters, H. F., Starkweather, C. W., & Hulstijn, W. (1993). Physiological differences between stutterers and nonstutterers in perceptually fluent speech: EMG amplitude and duration. *Journal of Speech and Hearing Research, 36*(1), 55–63.

Van Riper, C. (1954). *Speech correction: Principles and methods* (3rd ed.). New York: Prentice-Hall.

Van Riper, C. (1971). *The nature of stuttering*. Englewood Cliffs, NJ: Prentice-Hall.

Van Riper, C. (1973). *The treatment of stuttering*. Englewood Cliffs, NJ: Prentice-Hall.

Van Riper, C. (1975). The stutterer's clinician. In J. Eisenson (Ed.), *Stuttering, a second symposium* (pp. 453–492). New York: Harper & Row.

Van Riper, C. (1982). *The nature of stuttering* (2nd ed.). Englewood Cliffs, NJ: Prentice-Hall.

Van Riper, C. (1992). Stuttering? *Journal of Fluency Disorders, 17*, 81–84.

Van Riper, C., & Hull, C. (1955). The quantitative measurement of the effect of certain situations on stuttering. In W. Johnson & R. R. Leutenegger (Eds.), *Stuttering in children and adults* (pp. 199–207). Minneapolis: University of Minnesota Press.

Vanryckeghem, M., & Brutten, G. (1993). The Communication Attitude Test: A test–retest reliability investigation. *Journal of Fluency Disorders, 17*, 177–190.

Vanryckeghem, M., & Brutten, G. (1997). The speech associated attitude of children who do and do not stutter and the differential effect of age. *American Journal of Speech-Language Pathology, 6*, 67–73.

Virginia Department of Education. (2003). English standards of learning. Retrieved from www.doe.virginia.gov/VDOE/Superintendent/Sols/home.shtml

Vlasova, N. A. (1962). Prevention and treatment of children's stuttering in U.S.S.R. *Ceskoslovenska Otolaryngologie, 11*, 30–32.

von Sarbo, A. (1901). Statistik der an Sprachstorungen Leidenden Schulkinder Ungarns, *Medizinisch-padagogische Monatsschrift fur die gesamte Sprach-heilkundo*, 65–89.

Waddle, P. (1934). *A comparison of speech defectives among colored and white children* (Master's thesis). University of Iowa, Iowa City.

Wakaba, Y. (1983). Group play therapy for Japanese children who stutter. *Journal of Fluency Disorders, 8*, 93–118.

Wakaba, Y. (1992). Process of recovery from stuttering of a three year-old stuttering child. *Tokyo Gakugei University Research Institute for the Education of Exceptional Children, 41*, 35–46.

Wakaba, Y. (1999). *Research on remedial process of stuttering with early onset* (Unpublished doctoral dissertation). Nagoya University, Nagoya, Japan.

Walker, J., Archibald, L., & Cherniak, R. (1992). Articulation rate in 3- and. 5-year-old children. *Journal of Speech and Hearing Research, 35*, 4–13.

Walker, V. (1988). Durational characteristics of young adults during speaking and reading tasks. *Folia Phoniatrica, 40*, 13–20.

Wallach, G., & Butler, K. (1994). *Language learning disabilities in school-age children and adolescents*. New York: MacMillan.

Wallin, J. (1916). A census of speech defects. *School Sociology, 3*, 213.

Wallin, J. E. (1926). Speech defective children in a large school system. *Miami University Bulletin, 25*(4), 3–45.

Walnut, F. (1954). A personality inventory item analysis of individuals who stutter and individuals who have other handicaps. *Journal of Speech and Hearing Disorders, 19*, 220–227.

Waltzman, S., & Cohen, N. (2000). *Cochlear implants*. New York: Thieme.

Ward, D. (2006). *Stuttering and cluttering: Frameworks for understanding and treatment*. New York: Psychology Press.

Watkins, K., Smith, S., Davis, S., & Howell, P. (2008). Structural and functional abnormalities of the motor system in developmental stuttering. *Brain, 131*, 50–59.

Watkins, R. (2005). Language abilities of young children who stutter. In E. Yairi & N. Ambrose (Eds.), *Early childhood stuttering* (pp. 235–253). Austin, TX: Pro-Ed.

Watkins, R., & Johnson, B. (2004). Language abilities in children who stutter: Toward improved research and clinical applications. *Language, Speech, and Hearing Services in Schools, 35,* 82–89.

Watkins, R., & Yairi, E. (1997). Language production abilities of children whose stuttering persisted or recovered. *Journal of Speech, Language, and Hearing Research, 40*(2), 385–399.

Watkins, R. V., Yairi, E., & Ambrose, N. G. (1999). Early childhood stuttering: III. Initial status of expressive language abilities. *Journal of Speech, Language, and Hearing Research, 42,* 1125–1135.

Watkins, R. V., Yairi, E., Ambrose, N., Evans, K., DeThorne, L., & Mullen, C. (2000, November). *Grammatical influences on stuttering in young children.* Paper presented at the convention of the American Speech-Language-Hearing Association, Washington, DC.

Watson, B., & Alfonso, P. (1987). Physiological bases of acoustic LRT in nonstutterers, mild stutterers, and severe stutterers. *Journal of Speech and Hearing Research, 30,* 434–447.

Watson, B., & Freeman, F. (1997). Brain imaging contributions. In R. Curlee & G. Siegel (Eds.), *Nature and treatment of stuttering: New directions* (2nd ed.). Boston: Allyn & Bacon.

Watson, B., Freeman, F., Devous, M., Chapman, S., Finitzo, T., & Pool, K. (1994). Linguistic performance and regional cerebral blood flow in persons who stutter. *Journal of Speech and Hearing Research, 37*(6), 1221–1228.

Watson, B., Pool, K., Devous, M., Freeman, F., & Finitzo, T. (1992). Brain blood flow related to acoustic laryngeal reaction time in adult developmental stutterers. *Journal of Speech and Hearing Research, 35,* 555–561.

Watson, J., & Kayser, H. (1994). Assessment of bilingual/ bicultural children and adults who stutter. *Seminars in Speech and Language, 15,* 149–164.

Watts-Jackim, L. (2004). Is all the evidence in? *The Michigan Society for Psychoanalytic Psychology, 14*(1). Retrieved from www.mspp.net/jackimEBT.htm

Watzl, I. (1924). Statistics Erhenbungen uber das Vorkommen von Sprachstorungen in den Weiner Schulen. In *Proceedings of the First International Congress of Logopedics and Phoniatrics,* Vienna, Austria.

Weber, C., & Smith, A. (1990). Autonomic correlates of stuttering and speech assessed in a range of experimental tasks. *Journal of Speech and Hearing Research, 33,* 690–706.

Weber-Fox, C., & Hampton, A. (2008). Stuttering and natural speech processing semantic and syntactic constraints on verbs. *Journal of Speech, Language, and Hearing Research, 51,* 1058–1071.

Webster, L. M. (1977). A clinical note on psychotherapy for stuttering. *Journal of Fluency Disorders, 2,* 253–255.

Webster, R. (1979). Empirical considerations regarding *stuttering* therapy. In H. Gregory (Ed.), *Controversies about stuttering therapy* (pp. 209–240). Baltimore: University Park.

Webster, R. (1980a). *The precision fluency shaping program: Speech reconstruction for stutterers (Clinician's program guide).* Roanoke, VA: Communication Development.

Webster, R. (1980b). Evolution of target-based behavioral therapy for stuttering. *Journal of Fluency Disorders, 5,* 303–320.

Weiss, A., & Zebrowski, P. (1992). Disfluencies in the conversations of young children who stutter: Some answers about questions. *Journal of Speech, Language, and Hearing Research, 35,* 1230–1238.

Weiss, D. (1964). *Cluttering.* Englewood Cliffs, NJ: Prentice-Hall.

Weiss, D. (1967). Cluttering. *Folia Phoniatrica, 19,* 233–263.

Wells, G. (1979). Effect of sentence structure on stuttering. *Journal of Fluency Disorders, 2,* 123–129.

Wendahl, R., & Cole, J. (1961). Identification of stuttering during relatively fluent speech. *Journal of Speech and Hearing Research, 4,* 281–186.

West, R. (1958). An agnostic's speculations about stuttering. In J. Eisenson (Ed.), *Stuttering: A symposium* (pp. 167–222). New York: Harper & Row.

West, R., Nelson, S., & Berry, M. (1939). The heredity of stuttering. *Quarterly Journal of Speech, 25,* 23–30.

West, R., & Nusbaum, E. (1929). A motor test for dysphemia. *Quarterly Journal of Speech, 25,* 469–479.

West, T. A., & Bauer, P. J. (1999). Assumptions of infantile amnesia: Are there differences between early and later memories? *Memory, 7,* 257–278.

Wexler, K. B. (1982). Developmental disfluency in 2-, 4-, and 6-year old boys in neutral and stress situations. *Journal of Speech and Hearing Research, 25,* 229–234.

White House Conference Committee Report on Child Health and Protection. (1931). Section III, *Special Education: The Handicapped and the Gifted.* New York: D. Appleton Century.

White, A., Kraus, C., Flom, J., Kestenbaum, L., Mitchell, J., Shah, K., et al. (2005). College students lack knowledge of standard drink volumes: Implications for definitions of risky drinking based on survey data. *Alcoholism, Clinical and Experimental Research, 29,* 631–638.

White, E. (2002). Normal disfluency in young adults across three speech tasks (Unpublished master's thesis). University of Wisconsin-Milwaukee, Milwaukee, WI.

Wikipedia (2007). Psychotherapy. Retrieved from http://en.wikipedia.org/wiki/Psychotherapy

Williams, D. (1955). Masseter muscle action potentials in stuttered and nonstuttered speech. *Journal of Speech and Hearing Disorders, 20,* 242–261.

Williams, D. (1957). A point of view about stuttering. *Journal of Speech and Hearing Disorders, 22,* 390–397.

Williams, D. (1968). Stuttering therapy: An overview. In H. Gregory (Ed.), *Learning theory and stuttering therapy.* Evanston, IL: Northwestern University Press.

Williams, D. (1971). Stuttering therapy for children. In E. Travis (Ed.), *Handbook of speech pathology and audiology* (pp. 1073–1096). New York: Appleton-Century-Crofts.

Williams, D., & Brutten, G. (1994). Physiologic and aerodynamic events prior to the speech of stutterers and nonstutterers. *Journal of Fluency Disorders, 19*(2), 83–111.

Williams, D., & Kent, R. (1958). Listener evaluations of speech interruptions. *Journal of Speech and Hearing Research, 1,* 124–131.

Williams, D., Melrose B., & Woods, L. (1969). The relationship between stuttering and academic achievement in children. *Journal of Communication Disorders, 2,* 87–98.

Williams, D., Silverman, F., & Kools, J. (1968). Disfluency behavior of elementary school stutterers and nonstutterers: The adaptation effect. *Journal of Speech and Hearing Research, 11,* 622–630.

Williams, M. (2006). *Children who stutter: Easy, difficult, or slow-to-warm up?* Paper presented at the Annual Convention of the American Speech-Language-Hearing Association, Miami, FL.

Wingate, M. (1964a). A standard definition of stuttering. *Journal of Speech and Hearing Disorders, 29,* 484–489.

Wingate, M. (1964b). Recovery from stuttering. *Journal of Speech and Hearing Disorders, 29,* 312–321.

Wingate, M. (1970). Effect on stuttering of changes in audition. *Journal of Speech and Hearing Research, 13,* 861–873.

Wingate, M. E. (1972). Deferring the adaptation effect. *Journal of Speech and Hearing Research, 15,* 547–550.

Wingate, M. (1975). Expectancy as basically a short-term process. *Journal of Speech and Hearing Research, 18,* 31–42.

Wingate, M. (1976). *Stuttering: Theory and treatment.* New York: Irvington/John Wiley & Sons.

Wingate, M. (1979). The loci of stuttering: Grammar or prosody. *Journal of Communication Disorders, 12,* 283–290.

Wingate, M. (1986). Adaptation, consistency and beyond: I. Limitations and contradictions. *Journal of Fluency Disorders, 11,* 1–36.

Wingate, M. (1988). *The structure of stuttering.* New York: Springer-Verlag.

Wingate, M. (1997). *Stuttering: A short history of a curious disorder.* Westport, CT: Bergin & Garvey.

Wingate, M. (2001). SLD is not stuttering [Letter to the editor]. *Journal of Speech, Language, and Hearing Research, 44*(2), 381–383.

Wingate, M. (2002). *The foundations of stuttering.* San Diego, CA: California Academic Press.

Winkelman, N. (1954). Chlorpromazine in the treatment of neuropsychiatric disorders. *Journal of the American Medical Association, 155,* 18–21.

Wischner, G. (1950). Stuttering behavior and learning: A preliminary theoretical formulation. *Journal of Speech and Hearing Disorders, 15,* 324–335.

Wittke-Thompson, J., Ambrose, N., Yairi, E., Roe, C., Ober, C., & Cox, N. (2007). Linkage analyses of stuttering in a founder population. *Journal of Fluency Disorder, 32,* 33–50.

Wolery, M., & Dunlap, G. (2001). Reporting on studies using single-subject experimental methods. *Journal of Early Intervention, 24,* 85–89.

Wolk, L., Blomgren, M., & Smith, A. (2000). The frequency of simultaneous disfluency and phonological errors in children: A preliminary investigation. *Journal of Fluency Disorders, 25*(4), 269–281.

Wolk, L., Edwards, M., & Conture, E. (1993). Coexistence of stuttering and disordered phonology in young children. *Journal of Speech and Hearing Research, 36,* 906–917.

Wolpe, J. (1958). *Psychotherapy by reciprocal inhibition.* Stanford, CA: Stanford University Press.

Wolpe, J. (1990). *The practice of behavior therapy.* Tarrytown, NY: Pergamon Press.

Woods, S., Shearsby, J., Onslow, M., & Burnham, D. (2002). Psychological impact of the Lidcombe program of early stuttering intervention. *International Journal of Language and Communication Disorders, 37,* 31–40.

World Health Organization. (1977). *Manual of the International Statistical Classification of Diseases, Injuries, and Causes of Death* (Vol. 1, p. 202). Geneva: Author.

Wu, J., Maguire, G., Riley, G., Lee, A., Keator, D., Tang, C., et al. (1997). Increased dopamine activity associated with stuttering. *Neuroreport, 8,* 767–770.

Wyatt, G. L., & Herzan, H. M. (1962). Therapy with stuttering children and their mothers. *American Journal of Orthopsychiatry, 23,* 645–659.

Yairi, E. (1976). Effects of binaural and monaural noise on stuttering. *Journal of Auditory Research, 16,* 114–119.

Yairi, E. (1981). Disfluencies of normally speaking two-year-old children. *Journal of Speech and Hearing Research, 24,* 490–495

Yairi, E. (1983). The onset of stuttering in two- and three-year-old children: A preliminary report. *Journal of Speech and Hearing Disorders, 48,* 171–177.

Yairi, E. (1985). *Speech rate modification program for preschool-age children who stutter.* Unpublished manuscript.

Yairi, E. (1993). Epidemiology and other considerations in treatment efficacy research with preschool-age children who stutter. *Journal of Fluency Disorders, 18,* 197–220.

Yairi, E. (1997). Disfluency characteristics of early childhood stuttering. In R. F. Curlee & G. M. Siegel (Eds.), *Nature and treatment of stuttering: New directions* (2nd ed., pp. 49–78). Boston: Allyn & Bacon.

Yairi, E. (2006). The Tudor Study and Wendell Johnson. In Goldfarb R. (Ed.), *Ethics: A case study from fluency.* Plural Publishing.

Yairi, E. (2007). Subtyping stuttering I: A review. *Journal of Fluency Disorders, 32,* 165–196.

Yairi, E., & Ambrose, N. (1992a). A longitudinal study of stuttering in children: A preliminary report. *Journal of Speech and Hearing Research, 35,* 755–760.

Yairi, E., & Ambrose, N. (1992b). Onset of stuttering in preschool children: Selected factors. *Journal of Speech and Hearing Research, 35,* 782–788.

Yairi, E., & Ambrose, N. G. (1999a). Early childhood stuttering: I. Persistency and recovery rates. *Journal of Speech, Language, and Hearing Research, 42,* 1097–1112.

Yairi, E., & Ambrose, N. (1999b). Spontaneous recovery and clinical trials research in early childhood stuttering: A response to Onslow and Packman (1999). *Journal of Speech, Language, and Hearing Research, 42,* 402–410.

Yairi, E., & Ambrose, N. (2005). *Early childhood stuttering.* Austin, TX: Pro-Ed.

Yairi, E., Ambrose, N., & Cox, N. (1996). Genetics of stuttering: A critical review. *Journal of Speech and Hearing Research, 39,* 771–784.

Yairi, E., Ambrose, N., & Niermann, R. (1993). The early months of stuttering: A developmental study. *Journal of Speech and Hearing Research, 36*, 521–528.

Yairi, E., Ambrose, N., Paden, E. P., & Throneburg, R. N. (1996). Predictive factors of persistence and recovery: Pathways of childhood stuttering. *Journal of Communication Disorders, 29*, 51–77.

Yairi, E., & Carrico, D. (1992). Early childhood: Pediatricians' attitudes and practices. *American Journals of Speech-Language Pathology, 1*, 54–62.

Yairi, E., & Clifton, N. (1972). The disfluent speech behavior of preschool children, high school seniors, and geriatric persons. *Journal of Speech and Hearing Research, 15*, 714–719.

Yairi, E., Gintautas, J., & Avent, J. (1981). Disfluent speech associated with brain damage. *Brain and Language, 14*, 49–56.

Yairi, E., & Hall, K. D. (1993). Temporal relations within repetitions of preschool children near the onset of stuttering: A preliminary report. *Journal of Communication Disorders, 26*, 231–244.

Yairi, E., & Lewis, B. (1984). Disfluencies at the onset of stuttering. *Journal of Speech and Hearing Research, 27*, 154–159.

Yairi, E., Watkins, R., & Ambrose, N. (2001). What is stuttering? [Letter to the editor]. *Journal of Speech, Language, and Hearing Research, 44*(3), 585–592.

Yairi, E., & Williams, D. (1970). Speech clinicians' stereotypes of elementary school boys who stutter. *Journal of Communication Disorders, 3*, 161–170.

Yaruss, J. S. (1997a). Clinical implications of situational variability in preschool children who stutter. *Journal of Fluency Disorders, 22*, 187–203.

Yaruss, J. S. (1997b). Utterance timing and childhood stuttering. *Journal of Fluency Disorders, 22*, 263–286.

Yaruss, J. S. (2000). Converting between word and syllable counts in children's conversational speech samples. *Journal of Fluency Disorders, 25*, 305–316.

Yaruss, J. S., & Conture, E. G. (1993). F2 transitions during sound/syllable repetitions of children who stutter and predictions of stuttering chronicity. *Journal of Speech and Hearing Research, 36*, 883–896.

Yaruss, J. S., LaSalle, L., & Conture, E. (1998). Evaluating young children who stutter: Diagnostic data. *American Journal of Speech and Language Pathology, 7*(4), 62–76.

Yaruss, J. S., & Quesal, R. (2002). Research-based stuttering therapy revisited. *Perspectives on Fluency Disorders, 12*(2), 22–24.

Yaruss, J. S., & Quesal, R. (2004). Stuttering and the International Classification of Functioning, Disability, and Health (ICF): An update. *Journal of Communication Disorders, 37*(1), 35–52.

Yaruss, J. S., & Quesal, R. (2006). Overall Assessment of the Speaker's Experience of Stuttering (OASES): Documenting multiple outcomes in stuttering treatment. *Journal of Fluency Disorders, 31*, 90–115.

Yaruss, J. S., Quesal, R., Reeves, L., Molt, L., Kluetz, B., Caruso, A., et al. (2002). Speech treatment and support group experiences of people who participate in the National Stuttering Association. *Journal of Fluency Disorders, 2*, 115–134.

Young, M. (1961). Predicting ratings of severity of stuttering. *Journal of Speech and Hearing Disorders, Monograph Supplement, 7*, 31–54.

Young, M. (1964). Identification of stutterers from recorded samples of their fluent speech. *Journal of Speech and Hearing Research, 7*, 302–303.

Young, M. (1984). Identification of stuttering and stutterers. In R. Curlee & W. Perkins (Eds.), *Nature and treatment of stuttering: New directions* (pp. 13–30). San Diego, CA: College-Hill.

Young, M. (1985). Increasing the frequency of stuttering. *Journal of Speech and Hearing Research, 28*, 282–293.

Young, E., & Hawk, S. (1955). *Moto-kinesthetic speech training.* Stanford, CA: Stanford University.

Zebrowski, P. (1994). Duration of sound prolongation and sound/syllable repetition in children who stutter. *Journal of Speech and Hearing Research, 37*, 254–263.

Zebrowski, P., & Conture, E. G. (1989). Judgment of disfluency by mothers of stuttering and normally fluent children. *Journal of Speech and Hearing Research, 32*, 625–634.

Zebrowski, P., Weiss, A., Savelkoul, E., & Hammer, C. (1996). The effect of maternal rate reduction on the stuttering, speech rates and linguistic productions of children who stutter: Evidence from individual dyads. *Clinical Linguistics and Phonetics, 10*, 189–206.

Zimmermann, G. (1980a). Articulatory dynamics of fluent utterances of stutterers and nonstutterers. *Journal of Speech and Hearing Research, 23*, 95–107.

Zimmermann, G. (1980b). Articulatory behaviors associated with stuttering. *Journal of Speech and Hearing Research, 23*, 108–121.

Zimmermann, G. (1980c). Stuttering: A disorder of movement, *Journal of Speech and Hearing Research, 23*, 122–136.

Zimmerman, G., & Hanley, J. (1983). A cinefluorographic investigation of repeated fluent productions of stutterers in an adaptation procedure. *Journal of Speech and Hearing Research, 26*, 35–42.

Zimmermann, G., Liljebald, S., Frank, A., & Cleeland, C. (1983). The Indians have many terms for it: Stuttering among the Bannoch-Shoshoni. *Journal of Speech & Hearing Research, 26*, 315–318.

Zimmermann, G., Smith, A., & Hanley, J. (1981). Stuttering: In need of a unifying conceptual framework. *Journal of Speech & Hearing Research, 24*, 25–31.

Zimmerman, I., Steiner, V., & Pond, R. (1979). *Preschool Language Scale.* San Antonio, TX: The Psychological Corporation, Harcourt Brace Jovanovich.

Zwitman, D. (1978). *The disfluent child.* Baltimore: University Park.

Index